Springer Japan KK

K. Miyoshi, C.M. Shapiro
M. Gaviria, Y. Morita (Eds.)

Contemporary Neuropsychiatry

With 57 Figures, Including 3 in Color

Springer

Koho Miyoshi, Former Professor
Department of Psychiatry, Kyoto University Graduate School of Medicine
Sakyo, Kyoto 606-8397, Japan
Present address: Hyogo Institute for Brain Aging and Cognitive Disorders
520 Saisho-Koh, Himeji, Hyogo 670-0981, Japan

Colin M. Shapiro, Professor
The Toronto Hospital, Department of Psychiatry, University of Toronto
399 Bathurst Street, Toronto, Ontario M5T 2S8, Canada

Moises Gaviria, Professor
Division of Neuropsychiatry, Department of Psychiatry, University of Illinois at Chicago
912 S. Wood Street, Chicago, IL 60612, USA

Yoshio Morita, Professor
Department of Neuropsychiatry, Hyogo Medical University
1-1 Mukogawa, Nishinomiya, Hyogo 663-8501, Japan

ISBN 978-4-431-67992-9

Library of Congress Cataloging-in-Publication Data

Contemporary neuropsychiatry / K. Miyoshi . . . [et al.] (eds.)
p.; cm.
"Consists of selected papers from the 3rd International Congress of Neuropsychiatry, held in Kyoto April 9–13, 2000"—pref.
Includes bibliographical references and index.
ISBN 978-4-431-67992-9 ISBN 978-4-431-67897-7 (eBook)
DOI 10.1007/978-4-431-67897-7
1. Neuropsychiatry—Congresses. I. Miyoshi, Koho, 1935- II. International Congress of Neuropsychiatry (3rd: 2000 Kyoto, Japan)
[DNLM: 1. Mental Disorders—etiology—Congresses. 2. Brain—physiopathology—Congresses. 3. Brain Diseases—physiopathology—Congresses. 4. Neuropsychology—Congresses. WM 220 C761 2001]
RC327 .C765 2001
616.8—dc21

00-067934

Printed on acid-free paper

Originally published by Springer-Verlag Tokyo in 2001
Softcover reprint of the hardcover 1st edition 2001

Typesetting, printing, and binding: Best-set Typesetter Ltd., Hong Kong
SPIN: 10784672

Preface

On behalf of the editors, I would like to express my pleasure on the publication of *Contemporary Neuropsychiatry*. This monograph consists of selected papers from the 3rd International Congress of Neuropsychiatry, held in Kyoto April 9–13, 2000. I believe that the chapters in the book, contributed by leading psychiatrists and neurologists, provide us with a comprehensive perspective on neuropsychiatry.

The International Organization of Neuropsychiatry (ION) was formed by Spanish and American neuropsychiatrists in Seville in 1996, and its first congress was held as a satellite meeting of the World Psychiatric Association in Madrid. Approximately 200 people from around the world gathered to found this international neuropsychiatric organization.

Two years later, the second international meeting was held in Toronto. In conjunction with the Toronto meeting, the International Neuropsychiatric Association (INA), dedicated to promoting the study of the brain and behavior from a neuropsychiatric perspective, was established to supersede the ION. Twenty-four countries from Europe, North and South America, Asia, and Australia were represented. It was decided that the association would hold biennial meetings. Accordingly, the third congress was held in Kyoto in conjunction with the annual meeting of the Japanese Neuropsychiatric Association.

Neuropsychiatry endeavors to understand the complex interrelationship between behavior and brain function from a variety of perspectives, including those of psychology, neurology, and psychiatry. Neuropsychiatry aims especially to study the psychiatric symptoms of neurological disorders and to investigate psychiatric disorders as brain disorders.

According to the mission statement of the INA, we aim to prevent or reduce the suffering of people with brain–behavior disorders by increasing, integrating, and disseminating knowledge and understanding of the relationships between brain function and human behavior. The INA aims to accomplish this objective by providing a forum for interaction and exchange of ideas among a variety of professionals with an interest in neuropsychiatric issues. The INA endeavors to publicize and disseminate both clinical and academic advances in the field to bring about improved health for people throughout the world. Although rapidly advancing medical technology has greatly expanded the frontiers of neuropsychiatry, the INA will strive to preserve the humanistic values of medicine. The INA endeavors to raise awareness of neuropsychiatry particularly in those countries where it is not well known or recognized.

At the Kyoto meeting, we had approximately 700 participants from 31 countries and districts, namely, Australia, Belgium, Canada, Croatia, Egypt, France, Germany, Greece, Hong Kong, India, Israel, Italy, Japan, Korea, Lithuania, Macedonia, the Netherlands, the Philippines, Poland, Russia, Spain, Sweden, Switzerland, Taiwan, Thailand, Turkey, the United Arab Emirates, the United Kingdom, the United States, Uruguay, and Venezuela.

The Congress was fruitful and stimulating. I sincerely hope that this publication of its proceedings stimulates further development of neuropsychiatry in the future.

We would like to acknowledge support for the 3rd International Congress of Neuropsychiatry by the Japan National Tourist Organization (JNTO), the Osaka Pharmaceutical Manufacturers' Association, the Pharmaceutical Manufacturers' Association of Tokyo, the Takeo and Megumi Takayama Foundation, and the Uehara Memorial Foundation.

Koho Miyoshi, M.D.
Chairman, 3rd International Congress of Neuropsychiatry
Kyoto

Contents

Contributors

Worldwide Collaboration and the Future of Neuropsychiatry

The Future of Neuropsychiatry

Colin M. Shapiro, Madeline Li, Alan Ong, Ajmal Razmy, and Tonia Seli

Introduction

The coming era of neuropsychiatry will be one of unparalleled discovery. Advances in the realms of functional neuroimaging and molecular biology will be translated into greater understanding of, and improved therapy for, neuropsychiatric diseases. The clinical epidemiology of neuropsychiatric disorders will provide a more accurate measure of the global impact of these illnesses. With the aging population, neuropsychiatric disorders will become more prevalent. The understanding of what neuropsychiatry embraces will change as we learn more about the mind and the disorders that tread the line between traditional neurology and psychiatry. The appreciation of the relevance of diverse disciplines such as anthropology, psychology, and physiology to the conceptualization of neuropsychiatry will become more apparent.

The title of this chapter was the subject of a presentation by the first author at the Third International Neuropsychiatry meeting in Kyoto, Japan. The focus of that oral presentation was the scope of neuropsychiatry; the range of new issues that might be encompassed in a neuropsychiatric model, with special reference to the speaker's personal area of interest, i.e., fatigue and sleep disorders. Social ramifications and educational issues were highlighted. For the purpose of this chapter, an active decision was made to change the written format to include what the real future of neuropsychiatry is, namely the students that current neuropsychiatrists will attract into the field. At the present time, the first author is fortunate to have amongst his students a psychiatry resident with a PhD in genetics, a neurology fellow, a neuroscience student, and a psychiatry resident with an interest in neuroimaging. Collectively, we describe three key areas that will help in the development of this field—neuroimaging, genetics, and psychopharmacology.

Other developments in neuropsychiatry include deep brain stimulation in conditions such as movement disorders (Lang and Lozano 1998), but may enter areas such as appetitive behaviors and the management of obesity in the near future. These developments will add to our understanding of individual patients. Understanding the

Neuropsychiatry Programme, Department of Psychiatry, University of Toronto and University Health Network, Toronto, Canada molecular basis for numerous neuropsychiatric diseases will be a great challenge for the future. Knowing the pathogenesis of these disorders will be vital in developing treatments for them. Abnormal protein interactions and aggregations are involved in the development of numerous neurodegenerative disorders, including Alzheimer's disease, Parkinson's disease, and prion diseases. Other molecular scanning approaches are likely to be developed, and the further exploration of molecular defects in neuropsychiatric conditions may lead to treatments to inhibit or prevent these diseases.

The interplay between the biological and the experiential will be a key area of development. The notion that if words can harm then words can heal will be characterized in more biological terms based on a better understanding of the plasticity of the brain. A titration effect of potentially too much psychotherapy might be established based on biological changes and broader examples of the elegant studies by Baxter et al. (1996) in which both neuropharmacological and behavioral treatments were shown to induce similar effects in the brain as measured by metabolic changes. These will continue to inform us as to the range of treatments that are required in a comprehensive therapy.

The future of neuropsychiatry is as limitless as the human mind. Our learning about neuropsychiatric disorders will undoubtedly accelerate, and so too will our understanding of the mechanisms of the mind such as memory, learning, mood, emotions, fatigue, and sleep. This era will be an exciting one for neuropsychiatry.

Imaging in Neuropsychiatry

Can abnormalities of perception, cognition, emotion, and behavior be linked to brain dysfunction? One hundred years ago, there was little distinction between neurology and psychiatry, and since Freud's early observations as a young neurologist, the controversy continues over whether psychiatric disorders can be objectively diagnosed and ultimately localized in the brain. Since the technological developments in the 1970s, researchers and clinicians have had the ability to view the living brain, and this has had a major impact on our evolving theories, diagnoses, and treatment of brain-related disorders (Weight and Bigler 1998). First with computed tomography (CT) and then with magnetic resonance imaging (MRI), we can now see a slice of the human brain, offering precise structural and volumetric analyses. Functional imaging such as positron emission tomography (PET) and single photon emission computerized tomography (SPECT) provide an in vivo approach to examining physiological variables such as cerebral blood flow (CBF), brain metabolism (oxygen, glucose), and brain receptor distribution (Velakoulis et al. 1998). Furthermore, new technology such as functional MRI (fMRI) exploits the blood as an endogenous tracer to measure the natural hemodynamic response associated with neural activity (Longworth et al. 1999). Temporal resolution of the order of tens of milliseconds may ultimately be achievable (Menon et al. 1998). The prospect of molecular imaging as a new technology which will be as revolutionary as any of the preceding developments is on the drawing board. Discrete changes in signal can be mapped directly onto a high-resolution scan of the subject's anatomy, providing tremendous insight into brain function and *dysfunction*.

Current views of higher brain function emphasize two different perspectives. One is that processing occurs in discrete modules, easily identifiable on CT or MRI, which are anatomically circumscribed and referred to as *functional segregation* (Dolan et al. 1997). This is in contrast to the other dominant view that higher brain function is not strictly localized, but is a property of interactions between functionally specialized brain regions, i.e., *functional integration* (Dolan et al. 1997), and is therefore more amenable to PET, SPECT, or fMRI. Whether one favors a functional segregation or integrative approach, one's interpretations of imaging studies will be inherently affected by these basic assumptions of brain function. Intuitively, one may assume that functional segregation may be more relevant to elucidating the underlying brain function of specific symptoms, whereas functional integration may be more relevant to understanding fundamental disease mechanisms (Dolan et al. 1997). This assertion is evident in imaging studies in schizophrenia, which demonstrate abnormal frontotemporal activity which is independent of symptoms and stage of illness (Frith et al. 1995).

Additional theoretical challenges exist within the functional segregation approach when examining specific symptoms. Silbersweig and Stern (1997) state that specific symptoms such as hallucinations or delusions occur in different psychiatric disorders, and are more likely to map onto discrete locations than are heterogeneous syndromes (Silbersweig and Stern 1997). Furthermore, they argue that symptoms can be divided into symptom *traits* and symptom *states* (Silbersweig and Stern 1997). To examine traits, one must measure the symptom of interest with various rating scales, and then use *resting scans* (PET or SPECT) to find brain areas in which CBF correlates with symptom measures. Symptom states, on the other hand, entail eliciting the symptom of interest using an activation task, and capturing an image of the brain *as the symptom occurs* (fMRI). Both functional integration and functional segregation (trait and state) approaches have been used extensively in functional neuroimaging studies, and they address critical questions regarding both the localization and mechanisms of various psychopathologies. Bearing these theoretical and conceptual challenges in mind, we can begin to examine the contributions of imaging to various neuropsychiatric disorders.

Early imaging studies with CT scans demonstrated cortical atrophy and enlarged ventricles in psychotic disorders (Gerwitz 1994; Andreason 1988). Although much less expensive and more accessible, the use of CT in psychiatry has largely been surpassed by the use of MRI and functional imaging techniques such as PET, SPECT, and fMRI.

MRI provides higher-resolution images which are superior for structural and morphological analyses of the brain. MRI findings in obsessive compulsive disorder (OCD) include lesions in the caudate nucleus (Weilburg 1989), and a longer corpus callosum when compared with control subjects (Grachev et al. 1998). In posttraumatic stress disorder (PTSD), lateralized findings of reduced right hippocampal volume have been reported (Bremner 1995). Attention deficit hyperactivity disorder (ADHD) MRI studies have revealed right-sided dysfunction of the frontal striatal circuitry (Heilman et al. 1991), reduced total cerebral volume (Castellanos 1996), and smaller right-sided caudate nucleus, globus pallidus, and cerebellum (Castellanos 1996). In mood disorders, the most robust MRI finding involves cerebral white matter hyperintensities (WMHI). These WMHI volumes are significantly different when comparing patients with unipolar and bipolar disorders; with bipolar disorder patients showing a higher volume of abnormal white matter (Dupont 1995). MRI has been used extensively to replicate the findings of ventricular enlargement in acute and chronic schizophrenia (Gur 1994), and a reduction in the sizes of the hippocampus and amygdala, which are critical components of the limbic system (Hyde 1991). Further MRI studies have associated negative symptoms of schizophrenia with temporal rather than frontal lobe abnormalities (Turetsky 1995). Finally, in a 1996 MRI and PET study of medication-naïve patients with schizophrenia, volumetric analysis found that the thalamus of such patients was significantly smaller than that of controls (Buchsbaum 1996). This significant finding may provide a basis for perceptual abnormalities, as it is well known that the thalamus has extensive connections to the prefrontal cortex, which modulates sensory input (Buchsbaum 1996).

Functional brain imaging in neuropsychiatric disorders began with SPECT scans, and this technology is the only one used routinely in clinical care at present. SPECT scans measure CBF by detecting injected radiopharmaceuticals and their perfusion into different brain regions while the patient is at rest (Weight and Bigler 1998). They have increasingly been used in the investigation of dementia, movement disorders, epilepsy, and head injury (Velakoulis et al. 1998). Clinically, they have been most useful in evaluating dementia. Bilateral parietotemporal perfusion deficit is the most consistent finding in Alzheimer's disease (AD) (O'Brien et al. 1992), which can be clearly differentiated from the bilateral frontal hypoperfusion seen in frontotemporal dementia (FTD) (Velakoulis et al. 1998). Similarly, multiple "patchy" perfusion deficits can differentiate both AD and FTD from multiinfarct or vascular dementia. SPECT scans can also play an important role in the evaluation of mild to moderate head injury, especially when minimal or no structural imaging changes are evident (Velakoulis et al. 1998). SPECT findings in mood disorders have not been consistent, but some evidence suggests that depressed patients have decreased cortical and subcortical CBF (O'Connel 1995). Interestingly, SPECT data may provide a method of differentiating schizophrenia from psychotic depression. Both have hypofrontal blood flow, but this is more pronounced in the right inferior frontal lobe in patients with depression and psychotic features (Ebert 1993).

PET scans can be used to examine brain metabolism (with ^{18}F-fluorodeoxyglucase ([^{18}F]-FDG)), blood flow (with ^{15}O), and neurochemistry (with radioactively labeled ligands) but tissue resolution does not match that of CT or MRI (Weight and Bigler 1998; Silbersweig and Stern 1997). PET studies in PTSD have confirmed MRI findings of hypometabolism in both hippocampi (Markowitsch et al. 1998), which has been postulated to result from glucocorticoid toxicity and contribute to amnesia of the traumatic episode (Sapolsky and Pulsinelli 1985). In ADHD, PET scans have revealed significantly reduced glucose metabolic rates in the right thalamus, hippocampus, cingulate, and caudate (Zametkin 1990), which corresponds to the right-sided prefrontal striatal dysfunction seen in MRI studies. In one study of mostly bipolar patients, PET scans with [^{18}F]-FDG showed relative hypofrontality, with significantly lower metabolic rates in the basal ganglia compared with controls (Buchsbaum 1986). PET findings have not been able to differentiate reliably between unipolar and bipolar mood-disordered patients (Weight and Bigler 1998). Schizophrenia PET studies have replicated MRI findings of reduced thalamic metabolism (Buchsbaum 1996), which may disrupt complex thalamocortical circuits, and affect the patients' ability to filter, organize, and formulate concepts into meaningful experience.

Although still in its infancy, functional MRI joins the technologies of high-resolution MR scans with the ability to detect functional physiological changes. The most common form of fMRI is blood oxygenenation level-dependent (BOLD) imaging (Ogawa et al. 1990). The BOLD signal depends on the ratio of oxygenated to deoxygenated hemoglobin, with an increased ratio leading to an increased magnetic resonance signal, which is used as a marker of functional activation. Most fMRI involves measuring the BOLD signal while subjects are engaged in controlled tasks, during which changes in signal are mapped directly onto an MRI scan. This provides the opportunity of imaging brain function in vivo without the need for radioactive tracers (Longworth et al. 1999), and safely allows for repeated scans in the same patient to monitor the course of illness, and possibly its response to treatment.

Comparing brain activation recorded during emotionally sad or neutral film clips revealed that the left medial prefrontal cortex and the right anterior cingulate gyrus were activated more in depressed subjects than in controls (Beauregard et al. 1998). The investigators postulated that abnormal frontal activity in depression may disconnect the limbic system from normal modulatory influences (Beauregard et al. 1998). In schizophrenia, language tasks during fMRI have revealed specific hypoactivity in the frontotemporal cortex (Honey et al. 1998).

Functional MRI may help elucidate transient neuropsychiatric phenomena such as delusions, hallucinations, and mood. In Alzheimer's disease, a disorder with established neural correlates, fMRI has demonstrated temporoparietal hypoperfusion which correlates with the severity of the dementia (Sandson et al. 1996). Studies of brain activation in Alzheimer's disease using fMRI will continue to break barriers in our understanding of cognition, and of how the brain compensates in response to damage. Functional MRI shows promise as a diagnostic tool for the early detection of Alzheimer's disease. Different patterns of brain activation in patients at risk of developing Alzheimer's disease have been identified (Bookheimer et al. 2000). This is always a key factor with neurodegenerative conditions, and the principle treatments will involve arresting the process of abnormal protein accumulation to prevent the onset and onslaught of the disease.

Other new developments, such as real time fMRI, display the course of neural activation *during* the scan rather than processing the data after scanning. This will allow for an immediate assessment of brain function, and add to its possible applications, e.g., presurgical evaluation of lesions near critical cortical areas (Van Muiswinkle et al. 1999), and treatments based on biofeedback, which involves showing patients images of their own brain function while they are in the scanner (Longworth et al. 1999).

With continued advances in technology, fMRI appears to show the greatest potential, and should lead to an improved understanding of the relation between neural dysfunction and neuropsychiatric disorders. It will grow as a tool for earlier diagnosis of neuropsychiatric disorders, allowing treatment to be initiated sooner. Functional MRI has the ability to detect clinically silent evidence of neuronal dysfunction prior to detection using other tools. It has the ideal characteristics of a diagnostic tool, being noninvasive and nontoxic. The resolution of fMRI is greater than in techniques such as positron emission tomography (PET) or single photon emission computed tomography (SPECT). It will provide a more precise localization of areas of activation, and help in the understanding of the synchrony between multiple areas of the brain. The cost of fMRI will decrease as its use becomes more widespread.

In addition to examining specific symptoms and disease mechanisms, the future of imaging in neuropsychiatry will involve serial scans to temporally delineate the course of an illness and its response to treatment. The neuroimaging techniques discussed here are just beginning to extend the notion of neurological localization of psychiatric disorders, which were previously thought to be "psychological" owing to their apparent lack of associated structural lesions. With this in mind, we in neuropsychiatry continue to concern ourselves with the inexorably intertwined philosophical, dynamic, and social study of people's lives *in addition to* brain dysfunction.

Neuropsychiatric Genetics

Neuropsychiatric genetics is a rapidly expanding field which will ultimately have profound impacts on wide-ranging areas of neuropsychiatry—from etiology, diagnosis, and treatment, to public perception and medical ethics. Linkage analysis has been able to identify a genetic vulnerability for familial Alzheimer's disease (Drouet et al. 2000). Three causative genes, APP, PS1, and PS2, have been identified for the early-onset form of this disorder, while ApoE has been shown to be a susceptibility gene for later-onset disease. These findings have stimulated a wealth of neurobiological studies (Hardy and Israel 1999; Yu et al. 2000) which are beginning to translate from the bench back to the bedside, with new therapies targetting the molecular pathology of AD (Schenk et al. 2000).

However, as a newly emerging field, the recent explosion of published genetic associations with neuropsychiatric disorders has been fraught with inconsistent and nonspecific results (Owen et al. 2000; Stoltenberg and Burmeister 2000). With the exception of AD, simple linkage analysis has so far failed to unambiguously identify causative gene mutations for any neuropsychiatric disorder. What we have learned from these studies is that human behavior is genetically complex, and it is unlikely that single genes will be found which account for most genetic vulnerability to a neuropsychiatric disorder. Rather, such complex disorders more likely have a polygenic pathogenesis, involving the combined action of multiple vulnerability genes with small effects. Examples of consistent, but not unequivocal, associations include linkage to loci on chromosomes 5, 6, 8, 13, 18, and 22 for schizophrenia (Owen 2000), and 4, 6, 18, 21, and X for bipolar disorder (Pato et al. 1999). The report of the NIMH Genetics Workgroup summarizes recent genetic findings for ADHD, autism, bipolar disorder, depression, eating disorders, OCD, panic disorder, schizophrenia, and Tourette's syndrome (Moldin 1999). These results are complicated by the genetic heterogeneity present in different ethnic populations, co-morbidities among psychiatric diagnoses, and the fact that these diagnoses are based on clinical phenomenology and may not reflect distinct biological disease entities.

With respect to the latter, most neuropsychiatric disorders are really better described as syndromes comprised of a number of phenotypic symptoms. Particular phenotypic symptoms can overlap between disorders, which is consistent with the debate over whether schizophrenia and bipolar disorder are distinct entities or part of a spectrum. Rather than focusing on DSM-IV diagnostic categories, neuropsychiatric genetic studies are now beginning to be restricted to particular phenotypes which are common in affected individuals, but which are also present more often in unaffected relatives than in the general population. Examples include predisposing temperament traits, deficits in smooth pursuit eye tracking, quantifiable cognitive defects, electrophysiological measures, and specific neuroimaging correlates (Owen et al. 2000; Stoltenberg and Burmeister 2000).

With the completion of a working draft of the Human Genome Project in the summer of 2000, neuropsychiatric genetics has entered a new era. We will be able to take advantage of an unprecedented body of sequence information, and in conjunction with advanced technologies such as scoring single nucleotide polymorphisms on DNA microarrays (Sklar et al. 1999), it will be possible to perform detailed genome-wide association studies and simultaneously test thousands of candidate genes.

Association studies with candidate genes remains a fruitful approach to identifying susceptibility genes which can have early clinical utility. Homozygosity for low-activity allelic variants of a serotonin transporter promoter polymorphism (5-HTTLPR) has been associated with patients who are nonresponders to selective serotonin reuptake inhibitors (SSRIs) (Zanardi et al. 2000). Thus, genetic testing may lead to effective treatment matching.

Animal models for neuropsychiatric disorders would greatly assist the search for genetic determinants and the development of psychopharmacogenetics. Given the complexity of human behavior, it is unlikely that animal models can be developed that mimic the full spectrum of any neuropsychiatric disorders. However, animal models may be designed to exhibit particular neuropsychiatric phenotypes. Murine models have been engineered which develop the amyloid plaques of AD (Janus et al. 2000), and studies of emotionality in strains of mice are believed to model human anxiety (Flint and Corley 1996). Animal models are currently being developed for aspects of depression, hyperactivity, and schizophrenia. Such models may emerge from large-scale murine mutagenesis programmes aimed at generating novel phenotypes (MRC Mammalian Genetics Unit, Harwell, UK).

It is clear that neuropsychiatric disorders have a multifactorial pathogenesis, involving both environmental and genetic contributions. Elucidation of the genetic determinants of neuropsychiatric disease will facilitate the analysis of independent environmental factors. However, new statistical methods will have to be applied in order to account for co-morbidity, and multigenic and gene–environment interactions, and to correlate phenotypic associations with disease classifications (Sham 1998).

The potential benefits of neuropsychiatric genetics are numerous, but they are necessarily accompanied by sociological risks, and raise the specter of genetic discrimination or even neuropsychiatric eugenics (Farmer et al. 2000). Given the polygenic, multifactorial pathogenesis of neuropsychiatric syndromes, however, the actual predictive value of most neuropsychogenetic tests will be low. Reductionist determinism need not be invoked (Baron 1995). Instead, the future of neuropsychiatric genetics realistically has the power to clarify the age-old question of nature versus nurture, and the potential to revolutionize our diagnostic classifications and individualize patient treatment.

Neuropsychopharmacology

Without question, pharmacology has catalyzed the study and treatment of psychiatric disorders from a neuroscientific perspective. Aside from helping the mentally ill, discoveries of antipsychotics, antimanic agents, and antidepressants, found by a combination of serendipity and scientific ingenuity, have provided invaluable insight into the synaptic mechanisms of drug efficacy. Ironically, the development of these agents was predicated on results of successful pharmacological therapy that was viewed as a helpful aid to psychotherapy. Neuropharmacology is a driving force behind elucidating the mechanisms and treatment of mental disorders.

Although neuropharmacology has challenged psychodynamic explanations of mental illness, it has not led to a proliferation of new models to explain those disorders. However, an emerging approach that is providing new paradigms for basic research is a field called *cognitive neuropharmacology*. By definition, this field is a branch of neuropsychopharmacology which involves the design of drugs made to modify psychological functions. Such drugs are categorized into three groups: psycholeptics, psychoanaleptics, and psychodysleptics (Le Merrer and Nogues 2000; see Table 1) according to their effects on mental function.

Thus, the field of cognitive neuropharmacology targets the pharmacological investigation of cognition. According to this approach, understanding the mechanistic underpinnings of processes such as learning, memory, and attention will help clinicians to treat symptoms of mental disease and potentially reveal details of their etiology.

Much of the work incorporates animal models of cognition. According to Le Merrer and Nogues (2000), the investigation of cognition in animals via neuronal properties can be explained using both correlational and interventional approaches. Using a correlational model, animals are trained in specific cognitive tasks, and biochemical assays aimed at testing the involvement of molecular markers in the task are subse-

Table 1. Three categories of psychotropic drugs (from Le Merrer and Nogues 2000)

Drug category	CNS effect	Examples
Psycholeptics	Depress activity	Hypnotic or anxiolytic drugs
Psychoanaleptics	Increase activity	Amphetamine, caffeine
Psychodysleptics	Abnormal activity	Hallucinating substances or drugs of abuse

quently performed. The biochemical markers are compared relative to naïve animals, with the difference in pattern representing clues to the molecules involved in a particular task.

In contrast, the interventional model requires a comparison of the performance of control animals with that of animals treated with agents able to modify the target molecule. Two recent interventional methods are brain microdialysis and osmotic minipumps. The brain microdialysis technique (Westerink 1995) measures local neurotransmitter release *on-line* in correlation with animal behavior. By using an implanted guide cannula system tagged with a dialysis membrane, the extracellular concentration of neurotransmitters in the region of interest is determined. Osmotic minipumps (Ekman et al. 1998) are also a means to deliver drugs directly into the central nervous system (CNS). In this case, the drug can be administered by osmotic pressure through a catheter and a cannula directly into the relevant structure. Regardless of the approach used, cognitive neuropharmacology will help to refine current psychopharmacological treatment and provide critical insights into the mechanisms of drugs in mental functions.

For the most part, neuropharmacology has focused its mode of action on the synaptic cleft. Future intervention will elucidate brain mechanisms other than the classic processes of synaptic transmission. New classes of centrally acting agents are being discovered that behave differently than traditional transmitters.

Recent neuropharmacological research has focused experimentation on second-messenger systems. These systems regulate intraneuronal activity, the propagation of impulses down the neuron, and the configuration of receptor types (Schatzberg 2000). The link between neurotransmitters and second-messenger systems such as inositol phosphate is of particular interest. This type of approach has the potential to produce many new pharmacological agents that have not yet been fully described. Schatzberg (2000) recently commented,

> The identification of the key proteins involved in the so-called downstream effects and the genes that control them will allow development of treatment strategies or drugs that could affect these various subsystems without acting as agonists or reuptake blockers.

Another area which has gathered momentum over the past three decades is the investigation of neuropeptides in the pathogenesis of major psychiatric disorders (Nemeroff 1991). In particular, the identification of, often mulitple, receptor subtypes for each peptide, as well as the development of peptide antagonists, have opened a window to the study of the functional roles of neuropeptides. The modulatory role of neuropeptides is suggested by the fact that they are almost always stored with one or more classic transmitter types, although they are likely to be involved in many other types of function.

For instance, cholecystokinin (CCK) and its receptors have been implicated in anxiety, although this finding has not been replicated consistently in the literature, and this antagonist has also been variously reported to have analgesic effects (McCleane 1998; Price et al. 1985). It has been shown that CCK-4-induced panic attacks in humans can be attenuated by the CCKb antagonist CI-988 (Bradwejn et al. 1995).

Current research with regard to substance P and its receptor NK-1 implicate this peptidergic system in mood. Specifically, the NK-1 receptor antagonist MK869 has displayed antidepressant and anxiolytic properties (Kramer et al. 1998). MK869 was shown to be at least as effective as an SSRI prototype (paroxetine), with fewer side effects, in particular with regard to sexual dysfunctions and nausea. This has been claimed (Hokfelt 2000) as the first empirical evidence for dysregulation of a central neuropeptide system in a major mental disease. The recent demonstration of a melatonin analogue having clear antidepressant effects adds the opportunity of reconsidering the role of biological rhythms in depression.

In addition, the neuropeptide corticotropin-releasing factor (CRF) has also been described in relation to affective disorders such as anxiety and depression. Specifically, it is theorized that an increase in the secretion of CRF occurs in depressed patients. At a recent international congress on hormones, brain, and neuropsychopharmacology, Nemeroff (2000) cited four results that suggest that CRF is hypersecreted in patients with major depression. These are:

1. increased cerebrospinal fluid CRF concentrations in drug-free depressed patients;
2. increased numbers of cells expressing CRF in the hypothalamus of depressed patients in postmortem brain tissue;
3. reduced numbers of CRF receptor sites in the frontal cortex of depressed suicide victims compared with controls, presumably due to CRF hypersecretion;
4. a blunted adrenocorticotropin (ACTH) response to CRF receptor downregulation.

Thus, CRF antagonists may show potential for the treatment of depression. Nonpeptide antagonists acting on the CRF-1 receptor have been developed (McCarthy et al. 1999), opening up promising venues for clinical trials.

Recently, an important link between a peptidergic system and sleep disturbance has been revealed. The hypocretins/orexins, traditionally thought to be involved in feeding, are now linked to narcolepsy. Using a canine model of narcolepsy, Lin et al. (1999) have found a deletion in the transcripts of the hypocretin receptor 2 gene. Moreover, Chemelli et al. (1999) have described sleep abnormalities in narcoleptic mice with a deleted hypocretin/orexin gene. The significance of this genetic link between sleep regulation and a neuropeptide is pivotal, particularly if future research identifies any possible neuropsychiatric mediating factors (e.g., mood).

Finally, if one of the principle motives for the study of neuropharmacology is to uncover the circuitry behind human behavior and affect, then a truly integral investigation would be to evaluate the most fundamental human behavior: consciousness. Obviously an entirely pharmacological account of conscious experience would fail to account for the many spheres of consciousness, i.e., spiritual, affective, interpersonal, cognitive, and moral, to name a few, but what is it that "lights up" when you refer to consciousness, from a molecular point of view?

The race to solve the problem of consciousness is now in full flow (reviewed by Cotterill 1998; Crick 1994; Damasio 1999; Edelman 1989, 1992; Freeman 1995; Gazzaniga 1998; Greenfield 1995; Hobson 1999; Libet 1993; Searle 2000; Weiskrantz 1997). Perry et al. (1999) raised the issue that specific actions of acetylcholine (ACh) may represent previously unrecognized neural correlates of consciousness that are involved in integrating and defining the boundaries of the conscious "stream" of awareness. In support of their argument, these authors cite reports that cholinergic drugs, displaying muscarinic or nicotinic specificity, are involved in the regulation of levels of consciousness. These authors noted that in degenerative diseases of the brain, alterations in consciousness are associated with regional deficits in the cholinergic system. Noted in particular was that the loss of pedunculopontine cholinergic neurons in Parkinson's disease is likely to contribute to rapid eye movement (REM) sleep abnormalities. Critics have argued that Perry et al. (1999) took too much of a reductionist perspective in their analysis (Holscher 1999), or that they failed to look at consciousness at a finer molecular scale (Woolf, 1999).

The field of psychopharmacology has overtaken previous concrete, lock-and-key models of synaptic transmission. Mechanistic explanations of drugs are dynamic, taking into account the effects of multiple transmitter systems, interacting neuromodulators, and possibly the role of gases. Future work will continue to refine the success of available agents by the use of pharmacogenetics and neuroimaging as adjuncts to pharmacotherapy.

Conclusion

Decisions in the practice of neuropsychiatry will be shaped by developments in neuroscientific research. The 21st century neuropsychiatrist will need to be able to juggle the latest developments in the genetic and pharmacological spheres of basic science, and apply this knowledge to clinical studies.

In an excellent position paper, Price et al. (2000) suggest that three key questions should be the focus at the interface of neurology and psychiatry.

1. How do biological processes in the brain give rise to mental events?
2. How do environmental factors modulate the biological structure of the brain?
3. How can these forces be harnessed to promote mental health and recovery from brain injury?

We have very briefly alluded to facets of these questions in the comments concerning consciousness: the interaction between genes and the environment, and the development of new agents that take into account biological rhythms and processes, respectively.

Price et al. (2000) go on to recommend that the education of neurologists and psychiatrists should be revamped to give what, from the perspective of the current authors (Seli and Shapiro 1997), is the clearly neuropsychiatric stance that would be required for the full assessment of patients with brain behavior problems. We look forward to such developments, and anticipate an international organization, such as the INA, playing a key role.

References

Andreason NC (1988) Brain imaging: applications in psychiatry. Science 239:1381–1388
Baron M (1995) Neurogenetic determinism. Nature 375:351

Baxter LR, Schwartz JM, Bergman KS, et al (1992) Caudate glucose metabolic rate changes with both drug and behavior therapy for obsessive-compulsive disorder. Arch Gen Psychiatry 49:681–689

Beauregard M, Leroux JM, Bergman S, et al (1998) The functional neuroanatomy of major depression: an fMRI study using an emotional activation paradigm. Neuroreport 9:3253–3258

Bookheimer SY, Strojwas MH, Cohen MS, et al (2000) Patterns of brain activation in people at risk for Alzheimer's disease. N Engl J Med 343:450–456

Bradwejn J, Koszycki D, Paradis M, et al (1995) Effect of CI-988 on cholecystokinin tetrapeptide-induced panic symptoms in healthy volunteers. Biol Psychiatry 38:742–746

Bremner JD (1995) MRI-based measurement of hippocampal volume in patients with combat-related PTSD. Am J Psychiatry 152:973–981

Buchsbaum MS (1986) Frontal cortex and basal ganglia metabolic rates assessed by PET with [^{18}F] 2-deoxyglucose in affective illness. J Affective Disorders 10:137–152

Buchsbaum MS (1996) PET and MRI of the thalamus in never-medicated patients with schizophrenia. Am J Psychiatry 153:191–199

Castellanos FX (1996) Quantitative brain magnetic resonance imaging in ADHD. Arch Gen Psychiatry 53:607–616

Chemelli RM, Willie JT, Sinton CM, et al (1999) Narcolepsy in orexin knockout mice: molecular genetics of sleep regulation. Cell 98:437–451

Cotterill R (1998) Enchanted looms: consciousness networks in brains and computers. Cambridge University Press, Cambridge

Crick F (1994) The astonishing hypothesis: the scientific search for the soul. Scribner, New York

Damasio A (1999) The feeling of what happens: body and emotion in the making of consciousness. Harcourt Brace Jovanovich, New York

Dolan RJ, Friston KJ (1997) Functional imaging and neuropsychiatry. Psychol Med 27:1241–1246

Drouet B, Pincon-Raymond M, Chambaz J, et al (2000) Molecular basis of Alzheimer's disease. Cell Mol Life Sci 57(5):705–715

Dupont RM (1995) Magnetic resonance imaging and mood disorders: localization of white matter and other subcortical abnormalities. Dig Neurol Psychiatry 52:747–755

Ebert D (1993) A test-retest study of cerebral blood flow during somatosensory stimulation in depressed patients with schizophrenia and major depression. Eur Arch Psychiatry Clin Neurosci 242:250–254

Edelman G (1989) The remembered present: a biological theory of consciousness. Basic Books, New York

Edelman G (1992) Bright air, brilliant fire: on the matter of the mind. Basic Books, New York

Ekman A, Nissbrandt H, Heilig M, et al (1998) Central administration of dopamine D3 receptor antisense to rat: effects on locomotion, dopamine release and [^{3}H]spiperone binding. Naunyn Schmiedebergs Arch Pharmacol 358:342–350

Farmer A, Owen M, McGuffin P (2000) Bioethics and genetic research in psychiatry. Br J Psychiatry 176:105–108

Flint J, Corley R (1996) Do animal models have a place in the genetic analysis of quantitative human behavioral traits? J Mol Med 74(9):515–521

Freeman W (1995) Societies of brains: a study in the neuroscience of love and hate. Erlbaum, Hillsdale

Frith CD, Friston KJ, Herold S, et al (1995) Regional brain activity in chronic schizophrenic patients during the performance of a verbal fluency task. BMJ 167:343–349

Gazzaniga M (1998) The split brain revisited. Sci Am 279:35–39

Gerwitz G (1994) Results of computerized tomography during first admission for psychosis. Br J Psychiatry 164:789–795

Grachev ID, Breiter HC, Rauch SL (1998) Structural abnormalities of frontal neocortex in obsessive-compulsive disorder. Arch Gen Psychiatry 55:181–182

Greenfield S (1998) Brain drugs of the future. Br Med J 317:1698–1701

Gur RE (1994) Clinical subtypes of schizophrenia: differences in brain and CSF volume. Am J Psychiatry 151:343–350

Hardy J, Israel A (1999) Alzheimer's disease: in search of gamma-secretase. Nature 398:466–467

Hobson J (1999) Consciousness. Scientific American Lib./Freeman, New York

Holscher C (1999) Consciousness in mind: a correlate for ACh? Trends Neurosci 22:541–542

Honey GD, Soni W, Bullmore ET, et al (1998) Dissecting the components of linguistic processing in schizophrenia using functional MRI. Schizophrenia Res 29:65

Hyde TM (1991) Neuroanatomical and neurochemical pathology in schizophrenia. In: Tasman, Goldfinger (eds) Review of psychiatry. American Psychiatric Association Press, Washington, DC, pp 7–23

Janus C, Chisti M, Westaway D (2000) Transgenic mouse models of Alzheimer's disease. Biochim Biophys Acta 1502:63–75

Kramer MS, Cutler N, Feighner J, et al (1998) Distinct mechanism for antidepressant activity by blockade of central substance P receptors. Science 281:1640–1645

Lang AE, Lozano AM (1998a) Parkinson's disease. N Engl J Med 339:1044–1053

Lang AE, Lozano AM (1998b) Parkinson's disease. N Engl J Med 339:1130–1143

Le Merrer J, Nogues X (2000) Cognitive neuropharmacology: new perspectives for the pharmacology of cognition. Pharmacol Res 41:503–514

Libet B (1993) Neurophysiology of consciousness: selected papers and new essays. Birkhauser, Boston

Lin L, Faraco J, Li R, et al (1999) The sleep disorder canine narcolepsy is caused by a mutation in the hypocretin (orexin) receptor 2 gene. Cell 98:365–376

Longworth C, Honey G, Sharma T (1999) Functional magnetic resonance imaging in neuropsychiatry. BMJ 319:1551–1554

Markowitsch HJ, Kessler J, Van Der Ven C, et al (1998) Psychic trauma causing grossly reduced brain metabolism and cognitive deterioration. Neuropsychologia 36: 77–82

McCarthy JR, Heinrichs SC, Grigoriadis DE (1999) Recent advances with the CRF1 Receptor: design of small molecule inhibitors, receptor subtypes and clinical indications. Curr Pharmacol Design 5:289–315

McCleane GJ (1998) The cholecystokinin antagonist proglumide enhances the analgesic efficacy of morphine in humans with chronic benign pain. Anesth Analg 87:1117–1120

Menon RS, Luknowsky DC, Gati JS (1998) Mental chronometry using latency-resolved functional MRI. Proc Natl Acad Sci USA 95:10902–10907

Moldin S (1999) Report of the NIMH's genetics workgroup—summary of research. Biol Psychiatry 45:573–602

Nemeroff CB (1991) The neurobiology of neuropeptides: an Introduction. In: Nemeroff CB (ed) Neuropeptides and psychiatric disorders. American Psychiatric Press, Washington, DC, pp 3–11

Nemeroff CB (2000) Clinical studies on the role of CRF in mood and anxiety disorders. Neuropsychopharmacology 23(No. S2):S5

O'Brien J, Eagger S, Syed G, et al (1992) A study of regional cerebral blood flow and cognitive performance in Alzheimer's disease. J Neurol Neurosurg Psychiatry 55:1182–1187

O'Connel RA (1995) Single photon emission computerized tomography of the brain in acute mania and schizophrenia. J Neuroimaging 5:101–104
Ogawa S, Lee TM, Kay DW, et al (1990) Brain magnetic resonance imaging with contrast dependent on blood oxygenation. Proc Natl Acad Sci USA 87:9868–9872
Owen M (2000) Molecular genetic studies of schizophrenia. Brain Res Rev 2:179–186
Owen M, Cardno A, O'Donovan M (2000) Psychiatric genetics: back to the future. Mol Psychiatry 5:22–31
Perry E, Walker M, Perry GJ (1999) Acetylcholine in mind: a neurotransmitter correlate of consciousness? Trends Neurosci 22:273–280
Price BH, Adams RD, Coyle JT (2000) Neurology and psychiatry. Closing the great divide. Neurology 54:8–14
Price DD, van der Gruen A, Miller J, et al (1985) Potentiation of systemic morphine analgesia in humans by proglumide, a cholecystokinin antagonist. Anesth Analg 64:801–806
Roses AD (2000) Pharmacogenetics and the practice of medicine. Nature 405:857–865
Sandson TA, O'Connor M, Sperling RA, et al (1996) Noninvasive perfusion MRI in Alzheimer's disease: a preliminary report. Neurology 47:1339–1342
Sapolsky R, Pulsinelli W (1985) Glucocorticoids potentiate ischemic injury to neurons: therapeutic implications. Science 229:1397–1400
Schatzberg AF (2000) Psychopharmacology in the new millenium. In: Weissman S, Sabshin M, Eist H (eds) Psychiatry in the new millenium. American Psychiatric Press, Washington, DC, pp 179–192
Schenk DB, Seubert P, Leiberburg I, et al (2000) Beta-peptide immunization: a possible new treatment for Alzheimer disease. Arch Neurol 57:934–936
Searle JR (2000) Consciousness. Annu Rev Neurosci 23:557–578
Seli T, Shapiro CM (1997) Neuropsychiatry—the mind embrained? J Psychosom Res 43:329–333
Sham P (1998) Statistical methods in psychiatric genetics. Stat Methods Med Res 7:279–300
Silbersweig DA, Stern E (1997) Symptom localization in neuropsychiatry: a functional neuroimaging approach. Ann N Y Acad Sci 835:410–420
Sklar P, Altshuler D, Cargill M, et al (1999) DNA Microarrays for polymorphism detection and genotyping: utility in the understanding of complex neuropsychiatric diseases. CNS Spectrums 4(5):59–74
Stoltenberg S, Burmeister M (2000) Recent progress in psychiatric genetics—some hope but no hype. Hum Mol Genet 9:927–935
Turetsky B (1995) Frontal and temporal lobe brain volumes in schizophrenia. Arch Gen Psychiatry 52:1061–1070
Van Muiswinkle AC, van den Brink JS, Folkers PM (1999) Real-time fMRI on a clinical MR scanner. Neuroimage 9(2):S212
Velakoulis D, Lloyd JH (1998) The role of SPECT scanning in a neuropsychiatry unit. Aust N Z J Psychiatry 32:511–522
Weight DG, Bigler ED (1998) Neuroimaging in psychiatry. Psychiatr Clin N Am 21:725–759
Weilburg J (1989) Focal striatal abnormalities in a patient with obsessive-compulsive disorder. Arch Neurol 46:233–235
Weiskrantz L (1997) Consciousness lost and found. Oxford University Press, Oxford
Westerink BH (1995) Brain microdialysis and its application for the study of animal behaviour. Behav Brain Res 70:103–124
Woolf NJ (1999) Cholinergic correlates of consciousness: from mind to molecules. Trends Neurosci 22:540–541
Yu G, Nishimura M, Arawaka S, et al (2000) Nicastrin modulates presenilin-mediated notch/glp-1 signal transduction and beta-APP processing. Nature 407:48–54

Zametkin AJ (1990) Cerebral glucose metabolism in adults with hyperactivity disorder with childhood onset. N Engl J Med 323:1361–1366

Zanardi R, Benedetti F, Di Bella D, et al (2000) Efficacy of paroxetine in depression is influenced by a functional polymorphism within the promoter of the serotonin transporter gene. J Clin Psychopharmacol 20:105–107

Worldwide Collaboration in Neuropsychiatry

Moises Gaviria and Glorianna Montas

Modern neuropsychiatry is the psychiatric discipline that focuses primarily on the care of patients with major psychiatric disorders and with brain diseases that disrupt behavior. It requires clinical skills drawn from both psychiatry and neurology. Fundamentally, neuropsychiatric researchers explore the brain substrates of psychopathology, investigating the neurobiology of disordered emotion, cognition, and behavior (Coffey 1999).

The delimitation of the boundaries of neuropsychiatry as a clinical science is still not clear. In many places throughout the globe, researchers have studied the basis and connections between neurosciences, behavior, and psychopathologies. Although this field of study awakens new and innovational perspectives in some countries, in other countries many anniversaries of the beginnings of neuropsychiatry have been celebrated and commemorated. In fact, in several countries like Austria, Germany, and Russia, it is customary for physicians to become psychiatrists as well as neurologists if they wish to practice neuropsychiatry.

Neuroscience has come a long way since most Greek philosophers, as well as the ancient Egyptians, looked upon the heart as the seat of the soul and the organ responsible for many if not all mental functions. In the Roman Empire, the most influential physician was Galen, and his greatest works were on the nervous system. As far as he was concerned, the heart was not the organ of mind. He also numbered the cranial nerves, distinguished between sensory and motor pathways, and stated that "humoral" disorders were caused by vaporous influences that were carried by the arteries from the heart to the brain (Finger 1994).

Scholarship and new learning stagnated in the West during the Middle Ages; in the Dark Ages from about A.D. 800 to the twelfth century, little was accomplished. In the Middle East, however, philosophers such as Avicenna had access to the great Greek and Roman books of science. The Arabs and Christians translated the work of Hippocrates, Aristotle, and Galen. Western Europeans discovered much of this material only when they conquered Moorish Spain (1085–1248). The "new" scholarship soon spread to France, Italy, and others parts of Europe (Finger 1994).

Throughout the centuries, physicians used treatments such as potions, laxatives, ointments, gargles, baths, plasters, and bloodletting to treat the "loss of sense and

Division of Neuropsychiatry, University of Illinois at Chicago, Chicago, IL 60612, USA memory." In other periods, in the American colonies, supernatural and religious ideas about the mentally disturbed were stronger in the Puritan colonies. Satan was believed to have the power to drive or tempt a person into madness (Finger 1994).

The Renaissance is usually thought of as beginning in Italy in the midfourteenth century. One of the best recognized figures of this period was Leonardo da Vinci (1472–1519), who made more than 1500 anatomical drawings in his lifetime. About 1507, da Vinci conducted famous experiments on the ventricles of cattle to reveal their structure. Andrea Vesalius (1514–1564), a native from Brussels, published *De Humani Corporis Fabrica*, in which book IV dealt with the nerves and book VII with the brain (Finger 1994).

In 1664, Thomas Willis (1621–1675) published *Cerebri Anatome*. He proposed that cerebral gyri controlled memory, the will, and the imagination. Another important seventeenth-century figure was Niels Stensen (1638–1686), a Danish physician who emphasized the importance of studying the growth of the nervous system and suggested that the brain must be organized in parts to study its diverse functions (Finger 1994). In the eighteenth century, the first reasonable explanation was provided to account for damage on one side of the brain producing paralysis of the opposite side of the body. Both Charles Bell (1774–1842), from Scotland and François Magendie from France used experimental methods to study the spinal roots in dogs (Finger 1994).

According to Schiffer and Fogel, the first neuropsychiatric period started around the nineteenth century. In this period, there was a wealth of neurological symptoms among psychiatric patients. This therapeutics had originated with asylum-based reforms in France under Esquirol and Pinel, but found support from William Tuke and John Conolly in England. The principles of therapy included a reeducation of the patient in a humanistic enviroment, usually in a rural setting. Toward the middle of nineteenth century, the neurobehavioral side of the neuropsychiatric equation began to deepen. This change occurred because of diverse theories such as morbid heredity from France with Franz J. Gall in 1815 and Marie-Jean-Pierre Flourens in 1813, and neurobehavioral theories from the German laboratories of Frisch and Hitzig (Bechtel and Zawidzki 1988).

In post-Civil War years, because military patients presented both psychiatric and neurological conditions as the result of head trauma, neurology and psychiatry were taught together in the medical schools, and the early practitioners of neurology practiced both specialties. The same thing happened in other postwar periods throughout history (Bechtel and Zawidzki 1988).

Later on, clinical observations of Broca at the Salpetriere led to the development of early localizationist theories of neuropsychiatric function. Paul Broca presented his famous clinical case in 1861. His association between aphasia and damage to the frontal cortex became the first cortical localization that was widely accepted. Broca took a firm position about left-hemispheric dominance for articulate speech, but was careful to add that language was not the exclusive function of the left hemisphere (Finger 1994). About at the same time, the German neurologist Carl Wernicke investigated language functions other than speech. He proposed a model that could explain a number of different aphasic syndromes by lesions to different combination of centers and connections between centers.

In the 1870s, Emil du Bois-Reymond (1818–1896) had hypothesized that the transmission of the excitatory process from nerves to effector cells could take place either electrically via currents or chemically using excitatory substances liberated by nerve endings (Finger 1994). Other contributors to this field of study were Otto Selye and Korbinian Briedmann (1868) in Germany and Ramon y Cajal (1889) in Spain with several microscopic methods in neuroanatomy and basic principles of the functioning of neural connections (Bechtel and Zawidzki 1988).

In the beginning of the twentieth century, in the United States Walter Cannon (1911) conducted many experiments on the autonomic nervous systems and the problem of central regulation in the sympathetic nervous system. In 1919, Woodworth studied unusual rage responses in animals. In 1937, James Papez from Cornell University published a journal article in which he outlined a new circuit to account for emotion. He hypothesized that the hippocampus, the cingulate gyrus, the anterior thalamic nuclei, and the interconnections among these structures elaborated the function of central emotions (limbic system) (Finger 1994).

In the following years, subsequent biological therapies developed empirically. The true advent of biology in the treatment of psychosis was marked by the discovery of insulin therapy. Manfred Sakel (1937), like others before him, used the method during the withdrawal treatment of addicts. It was difficult to control the blood level and certain patients sometimes went into convulsions, whereas others fell into coma. During the same period, a Hungarian neuropsychiatrist, Laszlo von Meduna, was doing research in pathological anatomy of schizophrenia. He conceived the notion that inducing convulsions in schizophrenics could improve their condition. Later on (1938), Hugo Cerletti presented electroshock as a treatment for schizophrenia. It has been discovered, since 1945, that the target choice is depression (Pichot 1983).

Julian de Ajuriagerra (1945), who is considerated the founder of neuropsychology in Spain and France, developed a complete bibliography on child neuropsychiatry, dementias, and the cerebral cortex that he wrote along with his friend Henri Hecaen.

In Moscow, Aleksander Romanovich Luria in 1943 postulated his work about how higher cortical areas become associated through concrete activity and language; he also showed that our ways of thinking and reasoning are indeed culturally mediated and change when our lifestyles undergo historical transformations. Luria demonstrated that the brain is a flexible organ that, working together with cultural tools and signs, enables us to remediate our activities even when we are seriously impaired by injury, and developed a diagnostic system called syndrome analysis. He also carried out extensive research into the effects of brain injuries that had been sustained by people during World War II (Cole 2000).

In the United States, the pioneering writings of Norman Geschwind dramatically changed the way certain behavioral disturbances were viewed, imparting a radical neurological reductionism reminiscent of the previous century. When he described the disconnection syndromes in 1965, clinicians began to think for the first time in terms of a neuroanatomy of behavior; other discoveries were the existence of brain asymmetries, temporal lobe epilepsy syndromes, the aphasias, and the dyslexias.

Later on, new advances emerged because of biological treatments that developed in the early decades of the twentieth century (lithium in 1949, chlorpromazine in 1952, antipsychotic properties of reserpine in 1954, antidepressant properties of imipramine in 1957, and chlordiazepoxide in 1960). At this time biological psychiatry emerged as the result of diverse theories in genetics, molecular neurochemistry, imaging, and pharmachology. From that point of view almost every phenomenon could be explained with an objective and scientific base (Shiffer and Fogel 1996).

By midcentury, a paradigm shift of great consequence was beginning in the way psychiatrists viewed their patients—they were beginning to see major psychiatric disorders. This era of neuropsychiatry, as we see it today, emphasizes the neurological localization of the functions of the brain without underestimating interactions with the environment, genetics, and psychological issues (Shiffer and Fogel 1996).

In this past decade of technological advances, important developments have occurred such as neural networks and their applications to the development of artificial intelligence, therapeutic techniques of molecular biology, and neuroimaging. Understanding the brain offers the hope that we may eventually understand the mechanisms of major mental illnesses and ultimately develop methods for better treatment or perhaps even preventing them. Many symptoms of mental illness appear to represent distortions of normal brain functions. For example, hallucinations are abnormal perceptions whereas delusions are abnormalities in inferential thinking (Andreasen 1989). Brain imaging refers to a related group of techniques that permit us to study the structure and function of the human brain while people are still living. These techniques are noninvasive (Andreasen 1989).

Almost yesterday, it was unthinkable that we would, in fact, visualize the patterns of brain activity of normal, awake, behaving, thinking human beings without interfering in any way with it or with their behavior and mentation. Yet the unthinkable has happened. Functional imaging became a reality almost a decade ago. It revolutionized clinical diagnosis and has expanded tremendously the range of problems in the neurosciences that can be studied directly (Papanicolau 1998).

Before CT, we were able to see only the skull, using X-ray techniques, or at best to obtain an outline of the ventricles to make inferences about the brain through the complicated process of pneumoencephalography. Now, we can actually obtain clear pictures of the structures of the brain and observe it as it thinks and solves problems (Andreasen 1989).

Neuropsychiatric illnesses have become one of the major concerns in today's medical approaches. For example, in developed countries the quality of life is higher, people live longer, and the incidence and the prevalence of diseases such as dementia, Parkinson's disease, multiple sclerosis, and other degenerative illnesses is much higher than in those countries that are least developed (Privet 1996). On the other hand, in the less developed countries, or third world countries, where it is more common to have starvation, malnutrition, limited access to health care, developmental disorders such as mental retardation, epilepsy, meningitis, and other childhood illnesses are easier to find (Privet 1996). Because of the world's need to face these unquestionable and growing illnesses, more and more countries are unifying efforts to initiate fast and effective approaches to create consciousness in the medical communities.

Currently, there are many organizations and associations that encourage neuropsychiatry's growth in the world's medical society: in the United States, groups such as ANPA (American Neuropsychiatric Association), and in the international spectrum the INA (International Neuropsychiatric Association) (Coffey 1999). The first effort of ANPA in becoming a society took place in early May 1987, in Chicago, during the annual meeting of the American Psychiatric Association (APA). All physicians with dual certification in psychiatry and neurology and were invited to a reception. The second meeting of ANPA took place on April 18, 1988, in Cincinnati, hosting the annual meeting of the American Academy of Neurology (AAN). In the following year, Drs. Schiffer and Fogel formally established ANPA. Then on February 18, 1991, a newsletter announced that the directors had chosen the Journal of Neuropsychiatry and Clinical Neuroscience as their official founders (Coffey 1999). In July 1992, ANPA held its first international meeting, this in conjunction with British Neuropsychiatric Association (BNPA), in Oxford, England. The next 5 years marked an important period of growth, consolidation, and leadership in neuropsychiatry for the ANPA. In 1994, Jeffrey L. Cummings (professor of neurology and psychiatry, UCLA) became the first elected director of ANPA, beginning a 3-year term (Coffey 1999). Several annual meetings and congresses are held to update working professionals about the latest findings in recent studies. The First International Congress of the International Neuropsychiatry Association was established in Seville (1996). Following the first congress and the second one in Toronto (1998), this year the Third International Congress of Neuropsychiatry was held in Kyoto (2000). This last congress was held in conjunction with the 5th Annual Meeting of the Japanese Neuropsychiatric Association. In the year 2002, the Fourth Neuropsychiatry Congress will be celebrated in Israel.

Throughout the years, neuropsychiatry has been drifting from the biological side of sciences to the behavioral and more practical applications of its field. As an effort to priorize and differentiate one from the other, diverse writings led to the conclusion that it only depends on the field of study in which one is interested. However, in a time when the notion of interdisciplinary approaches to medical illnesses is so popular, mental health and neurology professionals have to embrace both points of view.

The boundaries that define the limits of neuropsychiatry are themselves only limited by the advances in new technologies that explore brain function. Because these are constantly changing, so too is the practice of neuropsychiatry. Twenty years ago, people would had thought that the techniques that are used today in modern neurosciences were no more than a science fiction novel. Today, an era of clinical neuroscience research is emerging that promises to provide a clearer definition of human brain–behavior relationships. With the consensus of the united efforts that are been reached by the world's largest countries, it is easy to predict that many changes will arrive in the upcoming decades as the new millenium unfolds.

References

Andreasen N (1989) Brain imaging: applications in psychiatry. American Psychiatric Press, Washington, DC

Bechtel W, Zawidzki T (1988) Biographies of major contributors to cognitive science. http://www.artsci.wustl.edu/-whechtel/ANAUT.html

Bentivoglio M (1999) Life and discoveries of Santiago Ramon y Cajal. Nobel Prize Foundation, Spain

Bigler D (1989) Neuropsychological functioning and brain imaging. Plenum Press, New York

Coffey E (1999) The American Psychiatric Association: ten years of progress and a great promise. J Neuropsychiatry Clin Neurosci 11:8–18

Cole M (2000) The making of a mind. http:/www.geocities.com/-nschmolze/luria.html

Corsi P (1991) The enchanted loom. Oxford University Press, New York
Finger S (1994) Origins of Neuroscience. Oxford University Press, New York
Papanicolau A (1998) Fundamentals of functional brain imaging. Swets & Zeitlinger, Houston, Texas
Pichot P (1983) A century of psychiatry. Dacosta, Paris
Privet M (1998) The world health report. http:/www.who.int/msa/mnh/ems/ratesold.htm

International Interaction in Neuropsychiatry: Vision of a Global Network

Eric Y.H. Chen

Introduction

Some issues concerning the possibilities for developing a more global framework of interaction in neuropsychiatry will be considered. Such interaction is made possible by advances in information technology, which has been evolving rapidly in the last few years and is likely to continue to do so in the coming years.

I shall first outline the basic arguments for collaborative work, as well as address the implications of information technology advances upon the nature of collaborative work. Then I shall consider the unique advantages offered by this new possibility, as well as ponder upon some of the potential difficulties that information technology has brought. Since the impact of information technology is likely to be increasingly pervasive, it is prudent to be considering how best to anticipate some potential problems and develop strategies for tackling them in advance. I shall be focusing in particular on activities that cross national boundaries. Although much of the focus is on research, I shall also cover aspects of education and service, which are all affected in very similar ways.

Rationale for Collaborative Work

After reviewing the processes involved in 20 of the most important technical advances made in the 20th century, Sir Alac Broers came to the conclusion that "We are in an era where the ideas of a single person alone seldom lead to fruition ...... If a researcher is not a part of the world technology network, he is unlikely to succeed." (Leadbeater 2000). Most of us would concede that the era of a lone scientist making a major breakthrough is largely over. Today, the remaining problems in science are perhaps of such a nature that progress is likely to rely on teamwork and cooperation between researchers.

Collaboration offers many competitive edges over working individually. Economy of scale is one of the most important principles leading to the success of large organizations. In contrast to working in a large number of small independent units, in one

Department of Psychiatry, University of Hong Kong, PRC

large program resources can be shared more effectively. In terms of research, this implies that a particular research protocol could be used by a larger number of groups. In addition, research instruments need to be developed and prepared once, and could then be shared by a larger number of participants. Often the most critical factor in good research is the availability of good ideas. Within a larger group, there is a better chance that a larger number of good research ideas emerge.

In addition, in research studies involving multiethnic collaboration, enhanced generalizability can be achieved if the findings are consistent across different ethnic groups. This can, to some extent, reduce the effort in later attempts to replicate the study in different populations. Such cross-ethnic validity of research result is important in many neuropsychiatric conditions and in clinical trials.

In neuropsychiatry, there are a number of interesting but rare syndromes or symptoms that up to now have only been captured in the form of single case studies or small case series. With the advent of the information revolution, there is now a real possibility of pooling these cases together in different sites and studying them with the same methodology. This should very substantially increase our knowledge of these rare disorders in a way that would have been impossible even 10 years ago.

Ethnic differences may also be one of the key features for understanding certain disorders. The need for international collaboration in studying these disorders is self-evident. The possibilities of further understanding ethnic differences will be powerfully enhanced with our ability to study the genetics of human ethnic variation, which has been made feasible by the genome project. Thus, the advantages associated with international collaboration are substantial, and the time is ripe for a significant increase in such effort. However, there are also other issues to be considered before collaborative relationships can become long-term and productive partnerships.

Ethics for Collaboration in an Age of Individualism

The drive towards cooperation is offset by an equally important instinct in the modern world, namely that of individualism and motivation by self-interest. In fact, most of our current market economy is based upon these principles. This will challenge the assumption that when a group of people work together, each person will honor the group objectives more than his own rewards. Often a very delicate balance is required to align individual goals with those of the group. Working in a group also involves concerns that others in the group might fail, either intentionally or unintentionally.

In general, the larger the scale of the cooperation, the more productive the group can be, but the risks involved are larger. This risk is somewhat reduced when we can choose who to work with. We therefore rely on our judgement, through past experience and interactions with our potential collaborator. In the age of information technology, there is going to be reduced social knowledge of the people we interact with and work alongside. Information technology offers us unprecedented opportunities to interact with a larger pool of people. The cost, however, is that the encounter between interacting individuals is going to be more limited in depth. In order to be successful in a collaboration, additional channels are required in order to allow individuals to meet. The function of scientific conferences may increasingly be weighted toward the provision of opportunities of personal encounter and face-to-face interaction rather than the conveyance of scientific content, which could be communicated much better through technology.

Potential Impacts of Information Technology

Information technology appears to be facilitating an increasing number of activities and productivity for scientific communities. It is becoming more widespread at an exponential rate, producing important changes in the way ordinary people run their lives. The arrival of the information age has already begun to affect the lives of many people, in many cases, in rather unexpected ways. For example, the arrival of e-commerce and banking is producing substantial challenges to traditional business and banking structures. The facilitation of global investment and the ability to shift resources around the world in an instant have contributed to the instability of the global economy. Thus, it is important to be aware of the potential opportunities it offers us, as well as some of the potential difficulties that it may bring.

Opportunities Offered by Information Technology

It is relatively easy to see what information technology offers. For instance, with just one keyword, "neuropsychiatry," within a minute one can access websites which offer a whole range of activities and information, including newsgroups, online journals, newsletters, etc.

Global Interaction in Research

It is not difficult to see that the technology could enhance our activities in research and education, as well as in clinical service. The coordination of international collaborative research is one area that would particularly benefit from such technology. A research team could be formed consisting of subunits operating in different countries. One of the units could take up the leadership role, but other units could share a lot of the work. The development of the protocol could largely be carried out by remote interactions. Each local team could monitor the feasibility of the protocol in their own setting, and suggest modifications. Changes would be negotiated between all teams. Statistical consultation, for example, could also be conducted in this way. Once a protocol is agreed, the preparation of the test procedures and instruments could be conducted at the various local sites, with feedback and clarifications being communicated efficiently via the Internet. Data collection could then be conducted at each local site. Data could be managed by a collective database with secure access by key individuals. Data analysis could also be carried out with extensive interaction through the Internet. Research team members could suggest perspectives and ways in which the data could be analyzed. An internet-mediated newsgroup could handle discussions between researchers, and should enhance the interpretation of results. Even the final preparation of the report could be a collective process. The process that I have been describing is a full, formal collaborative effort. There are also less formal ways of working. Groups may be drawn together because they share a common instrument, or ask a similar question, but use different ways to address that question. These groups could also benefit from the opportunities for discussion. For example, some of the more complex investigative techniques are usually set up in a process in which there is a long development period consisting of trial and error exploration. If different research groups could share their experience in this process, they could considerably shorten the learning curve for each other. Finally, even a network that only involves the exchange of ideas is offering the sort of stimulation and productivity that an entirely local setting could not compete with.

Global Interaction in Education

In terms of education, the development of a more global educational market is well underway, with the setting up of virtual libraries and electronic journals, as well as courses that can be taken via the Internet. This is particularly important for an area like neuropsychiatry, where the density of practitioners as well as of patient groups is rather low for some countries and in some conditions. Under such circumstances, the availability of an international network is particularly important for information, support, and professional development.

Global Interaction in Clinical Service

The possibility of offering Internet-based consultation and medical services is again a huge area under inevitable development (Zajtchuk and Gilbert 1999). This may take the form of the provision of information, consultations, and advise on treatment algorithms. This development has raised many concerns about the core competence in different areas of medicine, and the somewhat threatening question of the extent to which the physician could be replaced by self-help-type activity conducted through the Internet. Such developments challenge the monopoly of professional knowledge, and will have a profound impact on the way in which professional groups operate. Since this is a potentially threatening and sensitive issue, it could induce an attitude of defensiveness in the professionals if it is not dealt with properly.

Threats to Professional Knowledge in the Information Age

The key question is this: which part of our professional activity could be threatened? One important consideration is the nature of our professional knowledge. As is well characterized in cognitive psychology, there are at least two distinct kinds of knowledge. The first is explicit (declarative) knowledge. This type of knowledge can easily be expressed and communicated in language, flow charts, or algorithms. In contrast, implicit (tacit) knowledge is difficult to describe and define, and yet is essential for certain decisions. To carry out most complex tasks well, both explicit and tacit types of knowledge are required (Nonaka and Takeuchi 1995). Yet information technology selectively facilitates the propagation of the explicit type of knowledge. Ultimately, technology does not compensate for the lack of in-depth experiential knowledge. This differentiation between different types of knowledge can help us to reflect on the potential threat of the information revolution to our professional activities. The question then roughly translates into the extent to which our knowledge is explicit or tacit. The explicit part of our knowledge will be more easily replaced, and the tacit component will be relatively more valued, when information becomes open and cheap. Being more aware of the potential impact of the information revolution will help us to be less defensive, and in a better position to make the best use of the opportunities that it may offer.

Other Potential Difficulties in International Collaboration

The element that is most important to the protection of a professional boundary, i.e., tacit knowledge, may turn out to be the element that is most difficult to tackle amongst collaborators working through internet communication. One example is the elicitation of frontal lobe symptoms as well as the quantification of frontal lobe signs. Although much work has been done to try to operationalize these, the phenomenon is best observed in an unstructured setting, and rigid operationalization may pose inherent problems. Other obvious difficulties include the translation of instruments across languages, as well as studies in which language disorder is the focus. In such a case there may be fundamental languages differences which are not reconcilable by translation. One example is the "letter" fluency test, in which the subject has to produce as many words starting with a given letter as possible within a time limit. There is no real equivalent to this test in languages in which words do not consist of letters. In addition, one further serious problem exists in promoting international work. By making extensive use of information technology in mediating international collaboration, participants from the more deprived areas of the world are more likely to become excluded through lack of a good infrastructure. A number of solutions have been suggested, such as free access to databases and information, as well as aids to set up the basic equipment (Leadbeater 2000). In contrast, another problem is the potential shift of activities to areas with low labor costs. As commercial manufacturers have found out, more international exchange inevitably results in production being shifted to areas where labor costs are less expensive. There is no reason why this should not happen to scientific and medical activity as well. Once again, we need to foster a system of control and monitoring in advance, taking a lesson from industry.

Conclusions

In this chapter, I have explored a number of issue that could emerge as a result of more extensive international collaboration, made possible through information technology. I have addressed some new opportunities as well as some threats and pitfalls. If I have focused more on the problems than the opportunities, that is perhaps a reflection of the imminence of the impact. When a dream is far away, we tend to see the sunshine. When it is approaching closer, we begin to see the potential difficulties.

Having a clear awareness of the potential issues will help us to be ready, and more prepared to embrace the new technology as it begins to change the pattern of our work.

References

Leadbeater C (2000) Living on thin air: the new economy with a new blueprint for the 21st century. Penguin, Harmondsworth

Nonaka I, Takeuchi H (1995) The knowledge creating company. Oxford University Press, Oxford

Zajtchuk R, Gilbert GR (1999) Telemedicine: a new dimension in the practise of medicine. Dis Month 45:19997–262

Worldwide Collaborations in Psychiatry: The Role of Drug Trials in Schizophrenia in the Developing World

Sumant Khanna and K. Muthukumar

Summary. Drug metabolism differs significantly across ethnic populations due to various factors. One such factor is the genetic variability of the enzymes involved, and it is suggested that this genetic variation is a result of the interactions, in the remote past, of the ancestors and their environment. Ethnic groups also contrast markedly with regard to other pharmacokinetic factors. Some of these variations are the result of the respective environments of the ethnic groups in question. Data from drug trials illustrate differing placebo responses and side-effect reporting among groups, which are influenced by the prevailing cultural and related factors. In addition, serum drug concentrations, dose requirements, side effects, psychopathology, and the propensity to develop agranulocytosis are also found to differ among groups. Also, studies of certain ethnic populations were associated with various methodological issues, and factors other than biological were noted to influence the diagnosis and outcome studies of these populations. It is in this context of genetic and environmental differences markedly influencing the area of neuropsychopharmacology that the need for studies in various populations across the world is strongly felt.

Keywords. Schizophrenia, Drug trials, Ethnicity, Variability, Pharmacokinetics

The explosion that is occurring in the area of neuropsychopharmacology across the world is revolutionizing the treatment of neuropsychiatric disorders. In this presentation, an attempt is made to understand why newer psychotropic medication needs to be studied across the world and not only in developed countries.

Some of the genetically variable enzymes of drug metabolism include butyryl cholinesterase, serum paroxanase, cytochrome CYP 2D6, CYPmp, dopamine B-hydroxylase, catalase, superoxide dismutase, monoamine oxidase, alcohol dehydrogenase, aldehyde dehydrogenase, dihydropyrimidine dehydrogenase, *N*-acetyltransferase, glucuronyl transferase, thiol methyltransferase, phenol sulfotransferase, and glutathione-*S*-transferase (Lin and Poland 1995). These enzymes can result in ethnic differences in the metabolism of their target molecules.

The substrates for cytochrome CYP2D6 are the drugs clozapine, fluphenazine, haloperidol, perphenazine, risperidone, thioridazine, and trifluperidol, tricyclic

---

Department of Psychiatry, National Institute of Mental Health and Neurosciences, Bangalore 560029, India

antidepressants, SSRIs, monoamine inhibitors, antiarrhythmics, betablockers, and antihypertensives (Lin and Poland 1995). Regarding cytochrome CYP2D6, Lin et al. (1996) proposed that ethnic variation in alleles could be interpreted as the result of different environments to which ancestors were exposed, and that the unique pattern is the imprint of interaction between their ancestors and the prehistoric environment in which they lived.

Enzymes can be induced by different molecules: induction of cytochrome 3a is by glucocorticoids and carbamazepine, induction of cytochrome 2b and cytochrome 3a is by phenobarbitone, and induction of cytochrome 1a is by cruciferous vegetables, charbroiled beef, and cigarette smoking. Enzyme inhibition, on the other hand, can occur through three processes: competitive (reversible) inhibition, autocatalytic inactivation (irreversible), and repression of gene transcription.

Pharmacokinetic factors consist of drug metabolism, conjugation, volume of distribution, protein binding, etc. Yue et al. (1991) showed that slower glucuronidation of codeine occurs in Asians, leading to heightened sensitivity of the drug. Kumana et al. (1987) studied the volume of distribution, showing that the greater effect of diazepam in Asians depends on body build and body composition for lipophilic drugs. Studies on protein binding by Zhou et al. (1990) showed lower plasma alpha-1-acid glycoprotein but normal albumin in Asians. Kumana et al. (1987) showed lower albumin in Hong Kong Chinese, with Lin et al. (1993) finding higher drug-free fraction in Asians.

In an interesting study of pharmacokinetic factors, Branch et al. (1978) studied antipyrene in Sudanese living in Sudan or the UK and normal English subjects. Sudanese living in the UK and UK citizens were the same, whereas both groups differed from Sudanese residing in Sudan. Differences in environmental factors, especially dietary practices, were implicated.

Fraser et al. (1976) studied healthy Gambians in whom factors such as gender, cola nut consumption, hemoglobin (in women), and height (in men) were found to affect pharmacokinetics. Mahy (1977) studied black and white Barbadians treated with clomipramine. In this study, diet and climate were found to be important variables. Turner and Cooley-Quille (1996) reviewed existing studies to show that intragroup variance of a particular parameter can be greater than intergroup differences.

Drug trial data have shown that non-Caucasians are more responsive to placebo (Escobar and Tuason 1980). According to Lin et al. (1993), side-effect reporting was culturally determined and the role of stress, social support, and personality style affect response are important contributing variables.

Pharmacogenetics has classically been demonstrated in three areas of study, succinylcholine apnea, isoniazid-induced neurotoxicity, and primaquine hemolysis. Although these do not refer to the area of neuropsychopharmacology, probably examples in this area are needed.

Chang et al. (1993) showed that clozapine serum concentrations were significantly higher in Taiwanese schizophrenics as compared to Germans. Matsuda et al. (1996) studied Korean Americans in comparison with Caucasians and found that the Korean Americans received lower doses of clozapine, had greater change on the BPRS (Brief Psychiatric Rating Scale), had lower serum clozapine concentrations, and had more side effects. Higher risk for agranulocytosis was noted in the following populations: Finns (Amsler et al. 1977), Ashkenazi Jews (Lieberman et al. 1990), and American

Indians (Pfister et al. 1992). Caramikat et al. (1975) showed that African-Americans are more likely to have leukocyte counts below normal (benign leukopoenia).

Studies by Lin et al. (1988) showed larger prolactin responses to haloperidol in Asian normal volunteers as well as lower therapeutic ranges in Asian schizophrenic patients. Lin et al. (1988) compared Asian and Caucasian schizophrenics and found that Asians had higher plasma levels with fixed dose haloperidol. Also, they required lower doses, showed lower plasma concentrations, and had fewer side effects. Jann et al. (1989) demonstrated that Chinese have lower reduced haloperidol to haloperidol ratios, which suggests a lower rate of metabolism.

Studies on the pharmacology of schizophrenia by Jeste et al. (1996) showed no significant difference between African-American and Caucasian subjects in psychopathology or amount of neuroleptic therapy. Midha et al. (1988) compared African-American and Caucasian healthy males, finding wide interindividual variability in pharmacokinetic parameters of trifluperazine, but no significant differences were found between groups.

According to Lawson (1996), African-Americans are more likely to be diagnosed schizophrenic; also, poorer compliance, delays in seeking treatment, higher prescribed doses, and more prn usage confound racial differences in outcome. Adebimpe (1981) found that the diagnosis was influenced by social and cultural distance between patient and clinician, the stereotypes of psychopathology, false-positive symptoms, and biased diagnostic instruments. Strickland et al. (1991) reported that studies of African-Americans were characterized by various methodological issues such as diagnostic misclassification, presumed homogeneity, lack of age and gender controls, and minimal consideration of chronicity of illness.

Glazer et al. (1994) and Jeste et al. (1996) reported that African-American patients are at greater risk to develop tardive dyskinesia, probably due to unrecognized genetic or enzymatic defects. Although Pearlman (1984) reported no tardive dyskinesia in black patients in South Africa, Holden (1987) reported tardive dyskinesia in Zulu patients being comparable to Western figures.

In conclusion, it can be stated that pharmacodynamic and pharmacokinetic differences exist between racial groups and that biological and environmental factors appear to be important contributors to these differences. Hence, there is a need to have phase I, II, and III studies in different populations, especially in the emerging area of neuropsychiatry.

References

Adebimpe VR (1981) Overview: white norms and psychiatric diagnoses of black patients. Am J Psychiatry 133:706–709

Amsler HA, Teerenhovi L, Barth E, et al (1977) Agranulocytosis in patients treated with clozapine. A study of the Finnish epidemic. Acta Psychiatr Scand 56:241–248

Branch RA, Salih SY, Homeida M (1978) Racial differences in drug metabolizing ability: a study of antipyrine in the Sudan. Clin Pharmacol Ther 24:640–663

Caramikat E, Karayalcin G, Aballi G, Lunzowsky P (1975) Leukocyte count differences in healthy white and black children 1 to 5 years of age. J Pediatr 86:252–254

Chang WH, Chien CP, Lin SK, Chung MK (1993) Elevated Clozapine concentrations in Chinese patients. Neuropsychopharmacology 9:1178–1193

Escobar JI, Tuason VB (1980) Antidepressant agents: a cross-cultural study. Psychopharmacol Bull 16:49–52

Fraser HS, Bulpitt CJ, Khan C, et al (1976) Factors affecting antipyrine metabolism in West African villagers. Clin Pharmacol Ther 20:369

Glazer WM, Morgestern H, Doucette J (1994) Race and tardive dyskinesia among outpatients at a CMHC. Hosp Community Psychiatry 45:38–42

Holden TJ (1987) Tardive dyskinesia in long-term hospitalized Zulu psychiatric patients. S Afr Med J 71:88–90

Jann MW, Chang WH, Davis CM, et al (1989) Haloperidol and reduced haloperidol plasma levels in Chinese vs. non-Chinese psychiatric patients. Psychiatric Res 30:45–52

Jeste DV, Lindamer LA, Evans J, Lacro JP (1996) Relationship of ethnicity and gender to schizophrenia and pharmacology of neuroleptics. Psychopharmacol Bull 32:243–251

Kalow W (1990) Pharmacogenetics: past and future. Life Sci 43:1385–1397

Kalow W (1991) Interethnic variation of drug metabolism. Trends Pharmacol Sci 12: 102–107

Kumana CR, Lauder IJ, Chan M, et al (1987) Differences in diazepam pharmacokinetics in Chinese and white caucasians: relation to body lipid stores. Eur J Clin Psychopharmacol 32:211–215

Lawson WB (1996) Clinical issues in the pharmacotherapy of African-Americans. Psychopharmacol Bull 32:275–281

Lieberman J, Yunis J, Egea E (1990) HLA-B38, DR4 DQw3 and clozapine induced agranulocytosis in Jewish patients with schizophrenia. Arch Gen Psychiatry 47:945–948

Lin KM, Poland RE (1995) Ethnicity, culture and psychopharmacology. In: Bloom FE, Kupfer DJ (eds) Psychopharmacology: the fourth generation of progress. Raven Press, New York, pp 1907–1919

Lin KM, Poland RE, Lau J, Rubin RT (1988) Haloperidol and prolactin concentrations in Asians and Caucasians. J Clin Psychopharmacol 8:195–201

Lin KM, Poland RE, Lesser IM (1993) Psychopharmacology and psychobiology of ethnicity. American Psychiatric Press, Washington, DC, pp 11–26

Lin KM, Poland RE, Wan YJY, et al (1996) The evolving science of pharmacogenetics: clinical and ethnic perspectives. Psychopharmacol Bull 32:205–217

Mahy GE (1977) Clinical effects and plasma levels of clomipramine in depressed Barbadians. Postgrad Med J 53(suppl):87

Matsuda KT, Cho MC, Lin KM, et al (1996) Clozapine dosage, serum levels, efficacy, and side-effect profiles: a comparison of Korean-American and Caucasian patients. Psychopharmacol Bull 32:253–257

Midha KK, Hawes EM, Hubbard JW, et al (1988) A pharmacokinetic study of trifluperazine in two ethnic populations. Psychopharmacology 95:333–338

Pearlman T (1984) Different doses of neuroleptics for genetically different groups (letter). Am J Psychiatry 141:156–157

Pfister G, Hanson D, Roerig J, et al (1992) Clozapine-induced agranulocytosis in a Native American: HLA typing and further support for an immune mediated mechanism. J Clin Psychiatry 53:242–244

Strickland TL, Ranganath V, Lin KM, et al (1991) Psychopharmacologic considerations in the treatment of black American populations. Psychopharmacol Bull 27:441–448

Turner SM, Cooley-Quille MR (1996) Socioecological and sociocultural variables in psychopharmacological research: methodological considerations. Psychopharmacol Bull 32:183–192

Yue QY, Svensson JO, Sjoqvist F, Sawe N (1991) A comparison of the pharmacokinetics of codeine and its metabolites in healthy Chinese and Caucasian extensive hydroxylators of debrisoquin. Br J Clin Pharmacol 31:643–647

Zhou HH, Adedoyin A, Wilkinson GR (1990) Differences in plasma binding of drugs between Caucasians and Chinese subjects. Clin Pharmacol Ther 48:10–17

Behavioral and Psychological Symptoms in Turkish Alzheimer's Patients

Engin Eker and Turan Ertan

Summary. Studying behavioral and psychological symptoms of dementia (BPSD) across cultures allows the identification of similarities and differences that may be useful to determine the best approach to managing these symptoms in different populations. Although BPSD are not yet regarded as a main health issue in many developing countries, such as Turkey, these symptoms will undoubtedly become a management issue in the near future. There are also racial, ethnic, and cultural differences in dementia caregiving. There are some cross-national studies that use similar methodology in AD, and very few studies on BPSD that include developing countries or migrant populations. Although the BPSD constitute one of the major domains of symptomatology of age-associated dementia, Turkish family practitioners, residents in psychiatry and neurology, and even general psychiatrists and neurologists do not in general have sufficient experience to evaluate BPSD. Family members in Turkey are more likely to report behavioral and affective disturbances rather than memory problems. Caregivers in our community may underreport BPSD because of the fear the patient will be labeled or institutionalized, their need to maintain an acceptable social façade, their desire not to relinquish the caregiver role, and their religious values. Cultural influences must be considered in the studies of BPSD. Western countries should be able to compare results with different cultures. Therefore, joint studies are important.

Keywords. BPSD, Dementia, Turkish, Crosscultural

Alzheimer's disease and associated behavioral and psychological symptoms of dementia (BPSD) are already recognized as medical problems of the aging population in the Western world. Studying BPSD across cultures allows the identification of similarities and differences that may be useful to determine the best approach to managing these symptoms in different populations. An effective approach to management in one culture may not necessarily be effective in another, given the different prevalence of various BPSD and the level of tolerance for these within the community in which they occur. Although BPSD are not yet regarded as a main health issue in many developing

Department of Psychiatry, Section of Geriatric Psychiatry, Istanbul University Cerrahpaşa Medical School, Aksaray 34303, Istanbul, Turkey countries, such as Turkey, these symptoms will undoubtedly become a management issue in the near future (Cohen and Eisdorfer 1988). Because BPSD contribute most to the caregiver burden and interfere with patients' well-being, they are predictors of early institutionalization, especially in developed countries (Haupt and Kurz 1993).

There are some cross-national studies that use similar methodology in AD (White et al. 1996; Kua and Ko 1995; Chandra et al. 1998) and very few studies on BPSD that include developing countries or migrant populations (Binetti et al. 1998; Eker and Ertan, in press). On the other hand, there are racial, ethnic, and cultural differences in dementia caregiving (Connell and Gibson 1997; Eker and Ertan, in press; Chandra 1996; Mangone 1996; Youn et al. 1999).

Turkey has a young population with 40% of the total being under 20 years of age. According to the last census, people aged 60 years or older represented 6.9% of the total population and people 65 years or older represented 4.8%. In Turkey, demented patients mostly are cared for by their spouses or the eldest daughter in their homes and are only admitted to a specialist when BPSD are severe. Sleep disturbances and wandering are particularly upsetting to the patient's family. Although the BPSD comprise one of the major domains of symptomatology of age-associated dementia, Turkish family practitioners, residents in psychiatry, and neurology, and even general psychiatrists and neurologists do not in general have sufficient experience to evaluate BPSD. Knowledge and awareness of BPSD among the lay population are equally poor, and most demented patients' relatives regard cognitive impairment and BPSD as a natural consequences of aging.

The Outpatient Memory Clinics of the Istanbul University Cerrahpaşa Medical School, Department of Geriatric Psychiatry, has been serving patients since 1997. At this outpatient clinic, clinicians assess all elderly patients who report with memory disturbances and related psychiatric symptoms. The main areas of interest are the diagnosis of memory disorders and the assessment, treatment, and management of BPSD. All patients are evaluated according to the Diagnostic and Statistical Manual of Mental Disorders criteria for dementia (4th ed.) (APA 1994). The Turkish version of the Mini Mental State Examination (Folstein et al. 1975; Güngen et al. 1999) and the Global Deterioration Scale (GDS) (Reisberg et al. 1982) are routinely used for scoring the severity of clinical symptoms. All patients also undergo cranial MRI scanning and routine laboratory tests. The Behavioural Pathology in Alzheimer's Disease Rating Scale (Behave-AD) (Reisberg et al. 1987) is also routinely used to screen BPSD seen in our patients.

In a group of 123 patients (68.3% female) with probable AD admitted to our outpatient clinic between 1997 and the beginning of 2000, we examined data collected by using these scales. The mean age and years of education of the patients were 71.8 ± 8 (range, 48–95) and 7.1 ± 5 (range, 0–17), respectively. The mean Mini-Mental State Examination score was 13.7 ± 8 (range, 0–29). The most frequent BPSD among the patients in this study (Table 1) were delusion of "people stealing things" and "wandering," both reported in 45.5% of the study sample. In fact, delusions of "people stealing things" constitute the most common delusion in AD, occurring in approximately 40% of patients who have progressed to GDS stage 5 (Reisberg et al. 1982). Suspiciousness was seen in 24% of patients. This symptom has a considerable effect on caregivers, increasing their stress and possibly leading to institutionalization of the patient. "One's house is not one's home" was a delusion seen in 24% of the patients.

TABLE 1. Most frequent behavioral and psychological symptoms of dementia (BPSD) in Turkish Alzheimer's disease (AD) patients

Things are stolen, 45%
Wandering, 45%
Purposeless activity, 44%
Tearfulness, 40%
Inappropriate activity, 39%
Depressive mood, 37%
Fear of being left alone, 37%
Verbal outbursts, 37%
Diurnal disturbances, 35%
Anxiety with upcoming events, 31%
Visual hallucinations, 29%
Spouse (caregiver) being imposter, 27%
Agitation, 27%

Among the activity disturbances as we mentioned before, wandering was most common (45%), followed by purposeless activity (44%) and inappropriate activity (39.0%) such as hiding objects. Aggressiveness, including verbal outbursts (37%), physical threats or violence (21%), and agitation (27%) were common.

A considerable number of patients (37%) had depressed mood, and 40% showed tearfulness. We know that between one-quarter and one-third of patients with dementia are depressed (Cummings et al. 1995). Several authors claim that treatment of depression in demented patients is usually needed and that such treatment should focus not only on symptomatic relief but also on functional improvement. The rate of anxieties and phobias was fairly high; 37% of patients feared being left alone, and 31% had anxieties about upcoming events (Godot syndrome).

Analysis of scores on the Behave-AD indicated that behavioral disturbances were most severe in the moderate and moderately severe stages of AD. Nearly all symptoms in the study sample were most common in stage 6. Only 11% of the patients had no BPSD, with 89% having at least one symptom. The least frequent symptoms are seen in Table 2.

Conclusion and Recommendations

In Turkey, patients with Alzheimer's disease typically are seen by psychiatrists and neurologists at a late stage (in GDS stage 5 and 6) in outpatient clinics. These specialists take the history and provide a physical, psychiatric, and neurological examination. The DSM-IV criteria are widely used by all specialists interested in Alzheimer's disease. The Turkish version of the MMSE is the most widely used brief cognitive screening test, but only a minority of Turkish psychiatrists and neurologists use the GDS and Behave-AD.

Family members in Turkey are more likely to report behavioral and affective disturbances rather than memory problems. Caregivers in our community may underreport BPSD because of fear the patient will be labeled or institutionalized, their need

TABLE 2. Least frequent BPSD symptoms in Turkish AD patients

Suspiciousness, 24%
Physical threats, 21%
Anxiety, 20%
Delusion of infidelity, 18%
Auditory hallucinations, 15%
Phobias, 12%
Delusions of abandonment, 9%
Other delusions, 7%
Olfactory hallucinations, 6%
Tactile hallucinations, 5%
Other hallucinations, 2%

to maintain an acceptable social façade, their desire not to relinquish the caregiver role, and their religious values. The Turkish culture has traditionally emphasized paternal authority and family loyalty, and children are typically expected to care for parents in their old age even if they are demented. Relative caregivers of AD patients with BPSD do not want to place their patients in nursing homes. On the other hand, Turkey has no good quality services for AD (Eker 1995). Cultural influences must be considered in the studies of BPSD. Western countries should be able to compare results with different cultures. Therefore, joint studies are important. We need reliable instruments for the studies on cross-cultural differences in the presentation of BPSD.

References

APA (American Psychiatric Association) (1994) DSM-IV. Diagnostic and statistical manual of mental disorders, 4th edn. American Psychiatric Association, Washington, DC

Binetti G, Mega MS, Magni, et al (1998) Behavioural disorders in Alzheimer's disease: a transcultural perspective. Arch Neurol 36:885–889

Chandra V (1996) Cross-cultural perspectives: India. In: Finkel S (ed) Behavioural and psychological signs and symptoma of dementia: implications for research and treatment. Int Psychogeriatrics 8(suppl 3):479–483

Chandra V, Ganguli, Ratcliff G (1998) Practical issues in cognitive screening of elderly illiterate populations in developing countries. The Indo-US Cross-Cultural National Dementia Epidemiology Study. Ageing (Milano) 10(5):349–357

Cohen D, Eisdorfer C (1988) Depression in family members caring for a relative with Alzheimer's disease. J Am Geriatr Soc 36:885–889

Connell CM, Gibson GD (1997) Racial, ethic and cultural differences in dementia caregiving: review and analysis. Gerontologist 37(3):366–364

Eker E (1995) Services for elderly care in Turkey. In: Abstracts of the seventh congress of the International Psychogeriatrics Association, Sidney, Australia

Eker E, Ertan T. Behavioural and psychological symptoms of dementia in Eastern and South Eastern Europe and the Middle East. Int Psychogeriatrics 12(suppl 11) (in press)

Folstein MF, Folstein S, Meltugh PR (1975) Mini Mental State. A practical method for grading the cognitive state of patients for the clinician. J Psychiatr Res 12: 189–198

Güngen C, Ertan T, Eker E, et al (1999) The standardized Mini Mental State Examination in Turkish. In: Ninth congress of the IPA, 15–20 August, Vancouver, Canada

Haupt M, Kurz A (1993) Predictors of nursing home placement in patients with Alzheimer's disease. Int J Geriatr Psychiatry 8:741–746

Kua EH, Ko SM (1995) Prevalence if dementia among elderly Chinese and Malay residents of Singapore. Int Psychogeriatrics 7(3):439–446

Mangone CA (1996) Cross-cultural perspectives: Argentina. In: Finkel S (ed) Behavioural and psychological signs and symptoma of dementia: implications for research and treatment. Int Psychogeriatrics 8(suppl 3):473–478

Martin GM, Kukull WA (1996) Do cultural differences affect Alzheimer's disease? (editorial comment). JAMA 276(12):993–995

Reisberg B, Ferris SN, DE Leon MJ, et al (1982) The global deterioration scale for assessment of primary degenerative dementia. Am J Psychiatry 130:1136–1139

Reisberg B, Borenstein J, Salob SP, et al (1987) Behavioural symptoms in Alzheimer's disease: phenomenology and treatment. J Clin Psychiatry (Suppl):9–15

Richards M (1997) Cross-cultural studies of dementia. In: Holmes C, Howard R (eds) Advances in old age Psychiatry. Chromosomes to community care. Wrighton, London, pp 473–478

White L, Petroitch H, Ross GW, et al (1996) Prevalence of dementia in older Japanese-American men in Hawaii. The Honolulu-Asia Ageing Study. JAMA 276(12):955–960

Youn G, Knight BG, Jeong HS, et al (1999) Differences in familism values and caregiving outcomes among Korean, Korean American, and white American dementia caregivers. Psychol Ageing 14(3):55–64

MEG Functional Neuroimaging of Schizophrenic Patients and Comparison Subjects During Word Generation

Satoshi Ukai[1], Kazuhiro Shinosaki[1], Ryouhei Ishii[1], Yuko Mizuno-Matsumoto[1], Tsuyoshi Inouye[1], Norio Hirabuki[2], Toshiki Yoshimine[3], S.E. Robinson[4], and Masatoshi Takeda[1]

Summary. To investigate the abnormal functional interaction between language areas and prefrontal cortex in schizophrenic patients with auditory hallucinations, locations of significant change of neural activities between word generation and rest conditions were estimated using magnetoencephalography (MEG). Using MEG, five right-handed patients with auditory hallucinations and six normal volunteers were submitted to a spatial filtering analysis. In the normal volunteers, bilateral language areas including both posterior inferior frontal gyrus and posterior superior temporal gyrus, bilateral dorsolateral prefrontal cortex, and mid- to lower primary motor cortex showed significant changes. In four of the five schizophrenic patients, no language areas showed significant change in spite of the same performance level. These findings suggest the background hyperactivity of language areas in patients with auditory hallucinations that might be caused by the abnormal functional connectivity between language areas and prefrontal cortex.

Keywords. Schizophrenia, Language, Magnetoencephalography, Brain mapping, Hallucination

Introduction

During the experience of auditory hallucinations, delusions of control, and thought insertion, schizophrenic patients are supposed to be experiencing intrinsically generated activity as if it were extrinsically generated. Inouye et al. showed electromyogram discharge of the speech musculature during auditory hallucinations, suggesting auditory hallucinations can be associated with the patient's own subvocal speech or inner speech [1]. Recent functional neuroimaging studies have shown that increased activity in Broca's and Wernicke's areas occurs in schizophrenic patients with or during auditory hallucinations by using Xe CT [2], SPECT [3,4], or PET [5]. Ishii et al. showed abnormal activity in the left superior temporal area in a schizophrenic patient during auditory hallucinations by using MEG and a new analysis method, SAM (syn-

---

Departments of [1] Clinical Neuroscience, Psychiatry, [2] Radiology, and [3] Neurosurgery, Osaka University Graduate School of Medicine, Osaka, Japan
[4] CTF Systems, Inc., British Columbia, Canada

thetic aperture magnetometry) analysis [14]. These results are not sufficient to explain why patients with schizophrenia mistake self-generated neural activity for that extrinsically generated.

Abnormal functional interaction between language areas and prefrontal cortex is supposed to be the cause of the confusion in schizophrenia. Some neuroimaging studies of word generation tasks reported that activated neural network patterns in patients were different from those in normal subjects [6–8]. Frith et al. showed the failure of attenuation in the left superior temporal cortex during word generation in patients, while as much activation occurred in their dorsolateral prefrontal cortex (DLPFC) as in that of controls [6]. However, direct evidence of such disconnection between prefrontal and posterior brain areas is not yet available, possibly because of the low time resolution of PET and fMRI.

The aim of this study was to reveal abnormal patterns of neural activities in the language and prefrontal areas during the word generation task in schizophrenic patients by using magnetoencephalography (MEG). The locations of significant change in neural network activities were estimated by using a new functional neuroimaging method, SAM analysis [9,10].

Materials and Methods

Subjects and Tasks

Five patients (age 27 ± 5 years) with schizophrenia (according to DSM-IV) and six normal volunteers (28 ± 4 years) were studied. All subjects were right-handed according to the Edinburgh Inventory [11] and were native Japanese speakers. Before MEG recordings, they had been confirmed to be able to generate more than six nouns for 20 s. All patients suffered from auditory hallucinations despite of medication. All subjects gave their informed consent for the experimental procedures.

Subjects were instructed to play "capping" (called "Shiritori" in Japanese) silently, generating as many nouns and as quickly as possible during the task and to concentrate their breathing during the rest time while keeping their eyes open in both periods. Each trial set consisted of a 20-s task and successive 20-s rest period; eight trials were performed. Before and after the MEG recordings, subjects performed two 20-s overt "Shiritori" tasks respectively to count the amount of generated nouns.

MEG Recordings and Data Analysis

MEG recordings were obtained using a helmet-shaped 64-channel SQUID sensor array. MEG signals were digitized at 250 Hz, and filtered using a 60-Hz notch filter and 80-Hz low-pass filter. The tomographic distribution of neural activity was determined from the unaveraged MEG measurements, the SAM analysis. This analysis is classified as a special filter and estimates three-dimensional distribution of electrophysiological source currents from MEG measurements. Regions of significant cortical activation are determined by computing the Student's *t*-statistics from the source power of one state (the task) and another state (the rest) and their noise

TABLE 1. Activated areas (asterisks) per subject in normal volunteers

Subject no.	Left				Right				Total	
	DLPFC	Post-IFG	M1	Post-STG	DLPFC	Post-IFG	M1	Post-STG	L	R
1		*	*				*		2	1
2	*			*					2	0
3		*		*		*			2	1
4			*		*	*	*		1	3
5		*	*	*			*	*	3	2
6			*	*			*		2	1
Totals	1	3	4	4	1	2	4	1	12	8

DLPFC, dorsolateral prefrontal cortex; IFG, inferior frontal gyrus; M1, primary motor cortex; STG, superior temporal gyrus

TABLE 2. Activated areas (asterisks) in schizophrenic patients

Subject no.	Left				Right				Total	
	DLPFC	Post-IFG	M1	Post-STG	DLPFC	Post-IFG	M1	Post-STG	L	R
1	*								1	0
2		*	*			*			2	1
3			*						1	0
4			*						1	0
5	*								1	0
Totals	2	1	3	0	0	1	0	0	6	1

content, on a voxel-by-voxel basis. Finally, the SAM images are fused with each subject's MRI.

Eight trial sets were submitted to the SAM analysis. According to the results of our preliminary study, data were filtered into 8 to 25 Hz. The SAM analysis was used to generate a $16 \times 12 \times 12$ cm volumetric image of root-mean squared source activity from the filtered MEG signals, with a 5-mm voxel resolution.

When neural activity is elicited in a region, synchronization between neural cells in a frequency band decreases. Therefore, current source density as a mathematical model estimated by SAM analysis will decrease while neural activity is elicited. Thus, when the SAM analysis estimates that source current density decreases in one state compared with another, it is considered that the estimate reflects an increase of neural activity in that region.

Results

In the normal volunteers, the DLPFC, posterior inferior frontal gyrus (post-IFG, Broca's area), mid- to lower primary motor cortex (M1, cortical larynx area), and left posterior superior temporal gyrus (post-STG, Wernicke's area) were activated

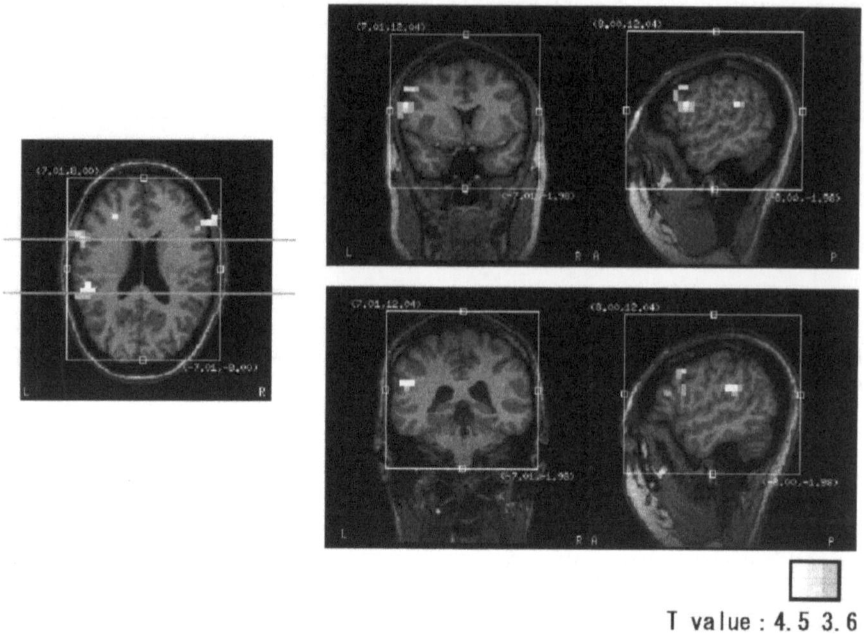

FIG. 1. Statistical parametric mapping (SPM) image of subject 3 of the normal volunteers. Bilateral post-IFG (inferior frontal gyrus) and left post-STG (superior temporal gyrus) were activated. *Gray color* shows significant activation where source current density during the task is significantly smaller than the rest; where the color is lighter, the *t*-statistic is larger

bilaterally. Activation was limited in these four (eight bilaterally) areas (Table 1). Post-STG was activated with left-side dominancy while DLPFC, post-IFG, and M1 were without apparent laterality. Table 2 summarizes the schizophrenic patients. Language areas including both post-IFG and post-STG showed no activation except in one patient. DLPFC and M1 showed activation only in the left hemisphere. Although the normal volunteers showed activation of bilateral hemisphere with left-side dominancy (left to right ratio, 12:8), only one schizophrenic patient showed activation in the right hemisphere (6:1).

Mean numbers of generated nouns for four 20-s overt tasks were 9.0 ± 1.5 in the schizophrenic patients and 9.2 ± 1.2 in normal volunteers, with no significant difference. Figures 1 and 2 show the statistical parametric mapping (SPM) images of subject 3 of the normal volunteers and subject 4 of the schizophrenic patients, respectively.

Discussion

Significantly activated areas in the neural network during the word generation task were located in bilateral Broca's areas, Wernicke's areas, DLPFC, and M1 in the

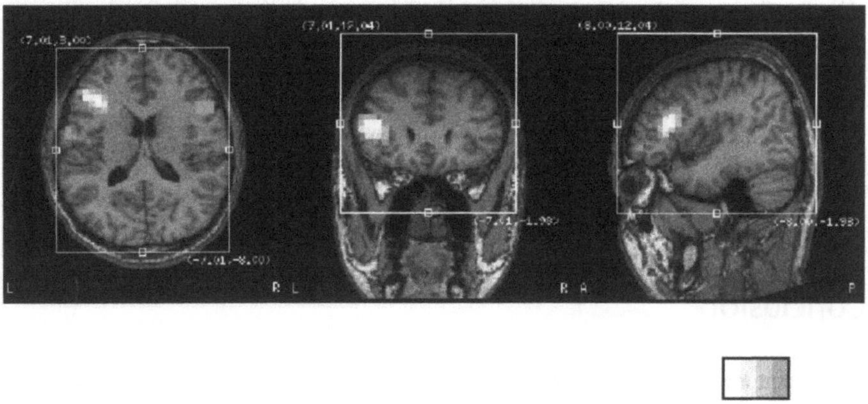

FIG. 2. SPM image of subject 4 of the schizophrenic patients. Bilateral post-IFG and left mid- to lower M1 were activated

normal volunteers. These results were in agreement with previous functional neuroimaging studies using fMRI [12,13]. In four of five patients, no language areas showed significant change in spite of the same word productivity, suggesting abnormal activity of the language areas in the patients. Previous studies reported that the patients with auditory hallucinations showed increased rCBF in left temporal areas [2,3] and that patients showed increased rCBF in the left superior temporal gyrus [4] and in Broca's areas [5], comparing when they had auditory hallucinations with no hallucinations. Our results would suggest that the language areas in the patients had been already hyperactivated, even in the rest period, instead of the failure of activation.

DLPFC was activated in two of the five patients and in two six of the normal volunteers, suggesting activation occurred to almost the same degree in both groups. However, the patients had a striking failure to show the normal pattern of increased activity in the language areas. Frith et al. speculated the disconnection between DLPFC and the language areas in schizophrenic patients from the following results by using PET during word generation: the marked activation of left DLPFC and anterior cingulate with reduction in activity of bilateral superior temporal cortex in normal volunteers, with failure of reduction in activity of the superior temporal cortex in schizophrenia [6]. Our results also suggest abnormal functional connectivity between DLPFC and the language association areas in patients.

Our word generation task, "Shiritori," requires the subject to generate a noun sequentially whose first syllable is coincident with the end syllable of the noun generated immediately previously. Broca's and Wernicke's areas are considered to subserve intrinsic word generation and linguistic process, respectively, so Wernicke's area is expected to be markedly activated by the "Shiritori" task compared with the conventional word generation tasks; e.g., generating words beginning with the alphabet (i.e., A-apple) and generating verbs for nouns (i.e., cake-eat). For this reason, post-STG showed as much activation as post-IFG by using the "Shiritori" task, while Cuenod et al. reported dominant activation in post-IFG by using the conventional task [13].

MEG and a new analysis method, SAM analysis, showed almost the same results as reported by PET or fMRI studies. For the next step, we can now begin to think about the dynamic temporal relationship between DLPFC and the language areas by using MEG characteristic of high temporal resolution.

Conclusion

Significant areas of change in MEG activities between word generation and rest conditions were revealed by using spatial filtering analysis in five schizophrenic patients with auditory hallucinations and six normal volunteers. Bilateral language association areas, including both post-IFG and post-STG and bilateral DLPFC and M1, showed significant changes in the normal volunteers, whereas bilateral language association areas did not show changes in the patients in spite of the same performance level. These results suggest the background hyperactivity of language association areas in the patients with auditory hallucinations, with abnormal functional connectivity between DLPFC and language association areas.

References

1. Inouye T, Shimizu A (1970) The electromyographic study of verbal hallucination. J Nerv Ment Dis 151:415–422
2. Kurachi M, Kobayashi K, Matsubara R, et al (1985) Regional cerebral blood flow in schizophrenic disorders. Eur Neurol 24:176–181
3. Matsuda H, Gyobu T, Hisada K, et al (1989) SPECT evaluation of auditory hallucination using ^{123}I-IMP. Adv Funct Neuroimaging 2:9–16
4. Suzuki M, Yuasa S, Minabe Y, et al (1993) Left superior temporal blood flow increases in schizophrenic and schizophreniform patients with auditory hallucination: a longitudinal case study using ^{123}I-IMP SPECT. Eur Arch Psychiatry Clin Neurosci 242: 257–261
5. McGuire PK, Shah GM, Murray RM (1993) Increased blood flow in Broca's area during auditory hallucinations in schizophrenia. Lancet 342:703–706
6. Frith CD, Friston KJ, Herold S, et al (1995) Regional brain activity in chronic schizophrenic patients during the performance of a verbal fluency task. Br J Psychiatry 167:343–349
7. Yurgelun-Todd DA, Waternaux CM, Cohen BM, et al (1996) Functional magnetic resonance imaging of schizophrenic patients and comparison subjects during word production. Am J Psychiatry 153:200–205
8. Curtis VA, Bullmore ET, Brammer MJ, et al (1998) Attenuated frontal activation during a verbal fluency task in patients with schizophrenia. Am J Psychiatry 155:1056–1063
9. Robinson SE, Rose DF (1992) Current source image estimation by spatially filtered MEG. In: Hoke M, Eme SN, Okada YC (eds) Biomagnetism: Clinical Aspects: Proceedings of the 8th International Conference on Biomagnetism. New York: Elsevier, pp 761–765

10. Ishii R, Shinosaki K, Ukai S, et al (1999) Medial prefrontal cortex generates frontal midline theta rhythm. Neuroreport 10:675–679
11. Oldfield R (1971) The assessment and analysis of handedness: the Edinburgh Inventory. Neuropsychologia 9:97–113
12. Hinke RM, Hu X, Stillman AE, et al (1993) Functional magnetic resonance imaging of Broca's area during internal speech. Neuroreport 4:675–678
13. Cuenod CA, Bookheimer SY, Hertz-Pannier L, et al (1995) Functional MRI during word generation, using conventional equipment: a potential tool for language localization in the clinical environment. Neurology 45:1821–1827
14. Ishii R, Shinosaki K, Ikejiri Y, et al (2000) Theta rhythm increases in left superior temporal cortex during auditory hallucinations in schizophrenia: a case report. Neuroreport 11:3283–3287

Brain Structures and Functions

Brain Laterality and Psychopathology

Guido Gainotti

Summary. The aim of this review is to evaluate if data on laterality of brain lesions producing various kinds of secondary psychopathology can help to choose between the two main models advanced to explain emotional lateralization, namely (a) the "Different Hemispheric Specialization for Positive and Negative Emotions" hypothesis and (b) the "General Right Hemisphere Dominance for Emotions" hypothesis. According to the first model, a major depression should usually result from disruption of the left-sided "center for positive emotions," whereas a manic syndrome should result from inactivation of the right-sided "center for negative emotions"; according to the second model, various forms of secondary psychopathology should prevail in patients with right-hemisphere damage. The results of this review are more consistent with the right hemisphere dominance than with the different hemispheric specialization hypothesis, because they show that some kinds of secondary affective disorders (namely mania and manic-depressive disorders), some forms of content-specific delusional syndromes, and some developmental social-emotional disorders are strongly linked to right-hemisphere lesions.

Keywords. Emotions, Hemispheric specialization, Poststroke depression, Misidentification–reduplication syndromes, Secondary psychopathology

Introduction

The hypothesis that a link may exist between psychopathology and hemispheric asymmetries is not a new one. About 30 years ago several investigations in this area have been prompted by the empirical observation that, in patients with temporal lobe epilepsy, a schizophrenia-like psychosis is mainly observed when the focus is on the left side, whereas an affective disorder is more frequently observed when the focus is on the right side [1]. Starting from these observations, several authors have tried to check if the two main psychiatric syndromes, namely depression and schizophrenia, may result from lateralized dysfunction of the right and left hemispheres.

My presentation differs from these previous investigations for two main reasons: (1) it starts from theoretical models, rather than from empirical findings, and (2) it

Neuropsychology Service, Catholic University of Rome, Largo A. Gemelli, 8-00168 Rome, Italy

assumes that lateralization of psychopathology, far from explaining the major psychiatric syndromes, may be the by-product of a more basic phenomenon, namely the lateralization of human emotions. To be sure, my presentation assumes that, because psychopathology relies on emotional disturbances, a link may exist between lateralization of emotions and lateralization of some forms of psychopathology. Data on laterality of lesions producing various kinds of secondary psychopathology should, therefore, help to choose among the main models advanced to explain emotional lateralization, namely the hemispheric specialization for positive and negative emotions hypothesis, and the general right hemisphere dominance for emotions hypothesis. The plan that I intend to follow, therefore, consists (a) in reviewing the clinical findings that have prompted these two main models of emotional lateralization; (b) in making a set of predictions on the lateralization of various aspects of psychopathology, based, respectively, on the model of a different hemispheric specialization for positive and negative emotions and on that of a general right hemisphere dominance for emotions; and (c) in seeing how the weight of data supporting the first and second models has changed in time. Some years ago, data obtained in stroke patients by Robinson and coworkers [2,3] seemed to support the first model, suggesting a link between major poststroke depression (PSD) and left-frontal lesions and between secondary mania and right-hemisphere lesions. In more recent years, however, the situation has changed, because the relationship between major PSD and left-frontal lesions has not been confirmed and a prevalence of right-hemisphere lesions in several forms of psychopathology has been found. These data support more the right hemisphere dominance rather than the different hemispheric specialization hypothesis. Finally, in the last part of my presentation (d) I survey laterality effects obtained in functional neuroimaging studies conducted either on clinical forms or in experimental models of psychopathology.

Clinical Data That Have Prompted the Two Main Models of Emotional Lateralization

The first data that have raised the problem of hemispheric asymmetries in emotional representation were gathered about 40 years ago by authors who observed a different emotional behavior in patients subjected to pharmacological inactivation of the right or left hemisphere [4,5]. These authors reported that injection of sodium amytal into the left carotid artery produces a "depressive-catastrophic reaction," characterized by bursts of tears and a sad attitude, whereas inactivation of the right hemisphere is followed by a "euphoric-maniacal reaction." These emotional manifestations were interpreted as resulting from disruption of neural mechanisms underpinning opposite aspects of mood (depressive catastrophic reactions being due to inactivation of a *center for positive emotions* located in the left hemisphere and euphoric-maniacal reactions to disruption of a *center for negative emotions* located in the right hemisphere).

Some years later, I could partly confirm these observations by analyzing the patterns of emotional behavior shown by right- and left-brain-damaged patients during a neuropsychological examination [6].

A catastrophic reaction was, indeed, typically observed in (aphasic) left-brain-damaged patients, whereas an indifference reaction was usually found in patients with right-hemisphere damage. However, a more careful analysis of the clinical context and of the qualitative aspects of these different emotional reactions caused me to refute the equivalence proposed by previous authors between catastrophic reaction and biological depression and between indifference reaction and euphoric-maniacal state. *Catastrophical reactions* were, indeed, usually observed in a context of severe Broca's aphasia and were triggered by repeated frustrating attempts of verbal expression. They were, therefore, considered as a dramatic, but psychologically appropriate form of reaction to a catastrophic event, rather than as a form of biological depression. On the other hand, right-brain-damaged patients with an *indifference reaction* were indifferent and unduly jocular rather than excited or euphoric. Furthermore, they often showed paradoxical behaviors, such as a tendency to deny or minimize their disabilities, sometimes coexisting with exaggerated expressions of hatred toward the paralyzed limbs. Overall, these patterns of behavior seemed to suggest an abnormal or inappropriate reaction to a dramatic event, rather than pointing to a mood shift toward the manic pole.

To explain the contrast between the different emotional reaction of left- and right-brain-damaged patients, I advanced the hypothesis that the right hemisphere may be dominant for emotional functions, just as the left hemisphere is dominant for language processing. According to this interpretation, the emotional reaction of a patient with left-brain damage is often dramatic but appropriate because the right hemisphere, which plays a critical role in emotional functions, is intact. This reaction can, on the contrary, be inappropriate in a right-brain-damaged patient if the lesion disrupts structures crucially involved in emotional processing.

Thus, the first clinical observations that have raised the problem of hemispheric asymmetries in emotional representation have also prompted the two models of emotional lateralization that are still considered as the most important models in this area and which can be labeled as the different hemispheric specialization and the general right hemisphere dominance hypothesis. To be sure, slightly different alternative versions of each of these models have been proposed by various authors. Thus, the model of a different hemispheric specialization for positive and negative emotions has been restricted to the level of emotional expression by Davidson [7,8], who in the most recent version of this model assumes that only the generation (and not the comprehension) of positive and negative emotions may be lateralized to the anterior parts of the left and the right hemisphere, respectively. On the other hand, various authors have proposed different versions of the general right hemisphere dominance hypothesis, assuming that specific components of emotions, such as nonverbal communication [9] or the vegetative component [10] may be specifically linked to the right hemisphere (see [11,12]). Nevertheless, these two models of emotional representation make rather different predictions for the lateralization of various aspects of psychopathology. A careful analysis of the laterality of lesions producing various aspects of psychopathology could, therefore, provide important data in support of either the different hemispheric specialization or the general right hemisphere dominance hypothesis.

Predictions Made by the Hemispheric Specialization and the Right Hemisphere Dominance Hypotheses for the Laterality of Lesions Producing Different Forms of Psychopathology

The model of a different hemispheric specialization for positive and negative emotions predicts that unilateral brain lesions should provoke a pattern of affective disorders similar to that reported after pharmacological inactivation of the right and left hemispheres. To be sure, a depressive syndrome, with the characteristics of a biological major depression, should result from disruption of the left-sided center for positive emotions, whereas a manic syndrome (due to inactivation of the right-sided center for negative emotions) should frequently be observed in right-brain-damaged patients. On the other hand, bipolar (manic-depressive) forms of affective disorders should be very rare and provoked only by bilateral lesions, whereas the other aspects of psychopathology should not be lateralized unless clearly linked to positive or negative emotions.

A very different set of predictions is made by the model of a general right hemisphere dominance for emotional functions. This model predicts, for example, that depression, being mainly caused by psychological rather than biological reasons, should not be strongly lateralized. Furthermore, this depression should have the characteristics of a motivated (reactive) depression rather than those of an unmotivated biological depression. As for the other forms of affective disorders, both secondary mania and secondary forms of bipolar manic-depressive disorders should prevail in patients with right-hemisphere injury because of the general dominance of this hemisphere for emotional functions. For the same reason, other forms of psychopathology should prevail in patients with right-brain damage because of the intimate links between psychopathology and emotional disturbances.

During the past 20 years there has been a shift from a first group of studies conducted on stroke patients by Robinson and coworkers, which seemed to support the different hemispheric specialization hypothesis, to a more recent group of data that are much more consistent with the right hemisphere dominance hypothesis. In this review, I therefore take into account first the model of poststroke depression (PSD) proposed by Robinson and coworkers and then discuss the more recent data, which have challenged this model and shown that a large array of psychopathological disorders are associated with a right-hemisphere injury.

Robinson's Model of Major Poststroke Depression and Its Consistency with the Hypothesis of a Different Hemispheric Specialization for Positive and Negative Emotions

At the beginning of the 1980s, Robinson and coworkers published an important series of papers on affective disorders of stroke patients and proposed an influential model of PSD that was consistent with the predictions based on the different hemispheric specialization hypothesis. According to this model, it is possible to distinguish, on the basis of DSM-III diagnostic criteria, two qualitatively different (a major and a minor) forms of PSD. The major form, considered as the most important form of PSD, was described as (a) undistinguishable from the clinicosymptomatological point of view from the endogenous forms of major depression [13] and (b) provoked by left-frontal lesions, which disrupt lateralized monoaminergic pathways relaying the brainstem to the neocortex [14]. The minor form of PSD was considered, on the contrary, as a dysthymic, reactive form of depression, less interesting from the clinical and theoretical point of view and with no specific anatomoclinical correlates.

Even if Robinson and coworkers did not make explicit reference to the different hemispheric specialization hypothesis, their description of the symptomatological and anatomoclinical aspects of major PSD was very consistent with this model. Furthermore, this consistency was further increased by their observation that a right-hemisphere lesion is usually found in the rare instances of secondary mania resulting from brain damage [23].

Robinson's model of major PSD has been very influential but has also raised important methodological and clinical objections. From the methodological point of view, it has been remarked that the distinction between major and minor forms of PSD (which plays a pivotal role in this model) was substantially based on DSM-III diagnostic criteria, but these criteria are not necessarily valid in stroke patients. A diagnosis of major depression requires, indeed, the presence (in addition to a depressed mood or to a loss of interest) of at least four of the following symptoms: loss of weight, sleep disorders, loss of energy, agitation, lack of concentration, guilt feelings, and thoughts of suicide. In stroke patients, however, some of these symptoms (e.g., lack of concentration and loss of energy) can be caused by the brain lesion per se and not by a major depression. From the clinical point of view, the most important objections have concerned (a) the symptomatological equivalence between major forms of PSD and of endogenous depression, because some of the most typical symptoms of endogenous depression (such as unmotivated self-blames, guilt feelings, or suicidal thoughts) are rarely observed in major PSD and (b) the anatomoclinical correlates of major PSD. Several authors [15,16] have, indeed, failed to confirm the relationship between major PSD and left-frontal lesions. In recent years these aspects of PSD have, therefore, been reconsidered by means of more methodologically correct clinical investigations.

Phenomenological and Anatomoclinical Data Inconsistent with Robinson's Model of PSD

To check the phenomenological equivalence between major forms of PSD and of endogenous depression and between minor PSD and dysthymic/reactive depression, Gainotti et al. [17] have constructed a new scale (the Post-Stroke Depression Rating Scale), specifically devised having in mind the symptoms and problems of depressed stroke patients. This scale, which tried to distinguish motivated (reactive) from unmotivated (biologically determined) symptoms, was administered to three groups of stroke patients, classified (as in Robinson's papers) on the basis of DSM-III diagnostic criteria as nondepressed, minor depression, and major depression. A group of patients with an endogenous form of major depression was also investigated, and the following predictions were made. (1) If Robinson's model is correct, then the symptomatological profiles should be very similar in patients with major forms of endogenous and of poststroke depression. In particular, both groups should obtain particularly high scores on the unmotivated aspects of depression, whereas motivated aspects should prevail in patients with minor (reactive) PSD. (2) If, on the contrary, no qualitative difference exists between major and minor forms of PSD, but both are due to the meaning that the patient attributes to the consequences of stroke, then a different symptomatological profile should be shown by patients with a major form of PSD and of endogenous depression. In particular, the unmotivated aspects of depression should prevail in patients with an endogenous form and the motivated aspects in those with a poststroke form of major depression. Furthermore, only a quantitative but no qualitative difference should be found between major and minor forms of PSD. The results of our research were not consistent with Robinson's model, because symptomatological profiles of patients with major PSD were more similar to those of patients with minor PSD than to profiles of patients with endogenous depression and because the immotivated aspects of depression prevailed in patients with endogenous depression, whereas the motivated (reactive) aspects prevailed in patients with a PSD.

If we pass, now, from the phenomenological to the anatomoclinical data, we see that almost all the recent studies conducted on this subject have failed to confirm the relationship between PSD and left-hemisphere (or left-frontal) lesions predicted by the different hemispheric specialization hypothesis. Thus, according to Agrell and Dehlin [18], who have reviewed 25 articles relevant from this point of view, only 8 of these studies have reported a higher frequency of depression after left-sided lesions, whereas 14 have shown no difference between right- and left-brain injury and 3 have reported a prevalence of depression after right-brain damage. Analogously, no relationship between PSD and side of lesion has been shown by the recent studies conducted on large groups of unselected stroke patients by Andersen et al. [19], Gainotti et al. [20], and Herrmann et al. [21].

Other Data on Psychopathology Secondary to Brain Damage Supporting the Right Hemisphere Dominance More Than the Different Hemispheric Specialization Hypothesis

In addition to phenomenological and anatomoclinical data contrasting with Robinson's model of major PSD, other recent observations concerning either different aspects of affective disorders or other forms of psychopathology resulting from brain damage are more consistent with the right-hemisphere dominance than with the different hemispheric specialization hypothesis. As a matter of fact, if we consider the laterality of lesion of affective disorders other than depression secondary to brain damage, we see that both secondary mania and secondary bipolar (manic-depressive) disorders are usually caused by bilateral or right-sided lesions. The strong lateralization to the right hemisphere of brain lesions provoking a secondary mania had already been noticed by Cummings and Mendez [22] and confirmed by Robinson et al. [23] and by Starkstein et al. [24,25]. This observation, however, can be explained both by the right hemisphere dominance and the different hemispheric specialization hypotheses because it can be considered either as a consequence of the critical role of the right hemisphere in emotional functions or as an affective imbalance resulting from the inactivation of the right-sided center for negative affects. Much more important, from the theoretical point of view, is the laterality of lesion in patients with secondary bipolar (manic-depressive) disorders because the predictions made on this subject by the two models of emotional lateralization are clearly divergent. The different hemispheric specialization hypothesis, assuming that an imbalance between lateralized centers for positive and negative emotions subserves both major depression and mania, can explain bipolar manic-depressive disorders only as a consequence of bilateral lesions. On the contrary, the right hemisphere dominance hypothesis predicts that these phenomena could be caused by right-hemisphere damage, owing to the critical role of this hemisphere in emotional functions.

Data of a recent study in which Starkstein et al. [25] have compared lesion location in patients who developed after a brain lesion mania only or a bipolar affective disorder clearly support the second hypothesis. These authors have shown that 6 of 7 manic depressive patients and 8 of 12 purely manic patients had lesions restricted to the right hemisphere and that only the intrahemispheric locus of lesion was different in the two groups. Bipolar patients had mainly subcortical lesions, whereas patients with purely manic states had a significantly higher frequency of cortical (fronto-orbital and basotemporal) involvement. These data are in contrast with the different hemispheric specialization and are consistent with the right hemisphere dominance hypothesis.

Content-specific delusions, involving the reduplication or the misidentification of persons or of elements of the environment, constitute a second area of psychopathology resulting from brain damage where the study of lesion laterality has clearly shown a critical role of the right hemisphere. The two main syndromes of delusional reduplication and misidentification described in patients with brain damage are (a) the Capgras syndrome, in which the patient maintains that a person well known to him (usually a family member) has been replaced by an impostor or by a double and that there are two versions of this person, and (b) the environmental reduplications (or reduplicative paramnesia), in which the patient maintains that there are two or more versions of a particular place (or room or building), the present place being usually closer to home than it is in fact the case. Several authors have recently shown that in these forms of content-specific delusions secondary to brain damage, lesions are usually bilateral or restricted to the right hemisphere. Thus, in an influential review of published cases of Capgras syndrome and of reduplicative paramnesias, Feinberg and Shapiro [26] found that about one-half of the reported cases had bilateral damage, but that in both conditions a lesion restricted to the right hemisphere was much more common than a lesion circumscribed to the left hemisphere (the ratio of right to left lesions was 4 to 1 in patients with a Capgras syndrome and 7 to 1 in those with a reduplicative paramnesia).

Similar results have been recently obtained by Murai et al. [27], using a standard questionnaire to detect environmental reduplications in unselected groups of brain-damaged patients, and by Malloy et al. [28], reviewing the recent literature on primary and secondary Capgras delusions. Furthermore, the relationship between content-specific delusions and right-hemisphere dysfunction has recently been confirmed by neuroimaging investigations that have studied the neuroanatomical correlates of these delusions in Alzheimer's disease patients. Using HMPAO-SPET, Staff et al. [29]

have clearly shown that content-specific delusions are associated with hypoperfusion of the anterior frontotemporal limbic structures of the right hemisphere. Several interpretations based on specific functions of the right hemisphere have been advanced to account for the special role played by this side of the brain in delusional misidentification syndromes. Feinberg and Shapiro [26], drawing on data showing that the right hemisphere plays a key role in producing the experience of familiarity and in distinguishing novel from familar stimuli, have suggested that delusional misidentifications could be caused by a defect of familiarity judgments. Cutting [30] has suggested, within his more general theory relating psychoses to right-hemisphere information processing abnormalities, that a failure of individual recognition could subserve content-specific delusional syndromes. Ellis [31] has assumed that a face recognition disorder due to a selective defect of the ventral visuolimbic route may cause the Capgras syndrome. In my opinion, all these interpretations consider only one aspect of the problem as they limit attention to the cognitive features of the right hemisphere, thus neglecting the emotional features, which certainly play an important role in the pathophysiology of the delusional misidentification syndromes. The selective involvement of the right hemisphere in delusional misidentification syndromes is probably caused by both the cognitive and the emotional characteristics of the right hemisphere. The laterality of lesions producing content-specific delusions is, therefore, also consistent with the right hemisphere dominance hypothesis.

A last area of research on laterality-specific aspects of psychopathology that seems consistent with the same right hemisphere dominance hypothesis concerns the laterality of lesions in developmental social-emotional processing disorders. This developmental syndrome is characterized by a history of deficient interpersonal relations, difficulties producing and interpreting nonverbal communication, impaired visuospatial processing, and poor emotional adjustment and psychiatric disorders. Previous authors [32] had associated this syndrome with a putative right-hemisphere dysfunction on the basis of neuropsychological profile and neurological examination findings. Manoach et al. [33] have recently confirmed this association with a more controlled study, showing that a poor development of social-emotional abilities is usually associated with early bilateral or right-sided hemispheric damage.

Taken together, recent studies that have shown a strong relationship between right-hemisphere lesions and some kinds of affective disorders (such as mania and bipolar manic-depressive disorders), some forms of (content-specific) delusional syndromes, and some developmental social-emotional processing disorders clearly suggest a relationship between the right hemisphere and various aspects of psychopathology and are consistent with the right hemisphere dominance hypothesis.

Functional Neuroimaging Studies That Have Found Laterality Effects in Psychiatric Patients or in Normal Subjects with Experimentally Induced Emotions or Psychopathology

Robinson's model of PSD influenced the first studies that about 10 years ago tried to investigate the neurobiological correlates of the functional forms of major depression with functional neuroimaging methods. As Robinson's model suggested a strong link between major PSD and left-frontal lesions, some authors assumed that a metabolic defect should also be present in the left-frontal areas in at least some forms of major endogenous depression. The first studies supported the model, showing a reduced metabolic rate in the left dorsolateral prefrontal cortex (DLPFC) both in unipolar [34,35] and in bipolar [34,36] forms of major depression. However, further more controlled studies have failed to confirm these data or have shown that the reduced glucose metabolism observed in previous investigations was the consequence, rather than the cause, of major depression. Thus, some studies of regional cerebral blood flow (CBF) have shown that both depressed and manic patients have a normal CBF [37] whereas other studies have even suggested that the CBF can sometimes be increased in the left prefrontal cortex [38]. This last finding has been interpreted as resulting from the activation that the (verbal) depressive ruminations of these patients provoke at the level of the left DLPFC, and this interpretation has suggested that symptoms associated with a given disease could play an important role in the pathophysiology of focal metabolic brain abnormalities usually considered as specific of that disease. Following this line of thought, Dolan et al. [39] have tried to check if the reduced metabolic rate reported by Baxter et al. [34], Martinot et al. [36], and Bench et al. [35] in the left DLPFC of depressed patients is a marker of major depression or results from the poverty of speech and of psychomotor activity often observed in these patients. To solve this problem, Dolan et al. [39] compared the profile of regional CBF measured under resting conditions in two groups of depressed and of schizophrenic patients (who had also shown a reduced metabolic rate in the left DLPFC), contrasting the profiles of patients showing and not showing a poverty of speech. Their results showed that reduction of CBF in the left DLPFC is a reflex of poverty of speech and of psychomotor activity, rather than a marker of the disesase because, independently of diagnosis, poverty of speech was strongly related to low levels of rCBF in the left DLPFC.

To minimize these methodological pitfalls, recent neuroimaging studies have tried to induce (with psychological or pharmacological procedures) mood changes in normal subjects, studying the resulting patterns of brain activation rather than analyzing the patterns of brain activity shown under resting conditions by various groups of psychiatric patients. Because many papers have been published on this problem, with inconsistent results by various investigators, and because a very high number of variables can influence the results obtained in these studies, I do not here enter into a detailed review of this issue. I limit myself to argue that the general picture that emerges from these investigations is more consistent with the right hemisphere dominance than with the different hemispheric specialization hypothesis. This claim is based on the fact that a rather consistent relationship has been found between induction of negative emotions (or of the corresponding experimental psychopathology) and increased activity of right frontotemporal limbic structures, whereas the relationship between induction of positive emotions and activation of left-sided limbic structures is much less consistent.

As for the first point, a prevalent activation of the right frontotemporal limbic structures has been observed by Rauch et al. [40,41] and by Shin et al. [42] by eliciting a phobic reaction with specific visual stimuli; however, Wik et al. [43] have obtained a decreased activity in the same structures with a similar technique. Analogously, a prevalent activation of the right amygdala has been provoked by Zald et al. [44] with an aversive gustatory stimulation, and an activation of the right frontal areas has been obtained by Hugdahl et al. [45,46] with an aversive conditioning procedure. As for the second point, two orders of data disconfirm the relationship between left hemisphere and positive emotions. (1) several authors [47–49] have observed a prevalent activation of the left hemisphere with stimuli inducing sadness or other negative affects. (2) Conversely, Paradiso et al. [49] and Lane et al. [50] have obtained a prevalent activation of the right temporolimbic structures provoking happiness with psychological methods, and a similar activation pattern has been observed by Breiter et al. [51] during the rush induced by cocaine administration.

Concluding Remarks

Data surveyed in this review approach from various aspects the problem of the relationships between brain laterality and psychopathology because they span from affective or delusional syndromes secondary to brain damage, to the focal metabolic defects observed in some major psychiatric syndromes, to the activation patterns observed in some experimental models of emotional or affective disorders. In spite of the very heterogeneous nature of the psychopathological manifestations taken into account in these different domains, the picture that emerges across these various lines of research is remarkably consistent and substantially in keeping with the predictions based on the right hemisphere dominance hypothesis. A clear prevalence of right-hemisphere lesions was, in fact, observed both in affective (mania and bipolar manic-depressive) disorders and in content-specific delusions (Capgras syndrome and reduplicative misidentifications) secondary to brain damage. Analogously, a prevalent activation of the right-hemisphere frontotemporal limbic structures has been observed in some experimental models of psychopathology and during experimental induction of negative emotions. Even if the most obvious implications of these data concern the models of hemispheric asymmetries in emotional representation, they also suggest some degree of hemispheric asymmetry (with a certain level of right-hemisphere dominance) also with respect to psychopathology. This right-hemisphere prevalence, however, does not equally concern all the aspects of psychopathology but only those that are more immediately linked to the field of emotions and affects (as in the case of affective disorders) or in which emotions interact with cognitive features mainly subserved by the right hemisphere (as in the case of content-specific delusions). Apart from these specific domains of psychopathology, there is no reason to think that the right hemisphere plays a crucial role in other more general aspects of psychatry.

References

1. Flor-Henry P (1969) Psychosis and temporal lobe epilepsy: a controlled investigation. Epilepsia 10:363–395
2. Robinson RG, Starkstein SE (1989) Mood disorders following stroke: new findings and future directions. J Geriatr Psychiatry 22:1–15
3. Starkstein SE, Robinson RG (1989) Affective disorders and cerebral vascular disease. Br J Psychiatry 154:170–182

4. Terzian H, Cecotto C (1959) Determinazione e studio della dominanza emisferica mediante iniezione intracarotide di Amytal sodico nell'uomo: I. Modificazioni cliniche. Boll Soc Ital Biol Sper 35:1623–1626
5. Rossi GF, Rosadini G (1967) Experimental analysis of cerebral dominance in man. In: Millikan CJ, Darley FL (eds) Brain mechanisms underlying speech and language. Grune and Stratton, New York, pp 167–174
6. Gainotti G (1972) Emotional behavior and hemispheric side of lesion. Cortex 8:41–55
7. Davidson RJ (1995) Cerebral asymmetry, emotion and affective style. In: Davidson RJ, Hugdahl K (eds) Brain asymmetry. MIT Press, Cambridge, pp 361–387
8. Davidson RJ (1998) Affective style and affective disorders: Perspectives from affective neuroscience. Cognition Emotion 12:307–330
9. Ross ED (1984) Right hemisphere role in language, affective behavior and emotion. Trends Neurosci 7:342–346
10. Wittling W (1995) Brain asymmetry in the control of autonomic-physiologic activity. In: Davidson RJ, Hugdahl K (eds) Brain asymmetry. MIT Press, Cambridge, pp 305–357
11. Gainotti G (1997) Emotional disorders in relation to unilateral brain damage. In: Feinberg TE, Farah M (eds) Behavioral neurology and neuropsychology. McGraw-Hill, New York, pp 691–698
12. Gainotti G (1999) Neuropsychology of emotions. In: Denes GF, Pizzamiglio L (eds) Handbook of clinical and experimental neuropsychology. Psychology Press, Hove, pp 613–633
13. Lipsey JR, Spencer WC, Robins PV, Robinson RG (1986) Phenomenological comparison of post-stroke depression and functional depression. Am J Psychiatry 143:527–529
14. Robinson RG, Kubos KL, Starr LB, et al (1984) Mood disorders in stroke patients: importance of lesion location. Brain 107:81–93
15. Sinyor D, Jacques P, Kaloupek DG, et al (1986) Post-stroke depression and lesion location: an attempted replication. Brain 109:539–546
16. House A, Dennis M, Warlow C, et al (1990) Mood disorders after stroke and their relation to lesion location. A CT scan study. Brain 113:1113–1130
17. Gainotti G, Azzoni A, Razzano C, et al (1997a) The Post-stroke Depression Rating Scale: a test specifically devised to investigate affective disorders of stroke patients. J Clin Exp Neuropsychol 19:340–356
18. Agrell B, Dehlin O (1994) Depression in stroke patients with left and right hemisphere lesions: a study in geriatric rehabilitation in-patients. Aging Clin Exp Res 6:49–56
19. Andersen G, Vestergaard K, Ingeman-Nielsen M, Lauritzen L (1995) Risk factors for post-stroke depression. Acta Psychiatr Scand 92:193–198
20. Gainotti G, Azzoni A, Gasparini F, et al (1997b) Relation of lesion location to verbal and nonverbal mood measures in stroke patients. Stroke 28:2145–2149
21. Herrmann N, Black SE, Lawrence J, et al (1998) The Sunnybrook Stroke Study. A prospective study of depressive symptoms and functional outcome. Stroke 29:618–624
22. Cummings JL, Mendez MF (1984) Secondary mania with focal cerebrovascular lesions. Am J Psychiatry 141:1084–1087
23. Robinson RG Boston JD, Starkstein SE, Price TR (1988) Comparison of mania and depression after brain injury: causal factors. Am J Psychiatry 145:172–178
24. Starkstein SE, Mayberg HS, Berthier ML, et al (1990) Secondary mania: neuroradiological and metabolic findings. Ann Neurol. 27:652–659
25. Starkstein SE, Fedoroff P, Berthier ML, Robinson RG (1991) Manic-depressive and pure manic states after brain lesions. Biol Psychiatry 29:149–158

26. Feinberg TE, Shapiro RM (1989) Misidentification-reduplication and the right hemisphere. Neuropsychiatry Neuropsychol Behav Neurol 2:39–48
27. Murai T, Toichi M, Sengoku A, et al (1997) Reduplicative paramnesia in patients with focal brain damage. Neuropsychiatry Neuropsychol Behav Neurol 10:190–196
28. Malloy P, Cimino C, Westlake R (1992) Differential diagnosis of primary and secondary Capgras delusions. Neuropsychiatry Neuropsychol Behav Neurol 5:83–96
29. Staff RT, Shanks MF, Macintosh L, et al (1999) Delusions in Alzheimer's disease: SPET evidence of right hemisphere dysfunction. Cortex 35:549–560
30. Cutting J (1990) The right cerebral hemisphere and psychiatric disorders. Oxford University Press, Oxford
31. Ellis HD (1994) The role of the right hemisphere in the Capgras delusion. Psychopathology 27:177–185
32. Weintraub S, Mesulam M-M (1983) Developmental learning disabilities of the right hemisphere. Emotional, interpersonal and cognitive components. Arch Neurol 40:463–468
33. Manoach DS, Sadson TA, Weintraub S (1995) The developmental social-emotional processing disorder is associated with right hemisphere abnormalities. Neuropsychiatry Neuropsychol Behav Neurol 8:99–105
34. Baxter LR, Schwartz JM, Phelps ME, et al (1989) Reduction of prefrontal cortex metabolism common to three types of depression. Arch Gen Psychiatry 46:243–250
35. Bench CJ, Friston KJ, Brown RG (1992) The anatomy of melancholia. Abnormalities of regional cerebral blood flow in major depression. Psychol Med 22:607–615
36. Martinot JL, Hardy P, Feline A, et al (1990) Left prefrontal glucose hypomethabolism in the depressed state: a confirmation. Am J Psychiatry 147:1313–1317
37. Silfverskiold P, Risberg J (1989) Regional cerebral blood flow in depression and mania. Arch Gen Psychiatry 46:253–259
38. Drevets WC, Raichle ME (1992) Neuroanatomical circuits in depression: implications for treatment mechanisms. Psychopharmacol Bull 28:261–274
39. Dolan RJ, Bench CJ, Liddle PF, et al (1993) Dorsolateral prefrontal cortex dysfunction in major psychoses: symptom or disease specificity? J Neurol Neurosurg Psychiatry 56:1290–1294
40. Rauch SL, Van der Kolk BA, Fisler RE, Alpert NM (1996) A symptom provocation study of post-traumatic stress disorder using positron emission tomography and script-driven imagery. Arch Gen Psychiatry 53:380–387
41. Rauch SL, Savage CR, Alpert NM (1997) The functional neuroanatomy of anxiety: a study of three disorders using positron emission tomography and symptom provocation. Biol Psychiatry 42:446–452
42. Shin LM, Kosslyn SM, McNally RJ, et al (1997) Visual imagery and perception in post-traumatic stress disorder: a positron emission tomographic investigation. Arch Gen Psychiatry 54:233–241
43. Wik G, Fredrikson M, Eriksson L, et al (1993) A functional cerebral response to frightening visual stimulation. Psychiatry Res Neuroimaging 50:15–24
44. Zald DH, Lee JT, Fluegel KW, Pardo JW (1998) Aversive gustatory stimulation activates limbic circuits in humans. Brain 121:1143–1154
45. Hugdahl K, Berardi A, Thompson WL, et al (1995) Brain mechanisms in human classical conditioning: a PET blood flow study. Neuroreport 6:1723–1728
46. Hugdahl K (1998) Cortical control of human classical conditioning: automomic and positron emission tomography data. Psychophysiology 35:170–178
47. George MS, Ketter TA, Parekh PI, et al (1995) Brain activity during transient sadness and happiness in healthy women. Am J Psychiatry 152:341–351
48. Lane RD, Reiman EM, Bradley MM, et al (1997) Neuroanatomical correlates of pleasant and unpleasant emotion. Neuropsychologia 35:1437–1444

49. Paradiso S, Robinson RG, Andreasen NC, et al (1997) Emotional activation of limbic circuitry in elderly normal subjects in a PET study. Am J Psychiatry 154:384–389
50. Lane RD, Chua PML, Dolan RJ (1999) Common effects of emotional valence, arousal and attention on neural activation during visual processing of pictures. Neuropsychologia 37:989–997
51. Breiter HC, Gollub RL, Weisskoff RM, et al (1997) Acute effects of cocaine on human brain activity and emotion. Neuron 19:591–611

Zen and the Brain: The Path

James H. Austin

Summary. The Path of Zen emphasizes the original teachings of the Buddha: human suffering is rooted in our longings, loathings, and ignorance. Zen training evolves during years of a restrained lifestyle that includes regular meditation, close relations with an authentic teacher and a support group, and regular meditative retreats. The Path evolves through the superficial "quickenings" and absorptions into more advanced, extraordinary, alternate states of consciousness. These brief experiences, conveying successively deeper levels of insight-wisdom, are moments of "awakening," of realizing the "way things *really* are." They are states described (imperfectly) using such terms as *kensho*, *satori*, and Ultimate Pure Being. Rarely—and usually in a monastic context—do the deepest transformations proceed to the advanced level of genuine "sage wisdom." This is an ongoing *stage* of enlightened traits.

During such a long training process, a person's egocentric maladaptions are dissolved, not only suddenly but also gradually. As these pejorative aspects of the *I-Me-Mine* drop off, the trainee's priorities become increasingly simplified, focused, and stabilized. The way is now open for this person to become a more actualized, buoyant, compassionate, humane being.

Keywords. Zen, Meditation, Psychophysiology, Enlightenment, Self-Transformation

> Once you realize that this flawless moon
> dwells deep and pure in each human heart,
> all dark nights dissolve into clear skies.
> Kojiju (1121–1201)

Historical Introduction

For neuropsychiatrists, the themes in this story are not new, nor are they isolated to one continent. Our narrative might begin in Nepal when young Siddhartha (563–483 B.C.E.) first saw life's harsh realities: a sick man, an old man, and a dead man. Deeply shaken, he later set out, age 29, on the age-old quest to find meaning in life.

Department of Neurology, University of Colorado Health Sciences Center, Denver, CO 80262, USA

Elsewhere, his contemporaries to the West were also being sorely troubled. Their distress echoes in Job's lament, voiced by an author of the Old Testament, around 400 B.C.E. "One thing alone I feared, and it befell me—the very thing I dreaded. No peace had I, no calm, no rest; but torments came."

And about the same time, Sophocles (496–406 B.C.E.) had his chorus express the Greek varieties of angst in these lines from Oedipus: "What is unwisdom but the lusting after longevity: that urge to grow older, and full of days! But this tide of years, so vast and unremitting, casts up to our view only sorrowful and joyless things. For once we've aged beyond our prime, our pleasures drift beyond reach, all washed away."

Not until Siddhartha was 35, and now living in North India, did he finally become fully enlightened, but only after a rigorous 6-year spiritual quest. His legendary awakening occurred only after he meditated intensively, and through a very "dark night." Suddenly, he saw with deep insight into the existential suffering of human beings. He realized: (1) what caused their anguish; and (2) how to prevent and relieve it. Indeed, after he died at the age of 80, his followers could distill his central message into these few words:

"Suffering I teach, and the Way out of suffering."

They called this man the Buddha, meaning the enlightened or awakened one. In simplified terms, his teachings focused on the three root causes of our sufferings and dissatisfactions: our *longings*, our *loathings*, and our *ignorance*. But how could we extinguish these self-centered desires, aversions, and illusions?

As both a teacher and a healer, the Buddha had a prescription for finding inner peace in a world of turmoil. His remedy was a course of action, still in use down to the present day. This Buddhist ethical approach still means following a sensible eightfold Path: a combination of right understanding, thought, speech, conduct, vocation, effort, mindfulness, and meditation.

In the old India of two and a half millennia ago, the Sanskrit word for meditation was *dhyana*. As Buddhism traveled north, dhyana then changed into the Chinese word *Ch'an*. In China, this meditation school evolved in the cultures of Taoism and Confucianism. Its influence peaked during the Tang Dynasty (618–907). Later, when Buddhist monks transplanted this Ch'an school to Japan, the Japanese would pronounce it Zen. The word, Zen, illustrates its history.

Zen Meditation

Included among the points of emphasis are the following:

1. Meditation serves not only as a way to enhance awareness and personal growth, but as the soil for the flash of enlightenment (insight–wisdom; *prajna*).
2. Zen values both this deepest intuitive understanding and the simplest direct act: the actual fact that one mindfully experiences the present moment.
3. For yes, you can learn about Zen in *zazen*, its system of meditation. But you do not just sit on a pillow. You also practice this mindful, mental-and-physical form of self-discipline during all the arts of everyday living.
4. Zen meditation develops and refines the arts of attention and introspection. The Way is long and difficult. Beginning with calmness and clarity, the path points

increasingly toward the further development of fruitful traits of character; in particular, toward simplicity, stability, gratitude, efficient action, and compassion.

Toward a Psychophysiology of Zen

Elsewhere, we have presented Zen not as an esoteric philosophy, nor in theological terms, nor as simple relaxation per se, nor as a set of psychoanalytical doctrines in the abstract (Austin 1998).

Instead, our approach focused on underlying psychophysiological mechanisms in the brain. Here, we propose to view Zen as (1) a subtle program of sustained brain training, one enhanced during meditative retreats; (2) a system that evolves, through a series of gradually calibrated adversities, into alternate state experiences; and (3) a long, humbling process of self-emptying. When advanced states of insight do thrust up into this more open, self-less setting, they now tend to transform the person along lines that can become affirmative and enduring.

An Outline of Zen

Zen training evolves during years of a restrained lifestyle (*sila*). The practice centers on an authentic teacher (the *roshi*), and on a support group of like-minded practitioners (the *sangha*). It involves decades of regular meditation (zazen) and repeated meditative retreats (*sesshin*).

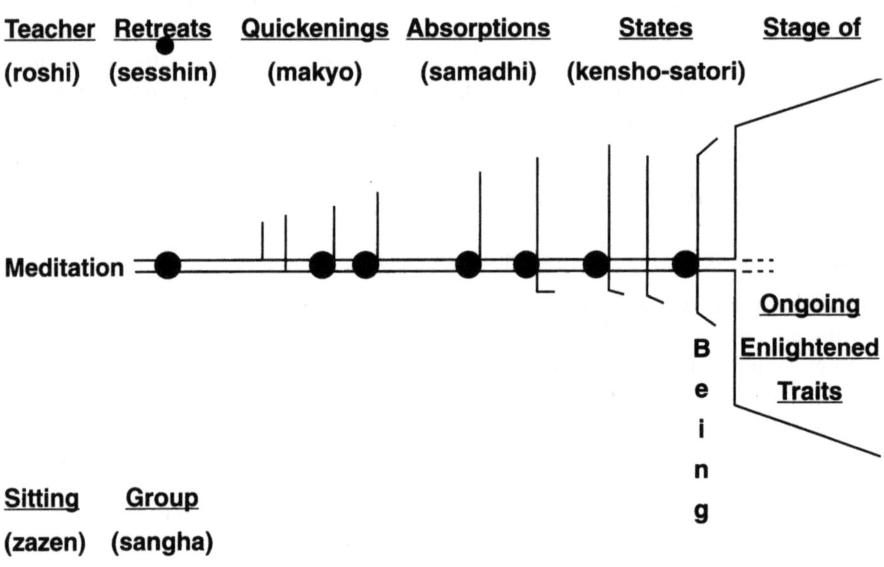

Let the previous diagram represent this decades-long timeline of practice. The solid round dots suggest this need for multiple retreats. Indeed, only during intensive retreats does the meditator usually arrive at levels of self-emptying sufficient to access advanced extraordinary alternate states of consciousness.

Quickenings

"Side effects" occur during the early months and years of meditating. Beginners are intrigued by these epiphenomena (emotional swings, unusual body sensations and perceptions, hallucinations). In formal Zen training, however, such "quickenings" (called *makyo*) are viewed as "by-products" of no spiritual significance, as merely signs that one is moving along the path.

Absorptions

Absorptions often arise in settings when concentrative meditative techniques are practiced, such as during a retreat. The several states of absorption have in common both a sustained, involuntary process of heightened attention and the sense that one's *physical* self has faded. One's attention feels held. Sometimes it is transfixed by some actual object that is perceived with senses open to the outside world (*external* absorption).

In contrast, other states turn inward (*internal* absorption). This field of greatly amplified internalized awareness contains neither thoughts, external sights, nor sounds. A vacuum opens up with no physical self inside, a vast space infused with a plenum of rapture and bliss (Austin 1998, Part VI, pp. 467–518).

States of Insight-Wisdom

These rare states develop later. The term *prajna* refers to the swordcut of their existential insights. It severs the sense of the *psychic* self. The cut subtracts not only its conceptual and affective roots but its roots into all other dualities. What happens when this flash of deep insight strikes into an awareness shorn of all prior subjective conditionings? The moonlight reveals "things as *they* really are." The salient impressions are of *ultimate reality*, of *eternity*, of *unity*, of *fearlessness*, and of a great sense of *release*.

A current trend is to label the initial insight experiences as *kensho* and to reserve the term *satori* for awakenings that plumb deeper levels. Although these two states of "enlightenment" are momentary, they tend to exert a positive transforming influence on the personality (Austin 1998, Part VII, pp. 519–624). So do those rarer states in this next category.

States of Ultimate Pure Being

These very rare states tap into primordial incomprehensibilities (Austin 1998, Part VIII, pp. 625–636). Experiential paradoxes abound. No word descriptions suffice when groundlessness coexists with an impression of infinite potential, nor when form and emptiness simultaneously coincide and equate (Austin 1999).

The Exceptional Stage of Ongoing Enlightened Traits

This long descriptive phrase refers not to a brief state but to a *stage*. It applies to that rare sage who—like the Buddha—continues to live selflessly, directly in touch with what goes on in the present moment (Austin 1998, Part VIII, pp. 636–697). Liberated from prior dysfunctional conditioning, this sage now leads a simplified life, yet adapts skillfully and compassionately to each new social complexity. Transformations at such depths reflect an amalgam of changes in traits, attitudes, thoughts, and behaviors. How can these arise?

Our Psychic Self and Its Dysfunctions

To William James, incoming sensory messages from our head and body were the perceptual nucleus for our usual sense of a *physical* self. Still other layers comprise our *psychic* self: our thoughts, concepts, emotions, and instincts. Basically nonsensory, these layers of our psychic self create a blend of cognitive and urgent affective properties.

Our fronto-temporal-limbic networks help contribute to many of these psychic layers, but their constructs have already been infused with emotional valences. Unconsciously, we have been positively (+) attracted or negatively (–) repelled. We have been polarized from the depths—been *overconditioned*—in countless unsuspected ways.

For purposes of discussion, we can visualize three main interactive components of selfhood—capitalized and italicized—in such operations:

I–Me–Mine

True, this triad serves useful constructive, adaptive ends. But our *I–Me–Mine* also has its covert, dysfunctional side. How does the sovereign *I* create problems? Because, if expressed in simple *a-b-c* terms, it is also *a*rrogant and *a*ggressive. Yet, it has a vulnerable partner: the fearful *Me*. This *Me* feels *b*esieged. It can get *b*attered. Finally, our *Mine* is readily *c*aptured by its greedy longings. It *c*lutches at other people, it *c*lasps onto material goods. Moreover, this *Mine* has another bad habit. It owns and *c*herishes each of its biased opinions.

Kensho's Impact on the Pejorative Self

These dysfunctional aspects are the main targets of the long training program just outlined. Yes, much of this brain training process is incremental, but the sudden entry of brief insightful states is essential. Only these insights expose how much the egocentric aspects of this triad had distorted reality. The way kensho cuts into maladaptive traits is summarized below. Only this *de*-conditioned brain can be said to experience "the original self."

THE DISSOLUTION OF	*MEANS SUBTRACTING*	*AND IS EXPERIENCED AS*
I	The aggressive "doing-self." Self-concepts in time.	Freedom from compulsive doing, from "shoulds and oughts." Timelessness . . .
Me	The besieged and fearful self.	Fearlessness. Deep Peace.
Mine	The clutching self that: 1. had possessed other persons and things. 2. had been captured by its dualisms.	The world as it really is, without self-referent attachments. Diversity, coherence, and Unity.

Further Dissolution of the Pejorative Self During the Long Training Process

This self that first emerges from kensho is humbled and awed. Both impressions linger for years. However, only several episodes of kensho and satori can remove the deepest, hidden roots of the dysfunctional self in ways that endure.

Meanwhile, does Zen training simply sponsor a series of "no mind" vacant meditative states? Not at all. A *mindful* process of introspection (Freud's "evenly hovering attention") keeps monitoring the meditator's thoughts and behaviors. This online self-analysis means (1) seeing deeply into one's lapses in daily living; (2) diagnosing what causes them, with unsparing clinical objectivity; and (3) then deliberately cultivating (willfully) a series of appropriate remedies.

Each self-analysis confirms the validity of the Buddha's first sermon. Much of the human predicament turns out to be self-inflicted. It reflects our personal liabilities and ignorance. But suppose one can accept that one's anguish is caused by one's excessive desires and longings. What remedy exists for such greedy impulses? Now, with greater clarity, the meditator understands the deep wisdom of *letting go*. So a partial remedy becomes deliberate generosity, skillfully applied, anonymously.

And how does one alleviate hatred, loathing, and anger (the other side of fear)? Now, the approach includes generous applications of forgiveness, tolerance, loving-kindness, and compassion. Finally, how can one repair basic ignorance and delusions? The remedy is to keep walking that ancient eightfold path. One keeps rediscovering, spontaneously, its inherent virtues. Further insights into reality arrive while celebrating one's blessings: the gift of being fully alive, in Nature's impermanence.

So, the transformations occur not only in sudden flashes—in insights of various kinds and sizes. They also evolve during a more glacial, erosive process involving forms of thoughtful intention. Over decades, changes finally occur in that former hard-edged arrogant, besieged, clutching *I-Me-Mine*. Those old italicized capital letters yield. A lower profile emerges, a softer and more humane being, an *actualized, buoyant, compassionate* person:

i-me-mine

Of course, the table and paragraphs merely outline, in an highly idealized form, the general nature of the many short-range and long-range transformations of the selfish (egocentric) self. Nothing happens easily. Backsliding occurs. Personalities resist change. Self-deceptions are legendary.

But this natural quest for larger meanings beyond the self is deeply established in human history. Zen is one of many paths in this direction. Should we be too surprised that the paths of such inspired endeavors are often called "spiritual"? For what do the old word-roots of "spiritual" reaffirm? Only how much our lives depend on respiration, on each breath in, and out. Indeed, for centuries, it has been a key element of Zen meditative practice to pay mindful attention to each inspiration and expiration. In, and out.

Using increasingly sophisticated tests, neuropsychologists may currently employ such terms as "autonoetic awareness." This term refers to those basic phenomena that link our privately experienced "knowing" to our existing constructs of a personalized "self" (Levine et al. 1998). But our real problems arise from our deeper *unconscious* self. Of this we are not aware. It is true that many psychic components of our omni-self (and these include its covert dysfunctions, which Zen aims selectively to dissolve) do appear normally to arise among the more rostral networks in our brains (Austin 2000). Among these, several of the more right-sided circuits do seem to sponsor many of our overt, testable forms of private, "self-knowing awareness," whereas still other kinds of general knowing seem referable to left-sided networks (Levine et al. 1998). But the axial roots of one's egocentric omni-self go deep (Austin 1998).

Thus far, whatever brief glimpse we have had of the subtle Path of Zen has been within the constraints that mere words impose upon softer psychological concepts. How else does Zen training proceed, in relation to the psychophysiology of the human brain? These issues are summarized in the author's companion chapter in this volume, entitled "The Brain and Zen."

References

Austin J (1998) Zen and the brain: toward an understanding of meditation and consciousness. MIT Press, Cambridge

Austin J (1999) Six points to ponder. J Consciousness Stud 6(2–3):213–216

Austin J (2000) Consciousness evolves when the self dissolves. J Consciousness Stud 7(11–12):209–230

Levine G, Black S, Cabeza R, et al (1998) Episodic memory and the self in a case of isolated retrograde amnesia. Brain 121:1951–1973

Functional Neuroimaging of the Human Brain

Hiroshi Shibasaki

Summary. In the functional neuroimaging of the human brain, the main effort so far has been put forward to cerebral localization of each function or functional specialization. Two examples based on the study by the author's group are presented: one on the cortical mechanism of pain perception in humans, which was studied by somatosensory evoked potentials as well as magnetic fields, blood flow activation by position emission tomography (PET), and functional magnetic resonance imaging (fMRI), and the other on central control of gait in humans, which was studied by single photon emission computed tomography (SPECT). Currently, increasing attention has been paid to the functional coupling among different cerebral areas, either cortical or subcortical, by combining multiple techniques; for example, PET-rCBF or fMRI activation studies combined with transcranial magnetic stimulation (TMS). It is expected that the transient impairment of local function caused by repetitive TMS, combined with fMRI or PET, will help in clarifying the network circuitry. Moreover, it is hoped that noninvasive imaging of various receptors such as dopamine, serotonin, benzodiazepine or GABA, and acetylcholine, of the uptake of neurotransmitters such as dopamine, and of transporters will become available for clinical as well as scientific investigation of neural functions.

Keywords. Functional neuroimaging, Human brain functions, Pain perception, Central control of gait

Introduction

The rapid advance of modern technologies in recent years has enabled us to investigate human brain functions noninvasively. Those techniques can be divided into four groups depending on the main principle: (1) electrophysiological techniques including analysis of electroencephalogram (EEG) and magnetoencephalogram (MEG), and transcranial magnetic stimulation (TMS); (2) techniques utilizing radionuclides consisting of positron emission tomography (PET) and single photon emission computed tomography (SPECT); (3) functional magnetic resonance imaging (fMRI); and (4)

Department of Neurology and Human Brain Research Center, Kyoto University Graduate School of Medicine, Kyoto, Japan

optical imaging. Generally speaking, the electrophysiological techniques provide us with sufficient temporal information of the order of milliseconds, while the neuroimaging techniques give spatial information on the order of several millimeters. Among those neuroimaging techniques, fMRI time-locked to a certain stimulus or event (event-related fMRI) is useful owing to its noninvasiveness, short time for data acquisition, and repeatability. In this chapter, advantages and disadvantages of these techniques are discussed by presenting some data related to pain perception and central control of gait that were recently reported by the author's group.

Cortical Mechanism of Pain Perception in Humans

In human pain perception, a role of the thalamus has been emphasized while cortical participation has remained unclarified. Therefore, we performed a functional activation study in normal subjects by using CO_2 laser stimulation and the measurement of regional cerebral blood flow (rCBF) with PET. This stimulus is known to activate the nociceptive receptors selectively. As the result, activation was detected, in addition to the contralateral thalamus, in the contralateral frontal lobe and bilateral second somatosensory areas (SII) and insula [1]. In the PET-rCBF study, ^{15}O-labeled water, with a half-life of about 2 min, is used as a radiotracer; it renders an image of summed activity over a period of 2 min. Thus, electrophysiological techniques can supplement the imaging study with sufficient temporal information time-locked to the stimulus presentation. Somatosensory evoked potentials (SEPs) recorded from the scalp following CO_2 laser stimulaion of the hand dorsum in normal subjects show at least three peaks: a small negative peak over the contralateral central area (N1) at a latency of around 150 ms, a relatively large negative peak (N2; 200 ms), and a large positive peak (P2; 300 ms) maximally at the vertex midline [2,3]. Because MEG is not influenced by a "shunt" effect of the structures surrounding the cerebral cortex such as spinal fluid and skull, studies of these evoked responses by MEG allow us to estimate generator sources of those SEP components with much higher accuracy. Our study using a whole-head planar type magnetometer showed at least three current sources: one in the contralateral postcentral gyrus (SI) at a latency of about 190 ms, and two others in bilateral SII (latency, 180 ms contralateral and 220 ms ipsilateral) [4]. The participation of SI in pain perception in human was substantiated by the first recording of pain SEP from the crown of the postcentral gyrus in a patient with medically intractable epilepsy [4]. It is most likely from these findings that the afferent nociceptive input reaches SI and SII in parallel, which is different from input of other somatosensory modalities that is characterized by the SI-to-SII sequential activation.

Event-related fMRI is particularly useful for investigating higher brain functions because it allows us to carry out an experiment on a single trial basis and thus to follow the temporal course of activation with an accuracy of seconds. Sawamoto et al. [10] addressed the question as to how the anxiety about pain modulates the somatosensory perception and compared two experimental conditions in normal subjects. In one condition, the subject was certain that the stimulus in all trials was nonpainful (CO_2 laser stimulus below the pain threshold), and in the other condition, either painful or nonpainful stimulus was presented randomly, depending on the trial, in which the subject was uncertain about the kind of the next stimulus. Thus, the hemodynamic change before and after the stimulus presentation was evaluated for each trial. In the anterior cingulate cortex and bilateral parietal operculum and posterior insula, activation started to increase several seconds before the stimulus presentation in all those three areas. After the stimulus presentation, the increased activation in the three areas was highest after the painful stimulus under the uncertain condition, lowest after the nonpainful stimulus under the certain condition, and intermediate after the nonpainful stimulus under the uncertain condition. It is concluded from these findings that anxiety about pain enhances the somatosensory perception in these cortical areas.

Central Control of Gait in Humans

In activation studies using PET-rCBF, the subject's head must be fixed throughout the scanning, thus making it impossible to apply the technique to motor tasks involving head movement such as walking and other daily behaviors. Fukuyama et al. [5] took advantage of SPECT-rCBF imaging, which enables us to measure the rCBF increase related to an experimental task after the actual task was finished, and applied this principle to the study of mechanism of urination in humans. They injected ^{99m}Tc-HMPAO into normal subjects while they were voiding, and the data were compared with the resting condition [5]. They further applied this technique to patients with Parkinson's disease while walking [6]. In normal subjects, the leg and trunk areas of the primary foot sensorimotor cortex, medial and lateral area 6, cingulate gyrus, superior parietal cortex, visual cortex, dorsal brainstem, and cerebellum were activated during walking [8]. In patients with Parkinson's disease who showed the typical parkinsonian gait with short step length and increased cadence (number of steps per minute), the same areas were activated during walking, but the level of rCBF increase was lower in the left supplementary motor area (SMA), right precuneus, and left cerebellar hemisphere as compared with age-matched healthy subjects [7].

It is well known that parkinsonian patients with frozen gait find it much easier to walk upstairs or by stepping across lines drawn transversely with respect to the walking direction (kinésie paradoxale). To elucidate the mechanism underlying the improvement of parkinsonian gait by certain visual stimuli, we carried out a SPECT-rCBF activation study while the patients walked on a treadmill that moved at a fixed speed, and compared the effects of transverse lines with those of the lines drawn parallel to the walking direction. In Parkinson's patients, the cadence decreased to normal level when walking across the transversely drawn lines whereas there was no difference between the two kinds of lines in normal subjects [8]. In Parkinson's patients and normal subjects, the gait-associated rCBF increase was greater with transverse lines as compared with parallel lines in the posterior parietal cortex and cerebellar hemispheres [8]. The only region where the difference in activation between the transverse and parallel lines was greater in Parkinson's patients compared with normal subjects was the right lateral premotor area [8]. In the Parkinson's group, the rCBF increase in the right lateral premotor area while walking with the parallel lines was smaller than that in the normal control, and it increased to normal level while walking with the transverse lines, indicating that the activation of this particular area by visual stimuli might play an important role in the improvement of parkinsonian gait [8]. This area is known to receive abundant visual input from the parietal cortex whereas the input from basal ganglia is relatively sparse; the more medial premotor area receives a strong facilitatory input from basal ganglia, and thus its function is decreased in Parkinson's disease.

Discussion

In functional neuroimaging of the human brain, the main effort put forward so far has been on cerebral localization of each function or functional specialization. Currently, increasing attention has been paid to the functional coupling among different cerebral areas, either cortical or subcortical, by combining multiple techniques, for example, PET-rCBF or fMRI activation studies combined with TMS. Using PET with fluorodeoxyglucose, Siebner et al. [9] recently disclosed increased glucose metabolism in the bilateral sensorimotor cortices and SMA even after repetitive TMS of the unilateral sensorimotor cortex with subthreshold intensity at 5 Hz for 12 min. It is expected that the transient impairment of local function caused by repetitive TMS, combined with fMRI or PET, will help in clarifying the network circuitry. Moreover, it is hoped that noninvasive imaging of various receptors such as dopamine, serotonin, benzodiazepine or GABA, and acetylcholine, of the uptake of neurotransmitters such as dopamine, and of transporters will become available for clinical as well as scientific investigation of neural functions.

References

1. Xu X, Fukuyama H, Yazawa S, et al (1997) Functional localization of pain perception in the human brain studied by PET. NeuroReport 8:555–559
2. Miyazaki M, Shibasaki H, Kanda M, et al (1994) Generator mechanism of pain-related evoked potentials following CO_2 laser stimulation of the hand: scalp topography and effect of predictive warning signal. J Clin Neurophysiol 11:242–254
3. Xu X, Kanda M, Shindo K, et al (1995) Pain-related somatosensory evoked potentials following CO_2 laser stimulation of foot. Electroencephalogr Clin Neurophysiol 96:12–23
4. Kanda M, Nagamine T, Ikeda A, et al (2000) Primary somatosensory cortex is actively involved in pain processing in human. Brain Res 853:282–289
5. Fukuyama H, Matsuzaki S, Ouchi Y, et al (1996) Neural control of micturition in man examined with single photon emission computed tomography using 99m-Tc-HMPAO. NeuroReport 7:3009–3012
6. Fukuyama H, Ouchi Y, Matsuzaki S, et al (1997) Brain functional activity during gait in normal subjects: a spect study. Neurosci Lett 228:183–186
7. Hanakawa T, Katsumi Y, Fukuyama H, et al (1999) Mechanisms underlying gait disturbance in Parkinson's disease. A single photon emission computed tomography study. Brain 122:1271–1282
8. Hanakawa T, Fukuyama H, Katsumi Y, et al (1999) Enhanced lateral premotor activity during paradoxical gait in Parkinson's disease. Ann Neurol 45:329–336
9. Siebner HR, Peller M, Willoch F, et al (2000) Lasting cortical activation after repetitive TMS of the motor cortex. A glucose metabolic study. Neurology 54:956–963
10. Sawamoto N, Honda M, Okada T, et al (2000) Expectation of pain enhances responses to nonpainful somatosensory stimulation in the anterior cingulate cortex and parietal operculum/posterior insula: an event-related functional magnetic resonance imaging study. J Neurosci 20:7438–7445

Psychological Dysfunction in Parkinson's Disease

HIROTARO NARABAYASHI[1] and AKIRA KANAZAWA[2]

Summary. Parkinson's disease is a slowly progressive disorder, starting from motor symptoms and later being added to and colored by psychological dysfunction. Psychological dysfunction is divided into two categories: one is of the cognitive sphere and the other of the emotional sphere. The former is often combined with motor symptoms and is therefore misinterpreted as motor symptoms, such as freezing of gait. Cognitive disturbance, which can be analyzed in the relatively early to middle stages of the disease (Hoehn–Yahr stage I–III), when the intellectual scale still remains in normal range, is markedly seen in execution of the internal cued responses and much less in the external cued responses or behavior. The latter emotional changes are interpreted as of change of mood or of limbic function, such as depressive mood, anxiety, hypochondriasis or tension state, and also inattention, loss of interest, inertia, or abulia. These two categories of symptoms are, working hypothetically, interpreted as relating to the caudate nucleus and the ventral striatum, respectively. Analysis based on neuropathological, clinical, and psychometric observations is discussed.

Keywords. Three DA projections, Freezing of gait, Cognitive dysfunction, Emotional function, Wisconsin Card Sorting Test (WCST)

Introduction

Parkinson's disease (PD) is a slowly progressive disease occurring in the relatively aged population. It starts by motor symptoms such as rigidity or tremor of unilateral extremities, and slowly and progressively worsens by involvement of other extremities and the trunk, causing various grades of difficulty of movement, posturing, and locomotion. This progression, finally leading to the bedridden state, is beautifully schematized by Hoehn–Yahr (H-Y) stages from I to V (Hoehn and Yahr 1967). With these motor difficulties, psychological changes also start to develop, which are often described as "akinesia" (Narabayashi 1993). Psychological and emotional changes such as depressive mood lead to a state of inertia or of abulia accompanying the severe

[1] Neurological Clinic, 5-12-8 Nakameguro, Meguro-ku, Tokyo 153-0061, Japan
[2] Department of Neurology, Juntendo University School of Medicine, Tokyo, Japan

motor difficulties during the progressive course; this is seen in PD that starts at an elderly age but much less often in younger-starting or juvenile cases (JP).

Pathological and Chemical Background

My (H.N.) working hypothesis is that the progressive worsening in the course of the disease may be related to the gradual spread of pathology within the three dopaminergic projections. It is well established that in the parkinsonian brain the severity of neuronal degeneration is more profound in the ventral tier of the substantia nigra zona compacta (SNc), which projects to the putamen, the motor part of the striatum, than in the dorsal tier projecting to the caudate nucleus or cognitive part (Fig. 1) (Goto et al. 1989; Gibb and Lees 1991). It is estimated that the pathology may first start at the ventral tier and then slowly spread to the dorsal tier within several years. It is estimated that progression of pathology might be much slower in JP than in PD (Gibb et al. 1991). Recent reports by Damier et al. (1999) also described neuropathological findings in a series of five cases, arrived at a similar interpretation. Neurochemical evaluation of the striatum has shown more severe deficiency of dopamine (DA) in the putamen than in the caudate (Hornykiewicz and Kish 1986). DA deficiency in the nucleus accumbens was a little slighter but varied case to case.

Such differences in pathology and chemistry with different divisions of the nigrostriatum lead us to consider the relationship to the progressive worsening of clinical picture. The underlying physiological mechanisms of motor symptoms have been intensively studied in the past 30 years through analysis of observation during careful stereotaxic surgery in human patients and also in animal experiments.

Psychological Changes

Psychological changes are described from the following two aspects. Cognitive changes are related to the nigrocaudal projection and the emotional changes to the paranigral DA neurons projecting to the ventral forebrain limbic system. The term

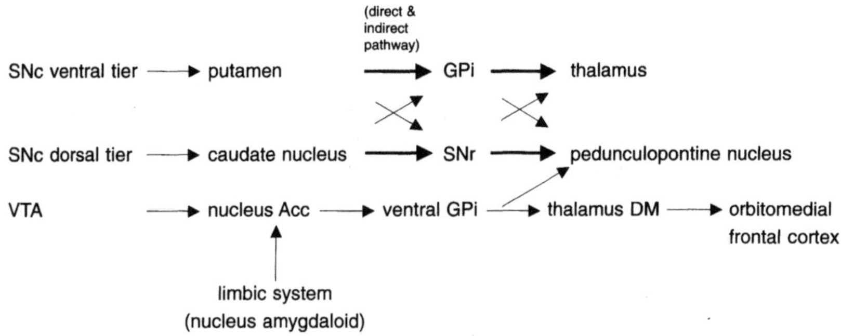

Fig. 1. Dopaminergic projections from the ventral tegmental area (VTA) and further projections proposed by the author (H.N.). *SNc*, substantia nigra zona compacta; *GPi*, internal segment of the globus pallidus; *SNr*, substantia nigra zona reticulata; *Acc*, accumbens; *DM*, dorsal medial nucleus

bradyphrenia (Rogers et al. 1986), which is frequently used to describe the psychological features of PD patients, is understood to indicate the mixture of disturbance of these two functional spheres.

Cognitive Sphere

With the spread of pathology to the nigrocaudal projection, cognitive function may start to be affected, especially in relation to motor performance. One such example is the so-called gait freezing, presenting the characteristic phenomenon of "kinésie paradoxale." The patient with this symptom can step up or down stairs without difficulty, but he or she shows severe difficulty in starting and stepping forward on a flat and smooth corridor floor. However, this difficulty is easily solved by asking the person to walk in response to visual signals, lines on the floor transverse to the direction of walking, or auditory signals such as a metronome sound below 2.5 Hz. Gait is normally performable under such signals. When these signals, or external cues, suddenly stop, freezing quickly returns, usually within several seconds. This observation may suggest that focused attention evoked by an external cue cannot be maintained for more than several seconds. Internal cues for initiating and maintaining the rhythmic movement seem not to work normally in such cases. Kinésie paradoxale may be the simplest example of sensory input working on peripheral rhythmic movement such as gait, speech, or finger-tapping, which is assumed to become effective on the basis of the short span of focused attention evoked by external cues.

Suzuki et al. (1994) reported one case of intracranial malignant lymphoma in the depth of the right frontal lobe, mostly involving the caudate nucleus, which presented severe freezing of gait and micrographia but without any other sign of motor disturbance. By treatment with betamethasone, the lymphoma shrank and disappeared. Both gait freezing and micrographia disappeared. At about 4 months after the cessation of treatment, the lymphoma started to grow again in the same area and the motor symptoms also recurred. This observation suggests that the caudate nucleus may be playing a key role in producing this specific symptom.

The common feature of cognitive disturbance is analyzed by psychological tests, which were carried out by one of the authors (A.K.). The Wisconsin Card Sorting Test (WCST) has frequently been used to detect disturbance in the cognitive sphere in PD (Lees and Smith 1983; Taylor et al. 1986). All 16 cases of PD and all 14 age-matched normal control subjects (NCS) presented a normal IQ, i.e., between 90 to 110 by the WAIS Test or over 25 by the Mini Mental Test (MMT). The 6 PD cases of H-Y stage I performed the WCST almost normally and correctly as the NCS. However, 10 cases of H-Y stage II to III presented a high-grade difficulty in performance and a marked increase in the number of errors and perseverations (Table 1).

Although statistical analysis is not yet available due to the small number of cases tested, clinical observations as described earlier indicate a clear difference in results between the earlier stage (H-Y stage I) and the middle stage (H-Y stages II–III). This difference may suggest that disturbance of cognitive function starts to appear when the pathology spreads to involve the nigrocaudate projection. However, we are not able to identify the elemental factor within the cognitive domain, such as difficulties in working memory, attention, visuospatial function, or executive function, that is

Table 1. Results of the Wisconsin Card Sorting Test (WCST): Milner version in PD in two groups of different H-Y stages

Case	Age/sex	Duration of disease (years)	H-Y stage (side of symptoms)	WCST	
				Categories achieved	Perseveration errors
1. H. T.	49/f	2	I (R)	6	0
2. G. I.	65/m	2	I (L)	6	0
3. M. Y.	65/f	7	I (R)	6	0
4. N. I.	46/f	0.5	I (R)	5	3
5. K. A.	55/m	6	I (L)	6	1
6. K. Y.	65/m	4.5	I (R)	6	1
7. K. E.	49/m	19	II (R < L)	4	2
8. S. O.	67/f	6	III (R > L)	3	8
9. R. K.	70/m	3	III (R > L)	2	8
10. U. K.	68/f	5	III (R > L)	0	9
11. A. K.	65/f	5	III (R < L)	0	13
12. K. F.	68/f	4	III (R < L)	2	5
13. Y. T.	70/m	9	III (R < L)	6	0
14. H. I.	64/f	2	III (R > L)	4	4
15. N. O.	63/f	5	III (R > L)	0	23
16. T. H.	60/f	12	III (R > L)	3	6

responsible for these disturbances. However, I (H.N.) am presuming a highly probable factor might be the disturbance of focused attention.

Emotional Sphere

Another important psychological change is in the emotional sphere, a depressed mood and lowered emotional response that, however, is not so severe as in cases of major depression. Loss of spontaneous activity, loss of interest, psychic asthenia, and lowered emotional expression, such as the lack of sadness for the death of a family member, are also common features in cases of long disease duration. Rarely, aggression or agitation caused by strong emotional stress can be observed. These emotional changes can be benefited sustainedly or at least transiently by lesions made in the internal segment of the globus pallidus (GPi) by posteroventral pallidotomy. This benefit is assumed to be due to direct partial involvement of the ventral GPi, which is an area receiving strong input from the ventral forebrain limbic structures, in cases of sustained benefit, and to transient postoperative swelling in cases of temporary benefit, as described in detail by Narabayashi et al. (1997).

Comment

A working hypothesis by the author (H.N.) on two divisions of psychological changes, cognitive and emotional, in PD has been described. The important question is what is the metabolic background for presenting these changes in addition to DA deficiency. A deficiency of norepinephrine (NE) in the brain of long-standing PD cases is suspected in the later stage of PD from the finding of severe lowering of dopamine-β-hydroxylase (NE-synthesizing enzyme) activity in the CSF. L-threo-3,4-dihydroxyphenylserine (DOPS), a synthetic precursor of NE, which is now on the market in Japan, is known to improve the depressive mood as well as the gait freezing (Narabayashi et al. 1986). In addition to NE, the role of serotonin (5-HT) has also become of interest.

References

Damier P, Hirsch EC, Agid Y, et al (1999) The substantia nigra of the human brain. I. Nigrosomes and the nigral matrix, a compartmental organization based on calbindin D28K immunohistochemistry. Brain 122:1421–1436

Gibb WRG, Lees AJ (1991) Anatomy, pigmentation, ventral and dorsal subpopulations of the substantia nigra, and differential cell death in Parkinson's disease. J Neurol Neurosurg Psychiatry 54:388–396

Gibb WRG, Narabayashi H, Yokochi M, et al (1991) New pathologic observations in juvenile onset parkinsonism with dystonia. Neurology 41:820–822

Goto S, Hirano A, Matsumoto S (1989) Subdivisional involvement of nigrostriatal loop in idiopathic Parkinson's disease and striatonigral degeneration. Ann Neurol 26:766–770

Hoehn MM, Yahr M (1967) Parkinsonism: onset, progression and mortality. Neurology 17:427–442

Hornykiewicz O, Kish SJ (1986) Biochemical pathophysiology of Parkinson's disease. In: Yahr MD, Bergmann KJ (eds) Advances in neurology, vol 45. Raven Press, New York, pp 19–34

Lees AJ, Smith E (1983) Cognitive deficits in the early stages of Parkinson's disease. Brain 106:257–270

Narabayashi H (1993) Three types of akinesia in the progressive course of Parkinson's disease. In: Narabayashi H, Nagatsu T, Yanagisawa N, et al (eds) Advances in neurology, vol 60. Raven Press, New York, pp 18–24

Narabayashi H, Kondo T, Yokochi F, et al (1986) Clinical effects of L-threo-3,4-dihydroxyphenylserine in cases of parkinsonism and pure akinesia. In: Yahr MD, Bergmann KJ (eds) Advances in neurology, vol 45. Raven Press, New York, pp 593–602

Narabayashi H, Miyashita N, Hattori Y, et al (1997) Posteroventral pallidotomy: its effect on motor symptoms and scores of MMPI test in patients with Parkinson's disease. Parkinsonism Relat Disord 3:7–20

Rogers D, Lees AJ, Trimble M, et al (1986) Concept of bradyphrenia: a neuropsychiatric approach. In: Yahr MD, Bergmann KJ (eds) Advances in neurology, vol 45. Raven Press, New York, pp 447–450

Suzuki T, Yamamoto M, Saitoh M, et al (1994) A case of intracranial malignant lymphoma with pure akinesia and repeated regression on CT scans. Brain Nerve 36:689–696

Taylor AE, Saint-Cyr JA, Lang AE (1986) Frontal lobe dysfunction in Parkinson's disease. The cortical focus of neostriatal outflow. Brain 109:845–883

Behavioral and Cognitive Changes Following Thalamic and Basal Ganglionic Lesions

Etsuro Mori

Summary. Subcortical small lesions involving the thalamus, caudate, and globus pallidus disrupt corticosubcortical circuits, resulting in cognitive dysfunction. Disruption of the frontosubcortical circuits leads to cognitive impairment with striking frontal lobe features, and disruption of the memory-related circuits leads to amnesia. Specific vascular lesions cause characteristic neurobehavioral syndromes: the syndrome of left polar thalamic artery territory infarction features amnesia accentuated for verbal materials, as compared with nonverbal ones, and emotional and motivational deficits; the syndrome of bilateral paramedian thalamic artery territory infarction features sudden onset of coma or confusion followed by a persistent amnesia of varying severity, with or without language impairment and frontal lobe dysfunction; and caudate or pallidal lesions lead to behavioral and cognitive changes including abulia, apathy, and depression in some patients, and disinhibition, hyperactivity, and inattention in others. These components are often the features of vascular dementia, and ischemic lesions in those strategic sites are often found in patients with vascular dementia. Studies of subcortical strategic lesions involving the neural circuits provide an important clue for understanding of vascular dementia. The effects of discrete ischemic subcortical lesions in the thalamus and basal ganglia on the neural circuits can be documented with high-resolution MR imagings and functional brain imaging.

Keywords. Thalamus, Basal ganglia, Behavior, Cognitive function, Vascular dementia

Introduction

Small lesions involving the thalamus, striatum, and pallidum, which are crucial components of the corticosubcortical circuits, often cause cognitive impairment and behavioral change. Disruption of the frontosubcortical circuits leads to behavioral impairment with striking frontal lobe features, and disruption of the memory-related circuits leads to amnesia. These impairments are the features of vascular dementia, and ischemic lesions in those strategic sites are often found in patients with vascular dementia. In this chapter, I document the effects of discrete ischemic subcortical

---

Divisions of Clinical Neurosciences and Neurology, Hyogo Institute for Aging Brain and Cognitive Disorders, 520 Saisho-ko, Himeji 670-0981, Japan

lesions in the caudate nucleus, pallidum, and thalamus on the neural circuits by using high-resolution MR imaging with stereotaxic techniques and functional brain imaging, and discuss the neuropsychological and behavioral correlates.

Bilateral Caudate Lesions

Caudate infarcts lead to behavioral and cognitive changes including abulia, apathy, disinhibition, hyperactivity, and major affective disturbance. Sometimes stereotyped and compulsive behaviors accompany the changes. A 65-year-old, right-handed, hypertensive man, who was previously a responsible bank branch manager, insidiously became lazy and slovenly. The patient engaged in repeated uninhibited sexual behavior, gambling, and shoplifting. MR imagings demonstrated that infarcts were confined to the head of the caudate nuclei. Results of MR angiography were unremarkable. In this patient, bilateral caudate infarcts caused a peculiar behavioral abnormality very similar to frontotemporal dementia. On examination, little neurological abnormality was noted. Memory and intelligence were preserved (ADAS, 12; WAIS-R full-scale IQ, 91). However, some of the executive functions were affected (Wisconsin Card Sorting test, 1 category achieved; phonetic cue verbal fluency, 2–6/min). In addition, he showed disinhibited and stereotyped behaviors, lack of insight, indifference, and euphoria. A PET demonstrated that glucose metabolism was decreased in the frontal lobes, basal ganglia, and thalamus. Hypometabolism was accentuated in the right lateral and medial prefrontal lobes, in the bilateral inferior lateral prefrontal lobes, and in the right thalamus.

The prototypic structure of the frontosubcortical circuits, like the motor and oculomotor circuits, has an origin in the frontal lobes, a projection to the striatum, a connection from striatum to the pallidum and substantia nigra, a projection from these to the thalamus, and a final link back to the frontal lobe (Fig. 1). The neuroimaging findings on this patient suggested that a disruption of the inferior prefrontal circuit leads to an orbitofrontal syndrome with prominent disinhibition, and a disruption of the lateral prefrontal circuit affects executive functions.

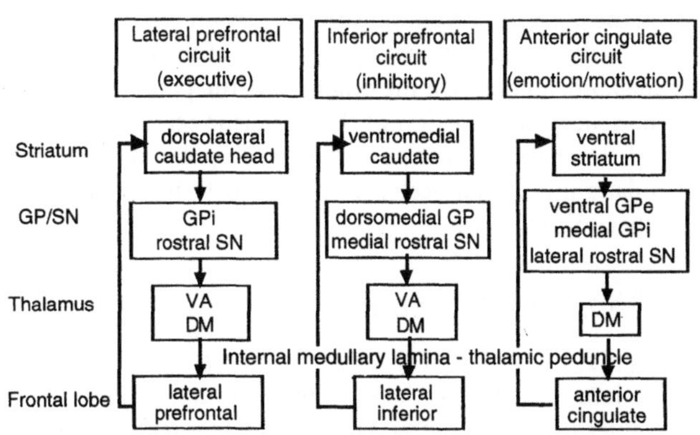

FIG. 1. Behavior-related frontostriatopallidothalamic circuits. *GPi*, Globus pallidus internus; *VA*, Nucleus ventralis anterior; *GP*, Globus pallidus; *SN*, Substatia migra; *GPe*, Globus pallidus internus; *DM*, Nucleus dorsomedialis

Bilateral Pallidal Lesions

Similarly, pallidal lesions lead to the behavioral and cognitive changes of frontal lobe features. Isolated pallidal damage is found following an anoxic event. A 40-year-old, right-handed man developed behavioral and personality changes 2 weeks after accidental carbon monoxide intoxication. The personality changes included apathy, indifference, placidity, and loss of drive. However, neither motor nor intellectual disturbance was noted. MR imaging demonstrated bilateral pallidal necrosis. There was neither neurological abnormality nor any cognitive impairment (WAIS-R full-scale IQ, 103; WMS-R general MI, 105; Wisconsin Card Sorting Test, 6 categories achieved). However, his personality change was striking. Apathy and placidity were remarkable. The patient completely lost desire, interest, initiative, and preference. On the Moudsley Personality Inventory, he scored 12, indicating intraversive. However, when it was applied as letting him pretend as if he were, he scored 44, which means very extraversive. Habib and Poncet (1988) coined the term athymhormia to describe such a syndrome. A stereotaxic analysis of high spatial resolution MR imagings demonstrated the lesions were confined in the ventrorostral globus pallidus, sparing the dorsocaudal part of the globus pallidus and the white matter in and outside the globus pallidus. A SPECT demonstrated bifrontal hypoperfusion. The hypoperfusion was accentuated in the mesial frontal lobe.

These findings substantiated the role of the anterior cingulate circuit in affect and drive in humans. A disruption of this circuit at the level of the ventrorostral globus pallidus dynamically depresses the mesial frontal lobe function, resulting in isolated athymhormia without affecting other parallel basal gangliathalamofrontal circuits (see Fig. 1).

Anteromedial Thalamic Lesions

The arterial supply of the anteromedial thalamus consists of two different systems: one is the polar artery and the other is the paramedian thalamic artery. The polar artery arises from the posterior communicating artery and irrigates the anterior thalamic nuclei and the adjacent structures. An occlusion of the polar artery leads to unilateral anterior thalamic infarcts. On the other hand, the paramedian thalamic artery arises from the mesencephalic portion of the posterior cerebral artery and irrigates the medial part of the thalamus just posterior to the polar artery territory. It often sends branches bilaterally, and an occlusion of the posterior cerebral artery leads to bilateral medial thalamic infarcts.

Left Anterior Thalamic Infarction

The syndrome of polar thalamic artery territory infarcts features amnesia and emotional and motivational deficits, but lacks other neurological deficits. Based on six patients with left anterior thalamic infarcts of polar artery territory, we elucidated the clinical and neuroimaging features of left polar artery territory infarcts. A verbal memory loss that is not accompanied by retrograde amnesia and disorientation, and language disturbance characterized by anomia, low verbal fluency, and difficulty with word definition, which is interpreted as a verbal semantic memory loss, are neuropsychological features of left anterior thalamic infarction. In addition, frontal lobe dysfunction including impairment of executive function, abulia, and either indifference or depression is characteristic. High-spatial resolution MR imagings were obtained in all six patients. The hypointensity area in each patient was cumulatively projected on Shaltenbrand and Wahren's (1977) stereotaxic atlas. The common lesion site included the mamillothalamic tract and internal medullary lamina and a part of ventroanterior and ventrolateral nuclei. We compared cerebral blood flow (CBF) by using the SPM software between the patients and six age/sex-matched healthy subjects. A significant reduction in CBF was noted in the anterior temporal cortices and amygdala and the medial prefrontal cortices and anterior cingulate gyrus of the left hemisphere, as well as in the left thalamus.

These results suggest that the intrathalamic white matter lesions are more important than the nuclear lesions. The mamillothalamic tract, which is a part of the hippocampal-related Papez circuit, and the ventral portion of the internal medullary lamina, which contains the ventroamygdalofugal pathway of the amygdala-related Yakovlev circuit, are the most likely candidates for the verbal memory loss (Fig. 2). This concept supports the model of the memory system proposed by Warrington and Weiskrantz (1982) and by Mishkin (1982). In addition, disruption of the frontostriatopallidothalamic circuits leads to apathy, abulia, and depression. Functional brain imaging actually demonstrates the disruption of the relevant circuits (Fig. 1). The left anterior temporal lobe is reportedly involved in verbal semantic memory. The finding of anterior temporal hypoperfusion likely explains the verbal semantic memory loss in patients with the left polar artery territory infarcts. However, the mechanism of the anterior temporal involvement remain to be elucidated. Although the thalamocortical projection to the anterior temporal lobe in human remains uncertain, our PET findings strongly suggest that there should be a direct projection to the anterior temporal lobe. We need to explore the relevant thalamic nuclei and pathway and their function in humans.

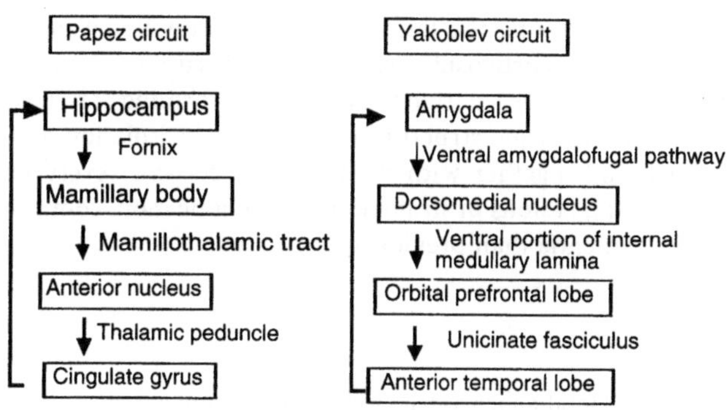

FIG. 2. Memory-related corticolimbothalamic circuits

Bilateral Paramedian Thalamic Infarcts

The syndrome of bilateral paramedian thalamic artery territory infarction features sudden onset of coma or confusion followed by a persistent amnesia of varying severity, with or without language impairment and frontal lobe dysfunction. Sometimes a disinhibition syndrome may be the main feature. A 57-year-old right-handed man developed hypersomnia, amnesia, and personality changes characterized by childlike speech and lack of spontaneity after a transient unconsciousness. MR imagings demonstrated bilateral paramedian thalamic infarcts. On examination, there were no neurological deficits. In addition to hypersomnia, inattention, loss of spontaneity, and lack of concern, euphoria, emotional lability, and disinhibited behaviors, childlike speech was characteristic. There was severe anterograde and retrograde amnesia. Intelligence and executive functions markedly declined. In an analysis of the exact extent of the lesion, by using high-resolution MR imagings and Shaltenbrand and Wahren's (1977) stereotaxic atlas, the lesions bilaterally affected the internal medullary lamina at the ventral portion and a part of the dorsomedial, centromedian, and ventral nuclei as well. The mamillothalamic tract was seemingly spared. A PET scan demonstrated decreased glucose metabolism in the frontotemporal lobes and thalmi.

The behavioral changes of frontal lobe feature and executive dysfunction would be attributable to a disruption of the frontostriatopallidothalamic circuits, most probably at the internal medullary lamina (see Fig. 1). In addition, hypersomnia was related to damage in the nonspecific thalamic nuclei; this appeared as a widespread hypometabolism on the functional brain imaging. Amnesia is attributed to the damage of the internal medullary lamina, a part of the amygdala-related Yakovlev circuit (see Fig. 2). Although the mamillothalamic tract seemed intact, the connection between the anterior nuclei and frontal lobe might be disrupted at the thalamic peduncle.

Conclusions

In conclusion, subcortical lesions may disrupt corticosubcortical circuits. A disruption of corticosubcortical circuits may lead to significant behavioral/cognitive changes without neurological deficits. Disturbances in emotion, motivation, executive function, and memory are the features. High-resolution MR imaging stereotaxic localization is helpful for identifying the lesion extent, and functional neuroimaging is helpful for documenting the corticosubcortical circuit disruption. A disruption of the corticosubcortical circuit plays an important role in forming vascular dementia. Lesions in a subcortical strategic structure rarely occur in isolation. However, such lesions were often found together with multiple infarcts and severe white matter changes, as in this patient. Lesions in strategic sites might be more common and more important cause for dementia than previously thought.

References

Cummings JL (1993) Frontal-subcortical circuits and human behavior. Arch Neurol 50:873–880

Eysenck HJ (1959) Manual of Maudsley personality inventory. University of London, London

Habib M, Poncet M (1988) Perte de l'élan vital, de l'intérét et de l'affectivité (syndrome athymhormique) au cours de lésions lacunaires des corps striés. Rev Neurol 144:571–577
Mishkin M (1982) A memory system in the monkey. Philos Trans R Soc Lond B Biol Sci 298:83–95
Mori E, Yamadori A, Mitani Y (1986) Left thalamic infarction and disturbance of verbal memory: a clinicoanatomical study with a new method of computed tomographic stereotaxic lesion localization. Ann Neurol 20:671–676
Mori E, Yamashita H, Takauchi S, Kondo K (1996) Isolated athymhormia following hypoxic biateral pallidal lesions. Behav Neurol 9:17–23
Mori E (1988) Acute behavioral derangement: impairments of awareness, attention, emotion, and motivation. In: Ginsberg M, Bogousslavsky J (eds) Cerebrovascular disease: pathophysiology, diagnosis, and management, vol 2. Blackwell, Cambridge, pp 1145–1148
Mori E, Ishii K, Hashimoto M (1999) The role of functional brain imaging in evaluation of vascular dementia. Alzheimer Dis Assoc Dis 13(suppl 3):S91–S101
Shaltenbrand G, Wahren W (1977) Atlas for stereotaxy of the human brain. Thieme, Stuttgart
Warrington EK, Weiskrantz L (1982) Amnesia: a disconnection syndrome? Neuropsychologia 20:233–248

Behavioral Manifestations of Alzheimer's Disease

Jeffrey L. Cummings

Summary. Neuropsychiatric manifestations are common in Alzheimer's disease (AD). Nearly all patients eventually exhibit some form of behavioral change. The Neuropsychiatric Inventory (NPI) is a valid and reliable means of assessing behavioral alterations in patients with AD and other dementias. The NPI assesses ten common types of behavioral changes evident in AD and has a caregiver distress scale allowing assessment of the amount of distress engendered by each of the behavioral changes. Investigations using the NPI and neuroimaging have demonstrated correlations between apathy and diminished medial frontal perfusion and psychosis and disproportionately reduced perfusion of left medial orbital frontal, left anterior cingulate, left and right dorsolateral frontal, left dorsal lateral parietal, left pulmonar, left ventral striatum, and left cerebellum. High scores on the dysphoria subscale of the NPI correlate with reduced metabolism in the left and right superior frontal gyrus, middle frontal gyrus, inferior frontal gyrus, and anterior cingulate gyrus. The NPI also allows assessment of the response of behaviors to psychopharmacological interventions. Reductions in behavioral pathology have been demonstrated with cholinesterase inhibitors (tacrine, donepezil, metrifonate, galantamine, and rivastigmine) as well as antipsychotic agents (olanzapine).

Keywords. Alzheimer's disease, Neuropsychiatric Inventory, Delusions, Depression, Agitation

Introduction

Alzheimer's disease (AD) is a complex neurodegenerative disorder with neuropsychological and neuropsychiatric manifestations. The typical neuropsychological features of AD include progressive amnestic type of memory impairment, language abnormalities with features characteristic of transcortical sensory aphasia, visuospatial abnormalities, impairment of calculation, and disturbances of executive function. These are the hallmark features of AD, and define the syndrome in most nosological schemas such as the Diagnostic and Statistical Manual of Mental Disorders [1].

Department of Neurology and Psychiatry and Biobehavioral Sciences, UCLA School of Medicine, 710 Westwood Plaza, Los Angeles, CA 90095-1769, USA

Neuropsychiatric and behavioral abnormalities also are common features of AD and are present in nearly all cases. This dimension of the illness produces distress in the patients, is responsible for a substantial proportion of the burden experienced by caregivers, frequently requires management with psychotropic medications, and may be the basis for abuse, neglect, or institutionalization of AD victims. The behavioral dimension of AD has been intensively studied in the past decade. It is increasingly well understood. Advances in methods for assessing neuropsychiatric and behavioral changes have facilitated research in this investigatory arena. The Neuropsychiatric Inventory (NPI) [2] is one of the instruments that has been used to explore the behavioral dimension of AD and other dementing disorders. This brief review describes the NPI and the results of descriptive imaging and pharmacological studies of AD in which the NPI was used as the principal assessment or outcome instrument.

Neuropsychiatric Inventory

The NPI is a scripted inventory that elicits information from caregivers familiar with the behavior of the patient being assessed. The NPI assess ten domains of behavior relevant to AD including delusions, hallucinations, agitation/aggression, depression/dysphoria, anxiety, euphoria/elation, apathy/indifference, disinhibition, irritability/lability, and aberrant motor behavior. For each of these domains, there is a screening question and if the caregiver indicates that behaviors described in the screening question are present, a series of subquestions are then asked. After confirming with the subquestions that the response to the screening question was accurate, the caregiver is then asked to score the frequency of the behavior (on a structured 1 through 4 scale) and the severity of the behavior (on a structured 1 through 3 scale). The total score for that domain is the product of multiplying the frequency times the severity. A total NPI score is generated by adding all the domain scores together.

After the caregiver has indicated the frequency and the severity of the behavior, they are then asked to judge the amount of distress that they experience as a result of the behavior (scored 0 through 5). A total caregiver distress score can be generated by adding all the individual distress scores together. The inquiry is based on the behaviors that have been present in the past 4 weeks and that were not present before the onset of the dementing disorder. The validity and reliability of the NPI have been demonstrated, and it has been translated into multiple languages for international application. An expanded version of the NPI is available with two additional elements assaying the presence of eating and appetite disturbances, as well as sleep and nighttime behavior disturbances. In addition, an NPI questionnaire (NPIQ) has been developed for rapid clinical assessment; it consists of the NPI screening question and the severity rating only. The subquestions and the frequency reading are deleted. A nursing home version of the NPI (NPI/NH) has been developed for use with institutional caregivers [3].

Neuropsychiatric Features of Alzheimer's Disease

The neuropsychiatric and behavioral disturbances of a clinical population of AD patients was investigated by Mega et al. [4]. Of the 50 patients in the clinical sample, only 12% did not evidence scorable behavioral abnormalities. The most common disturbance observed was apathy (72%), followed by agitation (60%), anxiety (48%), irritability (42%), aberrant motor behavior (38%), dysphoria (38%), disinhibition (36%), delusions (22%), hallucinations (10%), and euphoria (8%). Most behavioral disturbances worsened with disease progression, as manifested by declining Mini-Mental State Examination (MMSE) scores. For example, delusions increased from 12% to 25% to 31% of patients, progressing from Mini-Mental States of 30 to 21, 20 to 11, and 10 to 0. Likewise, agitation increased from 47% to 55% and then 85%; dysphoria increased from 2% to 45% to 62%; apathy increased from 47% to 80% to 92%; irritability increased from 35% to 40% to 54%; and aberrant motor behavior from 12% to 30% to 84%. Other behavioral disturbances were less predictable, although mild patients were less likely to exhibit any of the behavioral disturbances.

The percentages of occurrence of the behavior among patients were systematically related to the score so that behaviors that were more commonly exhibited among patients also tended to have the highest mean scores on the NPI subscales. Thus agitation, dysphoria, anxiety, apathy, and aberrant motor behavior all had systematically higher mean scores as the disease progressed from mild to moderate to severe.

The NPI has been factor analyzed in a sample of 162 AD patients into three identifiable syndromes, including a mood factor, a psychotic factor, and a frontal factor [5]. These factors accounted for 62% of the total variance. The mood factor includes anxiety and depression, the psychosis dimension includes agitation, hallucinations, delusions, and irritability, and the frontal factor includes disinhibition and euphoria. Two subscales did not fit this illusion, including aberrant motor behavior and apathy.

The caregiver distress scale portion of the NPI was studied in a separate sample of dementia patients, most of whom had AD. The mean total distress score was 8.7 (plus or minus 6.9), and the range was from 0 to 36. Nearly all the behavioral symptoms caused distress, and there was variability in the amount of distress experienced by caregivers in response to each behavior. Depression and irritability were the most distressing symptoms (mean score, 2.5 each); delusions(2.4), agitation (2.3), anxiety (2.2), and apathy (2.2) also produced substantial distress. Hallucinations (1.9), disinhibition (1.8), and aberrant motor behavior (1.5) were distressing but less so. Euphoria was the only symptom that produced relatively little distress (0.7). Then, caregivers were divided into low distress (NPI distress score 0–1), medium distress (2–3), and high distress (4–5) according to each subscale distress score, irritability, agitation, dysphoria, delusions, and hallucinations had the highest proportion of caregivers reporting high distress ratings. It is notable that in this study [6] total NPI scores correlated much more strongly than MMSE scores with an independent measure of caregiver distress.

Neurobiological Correlates of Neuropsychiatric Symptoms

The NPI has been used to investigate the neurobiological correlates of neuropsychiatric symptoms in AD. Functional neuroimaging studies including positron emission tomography (PET) and single photon emission computerized tomography (SPECT) have been employed to explore the regional metabolic and cerebral blood flow characteristics of patients with a variety of behavioral disturbances. Craig and colleagues

[7] demonstrated a significant correlation between the presence of apathy and reduced cerebral blood flow in the anterior cingulate, orbital frontal, dorsal lateral prefrontal, and anterior temporal regions. There were no significant differences in blood flow in parietal association, posterior temporal, or occipital primary visual cortex. Mega and colleagues [8] constructed two groups of patients matched for all behaviors except delusions and hallucinations, thus allowing psychotic patients to be contrasted with nonpsychotic patients. Differences in cerebral blood flow with lower perfusion in patients with psychosis were found for the following regions: left medial orbital frontal, left anterior cingulate, left and right dorsal lateral frontal, left dorsal lateral parietal, left pulvinar, left ventral striatum, and left cerebellum. Hirono and coworkers [9] examined correlations between dysphoria and regional glucose metabolism on PET scans. Significant correlations were found for left and right superior frontal gyrus, middle frontal gyrus, inferior frontal gyrus, and anterior cingulate gyrus.

The NPI has been employed to investigate the relationship between apolipoprotein-E genotype and the presence of behavioral disturbances. When correlations were controlled for the patients' level of cognitive impairment, there were no relationships between E4 dose and any of the ten cognitive symptoms assessed by the NPI [10].

Measuring the Response of Neuropsychiatric Symptoms to Treatment

The NPI has been used to investigate the relationship of neuropsychiatric symptoms to a variety of types of interventions in AD. Treatment with the cholinesterase inhibitor, tacrine, resulted in a significant decrease in apathy, disinhibition, and aberrant motor behavior and a nearly significant decrease in hallucinations [11]. There was a relationship between the severity of dementia and treatment response. All patients in the moderately severe group (MMSE 20–11) showed improvement in all NPI assessed symptoms. Mild subjects (MMSE 30–21) demonstrated improvement in delusions, hallucinations, agitation, apathy, disinhibition, and aberrant motor behavior but exhibited increases in the other four symptoms. Severe patients showed improvement in delusions, anxiety, apathy, and disinhibition and worsening of the other six symptoms assayed by the NPI. Morris and coworkers [12] demonstrated reduced scores on hallucination subscale of the NPI as well as total NPI score in patients treated with the cholinesterase inhibitor metrifonate.

The NPI has been used as an outcome assessment in studies of the use of psychotropic agents in patients with AD. Street and coworkers [13] used the NPI to demonstrate that olanzapine reduced the total of a core triad of NPI items (agitation, delusions, and hallucinations). A significant improvement was seen in patients receiving 5 or 10 mg of olanzapine.

Conclusion

Neuropsychiatric and behavioral disturbances are common in patients with AD. Nearly all patients exhibit behavioral and neuropsychiatric disturbances. The NPI has proven to be a useful instrument for assessing behavioral disturbances, investigating relationships between behavior in a variety of biological measures, and assessing treatment response. Further investigation of the neuropsychiatric aspects of AD would provide insights into the neurobiology of neuropsychiatric and behavioral disturbances in this disorder and may possibly guide investigations into these symptoms in other neurological and psychiatric conditions.

Acknowledgment. This project is supported by a National Institute on Aging Alzheimer's Disease Research Center grant (AG16570), an Alzheimer's Disease Research Center of California grant, and the Sidell-Kagan Foundation. The NPI described in this article is avoidable on request him the author.

References

1. American Psychiatric Association (1994) Diagnostic and statistical manual of mental disorders: DSM-IV, 4th edn. American Psychiatric Association, Washington, DC
2. Cummings JL, Mega M, Gray K, et al (1994) The Neuropsychiatric Inventory: comprehensive assessment of psychopathology in dementia. Neurology 44:2308–2314
3. Wood S, Cummings JL, Hsu M-A, et al (2000) The use of the Neuropsychiatric Inventory in nursing home residents. Am J Geriatr Psychiatry 8:75–83
4. Mega M, Cummings JL, Fiorello T, Gombein J (1996) The spectrum of behavioral changes in Alzheimer's disease. Neurology 46:130–135
5. Frisoni GB, Rozzini L, Gozzetti A, et al (1999) Behavioral syndromes in Alzheimer's disease: description and correlates. Dement Geriatr Cogn Disord 10:130–138
6. Kaufer D, Cummings JL, Christine D (1998) Differential neuropsychiatric symptom responses to tacrine in Alzheimer's disease: relationship to dementia severity. J Neuropsychol Clin Neurosci 10:55–63
7. Craig AH, Cummings JL, Fairbanks LEA (1996) Cerebral blood flow correlates of apathy in Alzheimer's disease. Arch Neurol 53:1116–1120
8. Mega MS, Lee L, Dinov ID, et al (2000) Cerebral correlates of psychotic symptoms in Alzheimer's disease. J Neurol Neurosurg Psychiatry (in press)
9. Hirono N, Mori E, Ishii K, et al (1998) Frontal lobe hypometabolism and depression in Alzheimer's disease. Neurology 50:380–383
10. Levy ML, Cummings JL, Kahn-Rose R (1999) Neuropsychiatric symptoms and cholinergic therapy for Alzheimer's disease. Gerontology 45(suppl 1):15–22
11. Kaufer DI, Cummings JL, Christine D, et al (1998) Assessing the impact of neuropsychiatric symptoms in Alzheimer's disease: The Neuropsychiatric Inventory Caregiver Distress Scale. J Am Geriatr Soc 46:210–215
12. Morris JC, Cyrus PA, Orazem J, et al (1998) Metrifonate benefits cognitive, behavioral, and global function in patients with Alzheimer's disease. Neurology 50:1222–1230
13. Street J, Clark WS, Mitan S, et al (1998) Olanzapine in the treatment of psychosis and behavioral disturbances associated with Alzheimer's disease. American College of Neuropsychopharmacology annual meeting. American College of Neuropsychopharmacology, Las Croabas, Puerto Rico

Brain Structures Subserving Componential and Hierarchical Aspects of Human Emotions

GUIDO GAINOTTI

Summary. The main similarities and differences existing between the "emotional" and the "cognitive" system are identified. Emotions as a multicomponent, hierarchically organized adaptive system are then described. The main components and the main levels of emotions that could be subserved by specific brain structures are next described. Within the emotional components are considered the appraisal of emotional situations, the emotional response, with its expressive-motor and autonomic components, and the control of the spontaneous emotional response. Within the levels of emotional functioning, a distinction is made between a level of automatic, spontaneous functioning and a level of conceptual, controlled processing of emotional information. The brain structures subserving the various components and levels of emotions and the emotional disorders risulting from injury to these brain structures are briefly discussed.

Keywords. Emotions, Amygdala, Hypothalamus, Fronto-orbital cortex, Hemispheric asymmetries

Introduction

The general adaptive nature of both the emotional and the cognitive systems has been stressed by Oatley and Johnson-Laird (1987). These authors have claimed that, to face a partially unpredictable environment and to select the most appropriate response patterns, the organism utilizes two operative systems: (1) the emotional system, considered as an emergency system, able to interrupt the ongoing action to rapidly select a new operative scheme; and (2) the cognitive system, considered as a more complex and evolved system, but needing much more time to carry out its work.

Both structural similarities and functional differences exist between the emotional and cognitive systems. The structural similarity stems from the fact that both systems base their activity on the integrated work of components that must (a) scan the external milieu; (b) analyze the ongoing information to compute its significance; (c) select the most appropriate response patterns; and (d) put all these data into appropriate

Neuropsychology Service of the Catholic University of Rome, Policlinico Gemelli, Largo A. Gemelli, 8-00168 Rome, Italy

memory systems. The functional differences (which concern the manner in which each system deals with sensory information and selects specific action schemata) ensue, on the other hand, from the general logic of the two systems

Main Components of the Emotional System

A different kind of analysis of sensory data is performed by emotional and cognitive systems as an exhaustive analysis of highly processed information is accomplished by the cognitive system whereas a quick computation of poorly processed sensory data is sufficient to decide if an external situation has an emotional (pleasant or dangerous) meaning for an individual.

Equally different are the action schemata activated by the process of emotional and of cognitive evaluation of the external data. The action schemata activated by the process of emotional computation are immediately selected from a small number of innate operative patterns, which typically include expressive-communicative components, and an important recruitment of the autonomic nervous system. On the other hand, actions selected by the cognitive system consist of controlled strategic plans, which usually do not include a communicative-expressive component and do not require (or are even disturbed by) a concomitant strong activation of the autonomic nervous system. Equally different are the learning mechanisms used by the emotional and the cognitive system, because the former is based largely on mechanisms of conditioned and unconscious learning, whereas the latter uses conscious and controlled mechanisms to store new information in declarative memory.

Hierarchical Structure of the Emotional System

The description of the emotional system that I have just given as an emergency system, independent from and parallel to the cognitive system, refers above all to the simplest forms of emotional behavior and to the earliest stages of emotional development. As a matter of fact, emotional and cognitive systems become more and more interconnected during both phylogenetic and ontogenetic development, and the complexity of emotions evolves accordingly. All these reasons have prompted the construction of hierarchically organized developmental models of emotions aiming to explain how complex emotions can be formed starting from the simpelst ones and how the highest (cognitively oriented) components of this structure keep under control the lowest and more primitive parts of the emotional system. In particular, Leventhal (1987) has put forward a developmental model which proposes that human emotions may be based on three functional levels: (a) the sensorimotor level, (b) the schematic level, and (c) the conceptual level. The sensorimotor level consists of a set of innate expressive-motor programs, which are triggered automatically by a certain number of stimuli and include components of motor and autonomic activation, as well as the corresponding subjective emotional feelings. During individual development, these basic programs are linked, by mechanisms of conditioned learning, to situations of the individual experience, building the "emotional schemata," which are the units of the second schematic level of emotional processing. These emotional schemata correspond to spontaneous emotions and are accompanied by the emotional feelings that give to these schemata the characteristics of a true emotion. The last stage of this model is the conceptual level, which is based on mechanisms of conscious declarative memory and does not store instances of concrete emotional experiences but rather abstract notions about emotions and about the social rules dealing with their expression. The activation of these representations is, therefore, not accompanied by the corresponding emotional feelings.

Brain Structures Subserving the Various Components and Levels of Emotions and Emotional Disorders Resulting from Injury to These Brain Structures

Emotional Evaluation

Several authors (see LeDoux 1996 for review) have proposed that the *amygdala* could be the structure in which the external stimuli are evaluated in terms of their emotional significance. Furthermore, LeDoux (1996) has recently shown that sensory signals coming from the outside world can be channeled through two different routes to reach the amydgala, where they acquire emotional meaning. The first route, which directly connects the thalamus with the amygdala, could trasmit to this structure the crude sensory data that are needed to make the quick and raw computation typical of the emotional processing of sensory information. The second route, on the other hand, reaches the amygdala after a more extensive processing of information in the sensory cortical areas. Some clinical and neuroimaging studies (e.g., Morris et al. 1996) have recently suggested that the role of the amygdala in emotional evaluation could be very selective because it could specifically concern the recognition of fearful expressions, but other authors have suggested that the amygdala could be involved in more general unpleasant emotional phenomena, such as the processes of fear conditioning (LeDoux 1996).

Emotional Response

The response programs triggered by the appraisal of emotionally laden stimuli include components of expressive-motor and of autonomic activation, which are probably subserved by different brain structures. The autonomic components of emotional reactions are probably generated by hypothalamic structures, whereas the expressive-motor and communicative aspects of the emotional response could be subserved by the ventral striatum. The major involvement of the *hypothalamus* in the generation of vegetative reactions is documented both by very old and by recent data. Among the former, the most important are perhaps the Karplus and Kreidl (1927) experiments, which showed that the electrical stimulation of the hypothalamus is followed by a strong activation of the orthosympathetic vegetative system, which is greatly involved in aggression/fear. Among the latter, we would quote Weddel's (1994) observations that, in patients with brain tumors selectively involving the hypothalamus, autonomic (and endocrinal) disorders are very frequent and survival/appetitive disorders (concerning eating, drinking, and sexual behavior) are less frequent but still common, whereas personality disturbances and disorders of social-emotional communication are very rare. The involvement of the *ventral striatum* (and of other parts of the basal ganglia) in the execution of stereotyped emotional action patterns is suggested by both anatomical and clinical data. From the anatomical point of view, these structures receive strong afferents from the amygdala and other limbic structures and send projections to cortical, subcortical, and brainstem components of the motor system (Nauta and Domesick 1984). From the clinical point of view, patients with a degenerative disease of the basal ganglia, such as Parkinson's disease, and stroke patients with lesions involving the basal ganglia show a marked reduction of spontaneous facial emotional expressions.

Control and Inhibition of Socially Unacceptable Emotional Responses

Some cortical executive structures, lying at the interface between the cognitive and the emotional system, exert a control over the output of the schematic level of emotional processing, inhibiting or modulating socially unacceptable emotional outbursts. The *ventromedial frontal cortex* plays a critical role from this point of view (see Damasio 1994 for review). Many well-studied patients with lesions restricted to these areas have, indeed, shown severe social-emotional disorders, in spite of having entirely normal profiles on standard neuropsychological measures and on cognitive tasks sensitive to frontal lobe damage. According to Damasio (1994), the inability to integrate the emotional response into an appropriate social and cognitive context could be caused by a defect in the activation of the "somatic markers"; i.e., of the autonomic and proprioceptive afferences that provide the subject with the feelings associated with a given response and which allow them to anticipate the personal consequences of their future behavior.

Different Hemispheric Involvement in Different Levels of Emotional Processing

The hypothesis of a right-hemisphere dominance for emotional functions is supported by a very large body of evidence (see Gainotti 2000 for review) and concerns components of emotional communication, autonomic response, and the subjective experience of emotions. The general dominance of the right hemisphere for the more basic negative emotions forms the basis for laterality effects observed in some domains of psychopathology, such as the manic-depressive disorders (Starkstein et al. 1987) and some forms of content-specific delusions (Feinberg and Shapiro 1989).

References

Damasio AR (1994) Descartes' error: emotion, research and the human brain. Avon, New York

Feinberg TE, Shapiro RM (1989) Misidentification-reduplication and the right hemisphere. Neuropsychiatry Neuropsychol Behav Neurol 2:39–48

Gainotti G (2000) Neuropsychological theories of emotions. In: Borod J (ed) The neuropsychology of emotions. Oxford University Press, New York, pp 214–236

Karplus JP, Kreidl A (1927) Gehirn und Sympathicus. VII. Uber Beziehungen der Hypothalamuszentren zu Blutdruck und innerer Sekretion. Pfleugers Arch Gesamte Physiol Menschen Teiere 215:667–670

LeDoux JE (1996) The emotional brain. Simon and Schuster, New York

Leventhal H (1987) A perceptual motor theory of emotion. In: Berkowitz L (ed) Advances in experimental social psychology. Academic Press, New York

Morris JS, Frith CD, Perrett DI, et al (1996) A differential neural response in the human amygdala to fearful and happy facial expressions. Nature (Lond) 383:812–815

Nauta WJH, Domesick VB (1984) Afferent and efferent relationships of the basal ganglia. CIBA Found Symp 107:3–23

Oatley K, Johnson-Laird P (1987) Toward a cognitive theory of emotions. Cognition Emotion 1:29–50

Starkstein SE, Pearlson GD, Boston J, Robinson RG (1987) Mania after brain injury: a controlled study of causative factors. Arch Neurol 44:1069–1073

Weddel RA (1994) Effects of subcortical lesion site on human emotional behavior. Brain Cognit 25:161–193

The Brain and Zen

James H. Austin

Summary. This chapter briefly touches on some plausible psychophysiological considerations involved in several large topics. Topics highlighted include the attentive aspects of meditation; meditative retreats and the momentary "quickenings" that can occur during them; the superficial states of absorption; the deeper states of awakening (*kensho-satori*) and of "Pure Being"; and the rare later advanced stage of ongoing enlightened traits. If we wish to understand how the Zen training process arrives at its transforming potentials, we need to clarify which brain functions are "let go of" during these various steps. The psychophysiology of triggering mechanisms and the dissociations during transitional intervals are useful points at which to begin.

Keywords. Zen mechanisms, Enlightenment, Thalamus, Limbic system, Neuromessengers

> With all your science can you tell how it is,
> and whence it is that light comes into the soul?
> Henry David Thoreau (1817–1862)

An outline of the Path of Zen is presented in my companion chapter in this volume. However, no such diagram suffices to answer Thoreau's question, nor could any of the speculations briefly advanced in these next few pages. For our challenge is (1) to "explain" meditation and quickenings; (2) next, to clarify the mechanisms underlying such diverse states as the absorptions, the awakenings (*kensho-satori*), and Being; and (3) finally, to explain how a sage's brain could mature into the rare stage of ongoing enlightened traits. Elsewhere, the following abbreviated comments receive a more detailed treatment (Austin 1998).

Zen Meditation as an Attentive Art

Starting from the foundations of calmness and clarity, two styles of meditation emerge. They tend to be used alternately.

Department of Neurology, University of Colorado Health Sciences Center, Denver, CO 80262, USA

Receptive meditation deploys an open awareness during "just sitting." Employing a light touch, it becomes a simple, bare, inclusive noticing of events, distracting or otherwise. Neither focused nor cultivated by struggle, it still notices when attention strays, then brings it gently back to the present moment. *Concentrative* meditation is a focused attentive process more willfully sustained and one-pointed. Finally, one may become more or less absorbed in it.

True, the right inferior parietal lobule and the right middle frontal gyrus help us "attend" to events in both sides of *extra*personal space (Johannsen 1997). Yet, attention remains an "associative" function. It draws on deep subcortical reservoirs, including the pulvinar of the thalamus. Moreover, most of our processing occurs subconsciously, effortlessly, preattentively, in less than $1/20^{th}$ of a second (Austin 1998, pp. 271–281).

Meditative Retreats Involve Somnolence, Stress Responses, Sensory-Motor Deprivation, and Self-Discipline

Yes, breathing out tends to dampen the firing rates of nerve cells in the amygdala, and theta waves in the EEG may correlate with the intervals of undistracted calmness and clarity reached during deeper levels of meditation. However, meditators struggle during prolonged retreats (Austin 1998, pp. 138–140). They struggle not only to remain attentive and to stay awake but also to endure major degrees of physical and psychic suffering (Austin 1998, pp. 355–358). During self-emptying (kenosis), one learns self-discipline.

Retreats, like "Outward Bound" experiences, are opportunities to find the "inner" self. Retreats become effective agencies of personal change, to the degree that they (1) evoke in the brain a calibrated series of physiological instabilities and stress responses; and (2) develop meditators' capacities to endure anguish and to find how much they create their own discomforts, resistances, and boredom.

"Quickenings" reflect a variety of corresponding surges in the activities of messenger molecules in the brain. Some of these varied phenomena tend to occur at the advancing tidal edges of conventional arousals. They arise either as part of circadian (daily) or of ultradian rhythms (every 90 min or so). Quickenings also seem to enter during the dynamic transitions between waking/drowsiness and sleep/REM sleep. Quickenings arise especially when the brain's own stress responses—releasing biogenic amines, peptides, acetylcholine, glutamate, and GABA—have gone on to destabilize and disrupt sleep cycles and other biorhythms.

States of Absorption, of "Awakening" (Kensho-Satori), and of "Pure Being"

These phenomena are extraordinary alternate states of consciousness. To understand Zen, it is essential to observe what they "let go" of, or subtract. In this regard, certain GABA, and peptide, inhibitory functions can help us understand how these three categories of states could express such selective "deletions" from consciousness.

For example, the reticular nucleus normally serves as a kind of "cap" on the thalamus. It blocks sensory impulses from being transmitted up to the cortex. Excessive activation of the back of this GABA cap offers a plausible explanation for two aspects of internal absorption: (1) for its blockade of exterior sensate impressions, and (2) for its loss of one's usual axial sense of a *physical* self. A delayed infusion of bliss can also occur in internal absorption. It suggests a release of endogenous opioid peptides, as part of a stress response.

The states of kensho-satori delete the *psychic* self of all former egocentric (self-referent) constructs. But note: these salient insights do not cut off sensate percepts from the outside world. Indeed, such *allocentric* (other-referent) percepts not only continue but become imbued with meaningful affirmative resonances. Thus, in kensho, an impression of basic "truth" arises, but it does not enter until one's previously intrusive, overconditioned, egocentric self drops out of the picture, for only with this "death" of the psychic self does the brain suddenly come to an ultimate, simplifying realization. Finally, it registers: "all things as THEY really are."

Two words emphasize the unique qualities of this awakening. The first is *anatta*. Buddhists use this technical term to refer to the anonymous state of no-self. It means non-I. In the writings of D.T. Suzuki, we find the second word: "suchness." It refers to this curious sense of "things as they *really* are." Suzuki concluded that suchness was "the basis of all religious experience" (Austin 1998, pp. 549–553).

A striking loss of fear occurs in kensho, which could represent inhibitions of primal fear circuits within and from the amygdala. For example, receptor mechanisms contributing to fearlessness could include the GABA and opioid receptors within relevant limbic and paralimbic regions and CRF_2 receptors in the lateral septum (Austin 1998, pp. 653–663; Radulovic et al. 2000).

Triggering events are noteworthy precipitants of kensho-satori. They raise the possibility that sudden stimuli can trigger the ascending cholinergic and glutamate systems in the brainstem to relay their activations to the rostral cerebrum above. One hopes that future studies will clarify how the rostral parts of the reticular nucleus then interact with these adjacent regions. Among them, the mediodorsal nucleus of the thalamus is of particular interest because it shares pivotal interrelationships with all three divisions of the prefrontal cortex.

The Stage of Ongoing Enlightened Traits

The earlier diagram (in this author's companion chapter in this volume) depicts this rare stage as arising only after decades of training and only after several prior transforming states of awakening. Moreover, it is represented as open ended.

The sage's low profile is one keynote of this stage. This liberated i-me-mine can act skillfully and compassionately, with great flexibility, because the genuine sage becomes free to navigate evenhandedly—and ethically—between such opposites as might previously have been labeled "good" and "bad" (Austin 1998, pp. 637–653).

How does a brain of the rare sage differ from that of a twin sibling? We might begin by inquiring which dysfunctional systems have been "subtracted" (Austin 1998, pp. 637–653). Obvious target systems include the "emotionalizing" networks of limbic and paralimbic regions. Of special interest are their links to ancient instincts for self-preservation; these center in that vital triad, the hypothalamus–amygdala–central gray. Can such nerve cells be selectively "pruned?" Potential mechanisms reside in the excitotoxic properties of glutamate and nitric oxide (NO$^{\cdot}$), and in apoptosis. Can fearlessness endure? Receptor levels can undergo long-term changes on cells in the amygdala and locus ceruleus in ways that stop their being overactivated (Caldji et al. 2000).

Still other innate circuits need to be selectively spared, reprogrammed, and rechanneled. Neuromessengers do set off a variety of delayed metabolic cascades, which can help to sponsor the emergence of a selfless sage's other adaptive functions.

References

Austin J (1998) Zen and the brain: toward an understanding of meditation and consciousness. MIT Press, Cambridge

Caldji C, Francis D, Sharma S, et al (2000) The effects of early rearing environment on the development of $GABA_A$ and central benzodiazepine receptor levels and novelty-induced fearfulness in the rat. Neuropharmacology 22:219–229

Johannsen P, Jacobsen J, Bruhn P, et al (1997) Cortical sites of sustained and divided attention in normal elderly humans. Neuroimage 6:145–155

Radulovic J, Fisher A, Katerkamp U, et al (2000) Role of regional neurotransmitter receptors in corticotropin-releasing factor (CRF)-mediated modulation of fear conditioning. Neuropharmacology 39:707–710

Neuropsychiatry in the Elderly

Sex Differences in Human Brain Aging

C. Edward Coffey

Summary. In humans, advancing age is associated with decreased brain tissue size and increased brain cerebrospinal fluid (CSF) volume. Although sex differences have been described in the size, symmetry, and function of several brain structures, only a few imaging studies have examined the effects of sex on brain aging in nonpatient samples of living humans. Using quantitative MR imaging, we found that age-related changes in brain size were significantly greater in males than females for the peripheral (sulcal) CSF volume, the lateral (Sylvian) fissure CSF volume, and the parieto-occipital region area. Main effects of age were observed for other brain regions, but these effects were similar in males and females. These findings suggest that brain morphology in humans is sensitive to the effects of both age and sex, and that these two variables may interact over the life span to influence brain size. These data should provide a useful context within which to interpret changes in regional brain structure associated with "abnormal" aging.

Keywords. Brain aging, Sex differences

Introduction

In humans, advancing age is generally associated with decreased brain tissue size and increased brain cerebrospinal fluid (CSF) volume. Although sex differences have been described in the size, symmetry, and function of several brain structures, only a small number of imaging studies have examined the effects of sex on brain aging in nonpatient samples of living humans (reviewed by Coffey 2000). Although the findings have been inconsistent, a few investigators have reported sex differences in the effects of age on some brain structures, and in most cases males showed greater aging changes than females. These studies are somewhat difficult to compare, however, given differences in subject samples (e.g., sample size, age range, exclusion criteria), imaging and data acquisition protocols (e.g., computed tomography [CT] versus magnetic resonance [MR] imaging), measurement technique, and statistical analyses.

Departments of Psychiatry and of Neurology, Henry Ford Health System, Detroit, MI 48202, USA

We recently employed quantitative MR imaging morphometry to examine the effects of sex on age-related changes in the size of regional brain matter and CSF spaces in a large sample of elderly volunteers living independently in the community (Coffey et al. 1998). We tested the hypothesis that such changes would be more dramatic in males than in females.

Methods

The sample was composed of 330 subjects, all of whom were participants in the Cardiovascular Health Study (CHS). There were 129 men and 201 women, ranging in age from 66 to 96 years (mean ± SD, 74.98 ± 5.09). All subjects were right handed, lived independently in the community, and were free of lifetime history of illness or injury referable to the brain, including psychiatric disorders. No subject was taking medication known to affect brain size.

Brain MR imaging was performed on either a General Electric 1.5-tesla scanner ($n = 248$) or a Toshiba 0.35-tesla scanner ($n = 82$) at one of two CHS field centers (Pittsburgh, PA, and Hagerstown, MD, USA, respectively). The brain images were transferred from magnetic tape to read/write magnetoptical disks. Data were analyzed on a Power Mac 8100 workstation with high-resolution color graphic monitor. The measurements of regional brain size were made on the recalled T_1-weighted axial images by one of two trained technicians blind to all subject characteristics. The following regions were defined for volume measurement: intracranial volume (IV), cerebral hemisphere volume, lateral ventricle volume, third ventricle volume, peripheral (sulcal) CSF volume, lateral (Sylvian) fissure CSF volume, frontal region area, temporoparietal region area, parieto-occipital region area, and intracranial area (IA).

Extensive reliability studies of our measurement techniques have indicated that area–volume measurements of these regions are highly reliable. Based upon a randomly selected sample of ten brains from the current study, intraclass correlation coefficients for interrater reliability of the two raters ranged from 0.85 (for small regions such as the third ventricle) to 0.99 (for large regions such as the cerebral hemisphere). Intraclass correlation coefficients for intrarater reliability ranged from 0.84 to 0.99.

Results

Linear regression analyses revealed significant age-by-sex interactions for the peripheral CSF volume, the lateral fissure CSF volume, and the parieto-occipital region area. For each of these regions, men showed greater age-related changes than women. For the peripheral CSF volume, the regression coefficient was 2.11 for men but only 0.06 for women ($P < 0.03$). For the lateral fissure CSF volume, the regression coefficient was 0.23 for men but only 0.10 for women ($P < 0.04$). For the parieto-occipital region area, the regression coefficient was −0.31 for men but only −0.09 for women ($P < 0.03$).

Age was significantly related to each of the remaining brain matter and CSF regions measured. Increased age was associated with decreased cerebral hemisphere volume (coefficient = −2.79, $P < 0.0001$), frontal region area (coefficient = −0.13, $P < 0.0001$), and temporoparietal region area (coefficient = −0.13, $P < 0.0001$). Increased age was also associated with increased volumes of the lateral ventricles (coefficient = 0.95, $P < 0.0001$) and the third ventricle (coefficient = 0.05, $P < 0.0001$). For all these regions, the age effects were similar in men and women.

Discussion

We found that age-related changes in brain size were significantly greater in men than women for the peripheral (sulcal) CSF volume, the lateral (Sylvian) fissure CSF volume, and the parieto-occipital region area. The main effects of age were observed for all the remaining brain regions examined, but these effects were similar in men and women.

Sex Effects on Age-Related Generalized Brain Atrophy

In our study, we found that from ages 65 to 95 years, men (of average IV) had an increase in peripheral CSF volume of approximately 32% compared to an increase of less than 1% in women. Gur et al. (1991) also found that the ratio of sulcal CSF volume to IV was greater for elderly (55 years and older) subjects and for men. Similarly, Blatter et al. (1995) found higher correlations between age and "subarachnoid" CSF volume (adjusted for IV) in males ($r = 0.653$) than in females ($r = 0.545$), although these correlations were not statistically compared. Other cross-sectional studies that examined peripheral CSF volume have found no sex effects on age-related increases (Sullivan et al. 1993; Murphy et al. 1996; Yue et al. 1997). In the longitudinal study of Mueller et al. (1998), females apparently showed greater age-related increases in total CSF volume than males (actual data not reported).

In contrast to the sex differences observed with regard to age-related increases in peripheral CSF, we found no sex differences in the age-related decrease in cerebral hemisphere volume. Similar negative findings have been reported (Yoshi et al. 1988; Gur et al. 1991; Coffey et al. 1992; Raz et al. 1993; Sullivan et al. 1993; Murphy et al. 1996; Raz et al. 1997). Although Condon et al. (1988) found that men, but not women, exhibited a significant correlation between age and the ratio of total brain volume to IV, these correlations were not statistically compared. Similarly, Blatter et al. (1995) observed higher correlations in males than females between age and the ratio of total brain volume/IV ($r = -0.675$ versus $r = -0.539$, respectively), but again these correlations were not statistically compared. Murphy et al. (1996) reported that males had a significantly greater age-related decrease in the ratio of cerebral hemisphere volume to IV than did females.

Our finding of a significant sex effect on the age-related increase in peripheral CSF volume, in the absence of a sex effect on age-related volume loss of cerebral hemisphere brain matter, is consistent with the observations of Gur et al. (1991). Taken together, these reports suggest that while peripheral CSF volume may show a greater age-related increase in males than females (likely as a result of cortical atrophy), such sex differences in cortical atrophy may not be apparent statistically when the size of the cortex is averaged in with a relatively larger structure such as the cerebral hemisphere. We are not aware of any studies that have examined sex effects on age-related tissue loss in the cortex per se.

Sex Effects on Age-Related Ventricular Enlargement

We found no sex effects on the age-related increase in lateral ventricular CSF volume or third ventricular CSF volume. Our results are in agreement with most other studies. Because age-related ventricular enlargement is presumed to occur as a result of shrinkage of periventricular brain matter, these results are also consistent with other studies that found no effect of sex on the age-related volume loss of structures that form the borders of the lateral ventricles (i.e., the caudate nuclei) (Krishnan et al. 1990; Murphy et al. 1996) or the third ventricle (i.e., the thalamus) (Murphy et al. 1996). In contrast, Grant et al. (1987) reported that men, but not women, exhibited a significant age-related increase in lateral ventricular volume, although this apparent gender difference was not tested. Likewise, Blatter et al. (1995) observed higher correlations in males than females between age and lateral ventricle volume (adjusted for IV) (r = 0.444 versus r = 0.218, respectively) and between age and third ventricle volume (adjusted for IV) (r = 0.634 versus r = 0.406, respectively), but again these correlations were not statistically compared. Kaye et al. (1992) reported that the precipitous age-related increases in lateral ventricular volume began about a decade earlier in males than females. Finally, Murphy et al. (1996) found that females actually had a greater age-related increase in the ratio of third-ventricle volume to IV than did males.

Sex Effects on Age-Related Differences in Regional Brain Size

We found that the age-associated increase in lateral fissure CSF volume, a marker of frontotemporal (and to a lesser extent, parietal) atrophy, was greater in men than women. For example, from ages 65 to 95 years, men (of average IV) had an increase in lateral fissure volume of approximately 80%, while women only had an increase of approximately 37%. Cowell et al. (1994) and Murphy et al. (1996) found that males exhibited greater age-related decreases in the ratio of temporal lobe volume to IV than did females. Similarly, Golomb et al. (1993) found that age-related hippocampal atrophy was more common in males than females, and Raz et al. (1997) observer greater age-related inferior temporal volume loss in males than females. In contrast, Murphy et al. (1996) actually observed greater temporal lobe atrophy in females than males. Despite differences in which sex is more affected, these published results suggest that sex may impact the age-related volume loss of the temporal lobe region. These findings may provide a neuroanatomical substrate for the sex differences in age-related verbal memory impairment.

The literature is also conflicting with regard to the effects of sex on age-related changes in frontal lobe size. Cowell et al. (1994) and Murphy et al. (1996) have both observed greater age-related frontal lobe volume loss in males than in females. In contrast, others have found no interactions between aging and sex effects (Coffey et al. 1992, 1998; Raz et al. 1993, 1997; Sullivan et al. 1993; Cowell et al. 1994). These discrepant results may reflect differences between studies in samples and brain measurement techniques (i.e., quantitative versus qualitative measures, area measures from a single slice versus volume measures from multiple slices).

With regard to more posterior brain regions, we found that the age-related decrease in parieto-occipital region area was greater for males than females. For example, from ages 65 to 95 years, men (of average IA) lost approximately 15% of their parieto-occipital lobe area, while women lost only 4% (Coffey et al. 1998). Using a somewhat different definition of this brain region, Cowell et al. (1994) did not find any sex effect on the age-related decrease in the ratio of the posterior cerebral hemisphere volume to IV. Murphy et al. (1996) likewise found no sex differences in the age-related decrease in parieto-occipital region volume/IV, although they actually observed worse atrophy in females for the ratio of parietal lobe volume/IV. Similarly, Raz et al. (1993) reported that females exhibited greater age-related volume loss in the visual cortex than did males. These widely divergent findings indicate a need for additional research.

Conclusion

In summary, brain morphology in humans appears to be sensitive to the effects of both age and sex, and converging data suggest that these two variables may interact over the life span to influence brain size. These data should provide a useful context within which to interpret changes in regional brain structure associated with "abnormal" aging. The neurobiological bases for these sex differences in brain aging are not known. Neuroendocrinological differences between sexes have been proposed as a possible explanation, given that gonadal steroids affect brain development and aging and that aging affects both the function and regional distribution of androgen and estrogen systems in the brain. Still, most studies of human brain aging at the cellular level have not examined sex effects.

The behavioral effects in humans of these sex differences in brain aging are likewise unknown. These findings may provide a neuroanatomical substrate for the sexually dimorphic effects of age on cerebral blood flow and metabolism, and it is possible that sex differences in brain aging could interact with a superimposed pathological process to produce sex differences in brain disorders such as Alzheimer's disease. In this regard, sex differences in brain aging are consistent with observed sex differences in some aspects of cognitive aging. Correlative neuropsychological investigations are currently under way in our laboratory to determine the potential functional significance of differences between the sexes in brain aging.

References

Coffey CE (2000) Anatomic imaging of the aging human brain. In: Coffey CE, Cummings JL (eds) Textbook of geriatric neuropsychiatry, 2nd edn. American Psychiatric Press, Washington, DC, pp 181–238

Coffey CE, Lucke JF, Saxton JA, et al (1998) Sex differences in brain aging: a quantitative magnetic resonance imaging study. Arch Neurol 55:169–179

Grant R, Condon B, Lawrence A, et al (1987) Human cranial CSF volumes measured by MRI: sex and age influences. Magn Reson Imaging 5:465–468

Condon B, Grant R, Hadley D, Lawrence A (1988) Brain and intracranial cavity volumes: in vivo determination by MRI. Acta Neurol Scand 78:387–393

Yoshi F, Barker WW, Chang JY, et al (1988) Sensitivity of cerebral glucose metabolism to age, gender, brain volume, brain atrophy and cerebrovascular risk factors. J Cereb Blood Flow Metab 8:654–661

Krishnan KR, McDonald WM, Doraiswamy PM, et al (1990) In vivo stereological assessment of caudate volume in man: effect of normal aging. Life Sci 47:1325–1329

Gur RC, Mozley PD, Resnick S, et al (1991) Gender differences in age effect on brain atrophy measured by magnetic resonance imaging. Proc Natl Acad Sci USA 88:2845–2849

Coffey CE, Wilkinson WE, Parashos IA, et al (1992) Quantitative cerebral anatomy of the aging human brain: a cross-sectional study using magnetic resonance imaging. Neurology 42:527–536

Kaye JA, DeCarli CD, Luxenberg JS, Rapoport SI (1992) The significance of age-related enlargement of the cerebral ventricles in healthy men and women measured by quantitative computed x-ray tomography. J Am Geriatr Soc 40:225–231

Golomb J, deLeon MJ, Kluger A, et al (1993) Hippocampal atrophy in normal aging: an association with recent memory impairment. Arch Neurol 50:967–973

Raz N, Torres IJ, Spencer WD, Acker JD (1993) Pathoclysis in aging human cerebral cortex: evidence from in vivo MRI morphometry. Psychobiology 21:151–160

Sullivan EV, Shear PK, Mathalon H, et al (1993) Greater abnormalities of brain cerebrospinal fluid volumes in younger than in older patients with Alzheimer's disease. Arch Neurol 50:359–373

Cowell PE, Turetsky BI, Gur RC, et al (1994) Sex differences in aging of the human frontal and temporal lobes. J Neurosci 14:4748–4756

Blatter DD, Bigler ED, Gale SD, et al (1995) Quantitative volumetric analysis of brain MR: normative database spanning 5 decades of life. AJNR Am J Neuroradiol 16:241–251

Murphy DGM, DeCarli C, McIntosh AR, et al (1996) Sex differences in human brain morphometry and metabolism: an in vivo quantitative magnetic resonance imaging and positron emission tomography study on the effect of aging. Arch Gen Psychiatry 53:585–594

Raz N, Gunning FM, Head D, et al (1997) Selective aging of the human cerebral cortex observed in vivo: differential vulnerability of the prefrontal gray matter. Cereb Cortex 7:268–282

Yue NC, Longstreth WT Jr, Elster AD, et al (1997) Clinically serious abnormalities found incidentally at MRI imaging of the brain: data from the Cardiovascular Health Study. Radiology 202:41–46

Mueller EA, Moore MM, Kerr DCR, et al (1998) Brain volume preserved in healthy elderly through the eleventh decade. Neurology 51:1555–1562

Neuropsychiatry in the Elderly

Jeffrey L. Cummings

Summary. The world's population is rapidly aging, and many countries will experience a rapid increase in the number of aged individuals. This increase in the aged population will occur disproportionately in countries with developing economies where the recent introduction of public health policies have led to greater longevity. Diseases of the aged are responsible for enormous financial burdens in all countries. Three neuropsychiatric disorders are common in the elderly: Alzheimer's disease, Parkinson's disease, and stroke. Each of these is accompanied by substantial neuropsychiatric morbidity, with behavioral manifestations being common in each of these illnesses. Recent strides in understanding the basic mechanisms of degenerative and vascular disorders has led to the introduction of new therapies and promise even greater therapeutic strides. A neuropsychiatric research continuum is critically important to ensure that basic science advances result in improved patient care. This continuum includes the basic sciences, clinical sciences, translational research (aimed at discovering optimal techniques for translating advances in basic and clinical science into improved patient care), and educational research.

Keywords. Alzheimer's disease, Cost, International, Translational research, Disease burden

Introduction

Neuropsychiatry is the discipline devoted to understanding the natural history, pathophysiology, and optimal treatment of brain disorders with behavioral manifestations. Brain diseases occur disproportionately commonly in the elderly, and therefore neuropsychiatry is an important dimension of care of elderly individuals. Neuropsychiatric expertise is important in caring for elderly individuals. Dementia syndromes, stroke, and Parkinson's disease all increase in frequency with aging. In addition, differences in drug metabolism, distribution, and receptor sensitivity in the elderly make it imperative that agents used in this population be specifically studied in aged individuals. Finally, many socioeconomic circumstances bear on aging that

---

UCLA Alzheimer's Disease Center, Department of Neurology and Psychiatry and Biobehavioral Sciences, UCLA School of Medicine, 710 Westwood Plaza. Los Angeles, CA 90095-1769, USA

create unique circumstances for elderly individuals. The occurrence of ill health and the coadministration of many medications, the increasing dependence on others for care, the likely occurrence of illness in one's spouse, exiting from the labor force and financial vulnerability, and changing relationships within the family all impact on manifestations of neuropsychiatric illness in the elderly and on the care that older individuals receive.

In this brief review of neuropsychiatry in the elderly, the changing demography of the world's population with an increase in the number of elderly individuals is reviewed. The spectrum of neuropsychiatric illnesses in the elderly is presented, and the economic impact of common acquired brain diseases of the aged is described. Advances in neuroscience relevant to understanding neuropsychiatric conditions in the elderly are presented, and new treatments for neuropsychiatric disorders in the elderly are discussed. A research continuum leading from advances in basic science to improved patient care is promoted.

The Changing Demography of the World Population

Life expectancy is increasing. For example, the life expectancy at birth in the Americas in 1970 was 65.7 years whereas life expectancy in 2025 in the Americas is anticipated to be 77.2 years of age. In Europe, a similar increase will occur, from a life expectancy of 69.5 years in 1970 to an anticipated expectancy of 78.1 in 2025. In Southeast Asia, the increase is more dramatic, from a life expectancy of 50.2 years in 1970 to that of 72.7 years in 2025 [1].

Countries with large populations and relatively high longevity have the highest absolute numbers of elderly individuals. For example, in 2025 it is anticipated that China will have 199.3 million individuals over the age of 65 in the population, that India will have 108.2 million, the United States 62.0 million, Japan 32.2 million, Russia 25 million, Indonesia 24.8 million, Brazil 21.1 million, Germany 20.4 million, France 14.3 million, and Italy 13.6 million [1].

Relative increases in size of elderly populations will be disproportionately large in countries with developing economies. For example, between 1985 and 2025, Guatemala will have a 350% increase in the number of aged individuals in the population, Singapore 348%, Mexico 324%, the Philippines 310%, Indonesia 301%, Brazil 292%, India 264%, China 238%, Hong Kong 219%, Canada 135%, Australia 125%, Japan 121%, the United States 105%, France 67%, and the United Kingdom 25% [2].

These figures on life expectancy, percent increases, and absolute numbers of elderly individuals in populations throughout the world reveal that there will be a substantial increase in the number of aged individuals and consequently a concomitant increase in the number of aged individuals with age-related brain diseases and neuropsychiatric manifestations.

Economics and Aging Relative to Neuropsychiatry

The cost of brain diseases including direct and indirect costs is extraordinary. The National Foundation for Brain Research [3] estimated that in the United States the annual expenditure on dementias was $113.2 billion, mental retardation $35.1 billion, multiple sclerosis $4.9 billion, head injury $48.3 billion, spinal cord injury $22.6 billion, stroke $17.9 billion, cerebral palsy $1.2 billion, epilepsy $609 million, and other neurological disorders $8.1 billion.

Insurance coverage for the elderly varies greatly around the world. Coverage is nearly universal in most highly industrialized countries; approximately 50% of elderly individuals are covered by some form of insurance in middle-income countries such as Argentina, Brazil, and Malaysia; 20% of the elderly have insurance coverage in lower-income countries such as Indonesia and the Philippines; and less than 10% of the elderly have insurance coverage in Sub-Saharan Africa [1]. The percent of the gross domestic product (GDP) spent on pension and health expenditures varies from 20.6% in Europe to 1.9% in Africa. The figure was 14.8% in the Americas, 9.2% in Southeast Asia, and 16.2% in the Western Pacific [1].

Thus, developing countries devote a substantial proportion of their GDP to caring for individuals with neurological disorders. Expenditures in countries with less well developed economies are substantially less, but individuals have reduced access to new medications and other health care resources.

Neuropsychiatric Disorders in the Elderly

Frequency of Neuropsychiatric Disorders

Neuropsychiatric disorders in the elderly include late-persisting early-onset disorders such as mental retardation; late-persisting conditions that begin in midlife such as depression, bipolar illness, and schizophrenia; late-onset disorders including depression and paraphrenia; and late-onset neurological disorders with neuropsychiatric manifestations including Alzheimer's disease, Parkinson's disease, and stroke. It is estimated that 6.1%–15.7% of individuals with mental retardation in the United States are currently over age 55; 40%–70% of these individuals have diagnosable psychiatric disorders. Thus, elderly individuals with mental retardation constitute a unique and important subgroup of aged individuals with neuropsychiatric disorders [4].

There is a complex relationship between depression and aging. Major depressive disorder may occur for the first time in elderly individuals or may persist as a chronic disorder in persons with young-onset depressive disorder. Major depression has been found in 20%–25% of older individuals with medical illnesses, and medical illnesses become more common with aging. Similarly, depressive symptoms occur in 40%–50% of individuals with Alzheimer's disease, and major depressive episodes are seen in 2%–10% [5].

Psychosis may also begin in the elderly or persist after onset in earlier life periods; 13% of schizophrenics have the onset of their syndrome after the age of 50, 7% in their sixties, and 3% in their seventies or later [6]. Psychosis also may occur with cerebrovascular disease and vascular dementia, Alzheimer's disease, and Parkinson's disease following treatment with dopaminergic agents.

Neuropsychiatric disorders contribute substantially to the global burden of disease [7]. Eight of the 15 illnesses contributing the greatest burden of disease as forecasted for 2020 included neuropsychiatric abnormalities such as unipolar major depression (ranked #2), road traffic accidents (ranked #3), cerebrovascular disease (ranked #4), war (ranked #8), human immunodeficiency virus diseases (ranked #10), conditions arising during the perinatal period (ranked #11), violence (ranked #12), congenital anomalies (ranked #13), and self-inflicted injuries (ranked #14). In addition, highly ranked disorders such as ischemic heart disease (#1), chronic obstructive pulmonary disease (#5), lower respiratory infections (#6), tuberculosis (#7), diarrheal diseases (#9), and tracheal, bronchial, and lung cancers (ranked #15) may have secondary neuropsychiatric aspects.

Alzheimer's Disease and Other Dementing Disorders

Alzheimer's disease is a highly age-related condition, doubling in frequency every 5 years after the age of 60. Thus, 1% of 60-year-olds are affected, 2% of 65-year-olds, 4% of 70-year-olds, 8% of 75-year-olds, 16% of 80-year-olds, and 30%–40% of those 85 and older suffer from a dementia syndrome, primarily Alzheimer's disease [8]. Neuropsychiatric disturbances are common in patients with Alzheimer's disease. In a recent study using the Neuropsychiatric Inventory [9], Mega and colleagues found that 88% of the 50 patients included in the study exhibited some form of scorable psychopathology; 72% exhibited apathy, 60% had periods of agitation, 48% manifested anxiety, 38% had aberrant motor behaviors such as rummaging and pacing, 42% were irritable, 36% exhibited disinhibition, 38% had dysphoria consistent with a depressed mood, 42% had delusions, 10% had hallucinations, and 8% had euphoric-type mood changes.

Stroke and Vascular Dementia

Stroke is also age related in incidence. The incidence among men rises from 0.8 per thousand in the age group 45–54 years, to 2.1 in the age group from 55 to 64, 4.5 among those 65 to 74, and 9.3 among those 75 to 84 years of age. Among women the incidence rises from 0.6 in the age group 45 to 54 to 1.2 in the 55 to 64-year-old range, 3.8 in the 65 to 74-year-old group, 7.4 in the 75 to 84-year-old group, and 7.9 per thousand among those 85 years and older [10]. Stroke is commonly accompanied by neuropsychiatric disturbances: major depression occurs in 10%–25% of poststroke patients and minor depression in 10%–40%. General anxiety with depression occurs in 20% and generalized anxiety without depression in 7%. Apathy is noted with depression in 11% and without depression in 11%. Anosognosia occurs in 24%–43% of patients, catastrophic reactions in 20% of patients, emotional lability in 20% of patients, and vascular dementia in 25% of patients [11]. Psychosis and mania are rare poststroke complications that occur with increased frequency among poststroke victims.

Parkinson's Disease and Parkinsonism

The incidence of Parkinson's disease increases with age. The frequency of Parkinson's disease increases from an annual incidence of approximately 2 per 100 000 in the 40 to 49-year-old age group, to 10–15 per 100 000 at age 50–59, 50–100 per 100 000 in the age group 60–69, and 75–125 per 100 000 in the age group 70–79 years. The average age of Parkinson's disease patients living in the community is 67–68 years, with 75%–80% of the patients between 69 and 79 years old [12]. Aarsland and coworkers

[13] used the Neuropsychiatric Inventory to determine the frequency of neuropsychiatric disease of Parkinson's patients living in a Norwegian community. In this sample, 16% of patients has delusions, 27% hallucinations, 16% agitation, 38% depression, 20% anxiety, 1% euphoria, 16% apathy, 6% disinhibition, 10% irritability, and 10% aberrant motor behavior.

Other Dementing Disorders

Neuropsychiatric syndromes have also been studied in other dementias. Patients with frontotemporal dementia manifest prominent disinhibition (68%) and euphoria (36%). Apathy is evident in 95%, aberrant motor behavior in 73%, anxiety in 47%, and delusions in 7% [16]. Litvan and colleagues [14] used the Neuropsychiatric Inventory to determine the prevalence of neuropsychiatric syndromes in patients with progressive supranuclear palsy. The two most common disturbances were apathy (91%) and disinhibition (36%). Fewer patients exhibited dysphoria (18%), anxiety (18%), irritability (9%), aberrant motor behavior (9%), and agitation (5%). Of patients with corticobasal degeneration, 73% had depression, 40% apathy, 20% irritability, 20% agitation, 13% anxiety, 13% disinhibition, 7% delusions, and 7% aberrant motor behavior [15].

Advances in Neuroscience: Relevance to Neuropsychiatric Disorders in the Elderly

Basic Neuroscience

Tremendous strides have been made in basic neuroscience relevant to neuropsychiatry, particularly in the areas of molecular biology and genetics of Alzheimer's disease, Parkinson's disease, and related neurodegenerative disorders. An evolving if incomplete consensus suggests that the accumulation of amyloid beta-protein is the central pathological feature of Alzheimer's disease. All the known mutations (chromosomes 21, 14, and 1) result in the overproduction of beta-amyloid protein, whereas sporadic disorders are associated with the excessive accumulation of amyloid beta-protein such as in individuals with the lipoprotein E4 genotype. The aggregation of the amyloid beta-protein or the intrinsic cellular processes that generate this product lead to nerve cell death in vulnerable regions of the cortex such as medial temporal lobes and the temporoparietal junction. Cell death in subcortical nuclear areas such as the nucleus basalis, locus coeruleus, and median raphe results in deficits in acetylcholine, norepinephrine, and serotonin, respectively. Neurochemical deficits, particularly the cholinergic abnormality, further exacerbate the dementia syndrome. The production of neurofibrillary tangles has not been fully explained or linked to the amyloidogenic cascade but may represent a less specific cellular response to injury associated with processes also responsible for amyloid generation. Thus, the pathogenesis of Alzheimer's disease is currently conceptualized as sequential steps leading from beta-amyloid protein production and aggregation to nerve cell death, neurochemical deficits, and an ensuing clinical syndrome [17]. This model provides a series of targets for therapeutic interventions.

The development of stains applicable to detection of Lewy bodies such as ubiquitin and alpha-synuclein has enhanced our knowledge of Lewy body diseases. Lewy bodies occur in the brainstem of patients with classical Parkinson's disease, and a small number are typically found in the cortex of Parkinson's disease patients. In patients manifesting dementia with Lewy bodies, these abnormally staining inclusions are found in the limbic and paralimbic cortex, particularly the cingulate gyrus and insula. The presence of cortical Lewy bodies and other unique neurochemical features of dementia with Lewy bodies—a marked dopaminergic deficit as well as a marked cholinergic deficit—produce an identifiable clinical syndrome characterized by visual hallucinations, fluctuating cognition, and parkinsonism [18].

Neuroimaging

Advances in neuroimaging technology have been among the most useful in aiding clinicians both in the diagnosis of disorders with neuropsychiatric manifestations in the elderly and in understanding the pathophysiology of these conditions. Patients with Alzheimer's disease, for example, exhibit reduced temporoparietal metabolism when studied with fluorodeoxyglucose (FDG) positron emission tomography (PET), and patients with agitation, depression, psychosis, or apathy exhibit distinctive syndrome-related changes when studied with FDG-PET or cerebral blood flow studies [19]. Studies with functional magnetic resonance imaging (fMRI), ligand-labeled PET, and magnetic resonance spectroscopy promise to provide additional insight into the pathophysiological changes underlying both primary neurological diseases of the elderly and their neuropsychiatric disturbances.

Advances in Treatment Relevant to Geriatric Neuropsychiatry

Improved understanding of the pathophysiology of disease has enlarged the spectrum of possible therapeutic interventions available in neuropsychiatry; where the pathophysiology is well understood, mechanism-based interventions are possible. In situations in which a neurochemical deficit has been identified, pharmacological replacement therapy is possible even when the underlying mechanisms of the deficiency remain to be revealed. Finally, psychotropic medications such as antipsychotics, antiagitation agents, and antidepressants may be used in conditions in which these behavioral manifestations are present and other types of interventions are unavailable or ineffective.

In Alzheimer's disease, progress has been made in defining disease-modifying therapies. Identification of the accumulation of beta-amyloid protein as a central feature of the disease suggested that antiamyloid therapies may be effective in preventing or deferring the onset or delaying the progress of the disease. Such agents are currently being studied but are not yet available for clinical implementation. Neuroprotective strategies offer another avenue of therapeutic intervention in neurodegenerative diseases. Vitamin E and selegiline have been shown to slow the progress of Alzheimer's disease [20]. Combined therapy had no benefit beyond that with selegiline or vitamin E alone, but combination therapy was associated with greater reduction of behavioral disturbances at the end of the trial compared to any other intervention. Nonsteroidal antiinflammatory drugs, hormonal interventions (estrogen, testosterone), and other antioxidant compounds are being tested for their possible disease-modifying utility.

Cholinesterase inhibitors have proven to be useful in improving cognition in Alzheimer's disease or reducing the rate of cognitive decline [21–24]. Recently these agents also have been shown to have psychotropic effects, reducing apathy and visual hallucinations predictably and having beneficial effects on other behavioral manifestations in some clinical circumstances [25].

Progress also has been made in investigating the utility of psychotropic compounds in patients with Alzheimer's disease and other neurodegenerative conditions. In many cases, application of psychotropic drugs approved for psychosis based on studies on schizophrenia has been extrapolated with the assumption that they would also prove to be efficacious in the psychosis or other behavioral disturbances associated with Alzheimer's disease. This assumption may be correct, but must specifically be proven because the plaque and tangle pathology of Alzheimer's disease as well as the cholinergic deficit may create a cerebral environment sufficiently different from that of schizophrenia to significantly alter efficacy. Recently, double-blind randomized controlled trials of risperidone [26,27] have shown this agent to be superior to placebo and somewhat better than haloperidol in reducing agitation and aggressiveness in patients with Alzheimer's disease and other dementias.

Studies with other atypical antipsychotics such as olanzapine and quetiapine are in progress. Similarly, a double-blind placebo controlled trial of clozapine demonstrated efficacy for drug-associated psychosis in patients with Parkinson's disease [28], and open-label studies with olanzapine [29] and quetiapine [30] indicate that these atypical antipsychotic agents may be useful in management of psychosis in Parkinson's disease. Randomized clinical trials of antidepressants and antiagitation agents (particularly antiepileptic drugs such as carbamazepine, valproate, and gabapentin) are being pursued.

A Neuropsychiatric Research Continuum

The principal aim of neuropsychiatric research is to improve patient care and patient quality of life. Thus, these outcomes must be directly measured as new therapies and management strategies are developed. A neuropsychiatric research continuum can be envisioned beginning with basic science research studying underlying pathophysiological mechanisms of the disease; transitional research extrapolating these basic observations to animal models of neuropsychiatric disorders; clinical research focused on behavioral characterization, neuroimaging, and clinical trials of emerging agents of neuropsychiatric importance; and translational research emphasizing how best to accomplish technology transfer, to change physician behavior to incorporate advances in neuroscience, and to develop patient-centered outcomes demonstrating changes in quality of life and patient self-efficacy following neuropsychiatric intervention. Once described, successful translation efforts can be the subject of education and globalization with cultural accommodation to make them culturally appropriate. This research continuum leading to improved patient quality of life can be promoted as the theme of all neuropsychiatric research.

Summary

The population of the planet is aging, and over the next five decades there will be an increase in the number and proportion of aged individuals in the population. A direct consequence of this change in demography is an increase in the number of individuals with age-related disorders. Brain disorders are among the most common of these. Neuropsychiatric disturbances accompany nearly all brain disorders associated with aging including the dementias, Parkinson's disease, and stroke. Substantial progress is being made in investigating the underlying pathophysiology of these disorders and new treatments are emerging. Implementation of a research continuum from basic through clinical and translational research will ensure that patients throughout the world will be the benefactors of this intensive neuropsychiatric research agenda.

Acknowledgment. This project was supported by a National Institute of Aging Alzheimer's Disease Research grant (AG16570), an Alzheimer's Disease Research Center of California grant, and the Sidell-Kagan Foundation.

References

1. World Health Organization (1998) World atlas of ageing. World Health Organization, Centre for Health Development, Kobe, Japan
2. Bureau of the Census (1987) International population reports series: an aging world. U.S. Department of Commerce, Washington, DC
3. National Foundation for Brain Research (1992) The cost of disorders of the brain. National Foundation for Brain Research, Washington, DC
4. Duffy JD, Hobbs E (2000) Mental retardation. In: Coffey CE, Cummings JL (eds) Textbook of geriatric neuropsychiatry, 2nd edn. American Psychiatric Press, Washington, DC, pp 463–476
5. Salzman C (2000) Mood disorders. In: Coffey CE, Cummings JL (eds) Textbook of geriatric neuropsychiatry, 2nd edn. American Psychiatric Press, Washington, DC, pp 313–328
6. Pearlson GD (2000) Late-life-onset psychoses. In: Coffey CE, Cummings JL (eds) Textbook of geriatric neuropsychiatry, 2nd edn. American Psychiatric Press, Washington, DC, pp 329–346
7. Murray CJL, Lopez AD (eds) (1996) The global burden of disease: a comprehensive assessment of mortality and disability from diseases, injuries, and risk factors in 1990 and projected to 2020. Harvard University Press, Boston
8. Jorm AF, Korten AE, Henderson AS (1987) The prevalence of dementia: a quantitative integration of the literature. Acta Psychiatr Scand 76:465–479
9. Cummings JL, Mega M, Gray K, et al (1994) The neuropsychiatric inventory: comprehensive assessment of psychopathology in dementia. Neurology 44:2308–2314
10. Babikian VL, Kase CS, Wolf PA (1954) Cerebrovascular disease in the elderly. In: Albert ML, Knoefel JE (eds) Clinical neurology of aging, 2nd edn. Oxford University Press, New York, pp 548–568
11. Starkstein SE, Robinson RG (2000) Stroke. In: Coffey CE, Cummings JL (eds) Textbook of geriatric neuropsychiatry, 2nd edn. American Psychiatric Press, Washington, DC, pp 601–620
12. Martilla RJ (1994) Epidemiology. In: Koller WC (ed) Handbook of Parkinson's disease, 2nd edn. Dekker, New York, pp 35–57

13. Aarsland D, Larsen JP, Lim NG, et al (1999) Range of neuropsychiatric disturbances in patients with Parkinson's disease. J Neurol Neurosurg Psychiatry 67:492–496
14. Litvan I, Mega M, Cummings JL, Fairbanks L (1996) Neuropsychiatric aspects of progressive supranuclear palsy. Neurology 47:1184–1189
15. Litvan I, Cummings JL, Mega M (1998) Neuropsychiatric features of corticobasal degeneration. J Neurol Neurosurg Psychiatry 65:717–721
16. Levy ML, Miller BL, Cummings JL (1996) Alzheimer's disease and frontotemporal dementias: behavioral distinctions. Arch Neurol 53:687–690
17. Cummings JL, Vinters HV, Cole GM, Khachaturian Z (1998) Alzheimer's disease: etiologies, pathophysiology, cognitive reserve, and treatment opportunities. Neurology 51(suppl 1):S2–S17
18. McKeith IG, Ballard CG, Perry RH, et al (2000) Prospective validation of Consensus criteria for the diagnosis of dementia with Lewy bodies. Neurology 54:1050–1058
19. Craig AH, Cummings JL, Fairbanks L, et al (1996) Cerebral blood flow correlates of apathy in Alzheimer's disease. Arch Neurol 53:1116–1120
20. Sano M, Ernesto C, Thomas RG, et al (1997) A controlled trial of selegiline, alphatocopherol, or both as treatment for Alzheimer's disease. N Engl J Med 336:1216–1222
21. Farlow M, Gracon SI, Hershey LA, et al (1992) A controlled trial of tacrine in Alzheimer's disease. JAMA 268:2523–2529
22. Rogers SL, Farlow MR, Doody RS, et al (1998) A 24-week, double-blind, placebo-controlled trial of donepezil in patients with Alzheimer's disease. Neurology 50:136–145
23. Morris JC, Cyrus PA, Orazem J, et al (1998) Metrifonate benefits cognitive, bahavioral, and global function in patients with Alzheimer's disease. Neurology 50:1222–1230
24. Corey-Bloom J, Anand R, Veach J (1998) A randomized trial evaluating the efficacy and safety of ENA 713 (rivastigmine tartrate), a new acetylcholinesterase inhibitor, in patients with mild to moderately severe Alzheimer's disease. Int J Geriatr Psychopharmacol 1:55–65
25. Cummings JL (2000) Cholinesterase inhibitors: a new class of psychotropic compounds. Am J Psychiatry 157:4–15
26. De Deyn PP, Rabheru K, Rasmussen A, et al (1999) A randomized trial of risperidone, placebo, and haloperidol for behavioral symptoms of dementia. Neurology 53:946–955
27. Katz IR, Jeste DV, Mintzer JE, et al (1999) Comparison of risperidone and placebo for psychosis and behavioral disturbances associated with dementia: a randomized, double-blind trial. J Clin Psychiatry 60:107–115
28. Parkinson Study Group T (1999) Low-dose clozapine for the treatment of drug-induced psychosis in Parkinson's disease. N Engl J Med 340:757–763
29. Wolters EC, Jansen ENH, Tuynman-Qua HG, Bergmans PLM (1996) Olanzapine in the treatment of dopaminomimetic psychosis in patients with Parkinson's disease. Neurology 47:1085–1087
30. Parsa MA, Bastani B (1998) Quetiapine (Seroquel) in the treatment of psychosis in patients with Parkinson's disease. J Neuropsychol Clin Neurosci 10:216–219

The Neuropsychiatry of Stroke

Robert G. Robinson

Summary. Although stroke represents a major public health problem throughout much of the world, relatively little work has been directed toward identifying and treating the common neuropsychiatric disorders that occur following stroke. Depression, anxiety disorder, catastrophic reactions, pathological crying, and psychosis have all been associated with stroke. Depressive and anxiety disorders have been shown to inhibit physical and cognitive recovery from stroke and lead to increase mortality. Although there are very few controlled trials examining the effectiveness of treatments for these disorders after stroke, both depression and pathological crying have been shown to be effectively treated with antidepressant medications.

Keywords. Stroke, Depression, Anxiety disorder, Treatment, Cerebrovascular disease

Introduction

The age-adjusted annual incidence rate for stroke in the United States is approximately 150 per 100 000, with very similar incidence rates reported in other industrialized nations [1]. Although stroke ranks as the third leading cause of death (behind heart disease and cancer), accounting for 150 000 fatalities/year in the United States, about 3 million stroke survivors are alive at any given time [2]. Of these survivors, two-thirds have some permanent disability requiring rehabilitation [3]. The emotional and psychopathological consequences of stroke have been examined in every continent in the world (Table 1).

Recent studies concluded that neuropsychiatric complications (i.e., emotional, behavioral, and cognitive disorders) may have a negative effect not only on the social functioning and overall quality of life of stroke survivors [4] but on the recovery of their motor functioning as well [5].

Department of Psychiatry, The University of Iowa College of Medicine, Iowa City, IA 52242, USA

Poststroke Depression

Although numerous neuropsychiatric disorders have been associated with stroke (Table 1), depression is probably the most common poststroke neuropsychiatric disorder.

Diagnosis

The diagnosis of poststroke depression (PSD) may be difficult or impossible to make in some groups of patients because of language or cognitive disorder. For instance, moderate to severe verbal comprehension impairment or severe cognitive impairment may prohibit the reliable assessment of symptoms of depression using the standard method of mental status examination [6].

In addition to not being able to diagnose depression in some patients with language comprehension deficits [7], some investigators have suggested that several symptoms used by DSM-IV for the diagnosis of major depression, such as loss of energy, loss of appetite, and insomnia, are also found among euthymic stroke patients secondary to the hospital environment, the use of medications, other associated medical conditions, or the stroke itself [8]. In 1991, Fedoroff et al. [9] examined the frequency of depressive symptoms among both depressed and nondepressed patients with acute stroke. This study found that, with the exception of morning awakening, all neurovegetative and psychological symptoms of depression were significantly more frequent among patients with depressed mood compared to patients without depressed mood. Even when the frequency of nonspecific symptoms among the nondepressed was taken into account, the frequency of major depression decreased only 2%, from 23% to 21%. Thus, although poststroke depression cannot be reliably diagnosed in patients with severe comprehension impairments, the DSM-IV diagnostic criteria for "depression due to stroke with major depressive-like episode" are applicable to patients with PSD [10].

Minor depression is a DSM-IV diagnosis requiring the presence of more than two but fewer than five major depressive symptoms including either a depressed mood or loss of interest. Although it excludes depressions "due to a general medical condition,"

Table 1. Neuropsychiatric disorders associated with stroke

Syndrome	Prevalence	Clinical features
Poststroke depression	35%	Depressed mood, appetite or weight loss, insomnia, social withdrawal
Mania	Rare	Elevated mood, decreased sleep, flight of ideas, pressured speech, grandiosity
Bipolar disorder	Rare	Alternating symptoms of depression and mania
Anxiety disorder	25%	Apprehensive expectation, restlessness, loss of energy, muscle tension
Apathy without depression	20%	Loss of interest and drives
Psychotic disorder	Rare	Delusions and hallucinations
Pathological affect	20%	Out-of-proportion emotional outbursts
Catastrophic reaction	20%	Burst of aggressive behavior, anxiety, crying

we have used this diagnosis to identify stroke patients with milder forms of depression. Our studies have validated this diagnosis by identifying differences between major and minor depression in the frequency of past personal history of depression [11], the association with cognitive impairment [12], and association with lesion location [13].

Prevalence

The frequency of poststroke depression (PSD) has been examined in numerous studies. The frequency depends upon whether patients are examined in hospital or in community surveys and whether they are studied during the acute poststroke period or many months following stroke (Table 2).

Using established diagnostic criteria, the mean prevalence of major depression in outpatient population studies was 21% and for minor depression 17%. The mean prevalence in hospitalized patients with acute stroke was 22% and 17% for major depression and minor depression, respectively, whereas in outpatient populations and rehabilitation hospital settings the mean prevalences were 23% for major and 35% for minor depression. Finally, the mean prevalence of major depression in community samples was 13% and 10% for minor depression.

Duration

The duration of depression has been examined in several longitudinal studies. Morris et al. [14] found that the mean duration of poststroke major depression was 34 weeks whereas the mean duration of minor depression was only 13 weeks. Åström et al. [15] also found that the majority of major depressions remitted by 1 year of follow-up. However, 30% of patients with in-hospital major depression remained depressed at 1 year of follow-up, 25% were depressed at 2 years of follow-up, and 20% were still depressed at 3 years of follow-up. Thus, although the mean duration of major depression appears to be about 9 months, there are a significant number of patients with major or minor depression in hospital who remain depressed for several years following their stroke (Fig. 1).

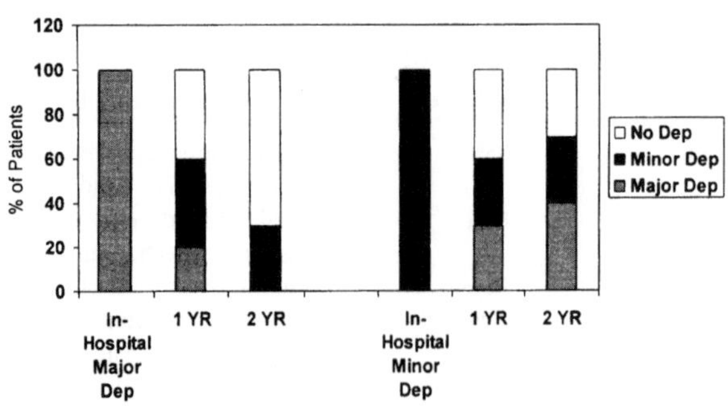

Fig. 1. The outcome of patients with in-hospital major or minor poststroke depression at 1 and 2 years follow-up. Note that the majority of patients with major depression are improved by 1 year while the majority of minor depression patients were still depressed at 2 years follow-up

TABLE 2. Prevalence studies of poststroke depression

Investigators	Patient population	n	Criteria	Major (%)	Minor (%)	Total (%)
Wade 1987 [36]	Community	379	Cutoff score			30
House 1991 [37]	Community	89	PSE-DSM-III	11	12	23
Burvill 1995 [38]	Community	294	PSE-DSM-III	15	8	23
Robinson 1983 [39]	Acute, hospital	103	PSE-DSM-III	27	20	47
Ebrahim 1987 [40]	Acute, hospital	149	Cutoff score			23
Fedoroff 1991 [9]	Acute, hospital	205	PSE-DSM-III	22	19	41
Castillo 1995 [30]	Acute, hospital	291	PSE-DSM-III	20	18	38
Starkstein 1989 [41]	Acute, hospital	80	PSE-DSM-III	16	13	29
Astrom 1993 [16]	Acute, hospital	80	DSM-III	25	NR	25[a]
Hermann 1993 [42]	Acute, hospital	21	RDC	24	14	38
Andersen 1994 [28]	Acute, hospital or outpatient	285	HDRS cutoff	10	11	21
Folstein 1997 [43]	Rehabilitation, hospital	20	PSE and items			45
Finklestein 1982 [44]	Rehabilitation, hospital	25	Cutoff score			48
Sinyor 1986 [45]	Rehabilitation, hospital	35	Cutoff score			36
Finset 1989 [46]	Rehabilitation, hospital	42	Cutoff score			36
Eastwood 1989 [47]	Rehabilitation, hospital	87	SADS-RDC	10	40	50
Morris 1990 [14]	Rehabilitation, hospital	99	CIDI-DSM-III	14	21	35
Shubert 1992 [48]	Rehabilitation, hospital	18	DSM-III-R	28	44	72
Schwartz 1993 [49]	Rehabilitation, hospital	91	DSM-III	40		40[a]
Feibel 1982 [50]	Outpatient (6 months)	91	Nursing evaluation			26
Robinson 1982 [51]	Outpatient (6 months–10 years)	103	Cutoff score			29
Collin 1987 [52]	Outpatient	111	Cutoff score			42
Astrom 1993 [16]	Outpatient					
	(3 months)	73	DSM-III	31	NR	31[a]
	(1 year)	73	DSM-III	16	NR	16[a]
	(2 years)	57	DSM-III	19	NR	19[a]
	(3 years)	49	DSM-III	29	NR	29[a]
Castillo 1995 [30]	Outpatient					
	(3 months)	77	PSE-DSM-III	20	13	33
	(6 months)	80	PSE-DSM-III	21	21	42
	(1 year)	70	PSE-DSM-III	11	16	27
	(2 years)	67	PSE-DSM-III	18	17	35
			Mean	20	21	34[a]

PSE, present state examination; SADS, schedule for affective disorders and schizophrenia; RDC, research diagnostic criteria; CIDI, composite international diagnostic interview; HDRS, Hamilton depression rating scale

[a] Because minor depression was not included, these values may be low

Source: Robinson RG (1998) The clinical neuropsychiatry of stroke. Cambridge University Press, Cambridge

Anatomical Correlates

Over the past two decades, numerous investigators have examined the relationship between lesion location and PSD to delineate a pathoanatomical basis for this disorder. We have found that during the acute poststroke period major depression is significantly more frequent among patients with left frontal or left basal ganglia lesions than any other lesion location. For example, one study of patients with acute stroke found that 14 of 22 patients with left-hemisphere lesions suffered either major or minor depression while these disorders occurred in only 2 of 14 patients with right-hemisphere lesions.

Although these findings have been replicated by several authors [16,17], several others have not found lateralized effects [18,19]. These studies that have failed to find an anatomical correlate of PSD have almost always examined patients more than 60 days and up to several years following their stroke. We have demonstrated that the anatomical correlates of PSD are found only during the first 1 or 2 months post stroke [20]. Thus, there appears to be a dynamic nature to the anatomical substrates of PSD, suggesting that the lateralized pathophysiological mechanism of PSD changes with time.

Association Between Physical Impairment and PSD

Although most stroke patients experience some natural recovery from their impairment in ability to perform activities of daily living (ADL), we have reported that, at 2 years of follow-up, patients with major or minor depression after acute stroke were significantly more impaired in their ADL than comparably impaired patients without depression. This finding held true even when we controlled for lesion size and location, age, education, and amount of rehabilitation therapy. In addition, however, we have also found that in-hospital impairment in ADL correlated with severity of depression at both 3 and 6 months of follow-up [21]. These findings suggest a reciprocal relationship between PSD and impairment in ADL. Depression influences ADL recovery, and severity of ADL impairment influences the duration and severity of depression.

Association Between Cognitive Impairment and PSD

Deficits in one or more domains of cognitive function are, along with motor impairment, the most common complications of stroke. We first reported a specific association between cognitive impairment and major depression in 1986 [22]. In this study, 38 patients who had single infarcts in the left hemisphere, as documented by either CT scan or clinical history, were grouped by depressive diagnosis. There were no significant differences in terms of background and neurological findings, but patients with major depression ($n = 11$) had significantly more cognitive impairments measured by the Mini-Mental State Exam (MMSE) [23] than minor depression or nondepressed patients ($n = 17$).

Using a comprehensive neuropsychological battery, we subsequently found that patients with major depression and left-hemisphere infarcts had significantly greater deficits in tasks involving language, temporal orientation, executive motor, and frontal lobe functions than patients with comparable lesions but without depression [24].

Longitudinal studies of the course of cognitive impairment and PSD found that this association tended to decline with time. House et al. [25], for example, found that the high correlation between depression measured with the Beck depression inventory (BDI) and cognitive impairment that was seen in 76 patients at 1 month after stroke failed to reach significance at the 1-year follow-up. In a 2-year longitudinal study of 103 stroke patients, we found that patients with in-hospital diagnosis of major depression following a left-hemisphere stroke had significantly greater cognitive impairment at the in-hospital, 6-month ($P = 0.03$) and 12-month ($P = 0.02$) follow-up but no difference in cognitive function at the 2 year follow-up [26].

Treatment

Currently, at least four double-blind placebo controlled studies have examined the efficacy of antidepressant medication in PSD. We conducted the first study, reported in 1984 [24], in which patients given nortriptyline showed a significantly greater improvement on the HAM-D Scale, the Zung Self-Rating Depression Scale, and the profile of depressive symptoms assessed by the Present State Examination than placebo-treated controls. It is worth noting that 3 of the original 14 patients treated with nortriptyline dropped out of the study. Two patients became delirious, and 1 had a sudden syncopal episode of unknown etiology.

In a controlled study by Reading et al. [27], seven PSD patients with an abnormal dexamethasone suppression test (DST) (i.e., failure to suppress serum cortisol for 24 h following a single dose of dexamethasone) treated with trazodone had a significantly greater improvement in activities of daily living over 5 weeks of treatment measured by the Barthel ADL scale compared to nine patients with positive PSTs treated with placebo.

Andersen et al. [28] assessed the efficacy and tolerability of the selective serotonin reuptake inhibitor (SSRI) citalopram in a controlled study of 66 patients with stroke. The HAM-D and Melancholia Scale (MES) scores were significantly better at both 3 and 6 weeks among the 33 patients on citalopram at 20 mg (under 65 years of age) or 10 mg (age 65 and over) compared to 33 patients given placebo.

We have recently reported, in a double-blind randomized study comparing nortriptyline with fluoxetine, that depression was significantly better among patients treated with nortriptyline ($n = 16$) than placebo ($n = 17$) or fluoxetine ($n = 23$). Approximately half the patients had major depression (the remainder had minor depression). Nortriptyline-treated patients had significantly lower Ham-D scores following 12 weeks of treatment of fluoxetine, and placebo-treated patients were not significantly different among themselves.

Poststroke Anxiety Disorder

Diagnosis

Anxiety disorder is a frequent neuropsychiatric complication of stroke. Although the spectrum of anxiety disorders includes generalized anxiety disorder (GAD), panic disorder, obsessive-compulsive disorder, and phobic disorder, most studies of poststroke anxiety disorder have focused on GAD.

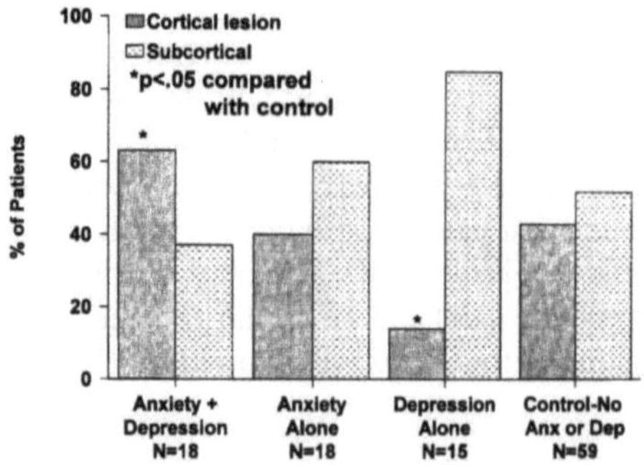

Fig. 2. The frequency of cortical and subcortical lesions of the left hemisphere among patients with depression (major or minor) and generalized anxiety disorder. Depression without anxiety was associated with subcortical left-hemisphere lesions whereas the combination of anxiety and depression was associated with left cortical lesions. (From Robinson RG [21] The clinical neuropsychiatry of stroke. Cambridge University Press, Cambridge, 1998, with permission)

The DSM-IV categorizes poststroke GAD as "anxiety disorder due to stroke with generalized anxiety." The criteria for primary GAD require the presence of sustained worrying or anxiety associated with at least three other symptoms including restlessness, decreased energy, difficulties in concentration, irritability, muscle tension, and sleep disturbance, for a period of at least 6 months. To study patients in the acute poststroke stage, most studies of poststroke GAD have not required the 6-month duration.

Prevalence

A significant comorbidity exists between poststroke anxiety and PSD (Fig. 2). In a study of 98 acute stroke patients, we [29] found that, although only 6 patients met modified DSM-III criteria for GAD (i.e., excluding the 6-month duration criteria) in the absence of any mood disorder, 23 of 47 patients with major depression also met criteria for GAD. In another study, we found that 78 (27%) patients of a population of 288 stroke patients met the modified DSM-III criteria for GAD (i.e., excluding the 6-month duration criteria). Major or minor depression, however, was present in most of them (i.e., 58 of 78 GAD patients) [30].

Comparable results were reported by Aström [31] in a 3-year longitudinal study of 80 patients with acute stroke. In this study, the prevalence of GAD in the acute stage was 28% with no significant decrease through the 3 years of follow-up. Criteria for major depression were met by 85% of poststroke GAD patients at some time during the 3-year follow-up period.

Using our overall group of 288 acute stroke patients, depression plus anxiety was associated with left cortical lesions; anxiety alone was associated with right-hemisphere lesions, and depression alone was associated with left basal ganglia lesions [29,30].

In the 3-year longitudinal study of stroke patients by Aström [31], similar findings were reported. In the acute poststroke period, pure GAD was significantly associated with right-hemispheric lesions, whereas comorbid anxiety or depression was significantly associated with left-hemispheric lesions. Another important finding of this study was that, at 3 years after stroke, GAD was significantly associated with both cortical and subcortical atrophy. Aström suggested that this atrophy might play a role in the prolonged existence of GAD after stroke.

Risk Factors and Effect on Recovery

Longitudinal studies of poststroke GAD have shown that functional recovery of patients with stroke was negatively affected by the presence of GAD. For example, in her 3-year longitudinal study Aström [31] found that ADL impairment was associated with GAD not only in the acute period but at all time periods after discharge from the hospital. Thus, anxiety was more than an immediate reaction to loss of function. In another study of 142 patients, we found that patients with GAD and depression ($n = 18$) who were matched for severity of impairment and severity of stroke had significantly greater impairment in ADL at 2-year follow-up than patients with PSD alone ($n = 9$) (40). We suggested one possible explanation was that the comorbidity of PSD and GAD produced a longer duration of depression than PSD alone; this prolonged depression might lead to more profound adverse physical and social functioning outcomes.

Treatment

Benzodiazepines are the medications most commonly prescribed for the treatment of GAD but tend to accumulate in older people. Given the fact that stroke patients constitute an older population, benzodiazepines should be used as a time-limited treatment.

Buspirone, an anxiolytic medication with partial serotonin agonist properties, has been reported [32] to have an efficacy similar to diazepam in the treatment of GAD but with a more tolerable side-effects profile. The utility of buspirone in this population has not been examined, however.

Other Poststroke Neuropsychiatric Disorders

Catastrophic Reaction

In 1939, Goldstein [33] created the term catastrophic reaction to describe a series of symptoms that may occur in patients with brain injury and appear to be caused by the "inability of the organism to cope with physical or cognitive deficits." Starkstein et al. [26] developed a scale (i.e., the Catastrophic Reaction Scale) for the assessment of the existence and severity of catastrophic reactions. Using this scale, catastrophic reactions were present in 19% of a consecutive series of 62 patients with acute stroke. Moreover, because catastrophic reactions were significantly associated with both major depression and basal ganglia lesions, we suggested that this phenomenon might represent the release of depressive emotions provoked by anterior subcortical damage.

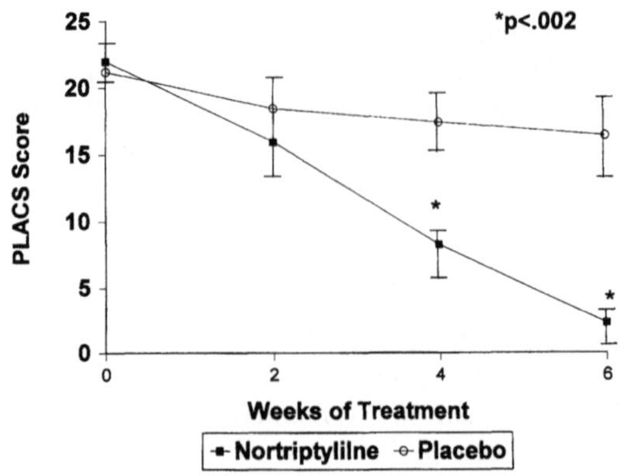

Fig. 3. Comparison of pathological laughter and crying scale (PLACS) scores during 6 weeks of double-blind treatment with nortriptyline or placebo. The nortriptyline was superior to placebo at both 4 and 6 weeks of treatment. (From Robinson RG [21] The clinical neuropsychiatry of stroke. Cambridge University Press, Cambridge, 1998, with permission)

Pathological Affect

Pathological affect is characterized by frequent and easily provoked episodes of crying or laughing that are not appropriate to the situation or are in excess of the underlying emotion. We demonstrated the reliability and validity of the Pathological Crying and Laughing Scale (PLACS) for the assessment of emotional lability in 54 patients with acute stroke [34]. Furthermore, in a double-blind drug trial of nortriptyline versus placebo, 14 patients receiving nortriptyline showed significantly lower PLACS scores (i.e., less pathological crying) at 4 and 6 weeks of treatment compared to 14 patients receiving placebo (Fig. 3).

Poststroke Psychosis

Psychosis (i.e., delusions and hallucinations) is a rare complication of stroke. Rabins et al. [35] screened all individuals 60 years of age or older who were admitted to a hospital during a 9-year period and identified five patients with poststroke psychosis. All of them had right frontoparietal lesions and showed a significantly greater degree of subcortical atrophy compared to five stroke patients matched for age and lesion size and location but without psychosis. Moreover, three of the five patients with poststroke psychosis had seizures whereas no seizures were seen in any of the five nonpsychotic patients.

Conclusions

There are numerous neuropsychiatric disorders that may occur following stroke (see Table 1). This review has examined only a few of these disorders. Depression and anxiety disorder are two of the most common poststroke neuropsychiatric disorders and frequently occur as comorbid conditions. In addition to producing a significant degree of psychological distress, both of these disorders have been shown to be associated with particular lesion locations and to adversely effect the physical recovery from stroke.

Similarly, catastrophic reactions, pathological affect, and poststroke psychosis are disorders that may occur following stroke and probably influence the course of recovery as well as quality of life following stroke. Given the frequent occurrence of these disorders and the magnitude of the public health problem produced by stroke, it is remarkable how few treatment studies have been conducted. Apart from the early treatment interventions to prevent infarction, treatment of the neuropsychiatric disorders following stroke appears to have the greatest potential to improve the outcome and quality of life for people who have suffered a stroke.

Acknowledgments. This work was supported in part by the following NIMH grants: MH-40355, MH-52879, and MH53592.

References

1. Bonita R (1992) Epidemiology of stroke. Lancet 339:342–344
2. American Heart Association (1989) Stroke facts. American Heart Association, Dallas
3. Bronstein KS (1991) Psychological components in stroke implications for adaptation. Nursing Clin N Am 26:1007–1017
4. King RB (1996) Quality of life after stroke. Stroke 27:1467–1472
5. Clark MS, Smith DS (1997) Abnormal illness behavior in rehabilitation from stroke. Clin Rehabil 11:162–170
6. Gustafson Y, Olsson T, Eriksson S (1991) Acute confusional states in stroke patients. Cerebrovasc Dis 1:257–264
7. Starkstein SE, Robinson RG (1989) Affective disorders and cerebral vascular disease. Br J Psychiatry 154:170–182
8. Harrington C, Salloway S (1997) The diagnosis and treatment of post-stroke depression. Med Health 80:181–187
9. Fedoroff JP, Starkstein SE, Parikh RM, et al (1991) Are depressive symptoms nonspecific in patients with acute stroke? Am J Psychiatry 148:1172–1176
10. American Psychiatric Association (1994) Diagnostic and statistical manual of mental disorders—DSM-IV, 4th edn. American Psychiatric Press, Washington, DC
11. Morris PLP, Robinson RG, Raphael B, Bishop D (1991) The relationship between the perception of social support and post-stroke depression in hospitalized patients. Psychiatry 54:306–315
12. Downhill JE Jr, Robinson RG (1994) Longitudinal assessment of depression and cognitive impairment following stroke. J Nerv Ment Dis 182:425–431
13. Paradiso S, Robinson RG (1999) Minor depression after stroke. An initial validation of the DSM-IV construct. Am J Geriatr Psychiatry 7:244–251
14. Morris PLP, Robinson RG, Raphael B (1990) Prevalence and course of depressive disorders in hospitalized stroke patients. Int J Psychiatry Med 20:349–364
15. Aström M, Olsson T, Asplund K (1993) Different linkage of depression to hypercortisolism early versus late after stroke: a 3-year longitudinal study. Stroke 24:52–57
16. Astrom M, Adolfsson R, Asplund K (1993) Major depression in stroke patients: a 3-year longitudinal study. Stroke 24:976–982

17. Morris PLP, Robinson RG, Raphael B, Hopwood MJ (1996) Lesion location and post-stroke depression. J Neuropsychiatry Clin Neurosci 8:399–403
18. House A, Dennis M, Warlow C, et al (1990) Mood disorders after stroke and their relation to lesion location. A CT scan study. Brain 113:1113–1130
19. Gainotti G, Azzoni A, Marra C (1999) Frequency, phenomenology and anatomical-clinical correlates of major post-stroke depression. Br J Psychiatry 175:163–167
20. Shimoda K, Robinson RG (1999) The relationship between post-stroke depression and lesion location in long-term follow-up. Biol Psychiatry 45:187–192
21. Robinson RG (1998) The clinical neuropsychiatry of stroke. Cambridge University Press, Cambridge
22. Robinson RG, Bolla-Wilson K, Kaplan E, et al (1986) Depression influences intellectual impairment in stroke patients. Br J Psychiatry 148:541–547
23. Folstein MF, Folstein SE, McHugh PR (1975) Mini-Mental State: a practical method for grading the cognitive state of patients for the clinician. J Psychiatric Res 12:189–198
24. Bolla-Wilson K, Robinson RG, Starkstein SE, et al (1989) Lateralization of dementia of depression in stroke patients. Am J Psychiatry 146:627–634
25. House A, Dennis M, Warlow C, et al (1990) The relationship between intellectual impairment and mood disorder in the first year after stroke. Psychol Med 20:805–814
26. Starkstein SE, Fedoroff JP, Price TR, et al (1993) Catastrophic reaction after cerebrovascular lesions: frequency, correlates, and validation of a scale. J Neurol Neurosurg Psychiatry 5:189–194
27. Reding MJ, Orto LA, Winter SW, et al (1986) Antidepressant therapy after stroke: a double-blind trial. Arch Neurol 43:763–765
28. Andersen G, Vestergaard K, Lauritzen L (1994) Effective treatment of poststroke depression with the selective serotonin reuptake inhibitor citalopram. Stroke 25:1099–1104
29. Starkstein SE, Cohen BS, Fedoroff P, et al (1990) Relationship between anxiety disorders and depressive disorders in patients with cerebrovascular injury. Arch Gen Psychiatry 47:785–789
30. Castillo CS, Schultz SK, Robinson RG (1995) Clinical correlates of early-onset and late-onset poststroke generalized anxiety. Am J Psychiatry 152:1174–1179
31. Aström M (1996) Generalized anxiety disorder in stroke patients: a 3-year longitudinal study. Stroke 27:270–275
32. Rickels K, Schweizer EE (1987) Current pharmacotherapy of anxiety and panic. In: Meltzer HY (ed) Psychopharmacology: the third generation of progress. Raven, New York, pp 1193–1203
33. Goldstein K (1939) The organism: a holistic approach to biology derived from pathological data in man. American Books, New York, p 35
34. Robinson RG, Parikh RM, Lipsey JR, et al (1993) Pathological laughing and crying following stroke: validation of measurement scale and double-blind treatment study. Am J Psychiatry 150:286–293
35. Rabins PV, Starkstein SE, Robinson RG (1991) Risk factors for developing atypical (schizophreniform) psychosis following stroke. J Neuropsychiatry Clin Neurosci 3:6–9
36. Wade DT, Legh-Smith J, Hewer RA (1987) Depressed mood after stroke, a community study of its frequency. Br J Psychiatry 151:200–205
37. House A, Dennis M, Mogridge L, et al (1991) Mood disorders in the year after first stroke. Br J Psychiatry 158:83–92
38. Burvill PW, Johnson GA, Jamrozik KD, et al (1995) Prevalence of depression after stroke: the Perth Community Stroke Study. Br J Psychiatry 166:320–327
39. Robinson RG, Starr LB, Kubos KL, et al (1983) A two year longitudinal study of post-stroke mood disorders: findings during the initial evaluation. Stroke 14:736–741

40. Ebrahim S, Barer D, Nouri F (1987) Affective illness after stroke. Br J Psychiatry 151:52–56
41. Starkstein SE, Robinson RG, Honig MA, Parikh RM, Joselyn P, Price TR (1989) Mood changes after right hemisphere lesion. Br J Psychiatry 155:79–85
42. Herrmann M, Bartles C, Wallesch C-W (1993) Depression in acute and chronic aphasia: symptoms, pathoanatomical-clinical correlations and functional implications. J Neurol Neurosurg Psychiatry 56:672–678
43. Folstein MF, Mairberger R, McHugh PR (1997) Mood disorders as a specific complication of stroke. J Neurol Neurosurg Psychiatry 40:1018–1020
44. Finklestein S, Benowitz LI, Baldessarini RJ, et al (1982) Mood, vegetative disturbance, and dexamethasone suppression test after stroke. Ann Neurol 12:463–468
45. Sinyor D, Jacques P, Kaloupek DG, Becker R, Goldenberg M, Coopersmith H (1986) Post-stroke depression and lesion location: an attempted replication. Brain 109:539–546
46. Finset A, Goffeng L, Landro NI, et al (1989) Depressed mood and intra-hemispheric location of lesion in right hemisphere stroke patients. Scand J Rehabil Med 21:1–6
47. Eastwood MR, Rifat SL, Nobbs H, et al (1989) Mood disorder following cerebrovascular accident. Br J Psychiatry 154:195–200
48. Schubert DSP, Taylor C, Lee S, Mentari A, Tamaklo W (1992) Detection of depression in the stroke patient. *Psychosomatics* 33:1–5
49. Schwartz JA, Speed NM, Brunberg JA, et al (1993) Depression in stroke rehabilitation. Biol Psychiatry 33:694–699
50. Feibel JH, Springer CJ (1982) Depression and failure to resume social activities after stroke. Arch Phys Med Rehabil 63:276–277
51. Robinson RG, Price TR (1982) Post-stroke depressive disorders: a follow-up study of 103 outpatients. Stroke 13:635–641
52. Collin SJ, Tinson D, Lincoln NB (1987) Depression after stroke. Clin Rehabil 1:27

Dementia and Poststroke Major Depression

ROBERT G. ROBINSON

Introduction

Numerous studies have identified depression as a frequent consequence of ischemic brain infarction [1–4], and several studies have identified greater cognitive impairment in depressed compared with nondepressed patients following stroke [5–7].

Clinicians have recognized for more than 40 years that patients with a variety of functional (i.e., no known neuropathology) psychiatric disorders, particularly depression, may show cognitive impairments [8]. The main clinical features of dementia of depression as identified by Wells [9] are the abrupt onset of intellectual impairment and rapid deterioration.

Caine [10] suggested that the diagnosis of pseudodementia or dementia of depression be based on four criteria: (1) intellectual impairment with primary psychiatric disorders; (2) features of neuropsychological abnormality resembling neuropathologically induced intellectual deficit; (3) reversibility of intellectual disorder; and (4) no apparent neurological process. Although these criteria exclude a primary neuropathological process from the causes of dementia of depression, there is growing evidence that major depression associated with a variety of neuropathological disorders might lead to cognitive impairment [11].

Cognitive Impairment Associated with Major Versus Minor Depression

We have recently examined cognitive impairment in a large group of patients (n = 309) whom we have examined following an acute stroke [12]. The mean age (±SD) for the group was 58.9 ± 13.4 years. The patients were 56.2% male, 43.2% married, 66.0% black, and 74.0% Hollingshead Social Class IV–V. The mean number of days between stroke and cognitive examination was 11.2 ± 3.9 days.

Based on symptoms elicited from the structured interview of the Present State Examination [13], patients were given a DSM-III diagnosis of major depression, minor

---

Department of Psychiatry, The University of Iowa College of Medicine, Iowa City, IA 52242, USA

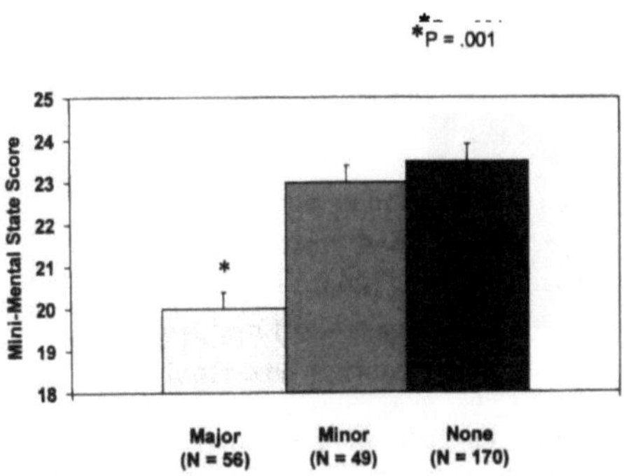

FIG. 1. Mean Mini-Mental State Exam (MMSE) scores of patients hospitalized with acute stroke divided in groups based on the existence of DSM-III *major* depression, *minor* (dysthymic) depression, or no mood disorder (*none*). Patients with major depression had significantly lower (more impaired) scores than the other two groups. *Bars* indicate standard errors of the mean

TABLE 1. Demographic information: in-hospital evaluation

	No cognitive impairment		Cognitive impairment	
	Nondepressed ($n = 122$)	Depressed ($n = 18$)	Nondepressed ($n = 94$)	Depressed ($n = 39$)
Age (years + SD)	57.47 + 13.5	49.9 + 14.8*	63.6 + 11.6**	57.3 + 15.48**
Education (years + SD)	10.3 + 3.8	11.3 + 3.3	8.3 + 4.3**	8.7 + 3.2**
Socioeconomic status, Hollingshead class III–IV (%)	93 (83)	15 (83)	79 (93)	34 (97)

* Depressed versus nondepressed, P < 0.05
** Cognitive versus noncognitive impairment, $P < 0.05$

depression (i.e., symptom criteria for dysthymic disorder but not 2 years in duration), or no depression. Mean scores on the Mini-Mental State Examination (MMSE) for patients with major depression, minor depression, and no depression are shown in Fig. 1. Patients with major depression had significantly lower (i.e., more impaired) MMSE scores than patients with minor depression ($P = 0.02$) or nondepressed patients ($P = 0.002$). Patients with minor depression were not significantly different in their MSME scores than nondepressed patients. Thus, cognitive impairment was associated with only one kind of depression, that is, major depression.

Clinical Variables Associated with Poststroke Cognitive Impairment

We divided our acute stroke group into patients with or without major depression and with or without cognitive impairment (i.e., MMSE scores < 24) (Table 1). Using a two-way analysis of variance (examining the factors of presence or absence of major depression and presence or absence of cognitive impairment), both major depression ($P = 0.0018$) and cognitive impairment ($P = 0.002$) were found to be significantly

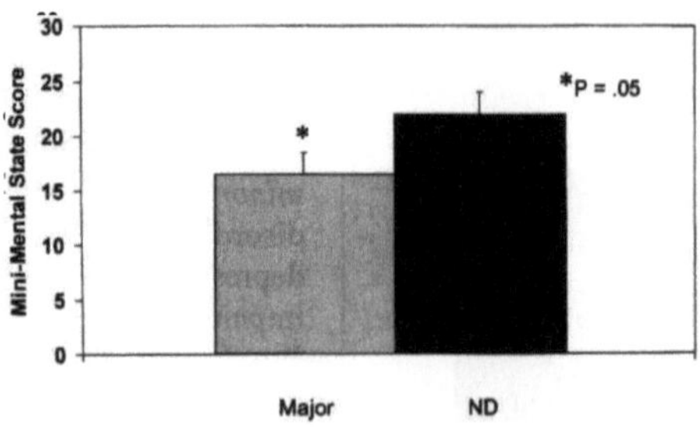

FIG. 2. Mini-Mental State Exam scores for 13 pairs of patients who were matched for lesion size and location. Patients with major depression (*Major*) were significantly more cognitively impaired than nondepressed (*ND*) patients. The groups were comparable in age and education as well as lesion characteristics. *Bars* indicate standard errors of the mean. (Data from Starkstein et al. 1988 [14])

related to age but without significant interaction. Patients with major depression, however, were younger than nondepressed patients, whereas patients with cognitive impairment were significantly older than the noncognitively impaired patients. Cognitive impairment but not depression was significantly related to fewer years of education ($P = 0.0003$).

A stepwise regression analysis to examine the influence of major depression, ethanol abuse, gender, age, and education on cognitive impairment as measured by MMSE showed that the greatest contribution to the variance was given by depression ($F = 23.5, P = 0.00002$) and age ($F = 12.7, P = 0.0004$).

Relationship to Lesion Location

Because brain lesions can affect cognitive function independent of depression, we have examined the separate effects of lesion location and depression. Using our overall group of patients with acute stroke [12], patients were divided into those with right- or left-hemisphere lesions based on computed tomography (CT) or magnetic resonance imaging (MRI) scan visualization (60%) or clinical diagnosis (40%). A two-factor ANOVA of MMSE scores (right- or left-hemisphere lesion was one factor and presence of absence of major depression was the other factor) demonstrated significant effects of depressive diagnosis ($P = 0.0001$) and site of injury ($P = 0.0017$) but no interaction ($P = 0.18$). Individual comparisons demonstrated that patients with major depression and left-hemisphere lesions were significantly more cognitively impaired than nondepressed patients with left-hemisphere lesions.

To determine whether differences in lesion location may explain why patients with major depression had greater cognitive impairment than patients with no depression, we examined patients with and without major depression who were matched for lesion size and location [14]. The study population consisted of 13 pairs of patients who were matched for lesion size, location, and hemisphere of injury; one patient of each pair had major depression while the other was not depressed. Patients were matched for location based on the existence of a brain lesion that involved the same brain regions (i.e., regions defined by Levine and Grek [15]).

Although no significant between-group differences were found in background characteristics, such as age, gender, years of education, and socioeconomic status, patients with major depression had significantly lower MMSE scores than nondepressed patients (Fig. 2) ($P = 0.001$). Of the 13 patients with major depression, 10 had lower MMSE scores than their respective lesion-matched controls, 2 had the same score, and only 1 nondepressed patient had a lower score than the lesion-matched patient with major depression ($P < 0.05$). We concluded from this study that although brain lesions frequently produce cognitive impairment as measured by the MMSE state examination, patients with major depression have a degree of cognitive impairment that cannot be explained based on the lesion alone.

We have also administered a comprehensive neuropsychological test battery [16] to 53 patients with single stroke lesions localized to the anterior or posterior region of the right or left hemisphere. Patients were comparable in age, education, and size and location of stroke lesion. There were 10 with major depression and 16 nondepressed left-hemisphere lesions, and 8 depressed and 19 nondepressed right-lesion patients.

Data analysis included in a two-way ANOVA of *Z*-scores (scores in each cognitive domain transformed to *Z*-scores to allow comparison between domains; factors in the ANOVA were presence or absence of depression and existence of right- or left-hemisphere lesions). There was a significant depression by side interaction ($P = 0.01$). The left-hemisphere depressed group performed significantly below the left-hemisphere nondepressed group ($P = 0.01$), the right-hemisphere depressed group ($P = 0.01$), and the right-hemisphere nondepressed group ($P = 0.01$). There were no significant differences among the depressed and nondepressed patients with right-hemisphere lesions or among the patients with left-hemisphere lesions who were nondepressed ($P = 0.3$ to 0.7). Within the left-hemisphere lesion group, the presence of depression was associated with significantly lower scores in orientation ($P = 0.02$), language ($P = 0.01$), executive motor function ($P = 0.01$), frontal lobe function ($P = 0.01$), and visual construction–visual perceptual ability ($P < 0.05$). In the right-hemisphere lesion group, there were no significant differences between the depressed and nondepressed groups in any of the nine cognitive domains.

We concluded from this study that, using a detailed neuropsychological battery that examined both right- and left-hemisphere cognitive functions, major depression was associated with cognitive impairment only following left-hemisphere lesions. In addition, the cognitive impairment involved a range of neuropsychological tasks generally associated with left- and right parietal as well as frontal lobe function.

Longitudinal Course of Cognitive Impairment

Of the patients evaluated with acute stroke, 140 patients were reexamined at 3, 6, 12, or 24 months following stroke. Because our previous data demonstrated that cognitive impairment was associated with major depression following a left-hemisphere lesion, we examined the effect of lesion location on follow-up cognitive status. The MMSE scores for patients with left-hemisphere stroke and in-hospital major depression (regardless of their diagnosis at follow-up) were compared to those of patients with left-hemisphere stroke but without in-hospital depression (regardless of their diagnoses at follow-up). There was a significant effect of depression on MMSE scores in-hospital, at 6 months ($P = 0.03$), and at 1-year follow-up ($P = 0.019$).

These findings indicate that the association of depression with cognitive impairment is strongest during the acute stroke period, but there is some effect for up to 1 year. At 2 years following stroke, however, major depression, even after a left-hemisphere stroke, is no longer associated with cognitive impairment.

Treatment

Based on the findings that treatment of depression significantly improves cognitive function in patients with functional depressive disorders [10,17], it would be predicted that treatment of depression should improve cognitive function in patients with stroke. Although this finding has been demonstrated in anecdotal cases [18], it has not been confirmed in a controlled treatment trial. Several double-blind, randomized treatment trials have demonstrated the effectiveness of antidepressant treatment for poststroke depression [19–21]. These trials, however, either have not examined the effect of treatment of depression on cognitive function [21] or have failed to show a significant improvement in MMSE scores associated with active treatment [21,22].

We have recently completed an analysis of data combining three of our published double-blind treatment studies of poststroke depression (20) plus 5 new patients (23). Change in MMSE scores among 15 patients with major depression and 9 with major depression who responded to treatment with nortriptyline (N = 16) or placebo (N = 9) (i.e., they had >50% reduction in Hamilton depression scores and no longer met criteria for depression) were compared with 18 patients with major depression and 5 with major depression who failed to respond to nortriptyline (N = 5) or placebo (N = 18). Among responders, there was a significantly greater improvement in MMSE score than among nonresponders (3.5 point improvement in responders vs 0.3 points in nonresponders) ($P = 0.005$) (23). This result indicates that cognitive improvement was related to remission of depression, not a specific cognitive effect of nortriptyline, and is the first time that cognitive dysfunction was found to be improved by antidepressant treatment in a double-blind controlled treatment trial.

Conclusion

In conclusion, cognitive dysfunction associated with poststroke depression is a specific phenomenon related to type of depression, lesion location, and time since stroke, suggesting that a specific pathophysiological mechanism (perhaps mediated by serotonergic dysfunction) produces the clinical syndromes of major depression and cognitive dysfunction. Future studies identifying the mechanism of this cognitive dysfunction may lead to the development of specific and rational treatments targeted at the pathophysiological processes disrupted by left-hemisphere stroke.

Acknowledgments. This work was supported in part by the following NIMH grants: MH-40355, MH-52879, and MH53592.

References

1. Astrom M, Adolfsson R, Asplund K (1993) Major depression in stroke patients: a 3-year longitudinal study. Stroke 24:976–982
2. Eastwood MR, Rifat SL, Nobbs H, Ruderman J (1989) Mood disorder following cerebrovascular accident. Br J Psychiatry 154:195–200
3. Morris PLP, Robinson RG, Raphael B (1990) Prevalence and course of depressive disorders in hospitalized stroke patients. Int J Psychiatry Med 20:349–364
4. Robinson RG, Starr LB, Kubos KL, Price TR (1983) A two-year longitudinal study of poststroke mood disorders: findings during the initial evaluation. Stroke 14:736–744
5. House A, Dennis M, Warlow C (1990) The relationship between intellectual impairment and mood disorder in the first year after stroke. Psychol Med 20:805–814
6. Robinson RG, Bolla-Wilson K, Kaplan E, et al (1986) Depression influences intellectual impairment in stroke patients. Br J Psychiatry 148:541–547
7. Anderson TS, Jenkins IH, Brooks DJ, et al (1994) Cortical control of saccades and fixation in man. A PET study. Brain 117:1073–1084
8. Kiloh LG (1961) Pseudo-dementia. Acta Psychiatr Scand 37:336–351
9. Wells CE (1979) Pseudodementia. Am J Psychiatry 136:895–900
10. Caine ED (1981) Pseudodementia. Arch Gen Psychiatry 38:1359–1364
11. Starkstein SE, Rabins PV, Berthier ML, et al (1989) Dementia of depression: evidence from neurological disorders and functional depression. J Neuropsychiatry Clin Neurosci 1:263–268
12. Downhill JE Jr, Robinson RG (1994) Longitudinal assessment of depression and cognitive impairment following stroke. J Nerv Ment Dis 182:425–431
13. Wing JK, Cooper JE, Sartorius N (1974) The measurement and classification of psychiatric symptoms: an instructional manual for the PSE and CATEGO programs. Cambridge University Press, New York
14. Starkstein SE, Robinson RG, Price TR (1988) Comparison of patients with and without poststroke major depression matched for size and location of lesion. Arch Gen Psychiatry 45:247–252
15. Levine DN, Grek A (1984) The anatomic basis of delusions after right cerebral infarction. Neurology 34:577–582
16. Bolla-Wilson K, Robinson RG, Starkstein SE, et al (1989) Lateralization of dementia of depression in stroke patients. Am J Psychiatry 146:627–634
17. Folstein MF, McHugh PR (1978) Dementia syndrome of depression. In: Katzman R, Terry RD, Bick KL (eds) Aging, vol 7. Alzheimer's disease: senile dementia. Raven, New York, pp 87–93
18. Fogel BS, Sparadeo FR (1985) Focal cognitive deficits accentuated by depression. J Nerv Ment Dis 173:129–134
19. Andersen G, Vestergaard K, Lauritzen L (1984) Effective treatment of poststroke depression with the selective serotonin reuptake inhibitor citalopram. Stroke 25:1099–1104
20. Lipsey JR, Robinson RG, Pearlson GD, et al (1984) Nortriptyline treatment of poststroke depression: a double-blind study. Lancet i:297–300

21. Reding M, Orto L, Willensky P, et al (1985) The dexamethasone suppression test: an indicator of depression in stroke but not a predictor of rehabilitation outcome. Arch Neurol 42:209–212
22. Lipsey JR, Robinson RG, Pearlson GD, et al (1985) Dexamethasone suppression test and mood following stroke. Am J Psychiatry 142:318–323
23. Kimura M, Robinson RG, Kosier JT (2000) Treatment of cognitive impairment after poststroke depression; a double-blind treatment trial. Stroke 31:1482–1486

Neuropsychiatric Significance of Subcortical Encephalomalacia: Implications for Mood Disorders*

C. Edward Coffey

Summary. Subcortical hyperintensity (foci of increased signal on T_2-weighted MR imaging) is associated with aging, vascular disease, and overall medical burden. Pathological data suggest that subcortical hyperintensity reflects the effects of brain hypoperfusion to subcortical regions. In otherwise healthy aging adults, the severity of subcortical hyperintensity is associated with dysequilibrium, cognitive dysfunction, and changes in brain function (decreased coherence, regional cerebral blood flow, and cerebral metabolism). Subcortical hyperintensity is also associated with mood disorders, particularly major depression in the elderly (especially of late-age onset) and possibly also major depression and bipolar disorder in nonelderly populations. In these patients, subcortical hyperintensity is predictive of cognitive dysfunction and possibly also treatment outcomes.

Keywords. Subcortical hyperintensity, Mood disorders

Numerous magnetic resonance (MR) imaging studies have demonstrated that aging is associated with an increased prevalence and severity of subcortical hyperintensity (foci of increased signal on T_2-weighted images) (see Coffey 2000 for review). In our study of healthy adults, subcortical hyperintensity was present in the deep white matter in 48 subjects (64.0%), in the periventricular white matter in 9 (12.0%), in the basal ganglia in 9 (12.0%), in the thalamus in 4 (5.3%), and in the pons in 16 (21.3%). The odds of subcortical hyperintensity increased by 5% to 9% per year of age, depending on the anatomical region involved.

A growing body of neuropathological evidence is beginning to define the pathophysiological significance of subcortical hyperintensity (Coffey 2000). Periventricular hyperintensities in the form of caps or rims are common in healthy individuals and do not appear to constitute pathology. Histological studies suggest that these periventricular caps and rims likely reflect increased water content resulting from various factors, including a loose network of axons with low myelin content, a patchy loss of

* This chapter is adapted from Coffey CE (2000) Anatomic imaging of the human brain. In: Coffey CE, Cummings JL (eds) Textbook of geriatric neuropsychiatry, 2nd edn. American Psychiatric Press, Washington, DC, pp 181–238, with permission.

Departments of Psychiatry and of Neurology, Henry Ford Health System, Detroit, MI 48202, USA

ependyma with astrocytic gliosis ("ependymitis granularis"), and the normal convergence of flow of interstitial fluid within the periventricular region. For the more severe changes of subcortical hyperintensity, however, a spectrum of histological changes may be present that range from vascular ectasia and dilated perivascular spaces to edema and demyelination and to frank lacunar infarctions. It has been suggested that these more severe changes are a consequence of chronic brain hypoperfusion stemming from some combination of advancing arteriosclerosis, hypertensive vascular disease, chronic recurrent hypotension, cerebral amyloid angiopathy, the presence of "senile" arteriolar hyaline lesions, age-related thickening of meninges, and impaired autoregulation of cerebral circulation associated with aging. Indeed, evidence on MR imaging of old cerebral "microbleeds" is reported in approximately 6% of neuropsychiatrically normal community volunteers and is associated with more extensive subcortical hyperintensity. The prevalence and severity of subcortical hyperintensity are thus increased in the presence of risk factors for vascular disease. As conceptualized by Awad, subcortical hyperintensity in otherwise healthy older subjects may reflect the "wear and tear" of brain parenchyma that accompanies aging and chronic cerebrovascular disease. Recent data in twins suggest that genetic factors may also contibute to individual differences in volume of subcortical hyperintensity.

Although a growing literature exists with respect to the relation between cognition and changes in subcortical white matter in normal aging, these results are conflicting and the studies are difficult to compare given methodological differences (Coffey 2000). Most studies find no relation between subcortical hyperintensity and scores on dementia rating scales. Positive findings have generally been more common among studies using more focal neuropsychological assessment batteries, with measures of frontal lobe function appearing to show the closest relation with subcortical hyperintensity.

In a recent study from our laboratory, we examined the relationship between subcortical hyperintensity and two specific neuropsychological instruments—the Benton Facial Recognition Test and the WAIS-R Digit Symbol. The former was chosen because it has yielded the highest level of significance of any test reported to be associated with subcortical hyperintensity, and the latter because it has been reported to be related to subcortical hyperintensity by two independent groups. In addition, both the Benton Facial Recognition Test and the Digit Symbol subtest of the Wechsler Adult Intelligence Scale—Revised (WAIS-R) were favored a priori, because subcortical pathology might be expected to disrupt visuospatial perception and visuomotor execution, respectively. We found that performance on both tests was highly related to age and education, but not to the presence of subcortical hyperintensity. The majority of our subjects had relatively mild findings of subcortical hyperintensity, however, and it thus remains possible that more severe changes might be associated with cognitive dysfunction in otherwise healthy adults. Indeed, extensive damage to subcortical white matter tracks would disrupt frontal-subcortical circuitry and possibly provide an anatomical substrate for the mental slowing and disturbed executive functioning seen with aging.

In 1987, we reported the presence of subcortical hyperintensity in older patients with severe depression referred for electroconvulsive therapy (ECT). Since then, numerous studies have confirmed an increased prevalence and severity of subcortical hyperintensity in patients with major depression, bipolar depression, or mania, even after controlling for cardiovascular risk factors (Campbell and Coffey, in manuscript). The imaging changes affect both the subcortical white matter and the gray matter nuclei (i.e., caudate, putamen, and globus pallidus), with no clear predilection for left versus right hemisphere predominance. In contrast, no association has been found between subcortical hyperintensity and patients with schizophrenia.

The association between depression and subcortical hyperintensity is particularly strong among older patients and may be related to late-age onset of the mood disorder. No clear association has been found between the presence of subcortical hyperintensity and clinical symptoms. On neuropsychological testing, however, depressed patients with subcortical hyperintensity have greater impairment of executive function, psychomotor speed, and possibly memory. Among elderly patients with depression, subcortical hyperintensity is associated with greater impairment of both physical and instrumental activities of daily living. The outcome of depressed patients with subcortical hyperintensity has not been well studied, but some data suggest a poorer response to antidepressant medications as well as a greater occurrence of cerebral side effects from somatic treatment. In particular, subcortical hyperintensity of the basal ganglia may predict risk of delirium from either ECT or antidepressant medication, as well as a greater risk of neuroleptic-induced parkinsonism. Finally, a 2-year follow-up study found that subcortical hyperintensity was associated with both functional and cognitive decline in older patients with depression.

In summary, subcortical hyperintensity is an abnormality on MR imaging that is believed to represent a range of pathological changes secondary to cerebral hypoperfusion. As such, subcortical hyperintensity increases in prevalence and severity with age and with the presence of vascular disease. Among elderly subjects with no lifetime cerebral or psychiatric illness, subcortical hyperintensity may be associated with mild impairment of frontal lobe and executive function on neuropsychological testing. Subcortical hyperintensity occurs with a greater frequency and severity among patients with mood disorders, especially the elderly, and it may be associated with late-age onset of illness, greater cognitive and functional impairment, poorer response to antidepressant medications, a greater risk of cerebral side effects from such medications, and poorer long-term outcome. It remains unclear whether subcortical hyperintensity is a cause or an effect of mood disorders.

Reference

Coffey CE (2000) Anatomic imaging of the aging human brain. In: Coffey CE, Cummings JL (eds) Textbook of geriatric neuropsychiatry, 2nd edn. American Psychiatric Press, Washington, DC, pp 181–238

Campbell J, Coffey CE. Neuropsychiatric implications of subcortical encephalomalacia. J Neuropsychiatry Clin Neurosci (in press)

Awad IA, Johnson PC, Spetzler RF, et al (1986) Incidental subcortical lesions an magnetic resonance imaging in the elderly, II: post mortem correlations. Stroke 17:1090–1097

Clinical Characteristics of Vascular Dementia

SHOTAI KOBAYASHI, NOBUO SUYAMA, and SHUHEI YAMAGUCHI

Summary. Vascular dementia (VD) is the most common type of dementia in elderly Japanese, but recently senile dementia of Alzheimer type (SDAT) has increased with the prolongation of average life span. We investigated the characteristics of VD using a neuropsychological battery, electrophysiological examinations, and neuroimaging. VD and SDAT were diagnosed by DSM-IV and ADDTC-92. The depressive state was evaluated by Zung's self-rating depression scale. Event-related evoked potential P3 was examined using the modified odd-ball task. Visuospatial attention was evaluated by eye camera, and Regional cerebral blood flow (rCBF) was examined by SPECT. Depressive state was observed to be significantly higher in the VD group than in the SDAT group (48% vs. 25%). Latency of novelty P3, which related frontal lobe function, was significantly prolonged in VD and that of target P3, which related temporoparietal lobe function, was prolonged in SDAT. Visuospatial attention was unstable against target in VD and fixed on central target in SDAT, and the rCBF study revealed frontal dominant reduction of CBF in VD and temporoparietal reduction in SDAT. We concluded that VD is mainly characterized by frontal dysfunction caused by subcortical disconnection.

Keywords. Vascular dementia, Dementia of Alzheimer type, Subcortical dementia, Neuroimaging, Cerebral blood flow

Introduction

Vascular dementia (VD) is the most common type of dementia in Japanese elderly, but recently dementia of Alzheimer type (DAT) has increased, especially in women, with prolongation of average life span. It has been known that the characteristic feature of VD was subcortical dementia, while that of DAT was cortical dementia. We investigated the characteristics of VD using neuroimaging, electrophysiological examinations, and a neuropsychological battery.

Department of Internal Medicine III, Shimane Medical University, 89-1 Enyacho, Izumo, Shimane 693-8501, Japan

Subjects and Methods

VD and DAT were diagnosed by DSM-IV and ADDTC-92. Cognitive function was evaluated by Hasegawa's dementia rating scale (HDRS; full score, 30). Karasawa's dementia stage (stage 1–4) was used for grading of dementia.

The regional cerebral blood flow (rCBF) pattern was qualitatively evaluated by SPECT (HMPAO) in 20 VD and 36 DAT patients. Event-related evoked potential target P3 was examined using a modified odd-ball task, and novelty P3, which reflected frontal function, also examined in 16 VD and 16 DAT patients. Visuospatial attention was evaluated by eye camera. Optic fixation and gaze shift were examined in 7 VD and 7 DAT patients. Depressive state was evaluated by Zung's self-rating depression scale (SDS) in 52 VD patients and 79 DAT patients. Apathy state was evaluated in 51 VD patients and 194 nondemented stroke patients by an apathy scale [1,2].

Results

In this study, VD of multilacunar infarcts with marked frontal confluent white matter lesions (Binswanger's type) was the most common type in VD patients. SPECT study revealed frontal dominant reduction of rCBF in VD of Binswanger's type. The pattern of bilateral frontal rCBF reduction was prominent with advanced dementia stage (Fig. 1). In contrast, DAT showed temporoparietoccipital (T-P-O) rCBF reduction at early to middle stage (stage 1–3). Unilateral T-P-O rCBF reduction was more common in stage 1 than in stages 2 and 3. Frontal rCBF reduction usually developed late (Fig. 2). ERP study revealed that amplitude, latency, and scalp topography of target P3 were comparatively affected by both VD and DAT. However, the amplitude of the novelty P3 was markedly reduced in VD but not in DAT. Target P3 latency was

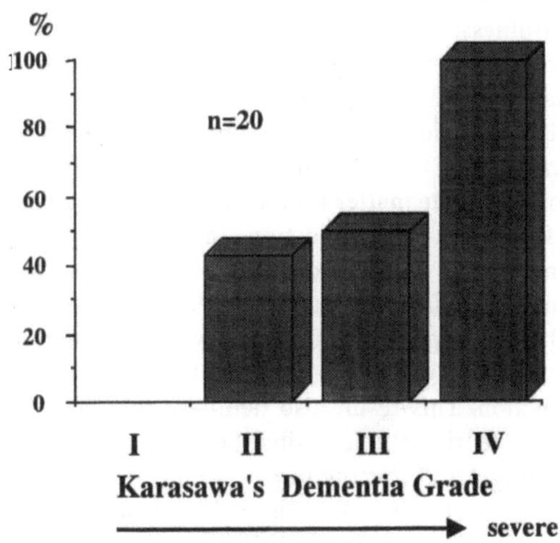

FIG. 1. Frontal cerebral blood flow (CBF) reduction in vascular dementia (VD)

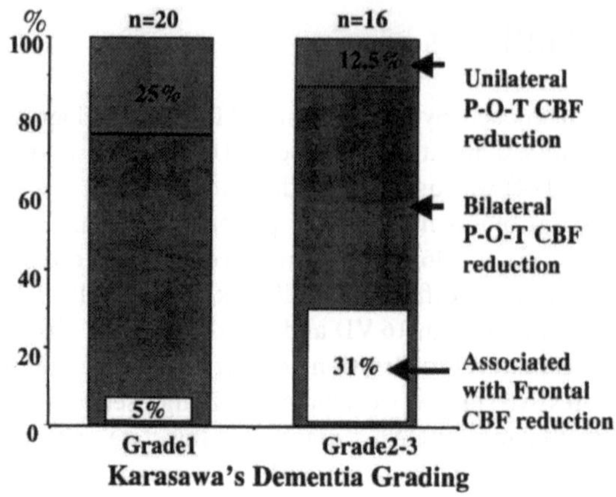

FIG. 2. SPECT pattern in dementia of Alzheimer type. *P-O-T*, parietoccipitotemporal

prolonged in both VD and DAT, whereas the novelty P3 latency was only prolonged in VD. Visuospatial attention detected by eye camera revealed hypooptic fixation for target in center and disturbance of gaze shift with fixation against shifting target in VD. In contrast, DAT showed normal on center target, but hyperfixation for shifting target. The depressive state was observed to be significantly higher in the VD group than in the DAT group (48% versus 25%). Incidence of apathetic state was significantly higher in VD than in nondemented stroke patients (68.6% versus 38.7%).

Discussion

VD is generally classified as subcortical dementia. Characteristics of subcortical dementia are forgetfulness, slowing of thought process, emotional or personality changes, and impaired ability to manipulate acquired knowledge. These disturbances are related to frontal dysfunction. In our SPECT study, VD with subcortical lesions showed frontal rCBF reduction, and this reduction pattern was prominent with advancing of dementia. This frontal rCBF reduction was thought to be caused by severe frontal subcortical white matter lesions. These lesions caused frontal hypometabolism due to functional dysconnection in the circuit between the basal ganglia/thalamus and frontal cortex. Most DAT patients showed rCBF reduction in temporoparietoccipital regions in the early to middle stage, and frontal rCBF reduction developed in the late stage. ERP studies showed low amplitude with prolonged latency of novelty P3 only in VD, not in DAT [3]. The novelty P3 is known to reflect frontal cognitive function. This result also demonstrated that VD had frontal dysfunction. Visuospatial attention studies using the eye camera showed optic hypofixation for both central target and shifting target in VD; this means that disturbance of attention and concentration exists in VD. These disturbances are known to be caused by frontal dysfunction. On the other hand, DAT showed hyperfixation on central target and disturbance of gaze shift. The extreme type of this disturbance, called the Balint syndrome, caused by bilateral temporoccipital cortical lesions. Neuropsychological study revealed that the depressive state was significantly more common in VD than in DAT. The apathetic state is also a common feature in VD. These emotional or personality changes are known to be characteristic in VD and to be related to frontal dysfunction.

We conclude that VD is characterized mainly by frontal dysfunction caused by subcortical disconnection.

References

1. Starkstein SE, Fedoroff JP, Price TR, et al (1993) Apathy following cerebrovascular lesions. Stroke 24:1625–1630
2. Okada S, Kobayashi S, Yamagata S, et al (1997) Poststroke apathy and regional cerebral blood flow. Stroke 28:2437–2441
3. Yamaguchi S, Tsuchiya H, Yamagata S, et al (1999) Event-related brain potentials in response to novel sounds in dementia. Clin Neurophysiol 111:195–203

Homocysteine as a Risk Factor for Cognitive Impairment in a Stroke Sample: Preliminary Results from the Sydney Stroke Study

PERMINDER SACHDEV, HENRY BRODATY, XING LI WANG, MICHAEL VALENZUELA, DAVID GILLIES, JEFFREY LOOI, LISA LORENTZ, DOROTA MONK, JULIANNE KINCH, LESLEY HOWARD, ALEXANDRA WALKER, RON SHNIER, ALESSANDRO ZAGAMI, and DAVID WILCKEN

Summary. It has been suggested that hyperhomocysteinemia, in addition to increasing the risk of stroke, may produce cognitive impairment independently of stroke. To determine if homocysteine levels were related to cognitive impairment that could not be accounted for by infarction, we examined stroke subjects ($n = 91$) soon after the stroke and performed detailed neuropsychological evaluations and MRI scans 3 months later. Control subjects ($n = 17$) were similarly assessed. Total homocysteine (tHcy) levels at baseline were significantly higher in the stroke sample, and had an inverse relationship with acute stage MMSE scores, which became stronger with higher tHcy levels, but not after accounting for other risk factors: B_{12} and folate levels, and stroke volume. When the stroke patients were divided into two groups (cognitively impaired and unimpaired) on the basis of the 3-month data, the former group had significantly more subjects with tHcy levels >20 µmol/l. Factor III from the analysis of the neuropsychological data, which was interpreted as a frontal-attentional factor, had a significant correlation with tHcy levels ($r = 0.47$, $P < 0.001$), and this correlation was significant after correction for age, folate levels, stroke volume, and white matter hyperintensity scores on MRI. Our findings suggest that hyperhomocysteinemia not only increases the risk of stroke but leads to greater cognitive impairment in stroke patients.

Keywords. Homocysteine, Stroke, Cognitive impairment, Vascular dementia

Introduction

Homocysteine is an amino acid in the intermediate metabolism of methionine, an essential amino acid in both animal and plant proteins. Hyperhomocysteinemia has recently been identified as an important risk factor for the development of atherosclerotic vascular disease (Mayer et al. 1996). The abnormality can be detected in up to 30% of patients with coronary artery disease (CAD) and 42% of patients with cerebrovascular disease (CVD) (Stein and McBride 1998). In the European Concerted

Schools of Psychiatry and Medicine, University of New South Wales; Neuropsychiatric Institute, Psychiatry of Old Age, Institute of Neurological Sciences, and Department of Cardiovascular Genetics, The Prince of Wales Hospital, & St George MRI Centre, Sydney, Australia

Action Project (Graham et al. 1997), the magnitude of increased risk for vascular disease associated with hyperhomocysteinemia (odds ratio, OR, highest to lower quintiles, 2.2) was higher than that of hypercholesterolemia (OR 1.4), less than that for hypertension (OR 3.9), and similar to that for tobacco use (OR 2.2). Homocysteine promotes atherosclerosis by producing endothelial cell injury, increasing platelet aggregation, and affecting the clotting cascade.

More recently, it has been argued that hyperhomocysteinemia may produce cognitive impairment independently of stroke. Clarke et al. (1998) demonstrated in 164 Alzheimer's disease (AD) subjects, 76 of whom were autopsy-confirmed AD, that elevated homocysteine levels and stable over time; 45% of AD subjects were in the top tertile of the control distribution (>14 μmol/l). In a study of elderly patients referred to a memory clinic (Lehmann et al. 1999), homocysteine was found to be an independent predictor of mini-mental state scores after correcting for age, B_{12}, and folate levels.

If homocysteine promotes cognitive impairment and is a risk factor for AD, it has important epidemiological implications, not only because abnormalities are common but also because treatment with folate, B_{12}, and pyridoxine can significantly lower plasma homocysteine levels. In this study, we examined plasma homocysteine levels in a sample of stroke patients who were investigated soon after the stroke and at 3 months; the examination included a detailed neuropsychological assessment and a brain MRI scan. The aim was to determine if there was an association between homocysteine levels and cognition and if this could be accounted for by infarct size or small vessel disease.

Methods

Sample

Subjects ($n = 91$) were consecutive admissions to the stroke units of two large general hospitals in Sydney who had recently suffered a stroke, did not have a diagnosis of dementia or other neurological disorder, and were well enough to consent to participate. They had a baseline assessment within 1 week of admission that included a detailed medical history and examination, history of risk factors for CVD and AD, a functional assessment, and laboratory investigations including total homocysteine (tHcy), serum B_{12} and folate levels, and plasma fibrinogen. Between 3 and 6 months after the stroke, they had a detailed neuropsychological assessment and the majority had a brain MRI scan. Healthy control subjects ($n = 17$) were recruited from the community and similarly assessed.

Homocysteine Measurement

Fasting blood was collected and centrifuged as soon as possible. The plasma was stored at −20°C for later analysis. Total Hcy was measured using a fluorescence-based immunochemical technique with demonstrated high repeatability.

MRI Scans

MRI was performed on a 1.5-T Signa GE magnet and the following protocol: a scout midsagittal cut (2-D, TR 300 ms, TE 14 ms; thk 5 mm, nex 1.5); 1.5-mm-thick T_1-

weighted contiguous coronal sections through whole brain using a FSPGR sequence and 3-D acquisition (TR 14.3 ms, TE 5.4 ms); 4-mm-thick T_2-weighted FLAIR coronal slices through whole brain (TR 8900, TE 145, TI 2200, FOV 25, 256 × 192).

Neuropsychological Test Battery

The following tests were used: WMS-R (Mental Control, Logical Memory I, Visual Reproduction I); WAIS-R (Block Design, Arithmetic, Digit Span, Similarities); WMS-R (Logical Memory II, Visual Reproduction II); BREAK (15 min); NART-R; Trail Making Test; Simple Copying; Reaction Time (simple and complex); Colour Form Sorting Test; Token Test; Ideomotor Apraxia; Boston Naming Test; FAS—Animals; Identities and Oddities; Sentence Repetition; Stereognosis, Finger Gnosis; and Symbol Digit Modality Test (oral).

Analysis

Hcy levels were first correlated with MMSE scores in the acute phase, both for the whole sample and for those with high levels. The model implying that tHcy affected MMSE scores not directly but through an increase in stroke volume, and the effect of tHcy independently of B_{12} and folate levels, was examined. Stroke volume was measured for each infarct and additive volume obtained. Stroke load was rated as follows: 0, nil; 1, single lacuna; 2, large lacuna or multiple small lacunae; 3, large stroke. The analysis was repeated for the 3-month neuropsychological performance. The neuropsychological data were reduced using a factor analysis, yielding a four-factor solution. The stroke sample was classified into vascular dementia (VaD), vascular cognitive impairment (VCI), and no cognitive impairment (NCI) groups based on test performance, and intergroup comparisons were made.

Results

The characteristics of the sample are described in Table 1. tHcy was significantly higher in the stroke sample. There was an inverse relationship between tHcy levels and acute stage MMSE scores, which became stronger with higher tHcy levels. For subjects in the top 50% of levels, $r = 0.4$, with the top 10% having a correlation coefficient of $r = 0.85$. In a regression model, tHcy levels were significant predictors of stroke load after B_{12} and folate levels, and CVD risk factor scores were added as covariates (R^2 change = 0.17, $P < 0.01$). However, when risk factor, B_{12}, and folate levels and stroke volume were entered, tHcy levels were not significant predictors of MMSE scores ($P = 0.52$). Although the stroke subjects had significantly higher tHcy levels than controls, the VaD (31%), VCI (23%), and NCI (46%) groups did not differ from each other. When the stroke patients were divided into two groups—impaired (VaD and VCI) and unimpaired (NCI)—the former group had significantly more subjects with tHcy levels >20 μmol/l. Factor III from the analysis of the neuropsychological data, which was interpreted as a frontal-attentional factor (Table 2), had a significant correlation with tHcy levels ($r = 0.47$, $P < .001$) (Fig. 1), and this correlation was significant after correction for age ($r = 0.43$, $P < 0.05$), folate levels ($r = 0.40$, $P < 0.05$),

TABLE 1. Characteristics of the sample

	Stroke	Controls
Socioemographic		
N	91	17
Age (years)	73.5	72.0
Gender (%M)	63	50
Education (years)	10.2	10.9
Blood assay		
tHcy	20.1 (7.8)	13.7 (3.6)*
B_{12}	270.8 (119.2)	274.2 (86.9)
Folate	20.2 (10.1)	23.4 (10.0)
Creatinine	0.10 (0.05)	0.14 (0.02)
Fibrinogen	4.87 (1.5)	4.14 (0.7)
Cognitive function		
MMSE	26.5	29.7*
Genetics		
MTHFR homozygote frequency	10%	—
Apo E4 frequency	24%	—

tHcy, total homocysteine; MMSE, Folstein's mini-mental state examination score; MTHFR, methylene tetra hydrofolate reductase
* $P < 0.05$

TABLE 2. Structural loading on factor III of neuropsychological function (global attention & frontal function factor)

Trails A, 0.89
Trails B, 0.86
Symbol digit, −0.73
Category fluency, −0.71
Logical memory II, −0.63
Picture completion, −0.61
Visual reproduction II, −0.61

Whole group correlation HCY and factor III = 0.47 ($P < 0.001$)

stroke volume ($r = 0.49$, $P < 0.05$) and white matter hyperintensity scores on FLAIR sequences ($r = 0.51$, $P < 0.05$).

Discussion

We have presented preliminary findings leading to the following conclusions: (i) tHcy levels are high in stroke patients; (ii) high tHcy levels are related to increased stroke volumes; and (iii) after accounting for confounding factors such as age, B_{12} and folate levels, and stroke volume, tHcy has a correlation with cognitive impairment. The risk with Hcy appears to be graded, with increased levels leading to greater dysfunction. The high-tHcy group (>14 μmol/l) were 2.6 times more likely to be in the worse half of cognitive performance. A limitation of our study was the small size of the control group, as further data are being collected. A further limitation was that blood

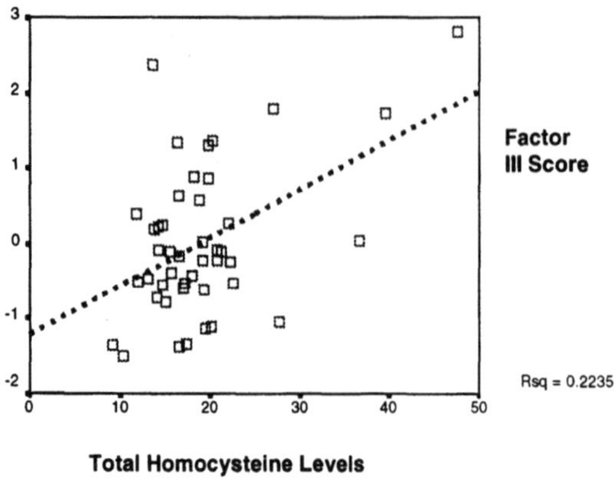

FIG. 1. Correlation of total homocysteine levels and factor III of neuropsychological performance for whole group

sampling was done at two sites, and although most samples were centrifuged within 1 h, there were occasional differences at one site (up to 2 h). The levels obtained in the subjects from the two sites did not differ significantly, however, thus suggesting a lack of systematic error.

If Hcy has a deleterious effect on cognition, what are the possible mechanisms? Hcy and its metabolite, homocysteic acid, are excitotoxic and lead to NMDA receptor activation and possibly cellular apoptosis. The mechanism may alternately be an increase in infarct size because of a large penumbra, which MRI may not be able to assess. It is also possible that high Hcy leads to small embolic infarcts that are hard to detect. Our study does not support the idea that Hcy is associated with in vivo microvascular disease as detected by signal hyperintensities on T_2-weighted MRI. Our findings need replication in view of the implications that folate and B_{12} supplementation may reverse a seemingly important cause of cognitive impairment.

Acknowledgments. The authors are grateful to Drs. M. Hersch, D. Pryor, R. Johnston, J. Enis and the neurologists at Prince of Wales Hospital for permission to study their patients; D. Hadzi-Pavlovic for statistical advice; and SEALS Laboratories for assistance in blood collection.

References

Clarke R, Smith AD, Jobst KA, et al (1998) Folate, vitamin B_{12}, and serum total homocysteine levels in confirmed Alzheimer disease. Arch Neurol 55:1449–1455

Graham I, Daly LE, Refsum HM, et al (1997) Plasma homocysteine as a risk factor for vascular disease: the European Concerted Action Project. JAMA 277:1775–1781

Mayer EL, Jacobsen DW, Robinson K (1996) Homocysteine and coronary atherosclerosis. J Am Coll Cardiol 27:517–527

Stein JH, McBride PE (1998) Hyperhomocysteinemia and atherosclerotic vascular disease: pathophysiology, screening and treatment. Arch Int Med 158:1301–1306

Neuroimaging and Pathological Correlates of Dementia Associated with Subcortical Ischemic Vascular Disease (SIVD)

HELENA CHUI[1], GEORGE FEIN[2], DANIEL MUNGAS[3], WILLIAM JAGUST[3], MIKE WEINER[2], and HARRY VINTERS[4]

Summary. Initial neuroimaging and neuropathological findings are reported from an ongoing, longitudinal study of dementia associated with subcortical ischemic vascular disease (SVID) and Alzheimer's disease (AD). Quantitative MRI studies identify hippocampal and neocortical atrophy, rather than subcortical lacunes and WML, to be the major determinants of dementia associated with SIVD. Autopsy findings suggest that hippocampal atrophy in SIVD results from a mixture of degenerative and ischemic pathologies. The cause of neocortical atrophy in SIVD remains unknown, correlates with the volume of WML, and does not necessarily reflect the presence of AD. For the practicing clinician, the presence of hippocampal and neocortical atrophy cannot be regarded as specific evidence for AD.

Keywords. Quantitative MRI, Atrophy, Hippocampus, Cortical, Vascular dementia

Introduction

The cause of cognitive impairment associated with subcortical ischemic vascular disease (SIVD) is subject to debate; inferences are often drawn from neuroimaging findings. Two obvious structural lesions appear as bright signals on proton density (PD) magnetic resonance imaging (MRI): discrete hyperintensities, ranging from 3 to 15 mm in diameter, are labeled lacunes (L); diffuse-confluent hyperintensities in the periventricular and deep white matter are labeled WML. According to the lacunar hypothesis, the number, size, and location of lacunes determine the likelihood, nature, and severity of cognitive impairment. A review of the literature suggests that when WML become confluent, slowing can be detected in cognitive and motor performance. Thus, lacunes in strategic locations and, to a lesser extent, confluent WML are important causes of cognitive impairment.

[1] Department of Neurology, University of Southern California, Los Angeles, CA, USA
[2] Psychiatry Research and Magnetic Resonance Unit, Department of Veterans Affairs Medical Center, and the Departments of Radiology and Psychiatry, University of California, San Francisco, CA, USA
[3] Department of Neurology, University of California, Davis, CA, USA
[4] Department of Pathology, University of California, Los Angeles, CA, USA

A definitive diagnosis of AD depends on the discovery of widespread neurofibrillary tangles and neuritic plaques at the time of autopsy. The absence of a specific premortem test for Alzheimer's disease (AD) also limits the accuracy of the clinical diagnosis of vascular dementia (VaD). Sudden onset, stepwise decline, focal neurological signs or symptoms, clinical stroke with temporal relation to onset of dementia, infarcts in strategic locations, or extensive WML are thought to increase the likelihood of VaD. Slowly progressive dementia, hippocampal atrophy, and cortical atrophy, on the other hand, are thought to increase the likelihood of AD. The specificity of the latter imaging features for differentiating AD from VaD, however, has not been adequately tested.

We report initial neuroimaging and pathological findings from an ongoing, multicenter, longitudinal study of cognitive impairment associated with SIVD. Three questions are addressed in the current report:

1. Among individuals with lacunes, what neuroimaging measures differentiate those who are cognitively normal (CN) versus those who are cognitively impaired (CI) versus demented (D)?
2. Among individuals with AD and SIVD, what neuroimaging measures predict severity and type of cognitive impairment?
3. Is cognitive impairment or dementia among patients with lacunes simply caused by concomitant AD?

Several of these findings have been accepted for publication as full-length manuscripts (Fein et al., 2000; Vinters et al., 2000). Key results are summarized here.

Materials and Methods

The sample comprises subjects with cognitive impairment attributed to either SIVD or AD and normal controls. Subjects were recruited from University-affiliated memory clinics; normal controls were recruited from the community. Inclusion criteria included age >55 years and Clinical Dementia Rating Score (CDR) ≤2 (Hughes et al. 1982). Subjects with dementia met National Institute of Neurological Communicative Disorders and Stroke—Alzheimer Disease and Related Disorders Association (NINCDS-ADRDA) criteria for probable or possible AD (McKhann et al. 1984) or ADDTC criteria for probable or possible SIVD (Chui et al. 1992). Exclusionary criteria included cognitive impairment due to causes other than AD or SIVD and evidence of cortical infarcts or intracerebral hemorrhage. Subjects were further classified into six groups, based on CDR score and the presence or absence of lacunes: cognitively normal (CN), cognitively normal with lacune (CN + L), cognitive impaired (CI), cognitively impaired with lacune (CI + L), demented (D), and demented with lacune (D + L). Neuropsychological and MRI are repeated prospectively. Final diagnosis incorporates autopsy findings when available.

MRI Variables

The following MR images were acquired on a 1.5 T (Siemens or GE Signa) system: axial proton density and T_2-weighted slices (3 mm thick); coronal T_1-weighted 3D MP RAGE (1.4 mm thick). Using automated segmentation software developed in house, followed by hand editing, intracranial content tissues were separated into the following six compartments: ventricular and sulcal cerebrospinal fluid (CSFv and CSFs), cortical and subcortical gray matter (GMc, GMsc), and normal and abnormal white matter (WM and WML). To estimate hippocampal volume (HV), the MP RAGE sequences were resliced perpendicular to the long axis of the hippocampus and the boundaries of the hippocampus were traced manually. Noncystic lacunes were defined as lesions 3–1.5 mm in diameter that are bright on PD MR. Lacunes were subcategorized by the following locations: caudate, putamen, thalamus, internal capsule, and white matter (Fein et al., 2000).

Neuropsychological Variables

The neuropsychological test battery included the Mattis Dementia Rating Scale (MDRS), Wechsler attention quotient, word learning list, Biber figural learning test, token test, Boston naming test, FAS and animal fluency tests, and finger tapping.

Neuropathological Diagnoses

At the time of death, the brain was removed, weighed, and fixed in 10% neutral buffered formalin. Two weeks later the brain was sectioned coronally into 0.5-mm-thick slices. Tissues were blocked, dehydrated, embedded in paraffin, sectioned at 10 μm, and stained with hematoxylin and eosin, cresyl violet, thioflavine, Bielschowsky silver, and antibodies against ubiquitin and glial fibrillary associated protein. Assessment of AD lesions was performed using Braak & Braak staging (Braak et al. 1993) and CERAD criteria (Mirra et al. 1991). Two scores were generated to rate the severity and distribution of ischemic brain injury: a CVD score reflects the severity of lesions throughout the brain, and an IVD score reflects the severity of lesions in brain regions considered important for behavior and cognition (Chui et al. 1999; Vinters et al., 2000).

Results

Question 1: Among Individuals with Lacunes, What Neuroimaging Measures Differentiate Those Who Are Cognitively Normal (CN) Versus Cognitively Impaired (CI) Versus Demented (D)?

The study sample comprised five groups (Fein et al., 2000). Three groups had lacunes or evidence of SIVD: CN + L ($n = 27$), CI + L ($n = 26$), and D + L ($n = 29$). Two groups without lacunes served as comparison groups: D (all met NINDCS-ADRDA criteria for probable AD, $n = 28$) and CN (cognitively normal controls). The comparison groups were matched to the corresponding SIVD groups by age, gender, and education; the AD group was also matched by Mini-Mental State Exam (MMSE score). HV, GMc, CSFv, and WML explained 38.1%, 17.9%, 35.8%, and 9.3% of the variance among the three SIVD groups and 49%, 42.7%, 31.6%, and 25.1% of the variance between the D + L and the CN groups. HV, GMc, and CSFv accounted for 62.3%, 24%, and 13% of the variance between the prAD and the CN groups. In SIVD, WML correlated with

GMc. Among the three SIVD groups, no significant differences were found in either the number or volume of lacunes.

Question 2: Among Individuals with AD and SIVD, What Neuroimaging Measures Predict Severity and Type of Cognitive Impairment?

Preliminary correlations were performed between brain volume and neuropsychological performance among 163 study subjects: CN = 51, CN + L = 34, CI = 10, CI + L = 25, D = 21, and D + L = 22 (D. Mungas, 2000, personal communication). There were 86 men and 77 women; their mean age was 74.2 ± 7.7 (range, 55–91) years. Mean education was 14.6 ± 3.2 years (range, 5–21 years). Table 1 shows the standardized beta values for multiple regression analyses in which gender, education, age, thalamic lacune volume, WML, GMc, and HV served as the independent variables. Education, but not age or gender, was an important predictor of neuropsychological performance. Both GMc and HV were strongly correlated with overall severity of dementia (total MDRS). HV, but not GMc, correlated with list recall and category fluency. WML was weakly correlated with letter and category fluency (both timed tests). No significant correlations were found for volume of thalamic lacunes.

Question 3: Is Cognitive Impairment or Dementia Among Patients with Lacunes Simply Caused by Concomitant AD?

Autopsies have been performed for 25 cases: 14 cases with lacunes (2 CN + L, 3 CI + L, 9 D + L) and 11 without lacunes (6 CN, 1 CI, 4 D) (Vinters et al., 2000). Of the 14 cases with clinical SIVD, all showed evidence of ischemic parenchymal brain injury. Some had evidence of hippocampal neurofibrillary tangles (Braak & Braak stage ≤4) or hippocampal sclerosis, but only 1 showed isocortical AD pathology (Braak & Braak stage ≥5). These preliminary findings confirm that cognitive impairment and dementia occur among patients with SIVD, without evidence of significant AD pathology in

TABLE 1. Multiple regression analysis: standardized beta values ($n = 163$)

	MDRS (total)	MDRS (I-P)	BNT	MAS (list recall)	Letter fluency	Category fluency
Gender	−0.4	−0.10	0.18*	−0.01	−0.06	0.00
Education	0.28****	0.22***	0.22**	0.21***	0.32****	0.27****
Age	0.04	0.10	−0.08	0.05	0.12	−0.03
Thalamic L	−0.11	0.19	−0.11	−0.03	−0.05	−0.06
WML	−0.02	−0.15	0.01	−0.06	−0.18*	−0.19*
GMc	0.38****	0.34***	0.28**	0.14	0.21	0.13
HV	0.33****	0.26**	0.26**	0.56****	0.11	0.33****

MDRS, Mattis Dementia Rating Scale; I-P, initiation and perseveration subtests; BNT, Boston naming test; MAS, Memory Assessment Scales; Thalamic L, thalamic lacune volume; WML, abnormal white matter volume; GMc, cortical gray matter volume; HV, hippocampal volume

* $P < 0.05$, ** $P < 0.01$, *** $P < 0.001$, **** $P < 0.0001$

From D. Mungas 2000 (personal communication)

the neocortex. A mixture of degenerative and vascular pathology, however, was frequently seen in the hippocampus.

Discussion

These initial findings identify hippocampal and cortical atrophy, rather than the more obvious subcortical lesions (i.e., lacunes and WML), as the predominant determinants of dementia associated with SIVD. Hippocampal atrophy correlates with impairment of secondary memory and may reflect a combination of ischemic and neurodegenerative pathologies. The cause of neocortical atrophy in SIVD remains unclear; it cannot be simply explained by concomitant AD pathology. In SIVD, WML predicts cortical atrophy and, to some extent, behavior (i.e., weakly correlated with impaired verbal fluency). Thus, it is possible that WML is a more useful marker for pathophysiological processes leading to widespread atrophy than for altered cognition.

The pathogenesis of dementia associated with SIVD may be complex and multifactorial. Dementia sometimes may reflect the multifocal effects of discrete lacunes (evidence coming from case studies in the literature, but not shown here). More often, it may be related to still poorly understood pathophysiological processes leading to hippocampal and diffuse neocortical atrophy. These findings complicate clinical diagnosis, as neither hippocampal nor cortical atrophy can be regarded as specific evidence of AD.

Acknowledgments. This work was supported by the National Institutes of Health (P01 AG12435) and the Alzheimer Program of State of California Department of Health Services.

References

Braak H, Braak E, Bohl J (1993) Staging of Alzheimer-related cortical destruction. Eur Neurol 33:403–408

Chui HC, Victoroff JI, Margolin D, et al (1992) Criteria for the diagnosis of ischemic vascular dementia proposed by the State of California Alzheimer Disease Diagnostic and Treatment Centers (ADDTC). Neurology 42:473–480

Chui H, Zarow C, Ellis W, et al (1999) Diagnosis of ischemic vascular dementia (IVD): clinical pathological correlations. In: Korczyn AD (ed) 1st international conference on vascular dementia. Monduzzi Editore, Bologna, pp 27–32

Fein G, Di Sclafani V, Tanabe J, et al (2000) Hippocampal and cortical atrophy, not lacunes correlate with dementia in subcortical ischemic vascular disease. Neurology 55:1626–1635

Hughes CP, Berg L, Danziger W, et al (1982) A new clinical scale for the staging of dementia. Br J Psychiatry 140:566–572

McKhann G, Drachman D, Folstein M, et al (1984) Clinical diagnosis of Alzheimer's disease: report of the NINCDS-ADRDA Work Group under the auspices of Department of Health and Human Services Task Force on Alzheimer's Disease. Neurology 34:939–944

Mirra SS, Heyman A, McKeel D, et al (1991) The Consortium to Establish a Registry for Alzheimer's Disease (CERAD). Part II. Standardization of the neuropathologic assessment of Alzheimer's disease. Neurology 41:479–486

Vinters H, Ellis W, Zarow C, et al (2000) Neuropathologic substrates of ischemic vascular dementia. J Neuropathol Exp Neurol 59:931–945

Clinical Variability of Frontotemporal Dementia

LARS GUSTAFSON[1], ULLA PASSANT[1], ANNE GRÄSBECK[1], and ARNE BRUN[2]

Summary. Frontotemporal dementia (FTD) is the second most common primary degenerative dementia with early onset and constitutes about 9% of dementia cases examined post mortem. The clinical picture is related to the distribution and severity of the degenerative changes. This chapter analyzes neuropathologically verified cases of Pick's disease (PiD) and frontal lobe degeneration of non-Alzheimer type (FLD) with regard to heredity and clinical features. When the two groups were compared, there was a female dominance in the PiD group, whereas the FLD group showed a stronger load of heredity concerning similar dementia disorders. A general impression was that symptoms were more prevalent and severe in the PiD group, which is consistent with the more severe atrophy in these cases. In frontotemporal dementia (FTD), as in other dementias, there is a need for a multidimensional classification system, keeping apart etiological, morphological, and clinical aspects. This approach allows flexibility and new combinations that facilitates study and understanding of the nature of FTD.

Keywords. Frontotemporal dementia, Pick's disease, Classification, Frontal lobe degeneration of non-Alzheimer type

The story of the syndrome of frontotemporal dementia (FTD) started when Arnold Pick (1892) pointed out the relationship between circumscribed lobar atrophy and aphasia and behavioral changes in dementia, thereby contributing to the evolution of modern neuropsychiatry. Arnold Pick's first cases showed mainly temporal lobe involvement, and the association with frontal lobe atrophy appeared in later publications. The histopathological account for lobar atrophy was given by Alzheimer (1911), and the clinicopathological entity of Pick's disease (PiD) was established in the 1920s by Onari and Spartz (1926) and Stertz (1926). A long series of researchers have elaborated on the clinical and pathological variability of this disease and its differentiation from Alzheimer's disease (AD). Van Mansfelt (1954) reviewed 196 cases of PiD reported in the literature and found an important variation of pathology with frontotemporal atrophy in 54%, mainly frontal atrophy in 25% and temporal atrophy in

Departments of Psychogeriatrics[1] and Pathology[2], University Hospital, SE-221 85 Lund, Sweden

17%. Cortical atrophy was asymmetrical with left-side predominance in 46% and right-side predominance in 17%.

One reason for the 1986 conference in Lund on "Frontal Lobe Degeneration of Non-Alzheimer Type (FLD)" was the recognition of the large number of cases with degenerative frontal lobe dementia lacking the specific histopathology of PiD and AD (Gustafson 1987). Frontotemporal dementia (FTD) was diagnosed post mortem in 9% of 400 consecutive cases in a prospective longitudinal study of dementia. The neuropathology was based on semiserial coronal sectioning of the whole brain, thus allowing the description of all types of pathology in the individual cases. So far we have included more than 140 FTD cases in our longitudinal study: 55 of these cases have been verified post mortem, 42 cases have been followed up until death but without postmortem examination, and the remaining 44 cases are still alive and being studied prospectively. Several research groups came to similar conclusions in the 1980s concerning the prevalence of degenerative dementia of frontal lobe type, and in 1994 the Manchester and Lund research groups published a consensus statement on clinical and pathological criteria for FTD (Brun et al. 1994). The consensus presents the most prevalent and typical clinical features in three neuropathological types of FTD: PiD, FLD, and motor neuron disease with dementia (MNDD). PiD is characterized by circumscribed lobar atrophy involving all cortical layers and the characteristic inflated neurons and argyrophilic globes called Pick bodies (Brun et al. 1994; Rossor 1999). In FLD, the degeneration is frontal or frontotemporal with neuronal loss, microvacuolization, and gliosis of cortical layers I to III (Brun 1987). These changes are similar to the frontal lobe pathology in MNDD.

An important question is to what extent clinical variability within the FTD group can be explained by differences in histopathology, topography, and genetics of the degenerative process. This chapter analyzes the clinical differences between PiD and FLD in 8 PiD and 32 FLD cases with neuropathologically verified diagnoses (Table 1). There were more female cases in the Pick group and an equal sex distribution in the FLD group. Age at onset was similar, but the duration of dementia was somewhat longer in PiD. Heredity of a similar dementia disorder was more common in the FLD group compared with the Pick group (53% and 38%, respectively), indicating that genetic factors are more important in FLD than in PiD. So far, no family with neuropathologically verified PiD and FLD has been described.

The early clinical symptoms were similar in FLD and PiD, although certain symptoms such as confabulation and disinhibition were more common in PiD; this is also the case for affective symptoms. Antidepressant medication, elated mood, and restlessness were somewhat more prevalent in PiD, whereas verbal aggressiveness as well as acts of violence were as prevalent in both patient groups. Delusions mostly of the paranoid type were reported in 38% and 28% of the FLD and PiD groups. Psychotic symptoms in general are badly controlled and are difficult to treat in FTD with psychological and pharmacological strategies. Progressive dynamic aphasia was observed in all patients in both groups and echolalia in 50% of PiD and 30% in FLD. Finally, all patients became mute but the ability to understand information often remained late, as did also practical abilities and spatial orientation. Hypomimia was a consistent late clinical feature in both patient groups. Components of the Klüver–Bucy syndrome such as hyperorality and bulimia were more prevalent in PiD, and utilization behavior was observed in about 35% of both groups. EEG remained normal in the

TABLE 1. Clinical characteristics in Pick's disease and frontal lobe degeneration of non-Alzheimer type (FLD) verified post mortem

	Pick's disease (*n* = 8)		FLD (*n* = 32)	
Sex (M/F)	1/7		15/17	
Age at onset (yr)	54.1 ± 9.6	(34–65)	53.2 ± 8.8	(35–70)
Age at death (yr)	65.1 ± 10.2	(42–72)	61.9 ± 9.1	(41–77)
Duration (yr)	11.0 ± 4.1	(5–17)	8.7 ± 4.5	(3–18)
Heredity for dementia (*n*)	3	38%	17	53%
Early features	*n*	%	*n*	%
Insidious onset	8	100	32	100
Loss of insight	8	100	26	81
Loss of social awareness	6	75	22	69
Disinhibition	6	75	19	59
Memory impairment	4	50	14	44
Confabulation	4	50	5	16
Depression	3	38	11	34
Antidepressant agents	5	63	11	34
Speech disorder	*n*	%	*n*	%
Decreased verbal output	8	100	29	91
Echolalia	4	50	11	34
Mutism	8	100	27	84
Klüver–Bucy Syndrome	*n*	%	*n*	%
Hyperorality	8	100	16	50
Bulimia	6	75	12	38
Hypersexuality	1	13	4	13
Utilization behavior	3	38	11	34
Physical signs	*n*	%	*n*	%
Normal EEG despite dementia	8	100	25	78
Dysphagia	3	38	15	47

majority of cases. Increased muscular tension was more common in PiD, and surprisingly many FTD patients developed dysphagia.

Thus, there were clinical similarities but also differences between individual cases and between the two most common histopathologically different types of FTD. The clinical differences could often be explained by variation in localization and severity of brain pathology against the background of a common pattern of cortical involvement. A general impression is, however, that symptoms were more prevalent and severe in the Pick group, which is consistent with the more severe atrophy. The clinical variation within the Pick group also seemed strongly related to the distribution of degenerative changes. Memory failure in PiD was most pronounced in cases with severe hippocampal degeneration, and parkinsonism, when present in PiD, showed strong correlation with nigral involvement. The dyspraxia and disorientation observed late in the course of PiD were associated with a more pronounced parietal lobe degeneration. The anterior–posterior gradient as well as laterality of degenerative brain changes influences the clinical picture in FTD. Consequently, left and right frontal variants (Gregory 1999) as well as left and right temporal clinical variants

(Edwards-Lee et al. 1997) of FTD have been described and related to brain dysfunction, as shown with functional and structural brain imaging.

There are important similarities between the progressive dynamic aphasia at an early stage of FTD and the clinical spectrum of progressive nonfluent aphasia (PA) as described by Mesulam (1982), Snowden and Neary (1993), and others. Language disturbances and relative preservation of memory and practical abilities characterize PA. This syndrome, also known as semantic dementia, has been included in the 1998 consensus on frontotemporal lobar degeneration (FTLD) by Neary et al. (1998). Ultimately, many PA cases developed FTD with the same degenerative process mainly restricted to the middle and anterior temporal gyri. In our study, 65% of the Pick cases and 40% of the FLD patients started with personality changes in combination with a disorder of expressive language. Other aspects of cognitive failure, although often present, were less pronounced.

MNDD has been described, mostly in Japan, by Mitsuyama (1979) and Morita et al. (1987) but also in the UK (Neary et al. 1990) and other countries. The prevalence of dementia in MND is difficult to determine because of insufficient clinical information and the presence of emotional reactions, dysarthria, and other neurological deficits in the individual case. The clinical picture is similar to that of FLD, and the diagnosis is based on recognition of a rapidly progressive dementia of frontal lobe type in combination with physical signs of anterior horn involvement. Functional brain imaging shows predominant precentral pathology whereas the EEG may remain normal.

The etiology of FTD is unknown, but there is strong evidence for genetic factors and linkage to chromosome 17 (Wilhelmsen and Clark 1998; Chow et al. 1999) and chromosome 3 (Brown et al. 1995; Ashworth et al. 1999). Several studies have identified families with FTDP (frontotemporal dementia with parkinsonism) linked to chromosome 17 and the tau gene (Hong et al. 1998; Hutton et al. 1998). Mutations in this gene have, however, also been linked to familial forms of progressive subcortical gliosis and progressive supranuclear palsy. Studies have also shown clinical heterogeneity within families with chromosome 17-linked dementia.

The analysis of clinical data from a Swedish family with FLD verified in five cases in the third generation has shown several common features but also individual traits (Passant et al. 1993). The pedigree contains 18 individuals in the second and the third generation; 2 of 6 men and 9 of 12 women developed FTD. Age at onset was 43 and 46 years in men and between 50 and 68 years among women. The average duration among females was 10 years, with a wide range from 3 to 21 years. The males were more similar in this respect with a duration of 15 and 17 years. The neuropathological examination showed frontotemporal or frontal and anterior cingulate involvement. The degeneration of hippocampus and substantia nigra varied markedly in accordance with the presence of memory failure and extrapyramidal features within the group. These findings strongly support the close association between the clinical picture and brain pathology.

The clinical classification of dementia, as that of mental disorder in general, is a controversial issue. It is based on our current knowledge of etiology, clinical manifestations, and brain pathology as shown with neuropathological, biochemical (Pasquier and Delacourte 1998; Procter et al. 1999), and neuroimaging techniques (Miller and Gearhart 1999) (Fig. 1). New classifications should, however, take into

Histopathology:
Frontal lobe degeneration of non-Alzheimer type (FLD)
Pick's disease
motor neuron disease with dementia

Biochemistry:
Neurotransmitter failure
Tau pathology

Topography:
Predominant localization frontotemporal, frontal, temporal, asymmetrical

Genetics:
Familial, sporadic
Mutations of chromosome 3, 17 (tau mutaitons, FTDP-17)

Early and/or predominant features and clinical course

FIG. 1. Clinical variability of FTD is related to these factors

consideration previous diagnostic principles and entities. On the other hand, it is important to encourage the search for new clinically relevant entities. Several clinical variants of FTD have been recognized and related to pathology and genetics. A problem is, however, that many patients with FTD present symptoms and signs for a period of 10, 20, and even more years before they die. They are passing through several clinical stages with a changing clinical picture, and the duration may vary markedly. The clinical variants we are talking of today are mainly based on the early clinical manifestations and less on symptoms and treatment problems appearing at later stages of the disease. These questions deserve more attention because of the increasing possibilities of early diagnosis and the development of new forms of treatment and care.

References

Alzheimer A (1911) Über eigenartige Krankheitsfälle des späteren Alters. Z Gesamte Neurol Psychiatr 4:356–385

Ashworth A, Lloyd S, Brown J, et al (1999) Molecular genetic characterisation of frontotemporal dementia on chromosome 3. Dement Geriatr Cogn Disord 10(suppl 1):93–101

Brown J, Ashworth A, Gydesen S, et al (1995) Familial non-specific dementia maps to chromosome 3. Hum Mol Genet 4:1625–1628

Brun A (1987) Frontal lobe degeneration of non-Alzheimer type. I. Neuropathology. Arch Gerontol Geriatr 6:193–208

Brun A, Englund B, Gustafson L, et al (1994) Clinical and neuropathological criteria for frontotemporal dementia. J Neurol Neurosurg Psychiatry 57:416–418

Chow TW, Miller BL, Hayashi VN, Geschwind DH (1999) Inheritance of frontotemporal dementia. Arch Neuro 56:817–822

Edwards-Lee T, Miller BL, Benson FD, et al (1997) The temporal variant of frontotemporal dementia. Brain 120:1027–1040

Gregory C (1999) Frontal variant of frontotemporal dementia: a cross-sectional and longitudinal study of neuropsychiatric features. Psychol Med 29:1205–1217

Gustafson L (1987) Frontal lobe degeneration of non-Alzheimer type. II. Clinical picture and differential diagnosis. Arch Gerontol Geriatr 6:209–233
Hong M, Zhukareva V, Vogelsberg-Ragaglia V, et al (1998) Mutation-specific functional impairments in distinct tau isoforms of heredity FTDP-17. Science 282:1914–1917
Hutton M, Lendom CL, Rizzu P, et al (1998) Association of missense and 5′-splice-site mutations in tau with the inherited dementia FTDP-7. Science 393:702–705
Mesulam MM (1982) Slowly progressive aphasia without generalized dementia. Ann Neurol 11:592–598
Miller B, Gearhart R (1999) Neuroimaging in the diagnosis of frontotemporal dementia. Dement Geriatr Cogn Disord 10(suppl 1):71–74
Mitsuyama Y (1979) Presenile dementia with motor neuron disease. Arch Neurol 36:592–593
Morita K, Kaiya H, Ikeda T, Namba M (1987) Presenile dementia combined with amyotrophy: a review of 34 Japanese cases. Arch Gerontol Geriatr 6:263–277
Neary D, Snowden JS, Gustafson L, et al (1998) Frontotemporal lobar degeneration. A consensus on clinical diagnostic criteria. Neurology 51:1546–1554
Neary D, Snowden JS, Mann DMA, et al (1990) Frontal lobe dementia and motor neuron disease. J Neurol Neurosurg Psychiatry 53:23–32
Onari K, Spatz H (1926) Anatomische Beiträge zur Lehre von der Pickschen umschriebenen Grosshirnrinden-Atrophie ("Picksche Krankheit"). Z Neurol 101:470–511
Pasquier F, Delacourte A (1998) Non-Alzheimer degenerative dementias. Curr Opin Neurol 11:417–427
Passant U, Gustafson L, Brun A (1993) Spectrum of frontal lobe dementia in a Swedish family. Dementia 4:160–162
Pick A (1892) Über die Beziehungen der senilen Hirnatrophie zur Aphasie. Prager Med Wochenschr 17:165–167
Procter AW, Qurne M, Francis PT (1999) Neurochemical features of frontotemporal Dementia. Dement Geriatr Cogn Disord 10(suppl 1):80–84
Rossor M (1999) Differential diagnosis of frontotemporal dementia: Pick's disease. Dement Geriatr Cogn Disord 10(suppl 1):43–45
Snowden J, Neary D (1993) Progressive language dysfunction and lobar atrophy. Dementia 4:226–231
Stertz G (1926) Über die Picksche Atrophie. Z Neurol 101:729–747
Van Mansfelt J (1954) Pick's disease. A syndrome of lobar, cerebral atrophy; its clinicoanatomical and histopathological types. Thesis. Enshede, Utrecht
Wilhelmsen KC, Clark LN (1998) Chromosome 17-linked dementias. In: Markesbery WR (ed) Neuropathology of dementing disorders. Arnold, London, pp 170–180

Dementia with Motor Neuron Disease: A Review

Yoshio Mitsuyama

Summary. Dementia associated with motor neuron disease has been described as a new clinicopathological entity, and more than 100 cases have been reported in Japan since 1964. The clinicopathological criteria in the diagnosis of dementia with motor neuron disease are (1) frontotemporal lobe-type dementia with insidious onset, mostly in the presenile period; (2) neurogenic muscular wasting during the course of the illness (ALS- or SPMA-like symptoms); (3) duration from the onset of illness to death, 2–5 years (average, 30.6 months); (4) both extrapyramidal symptoms and definite sensory deficits are less commonly present; (5) no characteristic abnormalities in the CSF or EEG in screening; (6) no known parental consanguinity or familial occurrence; and (7) nonspecific, mild to slight degenerative changes in the frontotemporal cortex, hypoglossal nuclei, spinal cord, and, frequently, in the substantia nigra. Dementia with motor neuron disease is characterized by ubiquitin-immunoreactive intraneuronal inclusions in cortical layer II and the hippocampal dentate granule cells.

Keywords. Frontotemporal dementia, Motor neuron disease, Ubiquitin

Introduction

Although reports of dementia lacking the distinctive non-Alzheimer type neuropathology have been increasing, the diagnosis is still far from distinct. It has become apparent that this population shows neuropathological heterogeneity, and some recent reports have been proposed a classification or criteria for these disease conditions. Frontotemporal lobe-type dementias may be associated with a variety of pathological entities and are complex disorders with a lack of distinctive histopathological markers. In addition, frontotemporal lobe-type dementias are the second most frequent degenerative-type dementia. Frontotemporal lobe-type dementias are a clinical syndrome corresponding to several histological entities, including the following: (1) Pick's disease, (2) nonspecific frontotemporal degeneration, (3) dementia with

Department of Psychiatry, Miyazaki Medical College, 5200 Kihara, Kiyotake, Miyazaki 889-1692, Japan motor neuron disease (MND), (4) progressive aphasia, (5) progressive subcortical gliosis, and (6) diffuse Lewy body disease. These disorders share similar outstanding neuropathological features with frontotemporal lobe degeneration. Dementia with motor neuron disease is a progressive neurodegenerative disorder with characteristic clinical and pathological features [1–3]. Dementia with MND is etiologically heterogenous; the causative factors have not yet been identified.

Clinical Symptomatology

The clinical symptomatology of dementia with MND is relatively similar between cases, including age of onset, rate of progression-pattern of neuropsychological deficits, and occurrence of noncognitive neuropsychiatric symptoms. The age at onset ranges from 38 to 75 years (average, 55.4 years). The initial symptom is dementia; i.e., uninhibited behavior and personality change occur in most patients. Other psychiatric symptoms include difficulties with memory loss, global impairment, emotional disorders, and adynamic spontaneous speech that culminates in mutism. This pattern of cognitive impairment implicates bilateral frontal lobe dysfunction. The patient does not show severe deterioration even in the late stage of the disease. The clinical features of MND may accompany or occasionally precede the onset of dementia. Both dementia and motor neuron involvement appear within 1 or 2 years of onset. No apraxia or agnosia, frequently seen in Alzheimer's disease, is found in cases of dementia with MND. All cases have clinical evidence of either an upper or lower motor neuron involvement. Neurogenic muscular atrophy and fasciculation are seen in all cases, and muscular wasting is prominent in the distal portion of the upper extremities, shoulder girdle, and face; the legs are less involved. Bulbar symptoms become evident with muscular atrophy and are progressive, causing death (Fig. 1). Pyramidal signs such as increased deep tendon reflex and Babinski's signs are rarely observed. The clinical picture of motor neuron disturbance is usually bulbar-type amyotrophic lateral sclerosis (ALS). Lower motor neuron are more prominent than upper motor neuron signs. Extrapyramidal signs such as rigidity, tremor, and myoclonic jerking are rarely observed. Neuroradiological studies show decreased frontotemporal lobe perfusion with hypometabolism on CT, MRI, single photon emission computed tomography, and positron emission computed tomography; such imaging results are suggestive of Pick's disease (Fig. 2) [4].

Neurological symptoms usually develop 6 to 12 months after the onset of psychiatric symptoms. There are no biological markers available for dementia with MND that allow presymptomatic detection or a definitive premorbid diagnosis. This disease should be suspected in patients with a normal EEG, with behavioral dyscontrol predating memory impairment, and who are also without spatial disorientation. Loss of personal awareness, hyperorality, stereotyped and perseverative behavior, progressive reduction of spontaneous speech, and MND are the criteria that clearly differentiate dementia with MND from Alzheimer's disease. Word fluency tasks are more sensitive measures of frontal lobe function; such tasks, if incorporated into imaging studies, may facilitate the recognition of subtle functional impairment in the frontal lobes in cases of dementia with MND. The emergence of MND with dementia is responsible for death within 3 years of onset.

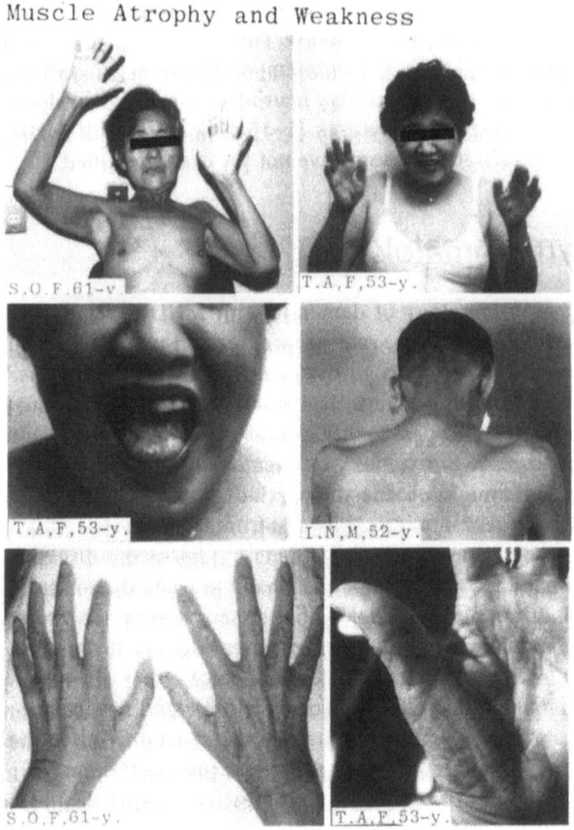

FIG. 1. Muscular wasting and atrophy of extremities and tongue

Neuropathology

In cases of dementia with MND, there is variable macroscopic atrophy and neuronal loss in the frontal and temporal lobes. The ventricles may be dilated and the blood vessels may appear healthy. Marked localized atrophy as seen in Pick's disease, or a marked diffuse atrophy, as seen in Alzheimer's disease, is not observed. A pattern of atrophy in the frontal lobes and hippocampal formation sparing the medial temporal lobe might be distinctive findings in cases of dementia with MND. Microscopically, all cases have cortical microvacuolation (spongy changes), which is limited to the superficial cortical layer II. Such cases are characterized by a mild to slight disappearance of neurons (Fig. 3) concomitant with lesions similar to those seen in MND. Fibrillary astrogliosis in the subcortical white matter of the cerebral hemisphere is frequently observed; severity varies from case to case. However, typically, the primary sensory and motor regions tend to be spared. Lesions in the cerebral cortex are less extensive than those seen in Alzheimer's disease or Creutzfeldt–Jakob disease.

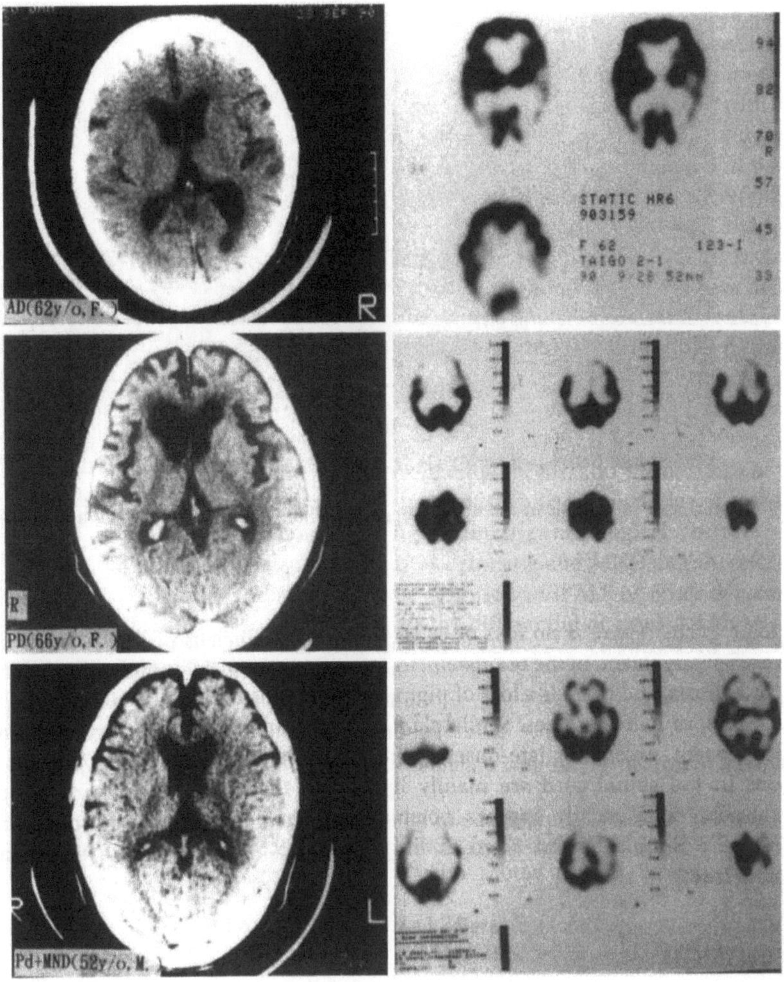

FIG. 2. CT and SPECT of Alzheimer's disease (*top*), Pick's disease (*middle*), and dementia with motor neuron disease (MND) (*bottom*)

Recently, a new ubiquitin-related abnormality, characterized by ubiquitinated inclusions in the neurites, has been found in some cases of frontotemporal dementia. Intraneuronal ubiquitin-immunoreactive inclusions, characteristic of the extramotor involvement of motor neuron disease, are also found in the hippocampal dentate granule cells and in the residual neurons remaining in the affected cortex. Inclusions are the most conspicuous in layer II, in contrast with the microvacuolation of the frontotemporal lobes [5]. Kinoshita et al. [6] have found that the ubiquitinated inclusions consist of abnormal filaments 10–15 nm in diameter. They also demonstrated a close relationship between ubiquitin and abnormal filaments in cases of dementia with MND. These changes are marked in frontal, insular, and anterior portions of the

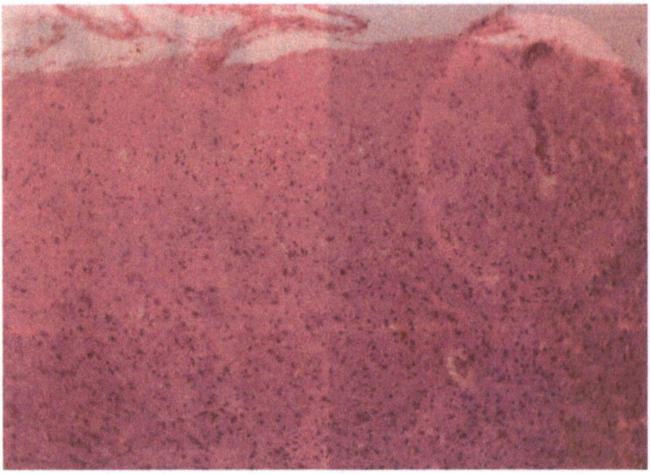

FIG. 3. Sponginess and gliosis in the upper layer of frontal cortex. Hematoxylm and eosin. ×99

cingulate gyrus. There is no loss of cells in the basal nucleus of Meynert, and Betz cells are usually intact. In the brainstem, the hypoglossal nuclei usually show neuronal loss and gliosis, and there is a loss of pigmented neurons in the substantia nigra, with astrogliosis, in half the cases. Senile plaques and granulovacuolar degeneration are usually absent, except for late-onset individuals who are more than 70 years old. Lesions in the spinal cord are mainly limited to the cervical and thoracic cord. The lumbar cord usually appears normal, and some preserved neurons contain eosinophilic Bunina bodies. There is little evidence of degeneration of the corticospinal tracts.

Discussion

The diagnosis of dementia with MND is highly dependent on the clinical symptomatology. Patients have been diagnosed as having amyotrophic lateral sclerosis (ALS) or spinal progressive muscle atrophy. These characteristic findings are not consistent with those of Alzheimer's disease or Pick's disease. The clinicopathological information associated with dementia with MND includes lesions similar to those observed in cases of frontotemporal lobe-type dementias described by the Lund and Manchester group [7]. Immunohistochemical studies have shown the presence of ubiquitin bodies in the frontal cortex and dentate gyrus of the hippocampus; there is severe involvement in the medial region of the temporal pole. Dendritic pathology as observed by the Golgi method reveals abnormal disconnections in the frontal cortex. Ubiquitin-positve and tau-negative inclusions in cortical, hippocampal, and motor neurons are found in cases of both dementia with MND and frontal lobe-type dementia [5]. These observations suggest a common pathogenesis for dementia with MND and frontotemporal lobe-type dementia.

Jackson et al. [8] reported some cases with intraneuronal ubiquitin-immunoreactive inclusions characteristic of MND in patients with frontotemporal dementias; in that report, no clinical or pathological evidence of motor system degeneration was observed. These findings extend the clinical spectrum of diseases associated with such inclusions. Hence, Jackson et al. [8] proposed the term motor neuron disease-inclusion dementia (MNDID) for these cases, according to their clinical and pathological characteristics. Typical and atypical cases could be classified. The presence of ophthalmoplegic sign, a long interval between dementia and MND, and the more dominant involvement of temporal lobes are commonly seen in atypical cases. A distribution of the frontal dopaminergic system might account for the cognitive deficits associated with frontotemporal lobe-type dementia. The behavioral symptoms of dementia with MND may improve after treatment with selective serotonine re-uptake inhilitors (SSRIs). Future neurochemical studies and controlled pharmacological trials may improve available treatment. It should be noted that dementia with MND differs from Pick's disease according to the preponderance of histological changes in the upper cortical layers, the scarcity of chromatolytic cells, and the absence of tau-positive Pick's bodies. The differential diagnosis of this disease includes of P-D-C of Guam, frontal lobe-type dementia lacking distinctive histological features, and Creutzfeldt–Jakob disease. The combination of dementia and MND can therefore be seen as a distinct disorder and should not be confused with ALS or other dementias. Clinicopathological studies should determine the differential diagnosis with MND.

References

1. Mitsuyama Y, Takamiya S (1979) Presenile dementia with motor neuron disease. Arch Neurol 36:592–593
2. Mitsuyama Y (1984) Presenile dementia with motor neuron disease in Japan; clinicopathological review of 26 cases. J Neurol Neurosurg Psychiatry 47:953–959
3. Mitsuyama Y (1993) Presenile dementia with motor neuron disease. Dementia 4:137–142
4. Beall DP, Martin D, Chin BB (1998) Decreased bilateral frontal lobe perfusion in dementia of amyotrophic lateral sclerosis. Clin Nucl Med 23:855–856
5. Bergmann M, Kuchelmeister K, Scmid KW, et al (1996) Different variants of frontotemporal dementia: a neuropathological and immunohistochemical study. Acta Neuropathol 92:170–179
6. Kinoshita T, Tomimoto H, Suenaga T, et al (1997) Ubiquitin-related cytoskeletal abnormality in frontotemporal dementia: immunohistochemical and immunoelectron microscopic studies. Acta Neuropathol 94:67–72
7. Lund and Manchester Group (1994) Clinical and neuropathological criteria for frontotemporal dementia. J Neurol Neurosurg Psychiatry 57:416–418
8. Jackson M, Lennox G, Lowe J (1996) Motor neuron disease-inclusion dementia. Neurodegeneration 5:339–350

Ubiquitinated Inclusions Link Amyotrophic Lateral Sclerosis with Frontotemporal Dementia

Carol F. Lippa[1], Terry Heiman-Patterson[1], Pierluigi Gambetti[2], Sidney Croul[3], and Sandra Koffler[4]

Summary. Although amyotrophic lateral sclerosis (ALS) is often viewed as a motor systems disorder, evidence has surfaced indicating that ALS patients may develop cognitive losses. In particular, clinical and histopathological studies suggest a predominance of frontotemporal pathology in some ALS patients. Pick-like ubiquitinated inclusions have been described in hippocampal dentate granule cells and in small cortical neurons of the frontal and temporal cortices. However, these inclusions are distinctive from those of Pick's disease because they do not contain tau protein and they lack argyrophilia. We report a case from a kindred with familial frontotemporal dementia (FTD) with identical ALS-like, ubiquitin-positive lesions. Tau-immunoreactive Pick bodies and other specific pathological changes were absent. This case lacked clinical signs of ALS and showed few histopathological features of ALS. We review the literature describing the clinical and pathological link between ALS and FTD, and propose that tau-negative, ubiquitinated inclusions similar to those of ALS may be seen in familial forms of FTD, even in the absence of typical clinical or pathological features of ALS. These ubiquitinated inclusions may be a common biological link underlying dementia in some ALS and FTD cases.

Keywords. ALS, Dementia, Frontotemporal dementia, Genetics, Ubiquitin

Introduction

Amyotrophic lateral sclerosis (ALS) was initially described as a pure motor disorder. More recently, however, it has been recognized that ALS patients may also develop cognitive losses. Some investigators consider these patients to be either atypical ALS cases or cases with coincidental concurrent diagnoses accounting for their cognitive losses [1]. However, it has become clear that frontotemporal syndromes occur more frequently in ALS subjects than would be expected by chance. Some ALS dementia cases show Pick-like ubiquitinated inclusions and neurites in the hippocampal dentate

Departments of Neurology[1], Pathology[3], and Psychiatry[4], MCP-Hahnemann University, 3300 Henry Ave, Philadelphia, PA 19129, USA
[2] Department of Pathology, Case Western Reserve University, Cleveland, OH, USA

gyrus and in the affected areas of cerebral cortex [2–4]. However, these inclusions are tau negative and are not argyrophilic, suggesting that they are not true Pick bodies [2–4]. Frontotemporal dementia (FTD) cases may show similar ubiquitinated, tau-negative pathology [5,6], which suggests that there may be a pathological spectrum between cases with ALS and those with FTD. This chapter uses a case report format to review the features of FTD cases with ubiquitinated, tau-negative inclusions. We describe the clinical, neuropsychological, neuroradiologic, and histopathological features of an affected individual from a kindred in which symptoms appear to be transmitted through an autosomal dominant mode of transmission.

Case Report

R.A.K was a solid member of her community and worked successfully as a secretary until the age of 46 when she was referred for neurological evaluation for her violent behavior. She had been fired from her job because she lost the ability to "work the phones or remember names or messages." In retrospect, her family and former coworkers noted the insidious onset of a personality change with socially inappropriate behavior as much as a decade before presentation. She had become withdrawn, started to hoard paper and photos, and spent hours sorting and resorting clothes. At the time of presentation, her driving became erratic, and this led to several arrests. At the time of the arrests, R.A.K would try to elude the police. When finally arrested, she assaulted the police officers. She then refused the aid of a lawyer stating that she had not done anything wrong. She was initially given the diagnosis of Borderline Personality Disorder.

At the time of her initial presentation, mental status testing showed R.A.K. to be alert and oriented, but inappropriate. Mild word-finding difficulties were noted. Aside from the frontotemporal features, R.A.K.'s general neurological examination was unremarkable. Cranial nerve examination showed smooth pursuit and saccades with no limitation of extraocular movements. There was no facial weakness, and no bulbar signs, such as dysarthria, or fasciculations or atrophy of the tongue were observed. Motor examination revealed normal muscle tone, bulk, and coordination. There was no tremor. Strength was intact, and there was no drift. No fasciculations of the extremities were present. R.A.K.'s gait was normal. Deep tendon reflexes were normoactive and symmetrical. No frontal release signs were present. Plantar responses were flexor bilaterally. Sensory testing was normal.

An MRI scan was remarkable for cerebral atrophy, which was marked in the right anterior temporal lobe, particularly in the superior temporal gyrus. There was also asymmetrical ventriculomegaly (right greater than left). Neuropsychological testing established that R.A.K had difficulty with frontotemporal functions. Although her language was nearly fluent, she had subtle difficulty naming objects. Her abstraction and judgment were poor, and she had little insight into her condition. R.A.K also showed mild memory impairment, and her orientation was slightly impaired. Mental calculations, visuospatial skills, and language comprehension were normal.

R.A.K started to believe that she lived in a "malevolent environment." She frequently sent air and water samples to toxicology laboratories for analysis. The laboratory personnel were unable to convince her that there were no contaminants in the

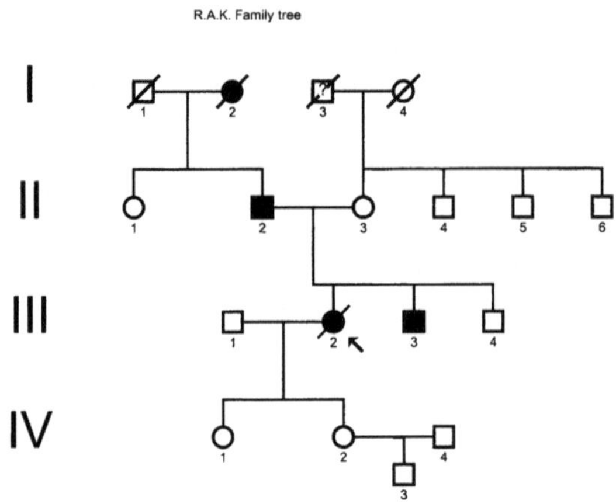

FIG. 1. Family tree demonstrating possible autosomal dominant transmission of dementia in this kindred

samples. She became paranoid about people she believed to be foreign. She also developed an interest in collecting garbage from public dumpsters.

Over several years, R.A.K's behavior and function continued to deteriorate. Mood problems developed. She then began to confabulate responses. Eventually, apathy replaced her troublesome behavior. Follow-up neuropsychological testing was limited by a severe expressive aphasia with echolalia and motor apraxia. During her last 2 years, R.A.K developed parkinsonism, particularly bradykinesia. However, no clear-cut upper or lower motor neuron signs developed. R.A.K died at age 53, after 7 or more years of symptoms.

Family history is remarkable for a brother with "dementia" at age 56. A second brother is cognitively normal at age 42. R.A.K.'s father and paternal grandmother had dementia, but developed symptoms at a later age (80 and 90, respectively; Fig. 1). A frontotemporal dementia with parkinsonism syndrome, linked to a tau mutation of chromosome 17, was suspected on the basis of her clinical features and strong family history.

At autopsy, the brain weighed 1026 g and showed marked anterior temporal lobe atrophy that was more prominent on the right than the left. There was knife-edge atrophy of the superior temporal gyrus, anteriorly. Other portions of the anterior temporal lobes were involved to a lesser degree. Frontal lobe atrophy was mild, and the more posterior brain regions were spared. Coronal sections showed the focal knife-edge atrophy and also right-sided ventriculomegaly and dilated temporal horns. There was thinning of the cortical ribbon and underlying white matter in affected regions.

The most striking histological feature was profound neuronal loss and gliosis of the cortex with loss of the underlying white matter in the cortical regions showing gross atrophy. No Pick bodies or Lewy bodies were observed. Neurofibrillary tangles were rare, and limited to the parahippocampal gyrus (mostly layer II) and the hippocampus. β-Amyloid plaques were almost nonexistent. Mild, focal spongiform degeneration was observed; however, inclusions suggesting other diagnoses were not present. Betz cells were identifiable in the motor strip.

Sections 6 µm thick cut from paraffin-embedded tissue blocks were stained using a panel of monoclonal and polyclonal antibodies raised to proteins that are abnormally expressed in CNS degenerative diseases. Tissue was stained with antibodies to the long- and short-tailed forms of β-amyloid (H. Mori), alpha-B-crystallin (H. Mori), and phosphorylated neurofilaments (SMI31; Sternberger-Meyer Immunocytochemicals, Jarrettsville, MD, USA). No immunoreactivity for any of these antibodies was observed. Staining with a panel of phosphorylation-independent (Tau-2, 1:750; Sigma, St. Louis, MO, USA; T14, 1:1000, V.M.-Y. Lee) and phosphorylation-dependent tau antibodies (PHF-6 [Thr-231], T3P [Ser-396], recombinant tau [17026], V.M.-Y. Lee) showed that the tissue was also not immunoreactive for these antibodies. Using antibodies to ubiquitin (H. Mori), numerous tau-negative, ubiquitin-positive intracellular inclusions were identified within neurons (Fig. 2A,B). Ubiquitin-positive neuropil dots and threads were also seen (Fig. 2B). Inclusions were most common in the hippocampal dentate granule cells, but were also observed in small neurons of affected frontal and temporal regions and in the striatum. Longer, threadlike ubiquitin-positive structures were also present in the affected regions of cortex (Fig. 2C). These inclusions were not observed in the precentral gyrus. Using glial fibrillary acidic protein immunohistochemistry, gliosis was demonstrated in the cortical regions with neuronal loss. Additionally, mild gliosis of the pyramidal tract was observed, but it was restricted to the level of the medulla.

Discussion

We have described the clinical, neuropsychological, neuroradiologic, and histopathological features of an affected member of a kindred with a familial FTD syndrome, possibly with autosomal dominant inheritance. Because she had frontotemporal symptomatology and developed parkinsonism (bradykinesia), the diagnosis of a frontotemporal dementia with parkinsonism (FTDP) syndrome resulting from a tau mutation was hypothesized. Instead, at autopsy, ubiquitinated neuronal inclusions in the hippocampal dentate gyrus and small, nonmotor cortical neurons were observed. This pathology has previously been described in ALS cases with dementia.

The differential diagnosis of familial FTD includes mutations of the tau gene on chromosome 17, but also genetic abnormalities linking to chromosome 3 and prion mutations. There are also kindreds not linking to these sites, indicating that there are other genes, as yet unidentified, implicated in these syndromes. Thus far, all FTDP cases linking to the tau gene have shown increased expression of hyperphosphorylated forms of tau. R.A.K. showed no tau immunoreactivity using several well-characterized antibodies. Linkage to exclude a tau mutation is ongoing with the current case. Interestingly, Kertesz et al. [6] also described a kindred with FTD, with similar ubiquitinated inclusions. Their family did not have a mutation of the tau gene. Mutations of the prion gene have also been associated with FTD [7]; however, biochemical analysis for the prion protein was negative, suggesting that a mutation of this gene is not likely. FTD kindreds linking to chromosome 3 have been described

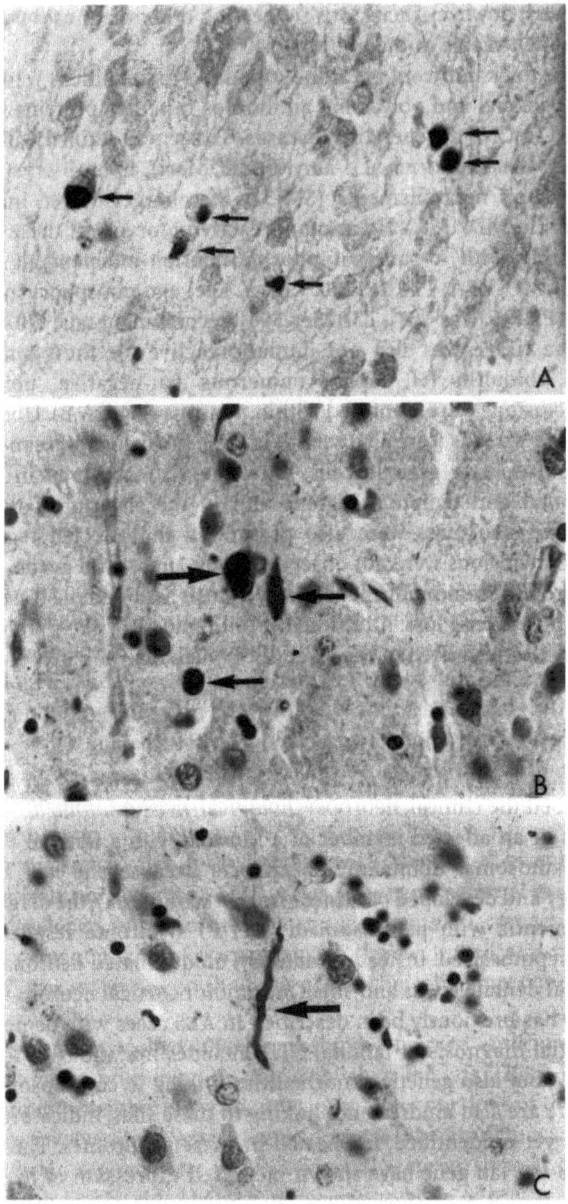

FIG. 2A–C. Photomicrographs of the dentate gyrus (**A**), basal ganglia (**B**), and orbitofrontal gyrus (**C**) after ubiquitin immunohistochemistry. In **A**, the *arrows* point to the frequent neuronal inclusions in dentate granule cells. In **B**, the *large arrow* points to a rounded inclusion in the cytoplasm of a small neuron; the *small arrows* point to the ubiquitin-positive neuropil dots and distended neurites. **C** shows the more elongated ubiquitin-positive neurites (*arrow*) that were common in the orbitofrontal region. ×60

[8,9], but they have shown diffuse β-amyloid plaques [9]. Our proband had virtually no β-amyloid plaques. However, interestingly, at least one chromosome 3 kindred showed genetic anticipation [8]. In the current kindred, anticipation cannot be excluded because the subject's father developed symptoms at age 80 and her grandmother at age 90. Anticipation usually occurs with trinucleotide repeat abnormalities. This type of genetic abnormality has not been conclusively identified in either FTD or ALS kindreds. Finally, as the histopathology paralleled that of ALS dementia cases, a genetic form of ALS should be considered. Mutations of the superoxide dismutase (SOD) gene have been described as a cause of familial ALS [10]. Moreover, familial ALS cases are more likely to develop dementia than sporadic ALS cases. However, cognitive dysfunction in this population may be difficult to assess due to the severe motor impairments; thus, the true incidence of FTD may be underestimated in familial and sporadic ALS. FTD cases associated with ALS have not yet shown linkage to the SOD gene. However, the range of phenotypic variability related to SOD mutations may be incompletely described.

Nonfamilial cases of FTD with similar pathological features have also been described. Iseki et al. described nonfamilial "atypical Pick's disease without Pick bodies" in 1998 [5]. This series of six cases showed ubiquitinated inclusions in the cytoplasm of small neurons of the dentate gyrus and cerebral cortex. These cases also showed threadlike inclusions in distal dendrites. Rossor et al. reported three cases with semantic dementia with similar inclusions.

A biological link between ALS and FTD is well established. In 1990, Neary et al. [3] described four patients with rapidly progressive frontal dementia that occurred in association with motor neuron symptomatology. Two years later, Wightman et al. [4] described ubiquitin-immunoreactive inclusions in dentate granule cells and superficial cortical neurons in these subjects. In 1994, Lowe [2] further described clinical and pathological findings in ALS, noting that ALS may present as a frontotemporal syndrome. His cases show identical ubiquitinated inclusions in nonmotor neurons of the frontal and temporal cortex. Lowe viewed ALS as a multisystems disorder with variable clinical manifestations. In this light, our kindred could be described as a frontotemporal variant of ALS even though she lacked overt clinical manifestations of the disease and had only medullary pathology.

Acknowledgment. We acknowledge Peter St. George-Hyslop, who is conducting the genetic analysis of the tau gene, and Richard Orrell, who is screening the *SOD* gene for mutations. We also thank Virginia Lee and John Trojanowski, who donated the tau antibodies, and Hiroshi Mori, who donated the ubiquitin antibody. We also acknowledge the family of R.A.K., who donated tissue for research. This work was supported by the National Institute on Aging of the National Institutes of Health (AG13623).

References

1. Cavalleri F, De Renzi E (1994) Amyotrophic lateral sclerosis with dementia. Acta Neurol Scand 89:391–394
2. Lowe J (1994) New pathological findings in amyotrophic lateral sclerosis. J Neurol Sci 124(suppl):38–51

3. Neary D, Snowden JS, Mann DM, et al (1990) Frontal lobe dementia and motor neuron disease. J Neurol Neurosurg Psychiatry 53:23–32
4. Wightman G, Anderson VE, Martin J, et al (1992) Hippocampal and neocortical ubiquitin-immunoreactive inclusions in amyotrophic lateral sclerosis with dementia. Neurosci Lett 139:269–274
5. Iseki E, Li F, Odawara T, et al (1998) Ubiquitin-immunohistochemical investigation of atypical Pick's disease without Pick bodies. J Neurol Sci 159:194–201
6. Kertesz A, Kawarai T, Rogaeva E, et al (2000) Familial frontotemporal dementia with ubiquitin-positive, tau-negative inclusions. Neurology 54(4):818;818–827
7. Nitrini R, Rosemberg S, Passos-Bueno MR, et al (1997) Familial spongiform encephalopathy associated with a novel prion protein gene mutation. Ann Neurol 42:138–146
8. Ashworth A, Lloyd S, Brown J, et al (1999) Molecular genetic characterisation of frontotemporal dementia on chromosome 3. Dement Geriatr Cogn Disord 10(suppl S1):93–101
9. Poduslo SE, Yin X, Hargis J, et al (1999) A familial case of Alzheimer's disease without tau pathology may be linked with chromosome 3 markers. Hum Genet 105:32–37
10. Ince PG, Shaw PJ, Slade JY, et al (1996) Familial amyotrophic lateral sclerosis with a mutation in exon 4 of the Cu/Zn superoxide dismutase gene: pathological and immunocytochemical changes. Acta Neuropathol (Berl) 92:395–403

Exclusive Mediotemporal Pathology Within the Spectrum of Frontotemporal Dementia

Rivka Ravid[1], Wouter Kamphorst[2], John C. van Swieten[3], Sonia Rosso[3], José Wouda[1], Michiel Kooreman[1], Anne Holtrop[1], and Thea Tadema[2]

Summary. We report here the recognition of a new distinctive small group of patients within the spectrum of frontotemporal dementia (FTD) pathology. We present three cases with the clinical diagnosis of frontotemporal dementia (FTD) and neuropathological changes restricted to the medial temporal lobe. The presenting symptoms of these cases were family history of dementia in two of the three cases (two sisters), agitation, apathy, dysphasia, and memory problems. Two of the three cases were clinically diagnosed as Pick's disease and the third with probable Alzheimer's disease. Pathologically, they resemble cases reported with hippocampal sclerosis, and ubiquinated inclusions were present in the hippocampus and ventral striatum. Our observations support the existence of a subgroup; we propose to call the cases with distinctive pathology as described in the present paper "Pick D", as they may be a restricted group who resemble PickC1 according to the division proposed by Constantinidis within Pick's disease.

Keywords. Frontotemporal dementia, Pick's disease, Pick bodies, Ubiquitin, Tau

In the past 10 years, the Netherlands Brain Bank (NBB) has performed rapid autopsies of 50 patients with the clinical diagnosis of Pick's disease, frontal dementia, or frontotemporal dementia. We encountered two cases in which the pathology was restricted to the medial temporal lobe and provisionally named them "Pick D" in honor of Constantinidis, who recognized four subtypes of Pick's disease: Pick A, Pick B, Pick C1, and Pick C2 (Constantinidis et al. 1974). Pick C1 is characterized by atrophy of the temporal pole, the amygdala-accumbens-stria terminalis complex, the temporal juxtaallocortex, the insula, and the orbital cortex; however, the hippocampus is normal. We assumed that "Pick D" might be a restricted form of cases resembling Pick C1. We wished to compare these two cases (the index group) with seven control cases: first, four cases (control group A) with similar mediotemporal pathology and in addition severe degenerative changes of the temporal neocortex, and second, (control group B) three cases with severe temporal neocortical pathology but without

[1] Netherlands Brain Bank, Meibergdreef 33, 1105 AZ, Amsterdam, Netherlands
[2] Department of Pathology, Free University Hospital, Amsterdam, Netherlands
[3] Department of Neurology, Erasmus University Rotterdam, Netherlands

mediotemporal changes. A third case has been added to the index group: case 1B, the sister of case 1A.

Tissue sections from 15 brain areas were stained with the classical histological stains, namely hematoxylin and eosin (H&E), Kluver, congo, Bodian, and methenamine silver, and the immunocytochemical (ICC) stains tau, beta-A4, ubiquitin, neurofilaments, and GFAP. Braak staging for tangles (Braak and Braak 1995) was scored on Bodian- and tau-stained slides. Braak scores for amyloid were determined on methenamine silver and beta-A4 stains.

Alzheimer's disease (AD) was the clinical diagnosis in one index case and in one control case. In both cases, memory problems were among the first symptoms as well as in two more control cases. The substantia nigra displayed cell loss in two cases in the index group and in one case in the control groups. In the index group, fine intracytoplasmatic ubiquitin-positive granules were present in the granular layer of the fascia dentata and some other areas. In the control groups, however, intracytoplasmic ubiquitine-positive crescentic and round bodies were found. In several cases Bodian staining resulted in a lower Braak score for neurofibrillary tangles than the immunoreaction for tau. Case 1B, who was clinically diagnosed as an AD patient, had higher scores than her sister, 1A, who was diagnosed as Pick's disease. Both sisters had few tau-positive glial cells in the white matter of the temporal lobe. A few of these cells also occurred in two control cases. In the neocortical and striatal neuropil of the control groups, few to moderate numbers of ubiquitin-positive thread-, splinter-, or clubshaped structures were observed in the neocortex, especially in layer 2, resembling the structures previously decribed (Kinoshita et al. 1997; Tolnay and Probst 1995).

The ICC staining for ubiquitin suggested that the study group is not a part of the spectrum of the control groups (= Pick C1 of Constantinidis). The ubiquitin-positive crescentic or round bodies were present in the hippocampus and ventral striatum of all contol cases and none of the index cases. Also, ubiquitin-positive neuropil structures were only seen in the control groups (Figs. 1–3).

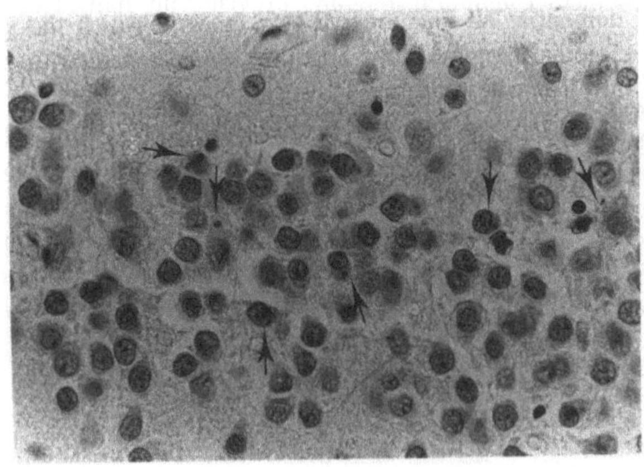

Fig. 1. Immunocytochemical (ICC) staining for ubiquitin shows fine granules (see *arrows*) in the cytoplasm of the granular cells of the hippocampus. Case 95–048. ×600

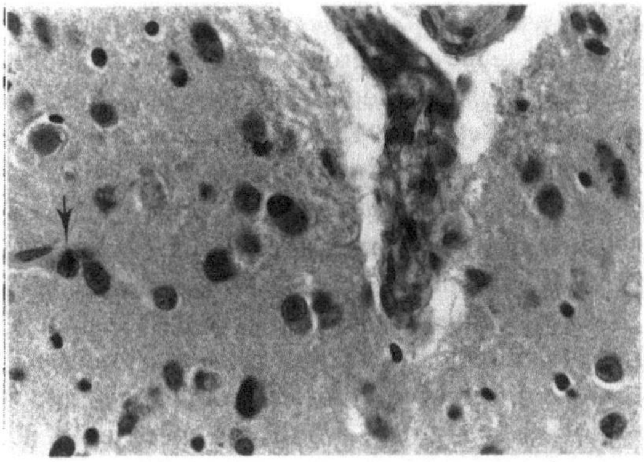

FIG. 2. Immunocytochemical (ICC) staining shows round bodies in the cytoplasm of the small neurons in the ventral striatum. Note that one of the bodies seems to emanate from the nuclear incisura (*arrow*). Case 96–041. ×600

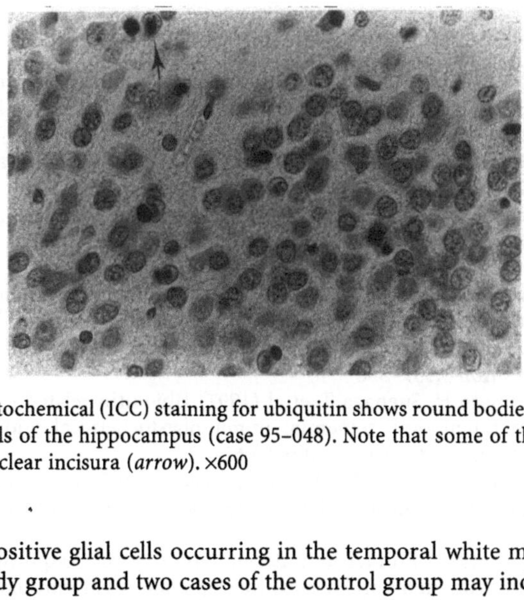

FIG. 3. Immunocytochemical (ICC) staining for ubiquitin shows round bodies in the cytoplasm of the granular cells of the hippocampus (case 95–048). Note that some of the bodies seem to originate in the nuclear incisura (*arrow*). ×600

The few tau-positive glial cells occurring in the temporal white matter of the two sisters in the study group and two cases of the control group may indicate that tau is involved in the pathogenesis of these cases. On the other hand, tau-positive glial cells may be aspecific indicators of degeneration (Odawara et al. 1995). The fact that patient 1B had high Braak scores for tangles and amyloid may indicate that the same pathological mechanism can enhance an Alzheimer-like process.

All control cases had mediotemporal degeneration and/or temporal neocortical degeneration and did not have motor neuron disease as described by Jackson et al. (1996), who did not mention ventral striatal inclusions and preferential temporal lobe degeneration. We wonder whether the ubiquitin pathology of the present cases is related to the involvement of the temporal lobe and whether ubiquitin-positive crescentic or round bodies are just as frequent in frontotemporal dementias with preferential frontal or mixed frontotemporal neocortical involvement. The present observation may support the existence of subgroups as Constantinidis observed, in this case of Pick C1. Our definition of the index group resembles the description of hippocampal sclerosis (Dickson et al. 1994). A Cerad study of 106 autopsies of clinical Alzheimer cases detected three "pure" hippocampal sclerosis cases, two of which had displayed frontal symptomatology (Gearing et al. 1995).

In conclusion, we have described three cases with mediotemporal pathology, two sisters, one of which was clinically diagnosed as Pick's disease and the other as AD. The third case was also diagnosed as Pick's disease. Pathologically, they resemble "pure" hippocampal sclerosis. It has been suggested previously that hippocampal sclerosis might belong to the group of frontotemporal dementias (Ala et al. 2000). As Constantinidis recognized four groups within the spectrum of Pick's diseases, we propose to refer to cases with clinically frontotemporal symptomatology and pathologically mediotemporal degeneration as "Pick D". The control group in this study resembling Pick C1 became important because ubiquitinated inclusions were present not only in the hippocampus of all cases but also in the ventral striatum.

References

Ala AT, Goffa O, Beh MD, et al (2000) Pure hippocampal sclerosis. Neurology 54:843–848

Braak H, Braak E (1995) Staging of Alzheimer's disease related neurofibrillary changes. Neurobiol Aging 16:271–278

Constantinidis J, Richard J, Tissor R (1974) Pick's disease. Histological and clinical correlation. Eur Neurol 11:208–217

Dickson DW, Davies P, Bevona C, et al (1994) Hippocampal sclerosis: a common pathological feature of dementia in very old (>80 years of age) humans. Acta Neuropathol 88:212–221

Gearing M, Mirra SS, Hedreen JC, et al (1995) The consortium to establish a registry for Alzheimer's disease (CERAD). Part X. Neurology 45:461–466

Jackson M, Lennox G, Lowe J (1996) Motor neuron disease-inclusion dementia. Neurodegeneration 5:339–350

Kinoshita M, Tomimoto H, Suenaga T, et al (1997) Ubiquitin-related cytoskeletal abnormality in frontotemporal dementia: immunohystochemical and immunoelectron microscope studies. Acta Neuropathol 94:67–72

Odawara T, Iseki E, Kosaka K, et al (1995) Investigations of Tau-2 positive microglia-like cells in the subcortical nuclei of human neurodegenerative disorders. Neurosci Lett 192:145–148

Tolnay M, Probst A (1995) Frontal lobe degeneration: novel ubiquitin-immunoreactive neurites within frontotemporal cortex. Neuropathol Appl Neurobiol 21:492–497

Dementia with Lewy Bodies: Clinical Management

Ian G. McKeith

Summary. Psychosis and associated behavioral disturbances are common features of dementia with Lewy bodies (DLB) and appear to be relatively independent of the severity of cognitive impairment or stage of disease. The occurrence of sensitivity reactions in 50%–60% of neuroleptic-treated patients is a major limitation to clinical management. Dopamine blockade may be an inappropriate pharmacological strategy for the core features of DLB, which postmortem studies have revealed to have an underlying neurobiological basis in cholinergic neurotransmitter deficits. In a double-blind, placebo controlled study, the cholinesterase inhibitor rivastigmine was administered to 120 patients clinically diagnosed as DLB according to Consensus criteria. A cluster of treatment-responsive DLB symptoms—apathy, hallucinations, delusions, and anxiety—was identified. Other neuropsychiatric features including aggression, agitation, and depression were unaffected. Cognitive performance also improved, the largest effects being observed for computer-based attentional performance tasks. Extrapyramidal motor features were not worsened.

Keywords. Dementia, Lewy body, Therapeutics, Cholinesterase inhibitor

Introduction

Dementia with Lewy bodies (DLB) accounts for 15%–20% of elderly demented cases reaching autopsy, making it the most common dementia subtype after Alzheimer's disease (AD). The neuropathological and clinical features of DLB have been described in some detail in an earlier chapter in this volume and are not repeated here. An important reason for making an accurate clinical diagnosis of DLB is that patients frequently require medication for psychiatric symptoms and associated behavioral disturbances. They are however particularly susceptible to severe adverse reactions to typical and atypical antipsychotics, and preliminary trials of cholinesterase inhibitors have suggested that they may provide a safer and more effective treatment strategy. Symptomatic control of extrapyramidal motor features also needs to be considered in managing patients with DLB.

Department of Old Age Psychiatry, Institute for the Health of the Elderly, Wolfson Research Centre, Newcastle General Hospital, Westgate Road, Newcastle upon Tyne, NE4 6BE, UK

The Neurobiological Basis of Symptoms in DLB

Pharmacological treatment strategies for managing DLB are based upon our knowledge of the neurochemical deficits underlying specific symptoms in DLB [1]. Activity of the cholinergic enzyme choline acetyltransferase (ChAt) is lower in DLB than AD, particularly in the temporal and parietal cortex [2]. Clouding of consciousness, confusion, and visual hallucinations are recognized effects of anticholinergic drug toxicity, and the summative effects of subcortical and cortical cholinergic dysfunction probably play a major role in the spontaneous generation of similar fluctuating symptoms in DLB. Reductions in ChAt are correlated with severity of cognitive impairment [3], and hallucinations may be related to hypocholinergic and (relatively) hypermonoaminergic neocortical neurotransmitter function [4].

Pharmacological Treatments

Antipsychotics

Managing psychosis is one of the most difficult challenges in the care of patients with DLB [5]. It is a major source of distress to patients, exacerbates caregiver burden, and is a major determinant of earlier transfer to institutional care and an increased mortality. Neuroleptic agents are usually the drugs of choice in most psychotic disorders, including those occurring in the course of AD and other dementias. The most important practice point, however, in the management of a patient with DLB is caution in, or preferably avoidance of, the use of neuroleptic medications [6]. Severe neuroleptic sensitivity reactions [6] can precipitate irreversible parkinsonism, further impair consciousness level, and induce autonomic disturbances reminiscent of neuroleptic malignant syndrome. These reactions occur in 40%–50% of neuroleptic-treated DLB cases (Fig. 1) and are associated with a two- to threefold increase in mortality [7].

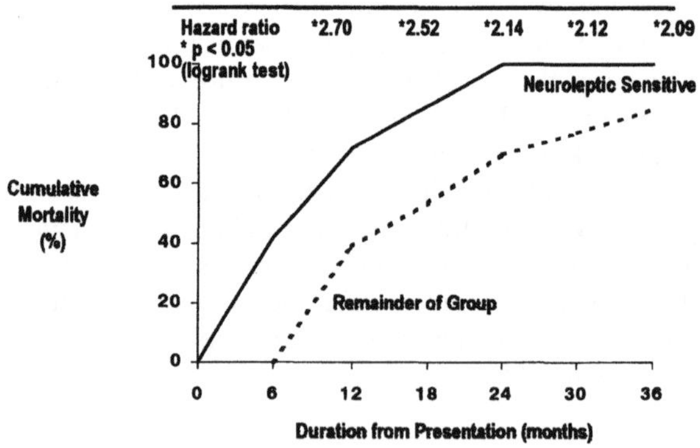

FIG. 1. Increased mortality curves for DLB patients sensitive to neuroleptics (*solid line*) comparedwith those either not exposed or tolerant of medication (*broken line*). Data from McKeith et al. 1992 [7]

Acute D_2 receptor blockade is thought to mediate these effects [8] and, despite some promising initial reports, atypical and novel antipsychotics such as risperidone [9] and olanzapine [10] seem to be about as likely to cause adverse reactions as older, "typical" drugs. Sedation, increased confusion, and worsening of parkinsonism are the most common side effects.

A randomized, double-blind study has reported the effects of clozapine in 60 patients with Parkinson's disease (PD) and psychosis, some of whom had cognitive impairment, a situation clinically analogous to DLB. A mean dose of approximately 25 mg daily (range, 6.25–50 mg) was associated with a fall in Brief Psychiatric Rating Scale score of 9.3 ± 0.3 points for those on placebo compared with 2.6 ± 0.2 points for those on placebo ($P < 0.001$). Clozapine treatment improved tremor and had no deleterious effects on either the severity of parkinsonism or cognition. There are no systematic reports about the use of clozapine in DLB, although its potent antimuscarinic effects might be expected to increase cognitive and attentional deficits.

Cholinesterase Inhibitors

There have been several reports that patients who respond well to cholinesterase inhibitor treatments are more likely to have DLB than AD at autopsy [12–14]. This evidence is consistent with the neurochemical profile of DLB and the fact that postsynaptic cortical muscarinic receptors are functionally intact. Case reports suggest that apathy, somnolence, hallucinations, and delirium are symptoms of DLB that improve substantially with cholinesterase inhibitors [15–17], and placebo controlled studies are in progress. Eleven DLB patients (mean age, 78.5 years) treated with rivastigmine in an open-label study over 12 weeks had reductions in delusions (73%), apathy (61%), agitation (52%), and hallucinations (31%). Six patients (55%) experienced very significant clinical improvement that had not previously been achieved with other treatments, including low-dose neuroleptics [18]. Medication was well tolerated, and no patient became more parkinsonian. A double-blind placebo controlled study of rivastigmine has broadly confirmed these findings, also demonstrating significant improvements in cognition, particularly in attention [19].

Other Medications

Limited levodopa response has generally been reported in DLB, only 40%–50% of patients improving significantly [20]. This finding may in part reflect a failure to treat, or to underdose, because of concerns about exacerbating psychotic symptoms. A randomized placebo controlled trial treatment in DLB is urgently needed. The monoamine oxidase-B inhibitor L-deprenyl has been proposed to slow disease progression in AD and PD and therefore might be thought to have a role in managing DLB. L-Deprenyl is however associated with an increased incidence of psychotic symptoms, possibly due to amphetamine-like effects, and is best avoided. There are no data available about the effects of antidepressants, anticonvulsants, or benzodiazepines. It has been suggested that clonazepam may be helpful in controlling the characteristic sleep disturbance of DLB with vivid dreams and a loss of normal REM sleep muscle atonia, leading to excessive jerking or complex vigorous movements [21].

Conclusion

Until safe and effective medications for DLB become available, there is no doubt that the mainstay of clinical management is to educate patients and their caregivers about the nature of their symptoms and suggest strategies to cope with them. The clinician must ascertain which symptoms are most troublesome for the sufferer and explain the risks and benefits associated with changes in medication [5]. In these circumstances in which the clinician is walking a therapeutic tightrope between parkinsonism and psychosis, the best outcome is invariably a compromise between a relatively mobile but psychotic patient and a nonpsychotic but immobile individual.

References

1. Perry EK, Perry RH (1996) Altered consciousness and transmitter signalling in Lewy body dementia. In: Perry R, McKeith I, Perry E (eds) Dementia with Lewy bodies. Cambridge University Press, New York, pp 397–413
2. Perry EK, Irving D, Kerwin JM, et al (1993) Cholinergic transmitter and neurotrophic activities in Lewy body dementia: similarity to Parkinson's and distinction from Alzheimer disease. Alzheimer Dis Assoc Disord 7:69–79
3. Samuel W, Galasko D, Masliah E, et al (1996) Neocortical Lewy body counts correlate with dementia in the Lewy body variant of Alzheimer's disease. J Neuropathol Exp Neurol 55:44–52
4. Perry EK, Marshall E, Kerwin J, et al (1990) Evidence of a monoaminergic-cholinergic imbalance related to visual hallucinations in Lewy body dementia. J Neurochem 55:1454–1456
5. Harrison RH, McKeith IG (1995) Senile dementia of Lewy body type—a review of clinical and pathological features: implications for treatment. Int J Geriatr Psychiatry 10:919–926
6. McKeith IG, Perry RH, Fairbairn AF, et al (1992) Operational criteria for senile dementia of Lewy body type (SDLT). Psychol Med 22:911–922
7. McKeith I, Fairbairn A, Perry R, et al (1992) Neuroleptic sensitivity in patients with senile dementia of Lewy body type. Br Med J 305:673–678
8. Piggott MA, Perry EK, McKeith IG, et al (1994) Dopamine D2 receptors in demented patients with severe neuroleptic sensitivity. Lancet 343:1044–1045
9. McKeith IG, Ballard CG, Harrison RWS (1995) Neuroleptic sensitivity to risperidone in Lewy body dementia. Lancet 346:699–699
10. Walker Z, Grace J, Overshot R, et al (1999) Olanzapine in dementia with Lewy bodies: a clinical study. Int J Geriatr Psychiatry 14:459–466
11. The Parkinson's Disease Study Group (1999) Low-dose Clozapine for the treatment of drug-induced psychosis in Parkinson's disease. N Engl J Med 340:757–763
12. Levy R, Eagger S, Griffiths M, et al (1994) Lewy bodies and response to tacrine in Alzheimer's disease. Lancet 343:176
13. Perry EK, Haroutunian V, Davis KL, et al (1994) Neocortical cholinergic activities differentiate Lewy body dementia from classical Alzheimer's disease. NeuroReport 5:747–749
14. Wilcock GK, Scott MI (1994) Tacrine for senile dementia of Alzheimer's or Lewy body type. Lancet 344:544
15. Aarsland D, Bronnick K, Karlsen K (1999) Donepezil for dementia with Lewy bodies: a case study. Int J Geriatr Psychiatry 14:69–74
16. Shea C, MacKnight C, Rockwood K (1998) Donepezil for treatment of dementia with Lewy bodies: a case series of nine patients. Int Psychogeriatrics 10:229–238

17. Kaufer DI, Catt KE, Lopez OL, et al (1998) Dementia with Lewy bodies: response of delirium-like features to donepezil. Neurology 51:1512
18. McKeith IG, Grace JB, Walker Z, et al (2000) Rivastigmine in the treatment of dementia with Lewy bodies. Int J Geriatr Psychiatry 15:387–392
19. McKeith I, Del Ser T, Spano P, et al (2000) Efficacy of rivastigmine in dementia with Lewy bodies: a randomised, double-blind, placebo-controlled, international study. Lancet 356(9247):2031–2036
20. Louis ED, Klatka LA, Liu Y, et al (1997) Comparison of extrapyramidal features in 31 pathologically confirmed cases of diffuse Lewy body disease and 34 pathologically confirmed cases of Parkinson's disease. Neurology 48(2):376–380
21. Boeve BF, Silber MH, Ferman TJ, et al (1998) REM sleep behaviour disorder and degenerative dementia. Neurology 51:363–370

Dementia with Lewy Bodies

Ian G. McKeith

Summary. Three main clinicopathological syndromes have been described in association with Lewy body (LB) disease: movement disorder, autonomic failure, and dementia. In elderly patients, these symptoms frequently coexist. Improved immunocytochemical stains reveal LB in the brains of 15%–20% of elderly demented cases reaching autopsy, making it the second most common dementia subtype. Alzheimer type and vascular pathology are additionally seen in a significant number of cases. The clinical presentation and course of DLB differs from Alzheimer's disease and other types of dementia. Neuropsychological testing, structural and functional brain imaging, and electrocortical mapping can all contribute toward the differential diagnosis of DLB, which includes other causes of delirium and dementia, other neurological syndromes, and late-onset psychiatric disorders.

Keywords. Dementia, Lewy body, Diagnosis

Introduction

The clinical presentation of Lewy body (LB) disease varies according to the site of LB formation and associated neuronal loss. Three main clinicopathological syndromes have been described: movement disorder, autonomic failure, and dementia. In elderly patients, these symptoms frequently coexist. LB disease was first described by Japanese workers and was initially considered to be a rare cause of dementia. In the late 1980s, improved immunocytochemical staining methods revealed LB in the brains of 15%–20% of elderly demented cases reaching autopsy, revealing it as the second most common dementia subtype. Alzheimer type and vascular pathology are additionally seen in a significant number of cases, but their relative contributions

Department of Old Age Psychiatry, Institute for the Health of the Elderly, Wolfson Research Centre, Newcastle General Hospital, Westgate Road, Newcastle upon Tyne, NE4 6BE, UK

to clinical features are not yet known. Accurate clinical diagnosis using standard methods and criteria is important because the clinical presentation and course of DLB differs from Alzheimer's disease (AD) and other types of dementia. Neuropsychological testing and structural and functional brain imaging can all contribute toward the differential diagnosis of DLB, which includes other causes of delirium and dementia, other neurological syndromes, and late-onset psychiatric disorders.

Neuropathology

Lewy Bodies and Lewy Neurites

Lewy bodies are spherical, intracytoplasmic, eosinophilic, neuronal inclusions that have a dense hyaline core and a halo of radiating filaments composed of abnormally truncated and phosphorylated intermediate neurofilament proteins [1]. They also contain ubiquitin, α-synuclein, and associated enzymes. Their presence in the brainstem nuclei of Parkinson's disease (PD) patients has long been recognized, and in 1961 Okazaki et al. [2] published case reports about two elderly men who presented with dementia and died shortly after with severe extrapyramidal rigidity. Autopsy showed LB in their cerebral cortex. Over the next 20 years, 34 similar cases were reported, [3]. Lewy body disease thus came to be considered as a rare cause of dementia until a series of studies in Europe and North America in the late 1980s identified LB in the brains of 15%–20% of elderly demented cases reaching autopsy [4,5], establishing it as potentially the second most common form of degenerative dementia in old age. Dementia with Lewy bodies (DLB) is now the preferred term [6] for such cases, which have, during the last decade, been known under a variety of names, including diffuse LB disease (DLBD) [3,7,8], dementia associated with cortical Lewy bodies (DCLB) [9], the LB variant of Alzheimer's disease (LBVAD) [5], senile dementia of LB type (SDLT) [4,10], and LB dementia (LBD) [11].

DLB is unlikely to be a newly occurring disorder. Its recent recognition is largely the result of the widespread use of improved neuropathological techniques that greatly enhance visualization of cortical LB [12]. Contrary to early reports, LB probably do not occur in normal aging. Their presence indicates neurological disease, the clinical presentation varying according to the site of LB formation and associated neuronal loss. In DLB, there is a consistent gradient of LB density as follows: substantia nigra > entorhinal cortex > cingulate gyrus > insula > frontal cortex > hippocampus > occipital cortex. Paralimbic and neocortical LB densities are highly correlated with each other but not with nigral pathology, suggesting that DLB should not be considered as just a severe form of PD [13]. A distinctive pattern of neuritic degeneration has additionally been identified in LB disease. "Lewy neurites" are seen in substantia nigra, hippocampal region CA2/3, dorsal vagal nucleus, basal nucleus of Meynert, and transentorhinal cortex. Ubiquitin immunocytochemistry and α-synuclein-specific monoclonal antibody stains are beginning to reveal the extensive nature of these neuritic changes [14], which are probably more relevant for symptom formation than the relatively sparsely distributed LB.

Additional Pathologies

A variety of additional pathological findings are also seen in addition to LB, and in particular the majority of DLB cases have β-amyloid senile plaques (SP) sufficient to qualify for a diagnosis of "plaque predominant" or "CERAD probable" AD. Neocortical NFT density is, by contrast, only slightly increased above age-matched normal control values and more than tenfold lower than the average in Alzheimer's disease [15]. The precise interpretation of these observations remains contentious. Some authorities regard them as evidence of coexistent Alzheimer's disease, which has an earlier clinical presentation than pure AD as a consequence of the additional burden of LB formation and associated neuronal loss [16]. Others regard the Alzheimer pathology in most cases merely to constitute "pathological ageing" rather than evidence of concomitant AD.

There is ongoing nosological debate on whether AD diagnostic criteria should be based on neocortical density of plaques or tangles or archicortical load of tangles according to CERAD [17], NIA/Reagan [18], or Braak staging [19], so the extent to which DLB cases mixed with AD pathologies should be classified as LB variant of AD has not been fully resolved [16]. Significant vascular pathology is additionally present in 30% of DLB cases [20,21], typically cortical or white matter infarcts combined with arteriosclerosis or congophilic angiopathy.

Clinical Features of DLB

Age at onset ranges from 50 to 83 years and age at death from 68 to 92 years, with a slight excess of men. Cognitive function appears to decline at approximately the same rate as in AD and parkinsonism at a rate similar to PD. Mean survival time is reported as similar to that for AD, although some DLB individuals show very rapid symptom progression and early death [22]. Twenty-six percent of clinical referrals to an old-age psychiatry service with dementia [23] and 24% of demented day hospital attenders met clinical criteria for DLB [24]. No estimates of prevalence and incidence in primary care- and community-based samples have been reported, although a community case register study [20], found 15% of elderly demented cases to have DLB at autopsy.

Dementia is usually, but not always, the presenting feature; a minority of patients present with parkinsonism alone, some with psychiatric disorder in the absence of dementia, and others with orthostatic hypotension, falls, or transient disturbances of consciousness [10,25]. Fluctuation in cognitive performance and functional ability, which is based on variations in attention and level of consciousness, is the most characteristic feature of DLB [6]. It is usually evident on a day-to-day basis, and often apparent within much shorter periods. The marked amplitude between best and worst performance distinguishes it from the minor day-to-day variations that commonly occur in dementia of any etiology. Repeated visual hallucinations are present in about two-thirds of patients. These take the form of vivid, colorful, and sometimes fragmented figures of people and animals, usually described in great detail. Emotional responses vary from intense fear to indifference or even amusement. Although patients may respond to their hallucinations, for example, as trying to feed an imaginary dog, they later often have good insight into their unreality. Others develop elaborate systematized delusions, usually persecutory or of a phantom boarder.

Auditory hallucinations are much less frequent and only a minority of patients have olfactory or tactile experiences. Depressive symptoms are common, and about 40% of patients will have a major depressive episode, similar to the rate in PD and significantly greater than in AD [26]. The frequency and severity of spontaneous motor features of parkinsonism varies greatly from one clinical setting to another. Up to 70% of patients have parkinsonian symptoms, with bradykinesia, limb rigidity, and gait disorder being the most common manifestations [27]. When present, these symptoms may be as severe in DLB as in PD, but it remains to be established whether they respond similarly to antiparkinsonian treatments. Recurrent falls and syncope occur in up to a third of DLB cases, reflecting autonomic nervous system involvement. Transient disturbances of consciousness in which patients are found mute and unresponsive for periods of several minutes may represent the extreme of fluctuation in attention and arousal and are often mistaken for transient ischemic attacks despite a lack of focal neurological signs [10]. REM sleep behavior disorder with nighttime restlessness, vivid dreaming, and motor overactivity is also associated with DLB as opposed to other dementia subtypes [28].

Diagnosis and Differential Diagnosis

There are four main categories of disorder that should be considered in the differential diagnosis of DLB. These are other dementia syndromes, other causes of delirium, other neurological syndromes, such as PD, progressive supranuclear palsy, multisystem atrophy or CJD, and other psychiatric disorders, such as late-onset delusional disorder, depressive psychosis, or mania. The most frequent clinical misdiagnosis of DLB patients is as AD [29]. Accurate diagnosis rests upon careful history taking and physical and mental state examination. There are no biological tests or markers currently available. Structural imaging in DLB reveals similar generalized atrophic changes to AD in many cases. Approximately 40% of DLB subjects, however, show preservation of medial temporal lobe structures, and this may help in the differentiation from AD [30]. DLB does not differ from AD in terms of degree of ventricular enlargement, frontal lobe atrophy, or presence of white matter changes on MRI [31]. Significant differences have been demonstrated between DLB and AD in striatal uptake of beta- and FP-CIT (ligands for the dopamine transporter), a difference that would be predicted from known anatomical and neurochemical differences in nigrostriatal pathology between AD and DLB [32,33].

Table 1 shows the Consensus criteria for clinical diagnosis of DLB. Particular emphasis needs to be given to recognizing the characteristic pattern of cognitive dysfunction with prominent attentional deficits, visuospatial impairment, and fronto-subcortical dysfunction [34,35]. In contrast to AD there is often a relative preservation of short-term memory, at least in the early stages [10,36], presumably reflecting less severe involvement of medial temporal lobe circuitry. Probable DLB is diagnosed if any two of the three core symptoms (fluctuation, visual hallucinations, spontaneous motor features of parkinsonism) are additionally present. If only one symptom is present, a possible DLB diagnosis is made.

Fluctuation is undoubtedly the most difficult symptom to establish. Some patients identify the variable cognitive state themselves, but generally the most productive

Table 1. Consensus criteria for the clinical diagnosis of probable and possible dementia with Lewy bodies (DLB)

1. The central feature required for a diagnosis of DLB is progressive cognitive decline of sufficient magnitude to interfere with normal social or occupational function. Prominent or persistent memory impairment may not necessarily occur in the early stages but is usually evident with progression. Deficits on tests of attention and of frontal-subcortical skills and visuospatial ability may be especially prominent.
2. Two of the following core features are essential for a diagnosis of probable DLB; one is essential for possible DLB.
   a. Fluctuating cognition with pronounced variations in attention and alertness
   b. Recurrent visual hallucinations that are typically well formed and detailed
   c. Spontaneous motor features of parkinsonism
3. Features supportive of the diagnosis are
   a. Repeated falls
   b. Syncope
   c. Transient loss of consciousness
   d. Neuroleptic sensitivity
   e. Systematized delusions
   f. Hallucinations in other modalities
4. A diagnosis of DLB is less likely in the presence of
   a. Stroke disease, evident as focal neurological signs or on brain imaging
   b. Evidence on physical examination and investigation of any physical illness, or other brain disorder, sufficient to account for the clinical picture

Source: McKeith et al. [6]

approach is to interview a reliable informant. Questions such as "Are there episodes when his/her thinking seems quite clear and then becomes muddled?" may be useful probes. Substantial changes in mental state and behavior may be seen within the duration of a single interview or between consecutive examinations. Parkinsonism and visual hallucinations pose fewer problems of identification [6].

Several autopsy validation studies [37] have examined the diagnostic accuracy of the Consensus criteria and find uniformly high specificity, usually 0.9–1.0, but sensitivity of case detection is more variable and generally lower (0.22–0.83). In summary, the current criteria for probable DLB can be applied with good specificity and can therefore be used in their current form for recruiting cohorts of DLB patients for research studies and clinical trials. These criteria are less useful for identifying cases in the clinic, although when a diagnosis is made it is likely to be correct. The index of suspicion for a diagnosis of DLB needs to be increased, not only in dementia assessment clinics but also in any setting where elderly patients may present with delirium, movement disorder, falls, or syncope [38].

Summary

DLB is a common form of dementia in the elderly that shares clinical and pathological characteristics with both AD and PD. Accurate clinical diagnosis can be achieved using operationalized diagnostic criteria supported by appropriate neuroimaging.

DLB patients may show catastrophic adverse reactions to antipsychotic medications, avoidance of which is one of the main reasons for correctly identifying DLB in the clinic. This and other management issues are discussed in the chapter immediately preceding this one.

References

1. Lowe JS, Mayer RJ, Landon M (1996) Pathological significance of Lewy bodies in dementia. In: Perry RH, McKeith IG, Perry EK (eds) Dementia with Lewy bodies. Cambridge University Press, New York, pp 195–203
2. Okazaki H, Lipton LS, Aronson SM (1961) Diffuse intracytoplasmic ganglionic inclusions (Lewy type) associated with progressive dementia and quadrapesis in flexion. J Neurol Neurosurg Psychiatry 20:237–244
3. Kosaka K, Yoshimura M, Ikeda K, Budka H (1984) Diffuse type of Lewy body disease: progressive dementia with abundant cortical Lewy bodies and senile changes of varying degree—a new disease? Clin Neuropathol 3:185–192
4. Perry RH, Irving D, Blessed G, et al (1990) Senile dementia of Lewy body type. A clinically and neuropathologically distinct form of Lewy body dementia in the elderly. J Neurol Sci 95:119–139
5. Hansen L, Salmon D, Galasko D, et al (1990) The Lewy body variant of Alzheimer's disease: a clinical and pathologic entity. Neurology 40:1–8
6. McKeith IG, Galasko D, Kosaka K, et al (1996) Consensus guidelines for the clinical and pathologic diagnosis of dementia with Lewy bodies (DLB): report of the consortium on DLB international workshop. Neurology 47:1113–1124
7. Dickson DW, Davies P, Mayeux R (1987) Diffuse Lewy body disease. Neuropathological and biochemical studies of six patients. Acta Neuropathol 75:8–15
8. Crystal HA, Dickson DW, Lizardi JE, et al (1990) Antemortem diagnosis of diffuse Lewy body disease. Neurology 40:1523–1528
9. Byrne EJ, Lennox G, Godwin-Austen RB, et al (1990) Dementia associated with cortical Lewy bodies. Proposed diagnostic criteria. Dementia 2:283–284
10. McKeith IG, Perry RH, Fairbairn AF, et al (1990) Operational criteria for senile dementia of Lewy body type (SDLT). Psychol Med 22:911–922
11. Gibb WRG, Esiri MM, Lees AJ (1987) Clinical and pathological features of diffuse cortical Lewy body disease (Lewy body dementia). Brain 110:1131–1153
12. Lennox G, Lowe J, Landon M, et al (1989) Diffuse Lewy body disease: correlative neuropathology using anti-ubiquitin immunocytochemistry. J Neurol Neurosurg Psychiatry 52:1236–1247
13. Gomez-Tortosa E, Newell K, Irizarry MC, et al (1999) Clinical and quantitative pathological correlates of dementia with Lewy bodies. Neurology 53:1284–1291
14. Trojanowski J (1998) Dementia with Lewy bodies: diagnostic accuracy using Consensus criteria. Neurobiol Aging 19(4S):S4
15. Harrington CR, Perry RH, Perry EK, et al (1994) Senile dementia of Lewy body type and Alzheimer type are biochemically distinct in terms of paired helical filaments and hyperphosphorylated tau protein. Dementia 5:215–228
16. Hansen LA, Samuel W (1997) Criteria for Alzheimer's disease and the nosology of dementia with Lewy bodies. Neurology 48:126–132
17. Mirra SS, Heyman A, McKeel D, et al (1991) The Consortium to Establish a Registry for Alzheimer's Disease (CERAD). Part II. Standardization of the neuropathological assessment of Alzheimer's disease. Neurology 41:479–486
18. Trojanowski JQ, Clark M, Schmidt ML, et al (1997) Strategies for improving the postmortem pathological diagnosis of Alzheimer's disease. Neurobiol Aging 18(4S): S75–S79

19. Braak H, Braak E (1991) Neuropathological staging of Alzheimer-related changes. Acta Neuropathol 82:239–259
20. Holmes C, Cairns N, Lantos P, Mann A (1999) Validity of current clinical criteria for Alzheimer's disease, vascular dementia and dementia with Lewy bodies. Br J Psychiatry 174:45–50
21. McKeith IG, Ballard CG, Perry RH, et al (2000) Prospective validation of consensus criteria for the diagnosis of dementia with Lewy bodies. Neurology 54:1050–1058
22. Papka M, Rubio A, Schiffer RB (1998) A review of Lewy body disease, an emerging concept of cortical dementia. J Neuropsychiatry Clin Neurosci 10:267–279
23. Shergill S, Mullan E, D'ath P, Katona C (1994) What is the clinical prevalence of Lewy body dementia? Int J Geriatr Psychiatry 9:907–912
24. Ballard CG, Mohan RNC, Patel A, Bannister C (1995) Idiopathic clouding of consciousness—do the patients have cortical Lewy body disease? Int J Psychogeriatrics 8:571–576
25. Byrne EJ, Lennox G, Lowe J, Godwin-Austen RB (1989) Diffuse Lewy body disease: clinical features in 15 cases. J Neurol Neurosurg Psychiatry 52:709–717
26. McKeith IG (1998) Dementia with Lewy bodies: clinical and pathological diagnosis. Alzheimer's Rep 1(2):83–87
27. Louis ED, Klatka LA, Liu Y, Fahn S (1997) Comparison of extrapyramidal features in 31 pathologically confirmed cases of diffuse Lewy body disease and 34 pathologically confirmed cases of Parkinson's disease. Neurology 48:376–380
28. Boeve BF, Silber MH, Ferman TJ, et al (1998) REM sleep behaviour disorder and degenerative dementia: an association likely reflecting Lewy body disease. Neurology 51(2):363–370
29. McKeith IG, Fairbairn AF, Perry RH, Thompson P (1994) The clinical diagnosis and misdiagnosis of senile dementia of Lewy body type (SDLT). Br J Psychiatry 165:324–332
30. Barber R, Gholkar A, Ballard C, et al (1999) Temporal lobe atrophy on MRI in dementia with Lewy bodies: a comparison with Alzheimer's disease, Vascular dementia and normal ageing. Neurology 54:1152–1158
31. Barber R, Gholkar A, Ballard C, et al (1999) White matter lesions on MRI in dementia with Lewy bodies, Alzheimer's disease, vascular dementia and normal ageing. J Neurol Neurosurg Psychiatry 67:66–72
32. Donnemiller E, Heilman J, Wenning GK, et al (1997) Brain perfusion scintigraphy with ^{99m}Tc-HMPAO or ^{99m}Tc-ECD and ^{123}I-beta-CIT-single-photon emission tomography in dementia of the Alzheimer type and diffuse Lewy body disease. Eur J Nucl Med 24:320–325
33. Walker Z, Costa DC, Ince P, et al (1999) In vivo demonstration of dopaminergic degeneration in dementia with Lewy bodies. Lancet 354:646–647
34. Salmon DP, Galasko D (1996) Neuropsychological aspects of Lewy body dementia. In: Perry RH, McKeith IG, Perry EK (eds) Dementia with Lewy bodies. Cambridge University Press, New York, pp 99–113
35. Ayre GA, Sahgal A, McKeith IG, et al. Distinct profiles of cognitive impairment in dementia with Lewy bodies and Alzheimer's disease. Neurology (in press)
36. Walker Z, Allen RL, Shergill S, Katona CLE (1997) Neuropsychological performance in Lewy body dementia and Alzheimer's disease. Br J Psychiatry 170:156–158
37. McKeith IG, O'Brien JT, Ballard C (1999) Diagnosing dementia with Lewy bodies. Lancet 354:1227–1228
38. McKeith IG, Perry EK, Perry RH (1999) Report of the second dementia with Lewy body international workshop. Neurology 53:902–905

Neuropathological Studies on Dementia with Lewy Bodies

KENJI KOSAKA and EIZO ISEKI

Summary. We review here some of our recent neuropathological studies of dementia with Lewy bodies (DLB). Using immunohistochemistry with anti-α-synuclein and other antibodies, we point out (1) the possibility of dying-back degeneration in hippocampal pathology, (2) more frequent coexistence of Lewy bodies and neurofibrillary tangles in the same neurons in the limbic areas than expected, and (3) the degeneration process of Lewy bodies, that the Lewy body degenerates slowly and appear extracellularly (ghost Lewy body) followed by microglias and astrocytes.

Keywords. Lewy body, Diffuse Lewy body disease, Dementia with Lewy bodies, α-synuclein, Immunohistochemistry

Introduction

In 1995, the term "dementia with Lewy bodies" (DLB; McKeith et al. 1996) was proposed as a generic term for dementia-causing illnesses associated with the presence of numerous cortical Lewy bodies (LB), including diffuse Lewy body disease (DLBD; Kosaka et al. 1984, Kosaka 1990). Since 1976, we (Kosaka 2000; Kosaka and Iseki 2000) have studied DLB from both clinicopathological and immunohistochemical aspects. In this chapter, we review some of our recent neuropathological and immunohistochemical studies on DLB.

Hippocampal Pathology Using Ubiquitin and α-Synuclein Immunohistochemistry

Ubiquitin-positive "Lewy neurites" in the CA2–CA3 areas of the hippocampus were also α-synuclein immunopositive. Various ubiquitin-positive structures, including granules, Lewy neurites, and spheroids, were found in the hippocampus of DLB brains (Iseki et al. 1997). The ubiquitin-positive granules and Lewy neurites were predominantly found in the CA2–CA3 areas, whereas the ubiquitin-positive spheroids were

Department of Psychiatry, Yokohama City University, School of Medicine, 3-9 Kanazawa-ku, Yokohama 236-0004, Japan

found in the stratum lacunosum-moleculare. Many of these structures may be caused by degeneration of terminal or distal axons of the nonperforant or perforant pathway from the entorhinal cortex. The nonperforant pathway degenerated more severely than did the perforant pathway in DLB brains; this was in contrast to Alzheimer-type dementia (ATD) brains (Iseki et al. 1997).

Both cortical and brainstem Lewy bodies are known to be specifically α-synuclein immunopositive. We examined hippocampal pathology in DLB brains using α-synuclein immunohistochemistry (Iseki et al. 1998). Ubiquitin-positive structures caused by degeneration of terminal axons of the perforant pathway were also α-synuclein-positive. These α-synuclein-positive degenerative terminals contained granulofilamentous or vesiculotubular components similar to those of Lewy bodies seen using immunoelectron microscopy, suggesting that α-synuclein may abnormally aggregate into filamentous or tubular cytoskeletal components. A "dying-back" degeneration caused by a blockage in axonal transport may explain why the degenerative terminals and Lewy bodies share similar α-synuclein-positive components.

Coexistence of Lewy Bodies and Neurofibrillary Tangles in the Same Neurons

We (Iseki et al. 1999) examined neurons with coexistent Lewy bodies and neurofibrillary tangles (NFTs) in DLB brains, using double immunostaining with anti-α-synuclein and anti-tau antibodies. Double-positive neurons were more frequently observed in the limbic areas than expected. These neurons mostly revealed the presence of intermingled α-synuclein- and tau-positive substances. Immunoelectron microscopy showed that the α-synuclein-positive components were contiguous with paired helical filaments (PHF). Some α-synuclein-positive Lewy bodies were surrounded by small PHF bundles, and randomly oriented PHF were also found within Lewy bodies. In the intermingled neurons, α-synuclein-positive nonfilamentous components were found among the large PHF bundles. These nonfilamentous components may represent the early stage of Lewy body formation (Iseki et al. 1999).

Degeneration Process of Lewy Bodies

The detailed degeneration process of Lewy body has not yet been clarified. In 1978, we (Kosaka 1978) reported the growth and degeneration process of cortical Lewy bodies by light microscopy. Very recently, we (Iseki et al. 2000) examined the degeneration process of brainstem Lewy bodies using the recent immunohistochemical method. According to the study, Lewy bodies degenerate very slowly and appear extracellularly (ghost Lewy bodies) followed by microglias and astrocytes.

References

1. Iseki E, Li F, Odawara T, Kosaka K (1997) Hippocampal pathology in diffuse Lewy body disease using ubiquitin immunohistochemistry. J Neurol Sci 149:165–169

2. Iseki E, Marui W, Kosaka K, et al (1998) Degenerative terminals of the perforant pathway are human α-synuclein immunoreactive in the hippocampus of patients with diffuse Lewy body disease. Neurosci Lett 258:81–84
3. Iseki E, Marui W, Kosaka K, Ueda K (1999) Frequent coexistence of Lewy bodies and neurofibrillary tangles in the same neurons of patients with diffuse Lewy body disease. Neurosci Lett 265: 9–12
4. Iseki E, Marui W, Kosaka K (2000) Degeneration process of Lewy bodies in the brains of patients with dementia with Lewy bodies using α-synuclein immunohistochemistry. Neurosci Lett 286:69–73
5. Kosaka K (1978) Lewy bodies in cerebral cortex. Report of three cases. Acta Neuropathol 42:127–134
6. Kosaka K (1990) Diffuse Lewy body disease in Japan. J Neurol 237:197–204
7. Kosaka K (2000) Diffuse Lewy body disease. Neuropathology 20:S73–78
8. Kosaka K, Iseki E (2000) Clinicopathological studies on diffuse Lewy body disease. Neuropathology 1:1–7
9. Kosaka K, Yoshimura M, Ikeda K, Budka H (1984) Diffuse type of Lewy body disease. Progressive dementia with abundant cortical Lewy bodies and senile changes of various degree. A new disease? Clin Neuropathol 3:185–192
10. McKeith IG, Galasko D, Kosaka K, et al (1996) Consensus guidelines for the clinical and pathologic diagnosis of dementia with Lewy bodies (DLB): report of the consortium on DLB international workshop. Neurology 47:1113–1124

Dementia with Lewy Bodies: What Is Its Relationship to Alzheimer's Disease?

Carol F. Lippa

Summary. The relationship between dementia with Lewy bodies (DLB) and Alzheimer's disease (AD) is poorly understood. In this chapter, the issue is discussed from a clinical and histopathological perspective, with an emphasis on early-onset familial forms of AD (FAD) related to identifiable genetic abnormalities. FAD cases frequently have Lewy bodies in the amygdala, and more widespread Lewy body formation is common. Overall, AD cases resulting from point mutations are more likely to develop Lewy bodies than cases with Down's syndrome. However, no specific point mutations of the amyloid precursor protein (APP) and presenilin-1 (PS-1) genes are consistently associated with Lewy body formation. FAD subjects with Lewy bodies inconsistently meet clinical consensus criteria for possible or probable DLB. Symptoms of DLB are more likely to be present when Lewy bodies occur in large numbers in multiple regions. However, some symptoms of DLB, such as spontaneous parkinsonism, occur in specific kindreds, including our C410Y PS-1 family. Here, parkinsonism occurs primarily in association with β-amyloid plaques and neuritic degeneration in the basal ganglia, rather than Lewy bodies. The frequent occurrence of Lewy bodies in early-onset FAD cases suggests that the genetic abnormalities leading to early-onset AD also may predispose individuals to developing Lewy bodies. Lewy body formation, particularly that which occurs in the amygdala, may be a manifestation of phenotypic heterogeneity seen in the AD process.

Keywords. Dementia with Lewy bodies, Down's syndrome, Alzheimer's disease, APP, Lewy body, Presenilin

Introduction

Kosaka et al. first proposed the term Lewy body disease in 1980 on the basis of their clinicopathological research indicating that a specific set of symptoms and neuropathological findings comprise such a disease entity [1]. Dementia with Lewy bodies (DLB) is now recognized as a common condition. It is the second most frequent diagnosis given to dementia patients after Alzheimer's disease (AD) in some centers [2–5]. However, despite its common occurrence, the clinical diagnosis cannot be made with

Department of Neurology, MCP-Hahnemann University, Philadelphia, PA 19129, USA certainty using established criteria. Some of this difficulty may arise because of overlap in the clinical and pathological features observed in DLB and AD subjects. For example, the majority of DLB patients have concurrent histopathological features of AD, and the reason for this is poorly understood. This report summarizes research exploring the relationship between DLB and AD with an eye toward assessing subjects with familial forms of AD.

Clinical features may help to distinguish pure AD from DLB but cannot distinguish pure DLB from DLB cases with concurrent AD pathology. The three cardinal symptoms of DLB are visual hallucinations, a fluctuating mental status, and spontaneous parkinsonism [6]. In sporadic AD cases without Lewy bodies (LBs), these symptoms infrequently occur early in the disease course. AD patients typically have memory loss as the most prominent early symptom [7]. However, clinicopathological correlation studies of DLB show variable correlations between the DLB triad of symptoms and the presence of LBs at autopsy.

We investigated the relationship between AD and LBs using antibodies directed against α-synuclein to determine how commonly LBs occur in familial AD (FAD) brains related to presenilin-1 (PS-1; $n = 58$), presenilin-2 (PS-2, $n = 7$), or amyloid precursor protein (APP; $n = 9$) gene mutations [8]. LBs were observed in 18% of FAD brains. These were most numerous in the amygdala where 63% of the FAD samples available for examination contained LBs. We then demonstrated the α-synuclein in LBs using immunoelectron microscopy [8] (Fig. 1). LBs were less often present in other regions of PS-1 or APP brains. The LBs occurred in cases with both APP and PS-1 mutations, but were not consistently present or absent in association with any specific mutation.

To determine whether the LBs identified in the amygdala had the same biochemical properties as those of LBs in Parkinson's disease and other cases of DLB, we performed Western blot analysis on amygdala extracts from two PS-1 cases with LBs in

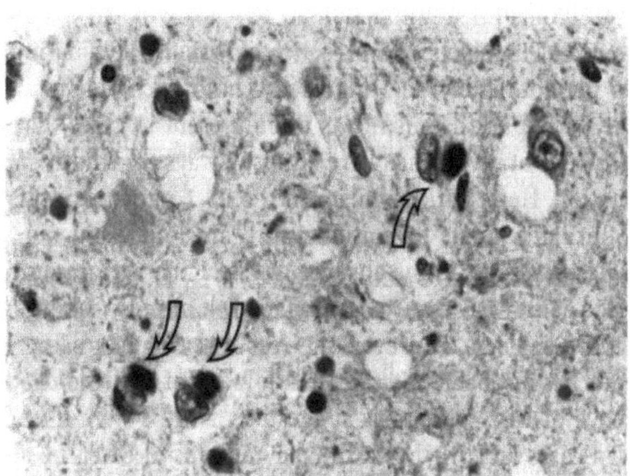

Fig. 1. High magnification photomicrograph showing Lewy bodies in the amygdala in a PS-1 Alzheimer's disease (AD) case. Note that Lewy bodies (*arrows*) are numerous in the amygdala. This patient has a mutation of the PS-1 gene (M146L). Clinically, he had a typical appearance of AD, lacking psychiatric symptomatology, fluctuation, or parkinsonism. ×60

TABLE 1. Frequency of Lewy bodies in the amygdala and other brain regions in our Alzheimer's disease (AD) patients

Region	PS-1 AD	PS-2 AD	APP AD	Down's syndrome	Sporadic AD
Amygdala	11/17	0/1	1/1	8/19	2/12
Other	10/58	1/7	1/9	6/19	1/12

the amygdala, one PS-1 case lacking LBs, and three age-matched normal control cases. The methods we used for Western blot analysis were previously described [9]. This biochemical analysis revealed similar amounts of α-synuclein in the soluble fractions of the extracts from all cases. However, formic acid-extractable extracts showed high molecular mass α-synuclein aggregates in the two PS-1 tissue samples that contained LBs. The FAD case without LBs and control brains lacked these aggregates. Thus, the increase in insoluble forms of α-synuclein in FAD cases with LBs suggests that LBs in DLB, Parkinson's disease, and PS-1 AD all are composed of insoluble forms of α-synuclein.

We then extended the immunohistochemical analysis to examine brain tissue from 20 Down's syndrome (DS) cases [10], and found that these amygdala also sometimes contained LBs. However, these were less commonly present, occurring in less than half the amygdala samples from elderly DS brains. LBs were never present in younger DS subjects, even if other AD-related pathology was present. These studies suggest that LBs may occur in several forms of early-onset FAD and that the tendency for LB formation may differ when the genetic etiologies differ (Table 1).

We then looked back to determine whether LBs in these patients were associated with any of the distinctive clinical features of DLB. We found that most often the FAD cases with LBs had typical features of AD, presenting with progressive memory loss. However, occasionally clinical features of DLB were evident early in the course of the disease. These symptoms and signs included psychosis or parkinsonism. Although uncommon in our FAD subjects, the presence of visual hallucinations or psychotic features early in the course of FAD indicated a high likelihood that LBs would be present. However, early parkinsonism was often present in cases that lacked LBs. In particular, rigidity and bradykinesia were almost always present in subjects with the C410Y PS-1 mutation. Here, parkinsonism in the PS-1 patients occurred in association with neurofibrillary tangle formation and β-amyloid plaques in the substantia nigra and other basal ganglia, in the absence of LBs. Early extrapyramidal symptoms have been reported as an early feature in other FAD kindreds. Generally, LBs have not been noted in these subjects. However, the frequency of LBs using more sensitive detection methods has not been documented in many of these kindreds. Thus, in our series, the presence of early psychosis suggested that LBs were likely. Also, because LBs are present in cases lacking the cardinal symptoms of DLB, the absence of clinical features indicative of DLB in these FAD cases cannot exclude the possibility that LBs are present.

LBs may occur for a number of reasons in the FAD brain. Our data from FAD brains suggest that LB formation may be inherent to the AD process. It is possible that some of the cases showed LBs as a nonspecific manifestation of end-stage disease. We do not believe that this explains the presence of LBs in all cases because the presence of LBs was not correlated with disease severity at death or disease duration. The clinical significance of LBs in these FAD cases may be dependent on quantitative factors, with the numbers of LBs in specific regions determining the clinical significance. Occasional LBs in an isolated region in an FAD brain from a patient with advanced disease or even large numbers of LBs in an isolated region may not produce typical symptoms and signs of DLB. LBs may be almost as numerous as neurofibrillary tangles in the FAD amygdala without a clinical accompaniment. In a more widespread distribution, LBs may be associated with specific symptoms, particularly psychiatric symptomatology in FAD. Overall, our findings indicate that LBs occur in FAD and that the clinical and biological importance of their presence is quantitative and reflects the distribution and number of LBs present.

Acknowledgment. The studies that are reviewed here were performed as a collaborative effort. Peter St. George-Hyslop conducted the genetic analyses on the familial AD cases. Linda Nee documented the inheritance and helped assess family members of these kindreds. Other investigators involved in the clinical characterization of these subjects include D. Pollen, R. Polinsky, and P. Frommelt. J.Q. Trojanowski, V.M.Y. Lee, and their associates performed the biochemical characterization of the α-synuclein in the FAD cases. Drs. Lee and Trojanowski also provided the α-synuclein antibody to C.F.L. for the immunohistochemical studies. T. Iwatsubo performed the immunoelectron microscopy on the FAD amygdala samples. Last, we wish to thank the families of our subjects with familial forms of AD who donated tissue for research. This work was supported by the National Institute on Aging of National Institutes of Health (AG13623).

References

1. Kosaka K, Matsushita M, Oyanagi S, Mehraein P (1980) A cliniconeurophathological study of the "Lewy body disease." Seishin Shinkeigaku Zasshi 82:292–311
2. Dickson DW, Ruan D, Crystal H, et al (1991) Hippocampal degeneration differentiates diffuse Lewy body disease (DLBD) from Alzheimer's disease: light and electron microscopic immunocytochemistry of CA2-3 neurites specific to DLBD. Neurology 41:1402–1409
3. Hansen L, Salmon D, Galasko D, et al (1990) The Lewy body variant of Alzheimer's disease: a clinical and pathologic entity. Neurology 40:1–8
4. Lennox G, Lowe J, Morrell K, et al (1989) Anti-ubiquitin immunocytochemistry is more sensitive than conventional techniques in the detection of diffuse Lewy body disease. J Neurol Neurosurg Psychiatry 52:67–71
5. Perry RH, Irving D, Blessed G, et al (1990) Senile dementia of Lewy body type. A clinically and neuropathologically distinct form of Lewy body dementia in the elderly. J Neurol Sci 95:119–139
6. McKeith IG, Galasko D, Kosaka K, et al (1996) Consensus guidelines for the clinical and pathologic diagnosis of dementia with Lewy bodies (DLB): report of the consortium on DLB international workshop. Neurology 47:1113–1124
7. McKhann G, Drachman DA, Folstein MF, et al (1984) Clinical diagnosis of Alzheimer disease: report of the NINCDS-ADRDA Work Group under the auspices of Health and Human Services task Force on Alzheimer's Disease. Neurology 34:939–944

8. Lippa CF, Fujiwara H, Mann DM, et al (1998) Lewy bodies contain altered alpha-synuclein in brains of many familial Alzheimer's disease patients with mutations in presenilin and amyloid precursor protein genes. Am J Pathol 153:1365–1370
9. Baba M, Nakajo S, Tu PH, et al (1998) Aggregation of alpha-synuclein in Lewy bodies of sporadic Parkinson's disease and dementia with Lewy bodies. Am J Pathol 152:879–884
10. Lippa CF, Schmidt ML, Lee VM, Trojanowski JQ (1999) Antibodies to alpha-synuclein detect Lewy bodies in many Down's syndrome brains with Alzheimer's disease. Ann Neurol 45:353–357

Brain Pathology of Dementias

Kenji Kosaka

Summary. Dementia is one of the most important chronic organic brain syndromes caused by variable brain lesions. We first introduce our classification of dementias from a clincopathological point of view, and then show clinical features of each dementia as well as some examples causing it. The most frequent and important dementia-causing disorders in the elderly are so-called aging-associated dementing illnesses. Among them, non-Alzheimer degenerative dementias (NADD) have recently received a great deal of attention. Then, we introduce our classification of NADD from a clinicopathological point of view and focus on dementia with Lewy bodies and dementia with neurofibrillary tangles.

Keywords. Dementia, Neuropathology, Non-Alzheimer degenerative dementias, Dementia with Lewy bodies, Dementia with neurofibrillary tangles

Introduction

Dementia is one of the most important chronic organic brain syndromes. We classify dementias as follows from the clinicopathological aspect: (1) cortical dementia, (2) white matter dementia, (3) limbic dementia including hippocampal dementia, and (4) subcortical dementia including thalamic dementia. Each dementia shows characteristic clinical features caused by variable pathological lesions in the brain. The main dementing illnesses in the elderly are classified into (1) degenerative dementias, (2) vascular dementias, and (3) mixed-type dementia. Degenerative dementias consist of Alzheimer-type dementia (ATD) and non-Alzheimer degenerative dementias (NADD) (Kosaka and Iseki 1998). In this article, we review clinical features and brain pathology of each dementia, and also the clinicopathological features of some NADD, focusing on dementia with Lewy bodies (McKeith et al. 1996; Kosaka 1998; Kosaka and Iseki 2000) and dementia with neurofibrillary tangles (Kosaka et al. 1997; Kosaka and Iseki 1998).

Department of Psychiatry, Yokohama City University School of Medicine, 3-9 Kanazawa-ku, Yokohama 236-0004, Japan

Variable Dementias and Their Neuropathological Substrates

Variable kinds of dementias have been classified by some researchers. We classify dementias from the clinicopathological point of view (Table 1). Cortical dementia is caused by various lesions widespread in the cerebral cortex. The representative disorders expressing this are ATD, Pick's disease, and dementia with Lewy bodies (DLB). On the other hand, Binswanger's encephalopathy and leukodystrophies show typical white matter dementia. Limbic dementia is typically detected in herpes simplex encephalitis. Hippocampal dementia is a subtype of limbic dementia that is observed in limbic neurofibrillary tangle dementia (LNTD) (Kosaka et al. 1997), which is described later. Lesions in subcortical nuclei without cortical and white matter pathology cause typical subcortical dementia. The examples showing this dementia are Huntington's disease, Parkinson's disease, and progressive supranuclear palsy (PSP). However, at the terminal stage of Huntington's disease, cortical degeneration may occur and cause cortical dementia. In PSP, numerous tau-positive glial tangles also appear in the cerebral cortex and white matter. The presence of these glial tangles might contribute to dementia. Thalamic dementia is an atypical type of subcortical dementia, which is caused by primary thalamus degeneration.

TABLE 1. Clinicopathological classification of dementias

Cortical dementia
Disturbance of various cortical functions
White matter dementia
Organic personality changes (euphoria, indifference)
Relatively preserved elementary intelligence
No disturbance of cortical function
Limbic dementia
Amnestic syndrome
Kluever–Bucy-like syndrome
Personality changes
Relatively preserved elementary intelligence
Hippocampal dementia
Amnestic syndrome
Mild dementia
Relatively preserved personality
Subcortical dementia
Forgetfulness
Slowing of mental processes
Impaired ability to manipulate acquired knowlege
Personality and affective changes (apathy and depression)
Thalamus dementia
Amnestic syndrome
Personality chages (apathy, aspontaneity)
Changes of alertness (hypersomnia)

Non-Alzheimer Degenerative Dementias

We have proposed NADD as a generic term for dementing illnesses caused by various degenerative brain pathology except for ATD (Kosaka and Iseki 1998). Then, we classified NADD as follows (Table 2): (1) dementia with Lewy bodies (DLB), (2) dementia with neurofibrillary tangles (NFT), (3) dementia with glial tangles, (4) frontotemporal dementia-parkinsonism linked to chromosome 17 (FTDP–17) (5) dementia with argyrophilic grains, (6) frontotemporal dementia, (7) dementia with predominant degeneration in subcortical nuclei, and (8) unclassified presenile dementia (Kosaka and Iseki 1998). In this article, only DLB and dementia with neurofibrillary tangles (DNFT) are introduced, based upon our recent clinicopathological studies.

Dementia with Lewy Bodies

DLB is a generic term proposed at the first International Workshop held in 1995 (McKeith et al. 1996), which includes diffuse Lewy body disease (DLBD; Kosaka et al. 1984; Kosaka 1990; Kosaka and Iseki 2000), senile dementia of Lewy body type (Perry et al. 1990), Lewy body variant of Alzheimer's disease (Hansen et al. 1990), and cerebral type of Lewy body disease (Kosaka et al. 1997). The CDLB guidelines for clinical and pathological diagnostic criteria (McKeith et al. 1996) were also proposed. However, not all cases with probable DLB meet the clinical diagnostic criteira.

Table 2. A classification of non-Alzheimer degenerative dementias (NADD)

1. Dementia with Lewy bodies (DLB)
   Diffuse Lewy body disease (DLBD)
   Senile dementia of Lewy body type (SDLT)
   Lewy body variant of Alzheimer disease
   Cerebral type of Lewy body disease
2. Dementia with neurofibrillary tangles (DNFT)
   Dementia–parkinsonism complex (PDC)
   Diffuse neurofibrillary tangles with calcification (DNTC)
   Limbic neurofibrillary tangle dementia (LNTD)
3. Dementia with glial tangles
   Progressive supranuclear palsy (PSP)
   Corticobasal degeneration (CBD)
4. Frontotemporal dementia–parkinsonism linked to chromosome 17 (FTDP-17)
5. Dementia with argyrophilic grains
6. Frontotemporal dementia (FTD)
   Pick's disease
   Progressive subcortical gliosis (PSG)
   Presenile dementia with motor neuron disease
   Unspecific frontotemporal dementia
7. Dementia with predominant degeneration in subcortical nuclei
   Huntington's disease
   Thalamus degeneration
   Dentatorubropallidoluysial atrophy (DRPLA)
8. Unclassified presenile dementia

We (Iseki et al. 1999) reexamined 23 pathologically verified DLB cases from the clinicopathological aspect. Eighteen of these cases were classified into neocortical type (10 cases), limbic type (7 cases), cerebral type (1 case), and the brainstem type (none) according to our pathological criteria, which were based on the regional incidence of Lewy bodies and the degree of neuronal loss in the substantia nigra. Each subtype of DLB was further divided into the common form and the pure form on the basis of the degree of concomitant Alzheimer pathology (Kosaka 1990). As the remaining 5 cases could not be classified into any type, they were designated as the SDAT type (2 cases) and the AD type (3 cases). Thus, the results of our study indicate that the neocortical common type, which is consistent with the common form of DLBD, is the major type of DLB, and that this type meets the CDLB clinical diagnostic criteria. However, new clinical diagnostic criteria for DLB should be devised on the basis of the new classification of DLB.

Alpha-synuclein is now one of the most important topics for the study of DLB. Our recent immunohistochemical studies have disclosed some important findings such as characteristic hippocampal pathology in DLB, frequent colocalization of Lewy body and NFT in the same neuron in the limbic region in DLB, and degeneration process of the Lewy body.

Dementia with Neurofibrillary Tangles

Dementia with NFT (DNFT) is a generic term for dementing illnesses caused by the presence of numerous NFT only. Parkinsonism–dementia complex (PDC) (Hirano et al. 1961), diffuse neurofibrillary tangles with calcification (DNTC) (Kosaka 1994) and limbic neurofibrillary tangle dementia (LNTD) (Kosaka et al. 1997) belong to this DNFT. Although some cases with frontotemporal dementia–parkinsonism linked with chromosome 17 (FTDP-17) can belong to this category, we categorize it as a single entity in this article.

Although PDC cases had been found only on Guam, recent cases with PDC have not been found there. It is, however, interesting that new cases with PDC were recently reported on the Kii Peninsula of Japan by Kuzuhara et al. (1998).

DNTC was proposed as a new disease entity by us (Kosaka 1994). About 20 autopsied cases have been reported in Japan, but only 2 cases were reported in Europe. Recently, we proposed clinical diagnostic criteria for DNTC: (1) presenile onset, (2) very slowly progressive dementia with personality changes, (3) temporofronal lobar atrophy on CT/MRI, (4) hypotemporofrontality on SPECT, and (5) Fahr-like calcification on CT. Since then, several clinical cases with DNTC have been reported in Japan. The pathology of DNTC was characterized by a temporofrontal lobar atrophy with diffuse occurrence of numerous NFT in the cerebral cortices as well as Fahr-like calcification.

LNTD is a term proposed by us (Kosaka et al. 1997). Yamada et al. (Yamada et al. 1996) call this disease senile dementia of neurofibrillary tangle type. LNTD is characterized by the following clinical features: (1) late senile onset (over 85 years old), (2) memory disturbance as the core symptom, (3) mild dementia, (4) relatively preserved personality, and (5) bilataral hippocampal atrophy on CT/MRI. Pathologically, the hippocampal and parahippocampal regions are atrophic. Marked neuronal cell loss and NFT are found there. No or rare senile plaques are found. This disease had been understood as atypical Alzheimer's disease. However, LNTD should be differentiated from ATD.

References

Hansen LA, Salmon D, Galasko D, et al (1990) The Lewy body variant of Alzheimer's disease: a clinical and pathological entity. Neurology 40:1–8

Hirano A, Malamud N, Kurland LT (1961) Parkinsonism-dementia complex. An endemic disease on the island of Guam. Brain 84:642–661, 662–679

Iseki E, Marui W, Kosaka K, et al (1999) Clinicopathological multiplicity of dementia with Lewy bodies. Neuropathology 19:386–394

Kosaka K (1990) Diffuse Lewy body disease in Japan. J Neurol 237:197–204

Kosaka K (1994) Diffuse neurofibrillary tangles with calcification. J Neurol Neurosurg Psychiatry 57:594–596

Kosaka K (1998) Diffuse Lewy body disease. Int Med 37:6–10

Kosaka K, Iseki E (1998) Recent advances in dementia research in Japan-non-Alzheimer-type degenerative dementias. Psychiatr Clin Neurosci 52:367–378

Kosaka K, Iseki E (2000) Clinicopathological studies on diffuse Lewy body disease. Neuropathology 1:1–7

Kosaka K, Yoshimura M, Ikeda K, Budka (1984) Diffuse type of Lewy body disease. Progressive dementia with abundant cortical Lewy bodies and senile changes of various degree. A disease entity? Clin Neuropathol 3:185–192

Kosaka K, Iseki E, Odawara T, et al (1997) Limbic neurofibrillary tangle dementia (abstract). Brain Pathol 7:1114

Kuzuhara K, Kokubo Y, Narita Y, et al (1998) Continuing high incidence rates and frequent familial occurrence of amyotrophic lateral sclerosis and parkinsonism-dementia complex (abstract). Neurology 50:173

McKeith IG, Galasko D, Kosaka K, et al (1996) Consensus guidlines for the clinical and pathologic diagnosis of dementia with Lewy bodies (DLB): report of the consortium on DLB international workshop. Neurology 47:1113–1124

Perry RH, Irving D, Blessed D, et al (1990) Senile dementia of Lewy body type. A clinically and neuropathologically distinct type of Lewy body dementia in the elderly. J Neurol Sci 95:119–139

Yamada M, Itoh Y, Otomo E, et al (1996) Dementia of the Alzheimer type and related dementias in the aged: DAT subgroups and senile dementia of the neurofibrillary tangles type. Neuropathology 16:89–98

Behavioral and Psychological Symptoms of Dementia (BPSD): A Current Focus for Clinicians, Researchers, Caregivers, and Governmental Agencies

SANFORD I. FINKEL

Summary. The behavioral and psychological symptoms of dementia (BPSD) are an area of clinical and research attention that has grown significantly during the past decade. It is now recognized that BPSD result in increased hospitalization and premature nursing home rates, increased suffering for both patients and their caregivers, excess disability, and significant financial costs. Many of the symptoms are well established, and in fact a psychotic syndrome recently has been described that differentiates Alzheimer's psychosis from other psychosis in late life. The etiology is multifactoral and complex with neurochemical, neuropathological, genetic, environmental, and psychosocial factors contributing. In the 1990s, significant numbers of clinical trials were conducted for the first time. These studies demonstrated efficacy and safety of novel neuroleptics.

Keywords. Behavior, Dementia, Geriatrics, Psychosis, Alzheimer's, BPSD

We are a rapidly aging world. In 1994, approximately 3% of the Japanese population was over the age of 80. By the year 2020, this proportion will increase to approximately 7.2%. In Italy, Germany, and France, 6% or more of the population will also be over the age of 80 by the year 2020 (United Nations 1998). In the United States, 3 million Americans were over the age of 85 in 1990, and this will increase to 8 million by the year 2020 and to between 15 and 20 million by the year 2050. Developing countries are only a few decades behind. By the year 2020, it is estimated that more than 250 million Chinese will be over the age of 60 and more than 125 million Indians over 60. The aging population is growing with special rapidity in countries such as Pakistan, Brazil, Indonesia, and Nigeria, with profound ramifications for their healthcare system.

Unless and until a cure or prevention of dementing illnesses is discovered, we will continue to have substantial increases in the number of demented elderly worldwide. An estimated 4 million Americans currently have Alzheimer's disease, and this number could increase sevenfold during the next half-century (Evans et al. 1989). Until very recently, most of the attention and research efforts worldwide have focused on the memory and cognitive deficits seen in dementing illnesses. It is only in the last

Geriatric Institute Council for Jewish Eldery, 3003 W. Touhy Ave., Chicago, IL 60645, USA

decade that more attention has been paid to behavioral and psychological symptoms of dementia (BPSD). BPSD is a term used to describe a heterogeneous range of psychological reactions, psychiatric symptoms, and behaviors resulting from dementia. Although it is a concept that is still emerging and developing, it has its origins in clinical descriptions that date back centuries. Esquirol (1838) described these symptoms in 1823 and Alzheimer (1906) described them in his first written case report almost 100 years ago. The woman whom he studied had not only memory problems but also paranoid delusions, delusions of sexual infidelity, visual and auditory hallucinations, and physical aggressivity.

We have come to learn that BPSD are associated with increased hospitalizations and emergency room visits, premature institutionalization in nursing home facilities, substantial increase in stress for both the Alzheimer's patient and the caregivers, excess disability, and substantial increase in financial costs (Colerick and George 1986; Morris et al. 1990; Stelle et al. 1990; O'Donnell et al. 1992; Deimling and Bass 1986; Burgio 1996; Rabins et al. 1982; Cohen-Mansfield 1995; Brody 1982).

The diagnosis and assessment of BPSD consists of direct interviews with the patients and also information derived from the caregiver and medical records. Some etiologies may be determined by laboratory and radiographic evidence. Further helpful evaluation can be obtained from a variety of measurements and scales. The most prominent and distressing symptoms include delusions, hallucinations, depressed mood, sleeplessness, and anxiety, as well as physical aggression, wandering, and restlessness. A second tier of distressing symptoms—usually not as severe but prominent—include misidentifications, agitation, pacing, and screaming. Less distressing symptoms include crying, cursing, apathy, shadowing, and hoarding.

Among the most common delusions are "that person is stealing from me" (Reisberg et al. 1989). Delusions of abandonment and sexual infidelity are also common. Misidentifications include accusing a loved one of being an impostor, believing that one's home is really not one's home, and interpreting one's reflection in the mirror as the presence of a stranger. Delusions are found in approximately 60% of all patients with Alzheimer's disease over the course of the illness (Reisberg et al. 1989). Recently, Jeste and Finkel (2000) proposed that there is a unique psychosis of Alzheimer's disease. It is differentiatable from schizophrenia in elderly patients. In patients with schizophrenia, bizarre or complex delusions are frequent, whereas they are rare in patients with Alzheimer's disease. Misidentification of caregivers is common with Alzheimer's but rare with schizophrenia. Patients with Alzheimer's disease are more apt to have visual hallucinations, those with schizophrenia auditory hallucinations. Schneiderian first-rank symptoms of active suicidal ideation and past history of psychosis are very common in schizophrenia but very uncommon in the psychosis in Alzheimer's disease. Patients with schizophrenia need many years of maintenance on antipsychotics, but this happens uncommonly in the psychosis of Alzheimer's disease. The average optimal daily dose of an antipsychotic for an older adult would be 40%–60% of that which a young adult needs in the case of schizophrenia but only 15%–25% of what a young adult with schizophrenia would need for those with Alzheimer's disease.

A diagnostic criteria for a psychosis of Alzheimer's disease has been proposed (Jeste and Finkel 2000) (Table 1).

TABLE 1. Diagnostic criteria for psychosis of Alzheimer's disease (AD)

A. Characteristic symptoms
 Presence of one (or more) of the following symptoms:
 1. Visual or auditory hallucinations
 2. Delusions
B. Primary diagnosis
 All the criteria for dementia of the Alzheimer type are met[a]
C. Chronology of the onset of symptoms of psychosis versus onset of symptoms of dementia
 There is evidence from the history that the symptoms in criterion A have not been present continuously since before the onset of the symptoms of dementia
D. Duration and severity
 The symptom(s) in criterion A have been present, at least intermittently, for 1 month or longer; symptoms are severe enough to cause some disruption in the functioning of patients or others
E. Exclusion of schizophrenia and related psychotic disorders
 Criteria for schizophrenia, schizoaffective disorder, delusional disorder, or mood disorder with psychotic features have never been met
F. Relationship to delirium
 The disturbance does not occur exclusively during the course of a delirium
G. Exclusion of other causes of psychotic symptoms
 The disturbance is not better accounted for by another general medical condition or direct physiological effects of a substance (e.g., a drug of abuse, a medication)
 Associated features: (*Specify* if associated)
 With agitation: when there is evidence, from history or examination, of prominent agitation with or without physical or verbal aggression
 With negative symptoms: when prominent negative symptoms, such as apathy, affective flattening, avolition, or motor retardation, are present
 With depression: when prominent depressive symptoms, such as depressed mood, insomnia or hypersomnia, feelings of worthlessness or excessive or inappropriate guilt, or recurrent thoughts of death are present

[a]*Note*: For other dementias, such as vascular dementia, criterion B needs to be modified appropriately

At a recent meeting at the Food and Drug Administration in Washington, D.C. (March 9, 2000), industry, national and international organizations, and individual researchers affirmed the belief that the psychosis of Alzheimer's disease is a unique syndrome and worthy of specific investigation and ultimately pharmacological labeling. Further, several other syndromes specific to Alzheimer's disease were proposed, including a syndrome of depression, as well as one for circadian rhythm abnormalities.

Other dementing illnesses may present with different behavioral and psychological symptoms. For example, estimates are 22% of patients with Alzheimer's disease develop depression, whereas for subcortical vascular dementia the percentage is 43% (Erkinjuntti 1987). Skoog et al. (1993) have found rates of psychosis in vascular dementia to be half of those in Alzheimer's, although Ballard et al. (1995) found rates of psychotic symptoms as high as 70% in vascular dementia compared to 47% with Alzheimer's disease. Rates of delusions and hallucinations are presented in Tables 2 and 3.

TABLE 2. Delusions in AD and vascular dementia (VaD)

	Sample size		Delusions (%)	
Study	AD	VaD	AD	VaD
Cummings et al. 1987	30	15	47	47
Binetti et al. 1993	61	31	45	38
Cohen et al. 1993	514	135	9	7
Skoog et al. 1993	64	69	3	4
Johansson and Gustafson 1996	19	27	63	56

TABLE 3. Hallucinations in AD and VaD

	Sample size		Delusions (%)	
Study	AD	VaD	AD	VaD
Cummings et al. 1987	30	15	3	27
Cohen et al. 1993	514	135	11	16
Ballard et al. 1995	88	20	25	60
Johansson and Gustafson 1996	19	27	53	22

In dementia of the Lewy body type, McKeith et al. (1998) found that 46% of patients suffered from visual hallucinations, 19% from auditory hallucinations, and 38% from depression. McKeith postulated that dementia of the Lewy body type may account for the following: hallucinations and delusions are associated with more rapid cognitive decline in AD (Drevets and Rubin 1989); psychotic symptoms are associated with extrapyramidal features in AD patients (Mayeux et al. 1985); and extrapyramidal features in AD (up to 30% of cases) are associated with reduced survival (Mayeux et al. 1985).

The behavioral and psychological symptoms of frontotemporal dementia frontotemporal (Picks Disease) are characterized by apathy, as well as irritability, restlessness, and aggression (Kertesz 2000). The etiology of many of these symptoms appears multifactorial. There is evidence (Holmes et al. 1998) that hallucinations are associated with 5-HT2A and 5-HT2C receptor polymorphisms. Sweet et al. (1998) have also found psychosis associated with DRD-1 and DRD-3 receptor polymorphisms. The association between apolipoprotein E and psychosis has demonstrated varied results, with positive findings by Ramachandran et al. (1996) but no association found in other studies (Holmes et al. 1996, 1997). There was also evidence of neurochemical (Zubenko 1996) and neuropathological (Bondareff 1996) contributants. Delusions in AD patients have been associated with lower blood flow in the left compared to right lateral frontal cortex (Kotrla et al. 1995), orbitofrontal/anterior cingulate hypometabolism (Mentis et al. 1995), and reduced perfusion in the superior and inferior temporal cortex (Starkstein et al. 1994). Binetti et al. (1995) utilized computerized tomography and found that isolated white matter lesions in the frontal lobes were significantly associated with delusions in dementia. Further, Smith et al. (1999) discovered amygdala volume correlated inversely with the noncognitive Alzheimer's Disease Assessment Scale (ADAS-noncog) score in Alzheimer's disease. Personality factors may also contribute (Meins et al. 1998). Finally, environmental and social contributors to BPSD are common. Increased hospitalization is often associated with change in social routine and environment, and demented patients are particularly sensitive to changes in the social environment. Clinicians believe that relocation can increase depressive behavior, agitation, and mortality and that caregiver distress and poor interpersonal relationship can exacerbate BPSD (Erickson 2000).

Until 1990, there were few pharmacological or nonpharmacological clinical trials for the behavioral and psychological symptoms of dementia. Schneider et al. (1990) reviewed the worldwide literature on double-blind placebo controlled studies with antipsychotic medications and discovered only seven; these dated back as far as 1960. Diagnostic criteria were prosaic by our current standards. Measurements and scales that were utilized were derived from the treatment of younger schizophrenic and bipolar patients. Research methodology was flawed; the duration of study was too short to determine differences, in general; and dosages were large by current standards. Some studies took place among chronically institutionalized demented people in state hospitals.

At the beginning of this decade, however, research began in earnest. Researchers were assisted by the development of the first scales in 1986–1987. The Cohen-Mansfield Agitation Inventory (1986) specifically measured a range of behaviors categorized as agitation in the nursing home setting. Reisberg et al. (1987) looked at behavior and other psychological constructs found commonly in Alzheimer's disease patients in the community, including delusions, hallucinations, activity disturbances, aggression, depression, anxiety, and sleep abnormalities. With the creation of these measurements and scales, the potential for conducting reliable clinical drug trials increased substantially. During the period from 1991 to 1999, the new medications shown in Table 4 have been studied, focusing on behavioral and psychological symptoms of dementia.

Finkel et al. (1995) studied 37 agitated, demented, nursing home elderly comparing thiothixene, at a flexible dose, with placebo. Following 11 weeks of treatment, there was a 1-week washout period followed by a 6-week crossover. In both regimens, thiothixene was superior to placebo. Side effects were nominal. Four patients died in the study, all on placebo. Devanand et al. (1998) conducted a placebo-controlled double

TABLE 4. Studies of Anti-Psychotic and other Psychotropic Medications for Treating Behavioral and Psychological Symptoms of Dementia

Drug (investigator)	Year	Sponsor
Thiothixene (Finkel et al. 1995)	1992	NIMH
Carbamazepine (Tariot et al. 1998)	1995	NIMH
Fluoxetine, haloperidol, thioridazine (Reisberg et al. 1987)	1995	NIMH
Buspirone (unpubished)	1995	BMS
Risperidone: international (De Dyn et al. 1999)	1996	Janssen
Olanzapine (Beasley 1997)	1996	Lilly
Risperidone: USA (Katz et al. 1999)	1997	Janssen
Haloperidol (Devanand 1998)	1998	NIMH
Olanzapine (Street 2000)	1998	Lilly
Aricept/Zoloft	1999	Pfizer/Eisai
Seroquel	1999	Zeneca
Valproate	1999	Abbott

blind study of haloperidol versus placebo and found significant improvement on the Brief Psychiatric Rating Scale on psychosis, as well as agitation inventories, favoring haloperidol over placebo. He concluded that haloperidol (2–3 mg daily) was moderately effective, superior to haloperidol (0.5–0.75 mg daily) or placebo. The low dose of haloperidol was no different than placebo. There was a trend toward more extrapyramidal symptoms (EPS) on the standard dose of haloperidol compared to placebo. In a 33-week study comparing fluoxetine, thioridizne, haloperidol, and placebo, Reisberg et al. (1987) found fluoxetine to be superior, with a better side-effect profile.

The first multisite study for agitation in the elderly took place in nursing home settings. Buspirone was compared to placebo. Although the study was completed 5 years ago, no data have yet been forthcoming. The newer antipsychotic medications, risperi-

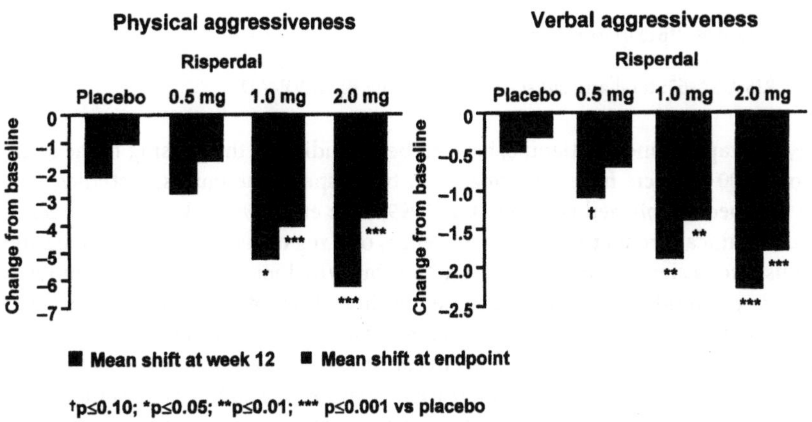

FIG. 1. RIS-USA-63: summary of efficacy results on the CMAI

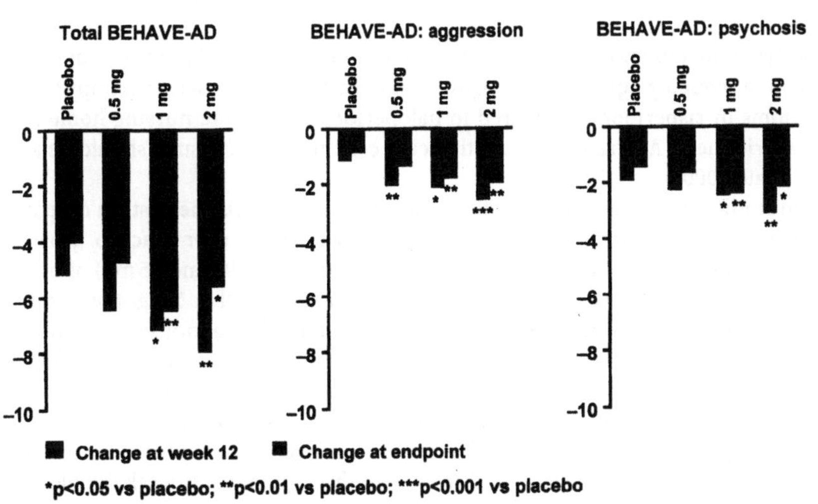

FIG. 2. RIS-USA-63: BEHAVE-AD scores in patients without somnolence

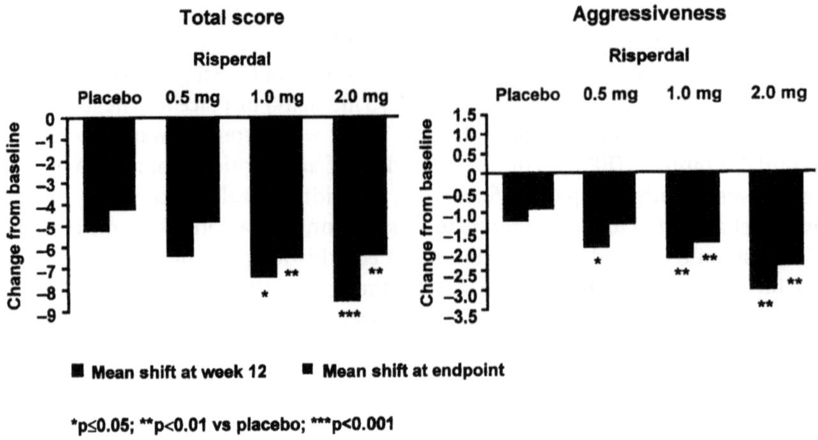

FIG. 3. RIS-USA-63: total and subscale scores on the BEHAVE-AD

done, olanzapine, and quetiapine, have all been studied in the nursing home setting. Almost 1000 subjects have participated in two risperidone multisite studies, which have now been published (DeDyn et al. 1999; Katz et al. 1999). Both studies demonstrated significant reduction of aggressiveness on 1 mg of risperidone. The Katz study demonstrates a significant difference on 2 mg, but with increased rates for somnolence and extra-pyramidal symptoms. In one study, three doses of risperidone—0.5, 1.0, and 2.0 mg—were compared to placebo. At 0.5 mg, there was little difference compared to placebo in terms of efficacy and side effects; at 1.0 mg, there was statistically significant improvement, but with some increase in somnolence and extrapyramidal symptoms; and at 2.0 mg, there was additional improvement but also additional side effects. Improvements took place in psychosis as well as in total aggression and physical aggression. Significance was sustained, even after controlling for somnolence. Subsequent follow-up with an open label design revealed an extremely low incidence of tardive dyskinesia.

DeDyn et al. (1999) found that both haloperidol and risperidone were superior to placebo in reducing agitation and aggression in that there were fewer extrapyramidal symptoms in risperidone compared to haloperidol. A multisite nursing home study on risperidone in Australia is currently being concluded, and results should be available in late 2000.

Two studies have been completed on olanzapine and BPSD. The first, an outpatient multisite placebo controlled study, revealed no advantage over placebo. However, doses were extremely low. A study utilizing higher doses (5, 10, and 15 mg) of olanzapine versus placebo was recently completed. Data showed that 5 mg, the preferred dose, substantially decreased agitation, delusions, and hallucinations; 10 mg was also statistically significant but less efficacious than 5 mg. There was little difference between 15 mg and placebo. Similar results were found with agitation as with delusions and hallucinations. The primary side effect was somnolence, occurring in 35% of the 15-mg sample and 25% of the 5-mg and 10-mg samples. Evidence for improvement occurred as early as week 3 and continued throughout the 6-week double-blind period. Both risperidone and olanzapine were found to be safe from the standpoint of vital signs, laboratory findings, and EKG. A multisite placebo controlled study of quetiapine compared to haloperidol has been completed in nursing home settings. Data should be forthcoming by the end of year 2000.

Selective serotonin reuptake inhibitors (SSRIs) have also been studied. Gottfries and Nyth (1991) have found that citalopram improved anxiety and depressive symptoms in demented elderly. In as yet unpublished data, Reisberg et al. found superiority to fluoxetine over conventional neuroleptics and placebo. A recent study has concluded comparing sertraline to placebo, and the results should be forthcoming by later in the year 2000.

Anticonvulsant medications have also been studied. Tariot et al. (1998) found superiority of carbomazapine to placebo in alleviating symptoms of agitation. However, side effects were common, and they concluded that adverse events might act as a deterrent for widespread use of carbomazapine. More recently, valproate has been studied in nursing home elderly in a placebo controlled study. Because of side effects associated with high doses, the study was stopped and a new study begun with lower doses. In the original study, however, agitation was reduced for those patients treated with medication.

In summary, the atypical antipsychotics appear to be the best drugs for alleviating the positive symptoms, as well as the negative symptoms, of the illness while significantly lowering the risk of tardive dyskinesia and other significant adverse side effects.

A paucity of nonpharmacological, placebo controlled studies have been conducted on managing the behavioral and psychological symptoms of dementia. Greater clinical understanding and a growing sophistication in understanding and decreasing dangerous wandering mark advances in the field. The use of electronic bracelets, special locks, dedicated walking areas, artificial partitions, etc., diminish the possibility of a demented older person wandering from the home and getting lost. Alterations in the environment to create a pleasant milieu, and the utilization of a wide range of activities that include music therapy, religious activities, pet therapy, art therapy, and movement therapy are all especially important. Background music has been demonstrated to alleviate anxiety in a number of medical conditions, and although not commonly studied this therapy can be helpful to those agitated elderly demented as well.

The caregivers of people with Alzheimer's disease and other dementias are of high risk for developing major depression or physical illness. They face many problems including restriction of their social life, increase in financial and other responsibilities, increasingly hard work taking care of their spouse, changes in interpersonal relationships, emotional and physical distress, financial hardship, and at times employment problems. They must contend with feelings of helplessness and hopelessness, loneliness and isolation, rage at the demented family member, and then guilt about having hostile feelings, periodic humiliation, and a sense of being stigmatized. Mittelman et al. (1993) found that caregiver support groups decrease rates of institutionalization of the demented patient. Three years after beginning a support group, more than three-quarters of demented family members remained in the community, compared to just over a third for those in the control group.

The International Psychogeriatric Association has taken special interest in BPSD. They have developed extensive educational materials and have published proceedings of symposia and international consensus conferences. The first consensus conference took place in 1996, with 60 experts representing 16 countries. The consensus was that the category of behavioral disturbances of dementia should be changed to behavioral and psychological symptoms of dementia. Further, a research agenda was prepared that has acted as a blueprint for the field for the last few years. As a result of the tremendous increase in activity between 1996 and 1999, a second international conference was held with 60 speakers from 17 countries and nine disciplines. Some of the conclusions and recommendations follow (Finkel et al. 2000):

1. BPSD are a distinct entity that can be differentiated from other late-life psychopathology and can be identified in different types of dementia.
2. Distinct target symptoms of BPSD can be identified.
3. The etiology of BPSD is often multifactorial, and the possible biopsychosocial pharmacological and nonpharmacological interventions need to be elucidated.
4. BPSD in AD and vascular dementia are similar and thus combined clinical trials of both are appropriate. The symptoms of other dementias, however, are different and thus separate clinical trials are necessary for these dementias.
5. The phenomenology of the psychosis of AD is sufficiently different from that of other late-life psychoses that there is justification for studying it as a syndrome.
6. The most important symptoms are aggression, delusions, misidentifications, agitation, wandering, insomnia, and hallucinations, and clinical and research resources should identify and prioritize these symptoms for investigation.
7. The atypical antipsychotics seems to show the most promise in managing psychotic and aggressive symptoms of BPSD, particularly agitation, physical aggression, and delusions. Ayptical antipsychotics appear to have much lower rates of tardive dyskinesia than conventional antipsychotics.
8. A number of diagnostic and outcome measures have been validated in multisite trials. However, those involved in the field should attempt to harmonize protocols where possible to facilitate comparison of results between studies.
9. Nonpharmacological and combined pharmacological/nonpharmacological clinical trials should be given priority.

Thus, behavioral and psychological symptoms of dementia are part and parcel of dementing illnesses. They are a legitimate concern of healthcare providers worldwide and present severe problems to caregivers and patients and also to society and its health services. However, treatment interventions and management are proving increasingly effective, and we can anticipate continued progress in this regard in the years ahead.

References

Alzheimer A (1906) Ueber einen eigenartigen schweren Er Krankungsprozeß der Hirnrinde. Neurol Centralbl 23:1129–1136

Ballard C, Bannister C, Graham C, et al (1995) Assocations of psychotic symptoms in dementia sufferers. Br J Psychiatry 167(4):537–540

Binetti G, Magni E, Padovani A, et al (1993) Delusions in Alzheimer's disease and multi-infarct dementia. Acta Neurol Scand 88(1):5–9

Binetti G, Padovani A, Magni E, et al (1995) Delusions and dementia: clinical and CT correlates. Acta Neurol Scand 91(4):271–275

Bondareff W (1996) Neuropathology of psychotic symptoms in Alzheimer's disease. Int Psychogeriatrics 8(suppl 3):233–237

Brody JA (1982) An epidemiologist views senile dementia—facts and figures. Am J Epidemiol 113:155–162

Burgio L (1996) Interventions for the behavioral complications of Alzheimer's disease: behavioral approaches. Int Psychiatry 8(suppl 1):45–52

Cohen D, Eisdorfer C, Gorelick P, et al (1993) Psychopathology associated with Alzheimer's disease and related disorders. J Gerontol 48(6):M255–M260

Cohen-Mansfield J (1995) Assessment of disruptive behavior/agitation in the elderly: function, methods and difficulties. J Geriatr Psychiatry Neurol 8(suppl 1):52–60

Cohen-Mansfield J, Billing N (1986) Agitated behaviors in the elderly: 1. A conceptual review. J Am Geriatrics Soc 34:711–721

Colerick EJ, George LK (1986) Predictors of institutionalization among caregivers of patients with Alzheimer's disease. J Am Geriatr Soc 34(7):493–498

Cummings JL, Miller B, Hill MA, Neshkes R (1987) Neuropsychiatric aspects of multi-infarct dementia and dementia of the Alzheimer type. Arch Neurol 44(4):389–393

DeDeyn PP, Rabheru K, Rasmussen A, et al (1999) A randomized trial of risperidone, placebo, and haloperidol for behavioral symptoms of dementia. Neurology 53(5):946–955

Deimling GT, Bass DM (1986) Symptoms of mental impairment among elderly adults and their effects on family caregivers. J Gerontol 41:778–784

Devanand DP, Marder K, Michaels KS, et al (1998) A randomized, placebo-controlled, dose comparison trial of haloperidol for psychosis and disruptive behaviors in Alzheimer's disease. Am J Psychiatry 155:1512–1520

Drevets WC, Rubin EH (1989) Psychotic symptoms and the longitudinal course of senile dementia of the Alzheimer type. Biol Psychiatry 25(1):39–48

Erickson S (2000). Impact of the environment on the behavioral and psychological symptoms of dementia. Int Psychogeriatrics 12(suppl 1):89–92

Erkinjuntti T (1987) Differential diagnosis between Alzheimer's disease and vascular dementia: evaluation of common clinical methods. Acta Neurol Scand 76(6):433–442

Esquirol JED (1838) Des maladies mentales.

Finkel SI, Burns A, Cohen G (2000) Overview of BPSD, a clinical and research update. Int Psychogeriatrics 12(suppl 1):13–18

Finkel SI, Lyons JS, Anderson RL, et al (1995) A randomized, placebo-controlled trial of thiothixene in agitated, demented nursing home elderly. Int J Geriatr Psychiatry 10:129–136

Food and Drug Administration (2000) March 9, 2000. Meeting of the Psychopharmacological Drugs Advisory Committee on the various psychiatric and behavioral disturbances associated with dementia. FDA, Washington, DC

Gottfries CG, Nyth AL (1991) Effect of citalopram, a selective 5-HT reuptake blocker, in emotionally disturbed patients with dementia. Ann N Y Acad Sci 640:276–279

Holmes C, Levy R, McLoughlin DM, et al (1996) Apolipoprotein E: non-cognitive symptoms and cognitive decline in late onset Alzheimer's disease. J Neurol Neurosurg Psychiatry 61(6):580–583

Holmes C, Fortenza O, Powell J, Lovestone S (1997) Do neuroleptic drugs hasten cognitive decline in dementia? Carriers of apolipoprotein E epsilon 4 allele seem particularly susceptible to their effects. Br Med J 314(7091):1411

Holmes C, Arranz MJ, Powell JF, et al (1998) 5-HT2A and 5-HT2C receptor polymorphisms and psychopathology in late onset Alzheimer's disease. Hum Mol Genet 7(9):1507–1509

Jeste DV, Finkel SI (2000) Psychosis of Alzheimer's disease and related dementias: diagnostic criteria for a distinct syndrome. Am J Geriatr Psychiatry 8(1):29–34

Johansson A, Gustafson L (1996) Psychiatric symptoms in patients with dementia treated in a psychogeriatric day hospital. Int Psychogeriatrics 8(4):645–658

Katz IR, Jeste DV, Mintzer JE, et al (1999) Comparison of risperidone and placebo for psychosis and behavioral disturbances associated with dementia: a randomized, double-blind trial. J Clin Psychiatry 60:107–115

Kotrla KJ, Chacko RC, Harper RG, et al (1995) SPECT findings on psychosis in Alzheimer's disease. Am J Psychiatry 152(10):1470–1475

Mayeux R, Stern Y, Spanton S (1985) Heterogeneity in dementia of the Alzheimer type: evidence of subgroups. Neurology 35(4):453–461

McKeith IG, O'Brien JT, Ballard C (1998) Diagnosing dementia with Lewy bodies. Lancet 354(9186):1227–1228

Meins W, Frey A, Thiesemann R (1998) Premorbid personality traits in Alzheimer's disease: do they predispose to noncognitive behavioral symptoms? Int Psychogeriatrics 10(4):369–378

Mentis MJ, Weinstein EA, Horwitz B, et al (1995) Abnormal brain glucose metabolism in the delusional misidentification syndromes: a positron emission tomography study in Alzheimer disease. Biol Psychiatry 38(7):438–449

Mittelman MS, Ferris SH, Steinberg G, et al (1993) An intervention that delays institutionalization of Alzheimer's disease patients: treatment of spouse-caregivers. Gerontologist 33(6):730–740

Morris RK, Rovner BW, Folstein MF (1990) Delusions in newly admitted residents of nursing homes. Am J Geriatr Psychiatry 147:299–302

O'Donnell BF, Drachman DA, Barnes HJ, et al (1992) Incontinence and troublesome behaviors predict institutionalization in dementia. J Geriatr Psychiatry Neurol 5:45–52

Rabins PV, Mace NL, Lucas MJ (1982) The impact of dementia on the family. JAMA 248:333–335

Ramachandran G, Marder K, Tang M, et al (1996) A preliminary study of apolipoprotein E genotype and psychiatric manifestations of Alzheimer's disease. Neurology 47(1):256–269

Reisberg B, et al (2000) Do many of the behavioral and psychological symptoms of dementia constitute a distinct syndrome: current evidence using the BEHAVE-AD. Int Psychogeriatrics 12 (suppl 1):155–164

Reisberg B, Borenstein J, Salob SP, et al (1987) Behavioral symptoms in Alzheimer's disease: phenomenology and treatment. J Clin Psychiatry 48(suppl):9–15

Reisberg BM, Frenssen E, Sclan S, et al (1989) Stage specific incidence of potentially remediable behavioral symptoms in aging and Alzheimer's disease: a study of 120 patients using the BEHAVE-AD. Bull Clin Neurosci 95:112

Schneider LS, Pollock VE, Lyness SA (1990) A metaanalysis of controlled trials of neuroleptic treatment in dementia. J Am Geriatrics Soc 38:553–563

Skoog I, Nilsson L, Palmertz B, et al (1993) A population-based study of dementia in 85-year-olds. N Engl J Med 328(3):153–158

Smith CD, Malcein M, Meurer K, et al (1999) MRI temporal lobe volume measures and neuropsychologic function in Alzheimer's disease. J Neuroimaging 9(1):2–9

Starkstein SE, Vazquez S, Petracca G, et al (1994) A SPECT study of delusions in Alzheimer's disease. Neurology 44(11):2055–2059

Stelle C, Rovner B, Chase GA, Folstein M (1990) Psychiatric symptoms and nursing home placement of patients with Alzheimer's disease. Am J Psychiatry 147:8

Sweet RA, Nimgaonkar VL, Kamboh MI, et al (1998) Dopamine receptor genetic variation, psychosis, and aggression in Alzheimer disease. Arch Neurol 55(10):1335–1340

Tariot PN, Erb R, Podgorski CA, et al (1998) Efficacy and tolerability of carbamazepine for agitation and aggression in dementia. Am J Psychiatry 155:54–61

United Nations (1998) Publication 106, Geneva

Zubenko GS (1996) Clinicopathologic and neurochemical correlates of major depression and psychosis in primary dementia. Int Psychogeriatrics 8(suppl 3):219–223

Recent Trends in Pharmacological Treatment of Dementia

Koho Miyoshi[1], Yoshio Morita[2], and Akinori Ueki[2]

Summary. Dementia is a syndrome with cognitive and noncognitive impairments caused by widespead and persistent degeneration of the brain. Although reversibility of cognitive symptoms is exceptional, pharmacological treatment with thymoleptics or antipsychotic drugs could ameliorate noncognitive impairment such as behavioral and psychological symptoms in dementia. The effects of various drugs, including calcium antagonists, prostaglandin, antioxidants, NMDA-receptor antagonists, coronary dilatators, and antithrombocytic drugs have been clinically evaluated recently in treatment of the cognitive and noncognitive symptoms of vascular dementia. For the treatment of cognitive impairment in Alzheimer's disease (AD), various cholinergic enhancers such as acetylcholinesterase inhibitor, muscarine or nicotinic agonist, and choline reuptake accelerator have been tried clinically. Significant effects of the cholinesterase inhibitors tacrine, donepezil, and rivastigmine for cognitive impairment of AD were proved in worldwide trials. New AchE inhibitors are designed to lessen the side effects and improve clinical efficacy. Clinical effects of neurotransmitter enhancers, neuropeptide enhancers, and neuroprotective drugs have been also evaluated recently in AD patients. Spontaneous alterations of cognitive impairment as well as variability in behavioral symptoms due to their surroundings cause difficulties in evaluating the effects of the drugs in demented patients. Limited results could be obtained without objective measures of evaluating cognitive functions and behaviors in clinical trials. The final purpose of the treatment of AD is slowing of the deterioration of AD pathology, such as amyloid deposit, tau formation, and neuronal loss. At this moment we lack predictive experimental models, excepting some transgenic mice, to test for neuroprotective effects.

Keywords. Dementia, Alzheimer's disease, Vascular dementia, Pharmacology, Animal model

---

[1] Hyogo Institute for Aging Brain and Cognitive Disorders, 520 Saisyo-Koh, Himeji, Hyogo, Japan
Previous address: Department of Psychiatry, Kyoto University Graduate School of Medicine, Sakyo, Kyoto, Japan
[2] Department of Neuropsychiatry, Hyogo College of Medicine, Nishinomiya, Hyogo, Japan

Introduction

Dementia is a syndrome with persistent cognitive impairment in which there is disturbance of the higher cortical functions, including memory, thinking, orientation, comprehension, calculation, learning capacity, language, and judgment (ICD-10; WHO 1991). This syndrome is often accompanied by noncognitive symptoms, such as decrease of motivation and drive, lack of spontaneity, irritability, and disinhibition of social behavior. Reversibilities of cognitive impairment of dementias are exceptional. In general, dementias, especially in neurodegenerative disorders and cerebrovascular disorders, take a downhill course in spite of intensive therapeutic efforts. On the other hand, noncognitive symptoms could be treated by pharmacological means.

Dementia usually occurs in pathological conditions with widespread and persistent degeneration of the brain and almost always is irreversible. However, dementias caused by reversible pathological processes, such as inflammation, metabolic disorders, intoxication, malnutrition, vitamin deficiency, and normal pressure hydrocephalus, could be ameliorated by treatments for the basic pathological processes. These types of dementias are known as treatable dementias.

Recently, various pharmacological treatments have been tried clinically on the dementia disorders, i.e., Alzheimer's disease and vascular dementia, that have been considered to be not treatable.

Vascular Dementia

Pathology of Vascular Dementia

Vascular dementia is a persistent cognitive impairment caused by ischemic, hemorrhagic, or hypoxic lesions resulting from cerebrovascular disorders. According to the NINCDS-AIREN Study (Roman et al. 1993), vascular dementias are classified as follows: multiinfarct dementia, strategic single-infarct dementia, small-vessel disease with dementia (multiple lacunar stroke, lacuna in frontal white matter, Binswanger's disease, cerebral amyloid angiopathy), hypoperfusion, hemorrhagic dementia, and others. Hypoxic-ischemic lesions, such as arterial territorial infarction, watershed infarctions, laminar necrosis, granular atrophy, subcortical leukoencephalopathy, and gliosis or incomplete ischemic necrosis are characteristic pathological feature of vascular dementia.

Among these pathologies, multiple infarctions and widespread degeneration of white matter are common pathological features in vascular dementia.

Clinical Symptoms and Treatment

Psychiatric and Behavioral Symptoms

Cognitive impairment is commonly accompanied by noncognitive symptoms, i.e., decrease of motivation and drive, lack of spontaneity, irritability, and disinhibition of social behavior. Hypochondria, depressive mood, inertia, visual hallucinations, and illusions are common symptoms in dementia of vascular origin.

Pharmacotherapy for psychiatric symptoms is essential to manage noncognitive symptoms in vascular dementia. Thymoleptics, including SSRIs such as fluvoxamine maleate, are widely used for treatment of depression. Aniracetam, an agonist of acetylcholine muscarinic receptor, was proved to significantly ameliorate behavioral and affective symptoms such as wandering, affect incontinence, depressive mood, anxiety, and agitation of the cerebrovascular disorders (Horikoshi et al. 1997; Bartolini et al. 1996). No significant effect of this drug is proved, however, on cognitive impairment of vascular dementia. Nefiracetam, an enhancing drug of the acetylcholine system, was reported to ameliorate psychiatric symptoms associated with cerebrovascular disorders (Hasegawa et al. 1994). Amantadine hydrochloride, originally known as an antiparkinsonian and antiviral agent, improves lack of spontaneity in the cerebrovascular disorders. Nicergoline, ergot alkaloid, activates brain metabolism and improves poststroke inertia. Nilvadipine, a calcium channel blocker, has an ameliorating effect on inertia in poststroke state. Vinpocetine, cinepazide maleate, and ibudilast improve cerebrovascular circulation and ameliorate affective symptoms.

Antipsychotic drugs such as risperidone, thioridazine, bromperidol, and haloperidol could be used for the treatment of psychotic and behavioral symptoms (De Deyn et al. 1999). The antidopaminergic drug tiapride hydrochloride is used especially for behavioral symptoms, such as aggression, psychomotor excitement, and wandering in vascular dementia. Anxiolytics like benzodiazepine are widely used for restlessness and anxiety.

Idebenone, a benzoquinone derivative, has an inhibitory effect on lipid peroxidation and has been widely used for the treatment of disturbance of emotion and volition in cerebrovascular disorders (Bergamasco et al. 1992). Indeloxazine was also commonly used in Japan to treat a memory impairment or emotional disturbance in patients who had suffered cerebral infarction, hemorrhage, or cerebral arteriosclerosis (Otomo et al. 1989). Placebo controlled clinical trials of these drugs had been performed at the request of the government. In 1998, the trials proved these drugs had no significant effect on the affective symptoms of cerebrovascular disorders. Since then, the government has stopped the use of these drugs in Japan.

Cognitive Impairment in Vascular Dementia

Diffuse cerebral lesions, such as multiple infarction with white matter degeneration due to cerebrovascular insufficiencies, cause dementia. Cognitive impairment in vascular dementia is closely related to the severity and extent of destruction in the cerebrum, especially in cerebral white matter (diffuse leukoaraiosis). However, impairment of recent memory in vascular dementia is usually less severe compared to that of Alzheimer's disease. Vascular dementia is called lacunar dementia because of the unevenness of severity of impairment of cognitive functions.

Prevention of Vascular Dementia

Prevention of the Cerebrovascular Disorders

To prevent cerebral infarction or hemorrhage, it is important to treat hypertension, diabetes mellitus, and hyperlipemia, which are known as the risk factors of cerebrovascular disorders. When warning signs of cerebrovascular insufficiency such as transient ischemic attack or asymptomatic cerebral infarction are noticed, antithrombocytic and vasodilatating drugs should be used to prevent further damage of the brain. Prevention of hypoperfusion in the cerebral white matter by blood pressure control or by administration of cerebrovascular dilatators, such as nicergoline and vinpocetin could delay the onset of vascular dementia.

Drugs on Clinical Trial for the Treatment of Vascular Dementia

Various compounds are now undergoing clinical trials for treatment of vascular dementia. The effects of muscarinic agonists, ACh releasers, D_2-receptor agonists, MAO-A-receptor inhibitors, NGF-activating drugs, TRH derivatives, calcium-antagonists, prostaglandin, antioxidants, NMDA-receptor antagonists, coronary dilatators, and antithrombocytic drugs have been clinically evaluated in the treatment of vascular dementia.

Alzheimer's Disease

Behavioral and Psychotic Symptoms of Alzheimer's Disease

The concept of behavioral and psychotic symptoms in dementia (BPSD) has been proposed by Finkel et al. (1996). Subjective symptoms, such as anxiety, depressive mood, hallucinations and delusions, and aggression, and objective symptoms, such as screaming, restlessness, agitation, wandering, culturally inappropriate behavior, sexual disinhibition, hoarding, cursing, and shadowing, are common symptoms of BPSD. These symptoms in dementia are usually treated by antipsychotic drugs such risperidone, thioridazine, bromperidol, and haloperidol (De Deyn et al. 1999). Tiapride hydrochloride is useful for behavioral symptoms, especially aggressive behaviors, in dementia disorders.

Recently, 5-HT2/D_2 receptor antagonists, initially used for treatment of schizophrenia, have drawn attention as convenient antipsychotic drugs for the elderly because of their negligible side effects.

Strategies for Treatment of Cognitive Impairment in Alzheimer's Disease

Exploration of Treatment of Cognitive Impairment

Animal Models for Learning Impairment

An animal model of dementia is necessary for screening the effects of new drugs. We could try to produce an animal model for studying certain aspects of cognitive disorders, even if they do not completely mimic dementia in humans. For example, basal forebrain-lesioned rats could be useful as a model of cognitive impairment and cholinergic alteration in Alzheimer's disease (Miyoshi and Ueki 1993). In Alzheimer's disease, the amount of acetylcholine and the activity of choline acetyltransferase decrease remarkably in the cerebral cortex, which correlates to the neuronal diminution of the basal forebrain, such as the nucleus basalis of Meynert, the diagonal band of Broca, and the internal septal nucleus. Furthermore, the diminution of central acetylcholine by the cholinergic inhibitor scopolamine could cause a transient decline of mental ability in humans. These facts suggest that disturbance of the central cholinergic system could induce cognitive dysfunction in Alzheimer's disease. The bilateral lesions of the basal forebrain cause a central cholinergic alteration and learning disability in rats. Two weeks after the injection of excitotoxin into the basal forebrain, two-thirds of the choline acetyltransferase-positive neurons disappear in the ventral globus pallidus, and acetylcholinestrase-positive fibers of the lesioned side reduce to approximately 36.7% of the control side in the cerebral cortex.

Morphometric examinations, using a computer image analyzer, revealed a slight but significant reduction in the size and number of neurons, especially in the third layer of the cerebral cortex of the lesioned side. Concentration of acetylcholine significantly decreased in the basal forebrain-lesioned side compared with the sham-operated rats. Rats with basal forebrain lesions show significant learning impairment, as evaluated with passive and active avoidance tests. These rats also show an acquisition and retention deficit in the passive-avoidance response test.

Oral administration of cholinesterase inhibitors increases acetylcholine in the cerebral cortex and antagonizes memory impairment induced by the basal forebrain lesion (Ueki and Miyoshi 1989). These cholinesterase inhibitors have been clinically tested for the ameliorating effects of cognitive impairment in Alzheimer's disease.

Animal Models for Alzheimer's Disease Pathology

Neuropathological hallmarks of Alzheimer 's disease are neurofibrillary tangles, senile plaques, and neuronal loss in the cerebral cortex. Neurofibrillary tangles consist of phosphorylated tau and ultrastructurally paired helical filaments. Senile plaques consist of amyloid deposits and degenerated neuronal processes. The mechanism of neuronal loss is still unknown. However, it is usually proportional to the severity of neurofibrillary tangles. The final purpose of the treatment of Alzheimer's disease is to prevent or slow the pathological alterations in the brain such as tau formation and amyloid deposition. For this purpose, animal models with Alzheimer neuropathology are essential for the exploration of pharmacological treatment of Alzheimer's disease. However, we lack the predictive experimental models to test for neuroprotective effects. At this moment, only transgenic mice, which overexpress mutant human APP, or mutant human tau, could be used for this purpose (Schenk et al. 1999).

Clinical Trials

Double-blind, placebo controlled trials should be performed to evaluate the efficacy and safety of drugs for Alzheimer's disease. Patients should be randomly assigned to treatment with placebo or the target drug after single-blind placebo washout. Efficacy to cognitive impairment is usually evaluated by the cognitive portion of the Alzheimer's Disase Assessment Scale (ADAS-cog), the Clinician's Interview Based Assessment of Change-Plus (CIBIC plus), and the Mini-Mental State Examination (MMSE). With these measurements, quality of life (QOL) or activity of daily life (ADL) are usually performed to evaluate behavioral changes. Only limited results could be obtained without objective measurement of evaluating cognitive functions and behaviors in clinical trials.

Spontaneous gradual alterations of cognitive impairment, as well as changeability of behavioral symptoms due to the surroundings cause difficulties in evaluating the effects of drugs for Alzheimer's disease patients.

Drugs for the Treatment of Alzheimer's Disease

Cholinergic-Enhancing Drugs

Cholinesterase Inhibitors

Cholinergic enhancers, cholinesterase inhibitors, have been clinically used for treatment of cognitive impairment in Alzheimer's disease. Tacrine, terahydroaminoacridine hydrochloride, is a reversible cholinesterase inhibitor. It acts by elevating acetylcholine concentrations in the cerebral cortex and by lowering the degradation of acetylcholine released by still intact cholinergic neurons. On clinical trials in the United States, administration of tacrine for 30 weeks caused significant improvement of cognitive function, as evaluated by ADAS cog. of AD patients (Davis et al. 1992; Knapp et al. 1994). However, the effect was modest and the side effects on hepatic function were severe and frequent.

Donepezil, methylpiperidine plus an acetylcholinesterase inhibitor, also provides significant effects on cognitive impairment in AD. This compound is less hepatotoxic and shows negligible adverse effects when administered clinically. Reports of clinical trials for 14–30 weeks indicated that the patients treated with donepezil showed dose-related improvements in the ADAS cog. and MMSE scores (Rogers et al. 1996). Significant effects of donepezil to cognitive impairment in Alzheimer's disease were approved in clinical trials in the United States, Europe, and Japan. In Japan, the efficacy and safety of donepezil were proven at 5 mg/day for patients with mild to moderately severe Alzheimer's disease for 24 weeks in a double-blind placebo controlled comparative trial (Homma et al., in press).

Rivastigmine, a selective acetylcholinesterase inhibitor, was proven to have a significant ameliorating effect on cognitive impairment in Alzheimer's disease patients (Corey-Bloom et al. 1998). In Europe, rivastigmine was licensed for the treatment of mild to moderately severe Alzheimer's disease in 1998.

The double-blind study of treatment for 26 weeks of Metrifonate, a cholinesterase inhibitor, demonstrated the efficacy and safety of the drug for Alzheimer's disease patients. Improvement in ADAS-Cog and the CIBIC, behavioral disturbances, and ADL of patients with mild and moderate Alzheimer's disease were proven in clinical trials (Cummings et al. 1998; Gelinas et al. 1998).

Other anticholinestrase agents are being tested. Galanthamine, a tertiary alkaloid originally isolated from bulbs of snowdrop and *Narcissus* species, a reversible AchE inhibitor, showed significant improvement of cognitive impairment in Alzheimer's disease patients in a placebo controlled study for 12 weeks (Bores et al. 1996; Wilcock and Wilkinson 1997).

Amiridin is a 4-aminopyridine derivative that has inhibitory effects on cholinesterase in vitro and in vivo. Originally, it had been tried for treatment of peripheral neuropathy and myasthenia gravis. Its hepatotoxicity is almost negligible. The ameliorating effects of amiridin to learning impairment in animals were almost at the same level as tacrine. Another cholinesterase inhibitor, phenylcarbamate, has been tried clinically on Alzheimer's disease patients. This compound shows fewer peripheral side effects on clinical trials. Benzazepine, a cholinesterase inhibitor, is less hepatotoxic and less effective in peripheral systems, and also has monoamine-activating effects. Experimentally, it has been proven to have ameliorating effects on learning impairment in animals. Velnacrine maleate, one of the metabolites of tacrine, has similar effects to those of tacrine in the treatment of Alzheimer's disease. It was expected to be much easier to use for Alzheimer's disease than tacrine. However, the pharmaceutical company stopped its development.

Cholinergic Receptor Agonists

Acetylcholine precursors, cholinesterase inbibitors, muscarinic receptor agonists, and choline reuptake accelerators have cholinergic-enhancing effects when administered orally. Quinuclidine, a selective M1 agonist, shows significant ameliorating effects on experimental learning impairment in rats. However, this compound has adversive effects such as hypersalivation, sweating, gastrointestinal disturbance, and urinary pain. Azaspirodekan is a selective M1-receptor agonist that shows a significant improvement on learning impairment in animal models. This compound is rather inconvenient for clinical use because of hypersalivation, sweating, and transient visual disturbances. Chenopyrimidine, a selective M1-receptor agonist, has a norepinephrine reuptake inhibitory effect. Nicotinic receptor agonists, ABT-418 (Potter et al. 1999), and choline reuptake accelerators are also on clinical trial. Nefiracetam is a pyroridone derivative and stimulates ACh, GABA, 5-HT, and NA systems in the brain. Recent clinical trials have revealed significant effectiveness on psychotic symptoms associated with cerebrovascular disorders.

Neurotransmitter-Enhancing Drugs

Some of the neurotransmitter-enhancing drugs have been tried clinically on Alzheimer's disease patients. A selective M1 receptor agonist, chenopyrimidine, also has a norepinephrine reuptake inhibitory effect. Ondansetron is a 5-HT-3-receptor antagonist. Benzothiophene derivative has acetylcholine- and monoamine-releasing effects. Nefiracetam is a cyclic GABA derivative that has enhancing effects on acetylcholine, GABA, 5-HT, and norepinephrine. Pyrroglutanamide is also a cylic GABA derivative and activates acetylcholine release. Aniracetam is a pyrrolidinone derivative and has an enhancing effect on the acetylcholine system. Citalopram is a 5-HT reuptake inhibitor. These drugs show an ameliorating effect on learning impairment in the animal model.

Neuropeptide-Enhancing Drugs

Some neuropeptide-enhancing drugs are also being clinically tested for Alzheimer's disease. Protirelin, TRH-SR, shows an ameliorating effect on learning impairment in animal models. Ebiratide is a polypeptide that shows an ameliorating effect on learning impairment in animals. Prorylendopeptidase, which is an inactivated enzyme of neuropeptide related to memory and learning, is inhibited by prorylendopeptidase inhibitors. Prorylendopeptidase inhibitors such as pyrrolidine and ebiratide were also tested clinically on Alzheimer's disease.

Neuronal Protecting Drug

One of the cytoskeleton-protecting drugs, sabeluzole, was evaluated for preventing the effects in Alzheimer's disease in long-term trials. *Ginkgo biloba*, which has antioxidant and free radical scavenger effects, has been reported to have an efficacy for cognitive functions in Alzheimer's disease (LeBars et al. 1997; Oken et al. 1998).

Other Agents

Oral administration of vitamin E (α-tocopherol) was reported to be helpful in delaying the progression of Alzheimer's disease (Sano et al. 1996). Selegiline, a selective MAO inhibitor, alone and combined in treatment with vitamin E, has also been tried for delaying the progression of Alzheimer's disease with moderate impairment. No evidence of the effect of selegiline was demonstrated on any clinical or neuropsychological measure after 2, 8, or 15 months (Burke et al. 1993). The benefits shown in these trials are modest at best.

Nonsteroidal antiinflammatory drugs (NSAIDs) have been tried for Alzheimer's disease patients (McGeer and Rogers 1992). Indomethacin was reported to protect mildly to moderately impaired Alzheimer's disease patients from the decline of cognitive functions (Rogers et al. 1993). However, the NSAIDs diclofenac and misoprostol showed no significant effect on cognitive declines in Alzheimer's disease (Scharf et al. 1999).

Estrogen replacement therapy has been reported to be beneficial in the treatment of dementia in postmenopausal women with Alzheimer's disease (Schneider et al. 1996). Recently, it was reported that estrogen replacement therapy for 1 year did not slow disease progression nor did it improve global, cognitive, or functional outcomes in women with mild to moderate Alzheimer's disease (Mulnar et al. 2000).

The chelating agent desferrioxamine has been tried for the treatment of Alzheimer's disease patients and showed no significant ameliorating effects.

It was reported that intracerebroventricular infusion of nerve growth factor (NGF) caused certain beneficial effects in Alzheimer's disease patients (Joenhagen et al. 1998). Immunophilin, FKBP12, a protein receptor for immunosuppressant drugs such as cyclosporin A and FK504, is neurotrophic and stimulates functional regrowth of damaged cortical cholinergic, dopaminergic, and 5-HT-nergic neurons (Snyder et al. 1998). FKBP 12 was reported to have an ameliorating effect on learning impairment in animals. Immunization against amyloid plaque-related proteins was reported to prevent the development of β-amyloid formation in young transgenic PDAPP mice (Schenk et al. 1999). Immunization with β-amyloid could be effective in preventing and treating Alzheimer's disease.

Discussion and Conclusion

Various pharmacological treatments have been tried clinically on vascular dementia and Alzheimer's disease. Vascular dementia is a persistent cognitive impairment due to lesions cused by cerebrovascular disorders. Antipsychotic drugs, as well as thymoleptics, are used for the psychotic symptoms of vascular dementia. Antithrombocytic drugs and drugs for improvement of cerebral circulation could be used for the prevention of vascular dementia.

The drugs now on clinical trial for Alzheimer's disease are mainly cholinergic enhancers, namely acetylcholinesterase inhibitors, muscarine or nicotinic agonists, and choline reuptake accelerators. The significant effects of cholinesterase inhibitors on cognitive impairment of Alzheimer's disease have been proven in worldwide trials. New acetylcholinesterase inhibitors and muscarinic receptor agonists are designed to lessen side effects and to improve clinical efficacy. Nicotinic receptor agonists and choline reuptake accelerators are also on clinical trial. As well as the cholinergic enhancers, clinical effects of neurotransmitter-enhancing drugs and neuropeptide-enhancing drugs have been assessed in Alzheimer's disease patients.

Evaluations of clinical effects of drugs are not easy in chronic neuropsychiatric disorders. Spontaneous gradual alterations of cognitive impairment, as well as changeability of behavioral symptoms due to the surroundings, cause difficulties in evaluating the effects of drugs in demented patients. Occasionally, a placebo can cause an improvement of behavioral symptoms in appearance, probably because of the initiation of intensive caregiving. Limited results could be obtained without objective measures of evaluating cognitive functions and behaviors in clinical trials.

The final purpose of the treatment of Alzheimer's disease is to slow the progression of pathological processes. We do not have the predictive experimental models to test for neuroprotective effects. It is necessary to have a animal model with Alzheimer pathology for screening the effects of drugs to prevent or ameliorate the pathological processes. At this moment, only transgenic mice that overexpress mutant human APP or mutant human tau could be used for this purpose.

References

Bartolini L, Casamenti F, Pepeu G (1996) Aniracetam restores object recognition impaired by age, scopolamine, and nucleus basalis lesions. Pharmacol Biochem Behav 53:277–281

Bergamasco B, Villardita C, Coppi R (1992) Idebenone in the treatment of multi-infarct dementia. A randomised double-blind, placebo controlled muticentre trial. Arch Gerontol Geriatr 15:271–278

Bores GM, Huger FP, Petko W, et al (1996) Pharmacological evaluation of novel Alzheimer's disease therapeutics. Acetylcholinestrase inhibitors related to galantamine. J Pharmacol Exp Ther 277:728–738

Burke WJ, Roccaforte WH, Wengel SP, et al (1993) L-Deprenyl in the treatment of mild dementia of the Alzheimer type: results of a 15-month trial. Am J Geriatr Soc 41:1219–1225

Burns A, Rossor M, Hecker J, et al (1999) The effects of donepezil in Alzheimer's disease: results froma a multinational trial. Dementia Geriatr Cogn Disord 10:237–244

Corey-Bloom J, Anand R, Veach J (1998) A randomized trial evaluating the efficacy and safety of ENA 713 (rivastigmine tartrate), a new acetylcholinesterase inhibitor, in patients with mild to moderately severe Alzheimer's disease. Int J Geriatr Psychopharmacol 1:55–65

Cummings JL, Cyrus PA, Ruzicka B, et al (1998) The efficacy of metrifonate in improving the hehavioral disturbances of Alzheimer's disease patients. Neurology 50:A251

Davis KL, Thal LJ, Gamzu ER, et al (1992) A double-blind, placebo-controlled multicenter study of tacrine for Alzheimer's disease. N Engl J Med 327:1253–1259

De Deyn PP, Rabheru K, Rasmussen A, et al (1999) A randomized trial of risperidone, placebo, and haloperidol for behavioral symptoms of demenita. Neurology 53:946–955

Finkel SI, Costa e Silva J, Cohen G, et al (1996) Behavioral and psychological signs and symptoms of dementia. A consensusu statement on current knowledge and implications for research and treatment. Int Psychogeriatry 8(suppl 3):497–500

Gelinas I, Gauthier S, Cyrus PA, et al (1998) The efficacy of metrifonate in enhancing the ability of Alzheimer's disease patients to perform basic and instrumental activities of daily living. Neurology 50:A90–A91

Hasegawa T, Sasao T, Maruyama K, et al (1994) Clinical evaluation of DM-9384 (Nefiracetam) in a long-term treatment of patients with sequelae of cerebrovascular disorders. Rinnsyo-Iyaku 10:2087–2106

Homma A, Takeda M, Imai Y, et al (2000) Clinical efficacy and safety of denepezil on cognitive and global function in patients with Alzheimer's disease: 24 week, multicenter, double-blind, placebo-controlled study in Japan. Dementia Geriatr Cogn Disord 11: (in press)

Horikoshi R, Niwa S, Takahashi Y, et al (1997) Clinical evaluation of aniracetam on chronic cerebral infarction with mental symptoms: evaluation by GBS scale and Hamilton rating scale (in Japanese). Geriatr Med 35:655–670

Joenhagen EM, Nordberg A, Backman L, et al (1998) Intracerebroventricular infusion of nerve growth factor in three patients with Alzheimer's disease. Dement Geriatr Cogn Disord 9:246–257

Knapp JM, Knopman DS, Solomon PR, et al (1994) A 3-week randomized controlled trial of high-dose tacrine in patients with Alzheimer's disease. JAMA 217:985–991

LeBars PK, Katz MM, Berman N, et al (1997) A placebo-controlled, double-blind, randomized trial of an extract of *Ginkyo biloba* for dementia. N Engl J Med 336:1216–1222

McGeer PL, Rogers J (1992) Anti-inflammatory agents as a therapeutic approach to Alzheimer's disease. Neurology 42:447–449

Miyoshi K, Ueki A (1993) The basal forebrain lesioned rat as a model of learning impairment. In: Bergener M, Belmaker RH, Tropper MS (eds) Psychopharmacology for the elderly. Springer, Tokyo, pp 153–169

Oken BS, Storzbach DM, Kaye JA (1998) The efficacy of *Ginkgo biloba* on cognitive function in Alzheimer's disease. Arch Neurol 55:1409–1415

Otomo E, Tohgi H, Hirai S (1989) Clinical effect of YM-08054 tablet (indeloxazine hydrochloride) in cerebrovascular disturbance (in Japanese). Igaku no Ayumi 136:535–555

Potter A, Corwin J, Lang J, et al (1999) Acute effects of the selective cholinergic channel activator (nicotinic agonist) ABT-418 in Alzheimer's disesase. Psychopharmacology 142:334–342

Rogers J, Kirbvy LC, Hempelman SR, Berry DL, et al (1993) Clinical trial of indomethacin in Alzheimer's disease. Neurology 43:1609–1611

Rogers SL, Friedhoff LT, Apter JT, et al (1996) The efficacy and safety of donepezil in patients with Alzheimer's disease: results of US multicentre, randomized, double-blind, placebo-controlled trial. Dementia 7:293–303

Roman GC, Tatemichi TK, Erkinjuntti T, et al (1993) Vascular dementia: diagnostic criteria for research studies. Report of the NINDS-AIREN international workshop. Neurology 43:250–260

Sano M, Ernesto C, Klauber MR, et al (1996) Rationale and design of a multicenter study of selegiline and α-tocopherol in the treatment of Alzheimer's disease using novel clinical outcomes. Alzheimer Dis Assoc Disord 10:132–140

Scharf S, Mander A, Ugoni A, Vajda F, et al (1999) A double-blind, placebo-controlled trial of diclofenac/misoprostol in Alzheimer's disease. Neurology 53:197–201

Schenk D, Barbour R, Dunn W, et al (1999) Immunization with amyloid-protein attenuates Alzheimer-disease-like pathology in the PDAPP mouse. Nature (Lond) 400:173–177

Schneider LS, Farlow MR, Henderson VW, Pogoda JM (1996) Effects of estrogen replacement therapy on response to tacrine in patients with Alzheimer's disease. Neurology 46:1580–1584

Snyder SH, Sabatini DM, Lai MM, et al (1998) Neural actions of immunophilin ligands. Trends Pharmacol Sci 19:21–26

Ueki A, Miyoshi K (1989) Effects of cholinergic drugs on learning impairment in ventral globus pallidus-lesioned rats. J Neurol Sci 90:1–21

WHO (1991) ICD-10 classification of mental and behavioural disorders. Churchill Livingstone, London

Wilcock G, Wilkinson D (1997) Galantamine hydrobrominde. Interim results of a group comparative, placebo-controlled study of efficacy and safety in patients with a diagnosis of senile dementia of the Alzheimer type. In: Iqbal K, Winblad B, Nishimura T, et al (eds) Alzheimer's disease. Biology, diagnosis, and therapeutics. Wiley, New York, pp 661–664

The Validity of Auditory Event-Related Potentials in Diagnosis of Dementia: Prospective Study

Yu-San Chang, Younger W-Y Yu, Kuan-Hung Yang, and Ming-Chao Chen

Summary. When predicting the probability of a patient's being demented, we found age and N200 and P300 latency to be the most important contributing factors. The probability equation is $1/1 + e^{-z}$; $Z = -93.22 + 0.42 \times \text{age} + 0.03 \times \text{N200 latency} + 0.14 \times \text{P300 latency}$. The overall rate of correct classification was 93.6% with 90.3% sensitivity and 95.4% specificity. We further collected information about 103 patients (57 nondementia versus 46 dementia) to evaluate the validity of this equation prospectively and to explore the relationship between mental deterioration and auditory event-related potentials (ERPs). The Mini-Mental State Examination (MMSE) and auditory ERPs (elicited by oddball paradigm, linked-ear reference) were performed on each patient. According to this equation, the results showed 87.0% sensitivity and 82.5% specificity. Mood disorder caused most of the false-positive rate. There was a negative correlation between P300 or N200 latency and the sum of MMSE, orientation, attention, recall, and language. This result shows that the greater the deterioration in mental function, the greater the values for N200 and P300 latency. We concluded that the sensitivity and specificity of our equation are satisfactory. Mental deterioration had negative correlation with variables in this equation, but further studies are needed to elucidate the relationship between mood disorder and dementia.

Keywords. Dementia, P300 latency, Sensitivity, Specificity, MMSE

Introduction

Dementia is characterized by a decrease in intellectual ability involving memory, abstract thinking, and other higher cortical functions. As the P300 component of event-related potentials (ERPs) is thought to reflect aspects of the cognitive processing of stimuli [1], an abnormal delay in its latency might be regarded as evidence of cognitive deterioration, which is one of the hallmarks of dementia. Goodin et al. [2] first reported in 1978 that an abnormal delay in the P300 latency component of ERP was a sensitive and perhaps specific marker of dementia. Since then, P300 latency had received considerable attention in dementia research. A number of studies found an

Kai-Suan Psychiatric Hospital, Kaohsiung, Taiwan, R.O.C.

abnormal delay of P300 latency (or N200 or both) in demented patients [3–6]. Because P300 latency is prolonged as patient age increase, however, a critical issue is exactly how normative P300 values are defined.

In our previous study [7], we tried to predict the probability of demented patients. We showed age, N200 latency, and P300 latency to be the most significant contributing factors that fit the model with the following equation: probability (dementia) = $1/1 + e^{-z}$; $Z = -93.22 + 0.42 \times \text{age} + 0.03 \times \text{N200 latency} + 0.14 \times \text{P300latency}$. The overall rate of correct classification was 93.6% with 90.3% sensitivity and 95.4% specificity. Because this study is retrospective, prospective studies that examine the predictive validity of diagnosing dementia are also needed.

Materials and Methods

This study collected information about 46 patients with dementia and 57 patients with nondementia (including 1 normal, 5 patients with schizophrenia, 26 patients with mood disorder, 8 patients with neurological disorder, 9 patients with other organic mental disorders, and 8 patients with other diseases such as delusional disorder or alcoholic psychosis). The demented group met the DSM-IV criteria for dementia, not subtyping in analysis. Mini-Mental State Examination (MMSE) and auditory event-related potentials (ERPs) were performed for each patient.

ERPs were recorded by using the linked-ear reference in an auditory oddball paradigm from the Brain Atlas III computer (Biologic System). The ERPs were elicited by tone pips of 50-ms duration (10-ms rise/fall times) using a stimulation rate of 1.3/s. The infrequent (16.7%) high-pitched tones (2000 Hz, 80 dB) were presented randomly, interspersed with frequent low-pitched tones (1,000 Hz, 80 dB) binaurally. The amplifier used was high filter, 30, low filter, 1.0, and gain, 20 000. Subjects were asked to focus their attention on the infrequent high-pitched tones and to ignore the frequent low-pitched tones.

Results

The demographic characteristic data of this study are shown in Table 1. There were no differences in gender, age, or education among the groups. The characteristics of the nondemented group are shown in Table 2. There was a negative correlation between P300 and N200 latency and the sum of MMSE, orientation, attention, recall, and language (Table 3). This result shows that the greater the deterioration in mental function, the greater the values for N200 and P300 latency. According to this equation, the results showed 87.0% sensitivity and 82.5% specificity. Mood disorder caused most of the false-positive rate.

Discussion

In most of the studies of diagnosis of dementia [3–6,8,9], P300 latency of a person was defined as falling outside 2 SE of the predicted P300 latency from normal adults of the same age; the results showed a high false-positive and -negative rate. In our

TABLE 1. Characteristics of the study group

Group	Demented group	Nondemented group
Case numbers	46	57
Gender		
Male	25	38
Female	21	19
Age (years)		
Mean ± SD	74.4 ± 8.0	69.1 ± 6.9
Range	(55–87)	(53–82)
Education (years)		
Mean ± SD	5.0 ± 4.7	6.4 ± 4.7
Range	(0–16)	(0–16)

TABLE 2. Characteristics of the nondemented group

Group	Schizophrenia	Mood disorder	Neurological disorder	OMD	Other
Number of cases	5	26	8	9	8
Gender					
Male	4	16	5	5	6
Female	1	10	3	4	2
Age (years), mean ± SD	67.8 ± 4.9	69.3 ± 6.6	68.6 ± 7.4	68.7 ± 7.5	69.9 ± 8.6
Education (years), mean ± SD	8.4 ± 4.3	5.9 ± 4.5	9.0 ± 5.7	4.3 ± 4.5	6.8 ± 4.5

OMD, organic mental disorder

TABLE 3. Relationship between MMSE and auditory event-related potentials

	Orientation	Registration	Attention and calculation	Recall	Language	Sum of MMSE
N100 latency (at Fz)	−0.029	0.026	0.012	−0.074	−0.048	−0.042
N100 amplitude	−0.022	0.178	−0.077	−0.096	0.062	−0.019
P200 latency (at Cz)	−0.169	−0.224*	−0.117	−0.107	−0.005	−0.137
P200 amplitude	−0.016	0.042	0.017	−0.025	0.005	0.010
N200 latency (at Cz)	−0.394**	−0.113	−0.392**	−0.415**	−0.301**	−0.441**
N200 amplitude	0.198*	0.107	0.211*	0.090	0.068	0.184
P300 latency (at Pz)	−0.409**	−0.231*	−0.407**	−0.393**	−0.338**	−0.470**
P300 amplitude	0.153	0.015	0.074	0.169	0.081	0.133

Pearson correlation: * $P < 0.05$, ** $P < 0.01$

previous study [10], we tried to evaluate the validity of P300 latency in the differential diagnosis of dementia by not using the outlying 2 SE of normal adults as the dementia classification criteria. The diagnostic accuracy of various cutoff points of P300 was evaluated by the receiver operating characteristic (ROC) curve [11]; the value of P300 latency is 392 ms, which may be the effective point in dementia diagnosis, and it provides a sensitivity of 80%, specificity of 81%, and an odds ratio of 4.2. Clinically, however, the delay of P300 latency is a nonspecific change in dementia; it can also be found in schizophrenia, depression, and other organic mental disorders [8]. Using the P300 latency increase as a diagnostic criteria of dementia is rather useless because of the high false-positive rate.

We added more study cases, then used logistic regression analysis to predict the probability. The analysis showed age, N200 latency, and P300 latency as the principal contributing factors that fit the model with the following equation: probability (dementia) $= 1/1 + e^{-z}$; $Z = -93.22 + 0.42 \times \text{age} + 0.03 \times \text{N200 latency} + 0.14 \times$ P300latency. However, the older the patient's age and the longer their N200 and P300 latency, the higher the probability there is of being a demented patient. Other studies [6,9] suggested that a combination of P300 latency and other ERP component measures might be more sensitive to dementia diagnosis. In this equation, not only ERP components but also the age factor were considered; this is reasonable because dementia is an age-related degenerative disorder—the older the age, the higher the incidence rate of dementia [12]. Thus, the equation improves specificity in dementia diagnosis by decreasing the false-positive rate. In this study, the results showed 87.0% sensitivity and 82.5% specificity; mood disorder caused the majority of the false-positive rate.

We concluded that the predictive equation model of dementia diagnosis shows both effective and objective results in clinical use; it provides a concrete probability value and a way to define a patient as being demented. The sensitivity and specificity of this probability equation are satisfactory. The mental deterioration had negative correlation with variables in this equation, but further studies are needed to elucidate the relationship between mood disorder and dementia.

References

1. Pritchard WS (1981) Psychophysiology of P300. Psychol Bull 89:506–540
2. Goodin DS, Squires KC, Starr A (1978) Long latency event-related components of the auditory evoked potential in dementia. Brain 101:635–648
3. Gordon E, Kraiuhin C, Harris A, et al (1986) The differential diagnosis of dementia using P300 latency. Biol Psychiatry 21:1123–1132
4. Polich J, Ehlers CL, Otis S, et al (1986) P300 latency reflects the degree of cognitive decline in dementing illness. Electroencephalogr Clin Neurophysiol 63:138–144
5. Goodin DS, Aminoff MJ (1986) Electrophysiological differences between subtypes of dementia. Brain 109:1103–1113
6. Patterson JV, Michalewski HJ, Starr A (1988) Latency variability of the components of auditory event-related potentials of infrequent stimuli in aging, Alzheimer-type dementia, and depression. Electroencephalogr Clin Neurophysiol 71:450–460
7. Yang KU, Yu YW, Lin CH, Chen MC (1998) The validation of auditory event-related potentials in differential diagnosis of dementia. Brain Topogr Today 569–573

8. Pfefferbaum A, Wenergrat BG, Ford JM, et al (1984) Clinical application of the P3 component of event-related potentials. II. Dementia, depression and schizophrenia. Electroencephalogr Clin Neurophysiol 59:104–124
9. Slaets JPJ, Fortbens C (1984) On the value of P300 event-related potentials in the differential diagnosis of dementia. Br J Psychiatry 145:652–656
10. Yu YW, Chen MC, Yang KU, Lin CH (1994) The value of auditory P300 in differential diagnosis of dementia (in Chinese). Chin Psychiatry 8:251–260
11. Mossman D, Somoza E (1991) ROC curves, test accuracy, and the description of diagnostic tests. J Neuropsychiatry Clin Neurosci 3:330–333
12. Gurland B (1996) Epidemiology of psychiatric disorder. In: Sadavoy J, Lazarus WL, Jarvik FL, Grossberg TG (eds) Comprehensive review of geriatric psychiatry, vol II. American Psychiatric Press, Washington, DC, pp 3–41

Quality of Life of Caregivers of Dementia Patients in India

Santosh K. Chaturvedi

Summary. Quality of life (QOL) of caregivers of 54 dementia patients was assessed using the WHOQOL-Bref scale, and psychological distress was assessed using the GHQ-12 scale. The caregiver's situation and behavior problems in the dementia patients were also noted. The subjective perception of QOL on WHOQOL had a mean score of 3.22 (SD, 0.42). QOL scores were higher for male caregivers (3.32) and for caregivers older than 60 years (3.60) as compared to younger ones. The QOL scores of caregivers did not vary significantly with gender, age, educational status, marital status, health, relationship with the dementia patients, type of residence, family type, or whether they received help; 37% had psychological distress as measured by GHQ-12. The correlation between WHOQOL total score and GHQ was found to be −0.39 ($P < 0.003$), confirming poor quality of life in relation to increasing psychological distress.

Keywords. Quality of life, WHOQOL, Caregivers, Dementia, India

Introduction

The longevity of life in India is gradually increasing. At the time of Independence from the British in 1947 it was 30 years; by 1980, it became 54 years, and by 1990 it was 62 years. The living conditions of the elderly in India are quite unique and distinct from many other cultures. In India, 77% of the elderly live with a joint family, 72% have a living spouse, 66% have a caring or understanding spouse, and 80% have social support. In the 1971 census, elderly formed nearly 4.5% of the general population, which increased in 1981 to 6% and in 1991 to 8% of the population. It is expected to increase by the year 2020 to 11%, and by 2025 it may constitute about 15% of the population. In terms of numbers there were nearly 40 million elderly in 1981, which increased in 1991 to 60 million and in 1998 to 70 million.

National Institute of Mental Health and Neurosciences, Nimhans Quarters, D.R. College P.O., Bangalore 560 029, India

Prevalence of Dementia in India

General Population

There are different figures available from different settings about the magnitude of dementia in India. A study on the rural aged above 60 years found a rate of 1.5 per 1000. Another study in the rural community in Bengal reported a rate of 1.6% whereas in a semiurban area it was 10%. Other studies have reported figures between 1% and 3.4%. The average prevalence of dementia seems to be between 0.15% and 6% (Nandi et al. 1997; Shaji et al. 1996; Kamath and Chaturvedi 1999). The Indian Council of Medical Research Taskforce (1987) studied 150 elderly of whom dementia was detected in 31 (20%): multiinfarct dementia in 20 and Alzheimer's disease in 11 subjects. The mortality was higher among people with dementia, as the 1-year follow-up noted 11 deaths of the 31 cases of dementia (Venkoba Rao 1989).

Behavioral Problems Among People with Dementia

A study by Khandelwal et al. (1992) noted that almost all subjects with dementia had some behavioral problems; the number of behavior problems ranged from 2 to 9. The commonest behavioral problems are psychotic symptoms (48%), purposeless activity (43%), aggression (40%), day–night disturbances (40%), depression (33%), and wandering (23%).

Burden on Caregivers of People with Dementia

This area has not been studied in the Indian setting. There are some indications that there is an increased risk of depression and medical problems, heightened use of psychotropics, and even changes in the immune system of the caregivers. This report pertains to the results of the center in India, which was a part of a multicenter international study The aims of this study were to study the quality of life (QOL) of caregivers of people with dementia (PWDem) in India and to compare caregiving situations, psychiatric morbidity, and quality of life of caregivers of people with dementia in India.

Instruments used were the WHOQOL BREF (26-item scale; WHOQOL 1998) to study QOL, and GHQ-12 (Goldberg and Williams 1988) was as a screening instrument to detect psychological distress and psychiatric morbidity among the caregivers. A semistructured interview pro forma was used to acquire information about the caregiver's demographic characteristics, facilities available for care of dementia patients, information about the sufferer (PWDem.), and behaviors and deficits in the PWDem.

At the Indian center, 54 caregivers were studied. Only 1 caregiver of the dementia patient was evaluated. When more than one person was involved in caregiving, the one involved more or who spends more time with the dementia patient was evaluated. If all were equally involved, any one caregiver was included in the study. Attempts were made to include caregivers from different social, economic, or rural–urban backgrounds, whenever possible. Also, attempts were made to include caregivers of dementia patients who were hospitalized or were at special centers for their care for a short period. Patients with a definite clinical diagnosis of dementia as per ICD-10 or DSM-

IV were identified. The key (or main) caregiver was also identified and included for the study. The purpose of the study was explained to the caregiver, and informed consent was sought.

The semistructured interview was administered first, and details of the caregiver and their relationship with the patient were recorded. Information about the PWDem and his/her behaviors, deficits, and abilities were assessed based on the semistructured interview pro forma. Service facilities available or received were enquired. The caregiver's opinion about the ability of their dementia patient was elicited as mentioned in the pro forma. The WHOQOL BREF and GHQ-12 were later administered. If the caregivers were illiterate, the items and possible responses were read verbatim to the caregiver and their responses recorded by the researchers. The SPSS program was used for data analysis.

Results

The total number of caregivers studied was 54. The mean age of the caregivers was 41.09 (SD, 13.92) and the mean age of the dementia patients was 65.04 (SD, 3.97). The quality of life (QOL) score was found to be 3.66 (SD, 0.37). The number of behavior problems ranged from 0 to 9 (mean, 3.65; SD, 1.92). The subjective perception of QOL on item 2 of WHOQOL had a mean score of 3.22 (SD, 0.42). These scores were higher for male caregivers (3.32) as compared to those of female caregivers (3.09) and for caregivers above 60 years (3.60) as compared to younger ones. However, these differences were not statistically significant.

These QOL scores did not vary significantly with the educational status of the caregivers, their marital status, health, relationship with caregivers, type of residence, family type, or whether they received help. Regarding psychological distress as measured by GHQ-12, there were 37% above the known cutoff point of above 3 for India who are probable cases. However, it can be seen that only 13% reported no distress and nearly 1 of 4 had moderate to severe distress (score 5 or more). The mean GHQ score for the Indian caregivers was 2.98 (SD, 2.14). The correlation between WHOQOL total score and GHQ was found to be –0.39 ($P < 0.003$), confirming poor quality of life in relation to increasing psychological distress. In relation to quality of life, one should perhaps also assess what is important for quality of life for caregivers of dementia patients, and whether spirituality and issues of personal significance are important and if so, how much (Chaturvedi 1991).

Acknowledgments. This report is based on the International Collaborative Study on Quality of Life of Caregivers of People with Dementia, which was coordinated by Professor Y. Nakane and Miyako Tazaki. The collaboration was supported partially by a fund from the Ministry of Education in Japan. Thanks are also due to all the participants and their families and to my research workers.

References

Chaturvedi SK (1991) What's important for quality of life for Indians in relation to cancer. Soc Sci Med 33:91–94

Goldberg DP, Williams PA (1988) Users guide to general health questionnaire, GHQ. NFER-NELSON, Windsor
Kamath K, Chaturvedi SK (1999) Psychogeriatric disorders in a developing country over a decade. Presented at the international conference of psychiatric epidemiology at Taipei
Khandelwal S, et al (1992) Behavioural symptoms in dementia: nature and treatment. Ind J Psychiatry 34:36–40
Nandi PS, et al (1997) A study of psychiatric morbidity of the elderly population of a rural community in West Bengal. Ind J Psychiatry 39:122–129
Shaji S, et al (1996) An epidemiological study of dementia in a rural community in Kerala, India. Br J Psychiatry 126:745–749
Venkoba Rao A (1989) Dementia. Neurology India 37:293–300
WHOQOL Group (1998) The World Health Organization Quality of Life Assessment (WHOQOL). Development and General Psychometric Properties. WHO, Geneva

The Neuropsychiatry of Mood Disorders

TMS in Mania and in Animal Models of Mania

NIMROD GRISARU, YURI YAROSLAVSKY, and R.H. BELMAKER

Summary. Transcranial magnetic stimulation (TMS) of the brain has been reported to be therapeutic in depression. Because it shares some properties with electroconvulsive therapy (ECT), and because ECT is effective in mania as well as depression, we started TMS in mania. A controlled double-blind trial of TMS as an add-on to ongoing medication treatment of mania showed significant benefit for TMS. In an amphetamine model of mania in rats, TMS reduced activity or enhanced activity, depending on length and frequency of TMS treatments.

Keywords. Transcranial magnetic stimulation (TMS), Mania, Animal models, Amphetamine

Introduction

Transcranial magnetic stimulation (TMS) is being studied as a novel method of stimulating brain neurons in conscious humans (Hallet and Cohen 1989). Uncontrolled (Grisaru et al. 1994; George et al. 1995) and controlled studies (George et al. 1997; Pascual-Leone et al. 1996) have reported antidepressant effects for TMS, especially left prefrontal repetitive TMS. In normal volunteers, TMS has also been reported to cause mood changes, specific to brain side, in two separate controlled studies (George et al. 1996; Pascual-Leone et al. 1996). Paradoxically, the studies of normals found subtle and subclinical increased sadness with left prefrontal stimulation and subtle and subclinical increased happiness with right prefrontal stimulation.

Electroconvulsive therapy (ECT) is effective in mania as well as in depression. TMS may have ECT-like properties (Belmaker and Fleischmann 1995), we decided to study TMS in mania. Because the studies in depression and normals suggested a laterality of TMS effects, we decided to compare left versus right prefrontal TMS in mania. We had no prior hypothesis, as it seemed possible that stimulation of the same lobe that benefits depression (the left) might benefit mania. However, it

Ministry of Health Mental Health Center, Faculty of Health Sciences, Ben Gurion University of the Negev, Beer-Sheva, Israel

seemed equally likely that stimulation of the lobe opposite that found to benefit depression might be of benefit in mania, because in normal volunteers opposite-lobe stimulation had opposite effects on affect. The extreme difficulties of drug free studies of mania are well known, and we designed our study on the basis of previous work in mania by our group as an add-on study of left versus right prefrontal TMS to ongoing unrestricted drug treatment. Based on reports of rapid response of mania to ECT (Small et al. 1988), we hypothesized that the effect of TMS would be apparent early enough and strongly enough to be measurable even against the background of ongoing pharmacotherapy (Grisaru et al. 1998).

TMS in Manic Patients

The first six patients were randomized to right or left stimulation (RHB) and then rated by an observer (NG) unblind to the site of stimulation as no hypothesis had yet been formed. As it became apparent that right stimulation seemed more therapeutic, a blind rater (YY) began to do all clinical ratings. Because there was no difference in the magnitude of the left versus right difference between the first six patients and the following ten blind patients, the results are presented for statistical analysis both combined and also separately for the ten blind patients only.

A Cadwell High Speed Magnetic Stimulator with a 9-cm-diameter circular coil was used. Each patient was assessed for motor magnetic threshold (Hallet and Cohen 1989) before the first treatment, and 80% of individual patient motor threshold was then administered for all treatment days (as per George et al. 1995). Mean patient motor threshold was 67% of maximum machine output for the left treatment group (range, 50%–80%) and 72% for the right treatment group (range, 55%–85%).

Patients were given 10 daily consecutive sessions, 20 trains per session. Frequency was 20 Hz for 2 s per train; intertrain interval was 1 min. Each of the participants was given the stimuli over the right prefrontal cortex or the left prefrontal cortex, as randomized (RHB).

The CGI improvement score at day 14 was significantly different for left-versus right-treated patients (median test, $P = 0.017$). Results at day 14 were significant even if only the ten blind patients were included for the Mania Scale ($P = 0.04$ at day 14 for post hoc Sheffe test after two-way ANOVA with covariance for baseline; $P = 0.057$), and for the CGI ($P = 0.02$ for interaction and post hoc Sheffe at day 14; $P = 0.03$) (Grisaru et al. 1998).

These results suggest that TMS stimulation in mania of the right prefrontal cortex has therapeutic effects. The effects of TMS in psychiatry may be complex, as certain stimulation patterns enhance neuronal activity and cause, for instance, a motor movement (Hallet and Cohen 1989), whereas other stimulation parameters can disrupt neuronal outflow and cause, for instance, speech arrest. Thus, further studies of frequency of the magnetic stimulus, its intensity, and location will be necessary before the contrast with ECT is proven. Animal studies may be useful to determine these parameters.

TMS in an Animal Model of Mania

To explore the effects of repetitive transcranial magnetic stimulation (rTMS) in an animal model of mania, we used the amphetamine-induced hyperactivity model (Shaldivin et al., in press). Amphetamine-induced hyperactivity is a well-investigated model of mania that includes reasonable face validity (increased activity, increase in secondary reinforcement value, increased aggression) and predictive validity because the effects are usually inhibited by lithium treatment and were also reported to be reduced by carbamazepine and valproate.

Three experiments were performed to evaluate the effects of subacute (two daily), daily chronic (7 days), and twice-daily chronic (7 days) rTMS treatment in the amphetamine-induced hyperactivity model. Subacute rTMS treatment produced a significant decrease in horizontal amphetamine-induced activity (ANOVA, treatment effect: $F(1) = 6.62$, $P < 0.02$). No significant effect was demonstrated for vertical activity, although a similar trend was observed. Daily rTMS treatment for 7 days significantly decreased amphetamine-induced horizontal hyperactivity (ANOVA, treatment effect: $F(1) = 5.46$, $P < 0.03$) with no significant effects on vertical activity. The effect of twice-daily treatment with rTMS was opposite to the effects of the previous treatment schedules. rTMS treatment augmented amphetamine-induced hyperactivity at both horizontal (ANOVA, treatment effect: $F(1) = 5.36$, $P < 0.04$) and vertical (ANOVA, treatment effect: $F(1) = 17.05$, $P < 0.001$) dimensions.

The results of the present study do not reveal a clear picture of TMS effects on amphetamine-induced hyperactivity. We hypothesized that TMS might reduce amphetamine-induced hyperactivity, as does lithium, and this effect was indeed apparent after two or after seven daily TMS treatments. However, TMS twice daily *enhanced* amphetamine-induced hyperactivity. The last effect may be similar to ECT effects, because chronic twice-daily ECS in rats was also demonstrated to increase amphetamine-induced hyperactivity, apparently in a manner similar to its enhancement of apomorphine-induced hyperactivity (Lerer and Belmaker 1982).

TMS effects on amphetamine-induced hyperactivity appear to depend on the treatment regimen, and such dependency was also demonstrated for ECS, in which acute treatment was reported to depress (Wielosz 1983) and repeated treatment to enhance (Ehlers et al. 1983; Nomikos et al. 1991) amphetamine-induced hyperactivity.

Conclusions

In humans, TMS stimulation of the brain has effects depending on the area stimulated (George et al. 1996). Reports suggest that left prefrontal cortex rapid stimulation is antidepressant and right prefrontal cortex stimulation is antimanic (George et al. 1997; Grisaru et al. 1998), although slow stimulation of the right prefrontal cortex may have antidepressant activity (Klein et al. 1999). In rats, available coils stimulate the whole brain, although a small region-specific coil in rats may be available in the future. The present results strongly suggest significant behavioral effects of varying schedules of TMS in interaction with amphetamine, but the direction of these effects may depend on the schedule of treatment in a similar way to EC effects in this model. The results support possible antimanic effects of TMS, but because localized stimulation is not available at present it is not yet possible to use the rat model to further examine the lateralization question.

References

Belmaker RH, Fleischmann A (1995) Transcranial magnetic stimulation: a potential new frontier in psychiatry (editorial). Biol Psychiatry 38:419–421

Ehlers CL, Indik JH, Koob GF, Bloom FE (1983) The effect of single and repeated electroconvulsive shock (ECS) on locomotor activity in rats. Prog Neuropsychopharmacol Biol Psychiatry 7:217–222

George MS, Wassermann EM, Williams WA, et al (1995) Daily repetitive transcranial magnetic stimulation (rTMS) improves refractory depression. NeuroReport 6:1853–1856

George MS, Wasserman EM, Williams W, et al (1996) Changes in mood and hormone levels after rapid-rate transcranial magnetic stimulation of the prefrontal cortex. J Neuropsychiatry Clin Neurosci 8:172–180

George MS, Wasserman EM, Kimbrell TA, et al (1997) Daily left prefrontal rTMS improves mood in depression: a placebo-controlled crossover trial. Am J Psychiatry 154: 1752–1756

Grisaru N, Yaroslavsky U, Abarbanel J, et al (1994) Transcranial magnetic stimulation in depression and schizophrenia. Eur Neurospychopharmacol 4:287–288

Grisaru N, Chudakov B, Yaroslavsky Y, Belmaker RH (1998) TMS in mania: a controlled study. Am J Psychiatry 155:1608–1610

Hallet M, Cohen LG (1989) Magnetism: a new method for stimulation of nerve and brain. JAMA 262:538–541

Klein E, Kreinin I, Chistyakov A, et al (1999) Therapeutic efficacy of right prefrontal slow repetitive transcranial magnetic stimulation in major depression: a double-blind controlled study. Arch Gen Psychiatry 56:315–320

Lerer B, Belmaker RH (1982) Receptors and the mechanism of action of ECT. Biol Psychiatry 17:497–511

Nomikos GG, Zis AP, Damsma G, Fibiger HC (1991) Effects of chronic electroconvulsive shock on interstitial concentrations of dopamine in the nucleus accumbens. Psychopharmacology 105:230–238

Pascual-Leone A, Rubio B, Pallardo F, Catala DM (1996) Beneficial effect of rapid-rate transcranial magnetic stimulation of the left dorsolateral prefrontal cortex in drug-resistant depression. Lancet 348:233–237

Shaldivin A, Alexander Kaptsan A, Belmaker RH, et al. TMS in an amphetamine hyperactivity model of mania Bipolar Disord (in press)

Small JG, Klapper MH, Kellams JJ, et al (1988) Electroconvulsive treatment compared with lithium in the management of manic states. Arch Gen Psychiatry 45:727–732

Wielosz M (1983) Effects of electroconvulsive shock on monoaminergic systems in the rat brain. Pol J Pharmacol Pharm 35:1–130

Comparison of Transcranial Magnetic Stimulation and Electroconvulsive Therapy in Depression

SAXBY PRIDMORE[1], MARZENA RYBAK[1], YVONNE TURNIER-SHEA[1], PHIL REID[1], RAIMONDO BRUNO[2], and NIMROD GRISARU[3]

Summary. Repetitive transcranial magnetic stimulation (rTMS) is a new technology that has an antidepressant effect superior to placebo in blind trials. Our group has demonstrated that rTMS can be safely applied concurrently with certain psychotropic medications, that it can normalize the abnormal dexamathasone suppression test response, that it can influence the facial expression in depression, and that it can be safely and usefully combined with electroconvulsive therapy (ECT). In this study we compared the antidepressant effects of rTMS and ECT in 32 patients suffering a major depressive episode (MDE). There was no limit to the number of treatment sessions that could be given, and treatment was continued until remission occurred or response plateaued. Blinded raters applied the Hamilton Depression Rating Scale (HDRS). A significant main effect for treatment type was found [Pillai Trace = 0.248, $F(3,28) = 3.076$, $P = 0.044$; Power = 0.656], reflecting an advantage for ECT patients on measures of depression overall. However, no differences between the rTMS and ECT groups in HDRS scores were found at entry or exit to the study. Additionally, no significant differences between the groups in percentage HDRS improvement or remission rates were shown. The rTMS group experienced fewer side effects than the rTMS group.

Keywords. Transcranial magnetic stimulation, Electroconvulsive therapy, Depression

Introduction and Update

The pioneers of transcranial magnetic stimulation (TMS) have been acknowledged by ourselves (Pridmore and Belmaker 1999) and others (George et al. 1999). All evidence points to TMS being safe (Pascual-Leone et al. 1992; Wassermann 1998). There is some evidence that it may facilitate cognition (Grafman and Wassermann 1999) and actuate a neuroprotective effect (Post et al. 1999).

[1] Department of Psychological Medicine, Royal Hobart Hospital, Hobart, Tasmania, Australia
[2] Department of Psychology, University of Tasmania, Sandy Bay, Tasmania, Australia
[3] Department of Psychiatry, Ben Gurion University of the Negev, Beersheva, Israel

There is clear evidence from blind placebo controlled trials (Pascual-Leone et al. 1996; George et al. 1997; Nahas et al. 1998; Klein et al. 1999; Berman et al. 2000) that TMS can provide an antidepressant effect in major depression.

There has been concern that TMS may provoke seizures, and early guidelines cautioned against the concurrent use of TMS and psychotropic medication. Our group (Turnier-Shea et al. 1999) has been able to report more than 1000 TMS treatments with no instance of seizure. The majority of our patients are receiving concurrent psychotropic medication. We are able to give details of 12 patients taking a tricyclic, 11 taking moclobemide, 14 taking sertraline, 12 taking fluoxetine, 8 taking paroxetine, 16 taking venlafaxine, and 18 taking an antipsychotic medication; 24% of patients experienced a headache on some occasion, and 10% took a mild analgesic for headache on some occasion during treatment.

Reid and Pridmore (1999) described a patient who had major depressive disorder and was a dexamethasone nonsuppressor. With the application of TMS, she experienced clinical improvement and converted to dexamathasone suppression test (DST) suppressor status on three separate occasions. She relapsed twice, but after the third treatment, she remained well to the time of writing (in excess of 2 years). Pridmore (1999) reported the response of 12 patients with major depressive disorder who were DST nonsuppressors to 12 to 16 sessions of rTMS. Six showed clinical improvement and converted to DST suppressor status.

Katsikitis et al. (1999) assessed the effect of repetitive TMS (rTMS) in major depression using a range of questionnaires and scored by one of the investigators and the Facial Expression Measurement System (FACEM; a computer-based objective indicator of mood status). Nine patients were examined before and after 10 to 14 rTMS treatments. There was significant improvement on questionnaire results. Analysis of FACEM revealed significant widening of the distance between the eyebrows, elevation of the eyebrows, and increase in the width of the mouth. These changes represent movement from the frowning, "long" face of depression to the smiling nondepressed countenance.

Walter et al. (in press) examined the experience, knowledge, and attitudes of recipients of rTMS that was provided as treatment of a drug-resistant major depressive episode. They interviewed 48 patient/recipients by telephone using a 60-item survey. Two-thirds had a history of electroconvulsive therapy (ECT), and almost three-quarters believed rTMS had been helpful. Most rated rTMS as more acceptable than ECT. The majority would have it again and recommend it to others.

Pridmore (in press) substituted rTMS treatments for ECT treatments in a course of ECT randomized, blind, controlled study. Two streams were conducted. One stream received nondominant unilateral (UL) ECT only, treatments being given three times per week for 2 weeks. The other stream received a combination of treatments: one UL ECT on day 1 and rTMS on the following 4 days, all repeated once, after a 2-day respite. Of the 22 patients recruited, 11 were allocated to each stream. There was no evidence that the antidepressant effect of the ECT-only stream was superior to that of the ECT-plus-rTMS stream. There was no increase in subjective side effects in the ECT-plus-rTMS stream. On the contrary, this stream was accompanied by fewer side effects than the ECT-only stream in this study. The conclusion was that it is possible to substitute rTMS treatments for ECT treatments in a course of ECT without loss of antidepressant effect or an increase in subjective side effects.

Grunhaus et al. (1999) compared rTMS and ECT in an open study. They treated 20 patients with ECT and 20 patients with rTMS for as many as 20 treatments. They found significant treatment effects for both groups. When the total group was split into psychotic and nonpsychotic subgroups, ECT was superior to rTMS in the psychotic group, but for those without psychosis, the response to ECT and rTMS was similar.

Aims

The aims of the study were (1) to compare the maximum antidepressant response to rTMS and ECT achievable with courses of treatment of unlimited length and (2) to compare the side-effect profile of the two treatments.

Method

Patients suffering major depressive episode who scored 18 or above on the 17-item Hamilton Depression Rating Scale (HDRS) and who had failed to respond to a 4-week trial at maximum recommended doses of medication from at least one family of antidepressants and for whom, on clinical grounds, a physical treatment was considered to be the next appropriate step, were invited to participate. They were randomly assigned to groups according to order of presentation. Medication was tapered and ceased where possible; no new medication was commenced in the 2 weeks before entry into the study. Blind raters conducted the 17-item HDRS at entry and exit. A side-effects scale was developed for this study and administered at entry and exit. It rated "headache," "memory problems," "muscle stiffness," "dry mouth or blurred vision," "nausea, abdominal discomfort or bowel problems," "tremor," and "weakness, tiredness or sleepiness" on a four-point severity scale.

To allow maximum response to these forms of treatment, there was no upper limit of treatment sessions that could be provided. rTMS was provided using a Magstim Super Rapid Stimulator. Treatments were given 5 days per week, applied to the left prefrontal cortex (LPFC) at the following parameters: 100% of motor threshold (MT), 20 Hz, 2-s trains, 30–35 trains per day separated by 28-s rest periods. ECT was provided using a Thymatron DGx and Thymapad electrodes (Somantics). Treatments were given 3 days per week, applied to the nondominant hemisphere using 100% of machine output (504 mC) with the stimulus width at 0.5 ms.

Results

There were no significant differences between the groups with respect to demographic or historical data. The mean number of treatments for the rTMS group was 12.2 (SD = 3.4) and for the ECT group 6.2 (SD = 1.6). Data were analyzed following a doubly multivariate design with the independent variables of time (entry, exit) and treatment (rTMS, ECT), and the dependent measures comprising the HDRS and VAS. Multivariate tests show a significant main effect for time [Pillai Trace = 0.824, F (3,28) = 43.749, $p < 0.001$], reflecting the improvement in all measures of depression during the subject's hospital stay. A significant main effect for treatment type was also found

[Pillai Trace = 0.248, F (3,28) = 3.076, P = 0.044; Power = 0.656], reflecting an advantage for ECT patients on measures of depression overall. There was no significant interaction between treatment and time [Pillai Trace = 0.151, F (3,28) = 1.663, P = 0.198], reflecting that the improvement in depression ratings over time was common for both ECT and rTMS treatment groups.

HDRS Comparisons

Repeated-measures ANOVA for the effect of time and treatment type showed a significant main effect of time: F (1,30) = 102.066, $P < 0.001$, referring to the improvement in HDRS scores over the course of treatment for both groups. No significant main effect of treatment type [F (1,30) = 0.579, P = 0.452] or treatment by time interaction [F (1,30) = 1.220, P = 0.278] was found. This result reflects the fact that no differences between the rTMS and ECT groups in HDRS scores were found at entry or exit to the study. Additionally, no significant differences between the groups in percentage HDRS improvement or remission rates were shown.

Side-Effects Comparisons

Repeated-measures ANOVA for side-effect ratings showed a significant main effect of time: F (1,30) = 9.190, P = 0.005, indicating that, overall, reported side effects reduced over time in treatment. There was no difference in side-effect ratings for the marginal means of the two groups [F (1,30) = 0.111, P = 0.742]. Additionally, a significant time by treatment interaction appeared [F (1,30) = 4.187, P = 0.050], reflecting the "crossover" in the side-effect data, in that TMS patients started the study with non-significantly higher side-effect ratings than ECT patients and exited with slightly lower ratings.

Discussion

This study compared an experimental treatment (rTMS) and the most effective treatment of depression (ECT). We are reporting a 55.6% improvement in HDRS with rTMS. This result is slightly higher than those reported previously. Our study design allowed continuation of rTMS while improvement continued. Those who went on to remission received a mean number of 13.1 (SD = 3.1) treatments whereas those who did not achieve remission received a mean number of 10.6 (SD = 3.8) treatments. This flexibility is unique among the studies and may have contributed to the high remission rate.

References

Berman R, Narasimhan M, Sanacora G, et al (2000) A randomized clinical trial of repetitive transcranial magnetic stimulation in the treatment of major depression. Biol Psychiatry 47:332–337

George MS, Wassermann E, Kimbrell T, et al (1997) Mood improvement following daily left prefrontal repetitive transcranial magnetic stimulation in patients with depression: a placebo-controlled crossover trial. Am J Psychiatry 154:1752–1756

George M, Lisanby S, Sackheim H (1999) Transcranial magnetic stimulation. Arch Gen Psychiatry 56:300–311

Grafman J, Wassermann E (1999) Transcranial magnetic stimulation can measure and modulate learning and memory. Neuropsychologia 37:159–167

Grunhaus L, Dannon P, Schreiber S, et al (1999) Repetitive transcranial magnetic stimulation is as effective as electroconvulsive therapy in the treatment of nondelusional major depressive disorder: an open study. Biol Psychiatry 47:314–324

Katsikitis M, Pridmore S, Marzullo M (1999) The facial expression measurement system in the assessment of the efficacy of transcranial magnetic stimulation in the treatment of depression. Eur Rev Appl Psychol 49:123–128

Klein E, Kreinin I, Chistyakov A, et al (1999) Therapeutic efficiency of right prefrontal slow repetitive transcranial magnetic stimulation in major depression: a double blind controlled trial. Arch Gen Psychiatry 56:315–320

Nahas Z, Speer A, Molloy M (1998) Preliminary results concerning the roles of frequency and intensity in the antidepressant effect of daily left prefrontal rTMS (abstract). Biol Psychiatry 43(94s):315

Pascual-Leone A, Houser CM, Reese K, et al (1992) Safety of rapid-rate transcranial magnetic stimulation in normal volunteers. Electroencephalogr Clin Neurophysiol 89: 120–130

Pascual-Leone A, Rubio B, Pallardo, Catala D (1996) Beneficial effect of rapid-rate transcranial magnetic stimulation of the left dorsolateral prefrontal cortex in drug-resistant depression. Lancet 348:233–238

Post A, Muller M, Keck M (1999) Repetitive transcranial magnetic stimulation in rats: evidence for a neuroprotective effect in vitro and in vivo. Eur J Neurosci 11:3247–3254

Pridmore S (1999) Rapid transcranial magnetic stimulation (rTMS) and normalization of the dexamethasone suppression test (DST). Psychiatry Clin Neurosci 53:33–37

Pridmore S (2000) Substitution of rapid transcranial magnetic stimulation treatments for electroconvulsive therapy treatments in a course of electroconvulsive therapy. Anxiety Depression 12:118–123

Pridmore S, Belmaker R (1999) Transcranial magnetic stimulation in the treatment of psychiatric disorders. Psychiatry Clin Neurosci 53:541–548

Reid P, Pridmore S (1999) Dexamethasone suppression test reversal in rapid transcranial magnetic stimulation treated depression. Aust N Z J Psychiatry 33:274–277

Turnier-Shea Y, Rybak M, Pridmore (1999) Update on psychotropic medication used concurrently with transcranial magnetic stimulation. Ger J Psychiatry 2:46–59

Walter G, Martin J, Kirkby K, Pridmore S (2001) Transcranial magnetic stimulation: experience, knowledge and attitudes of recipients. Aust N Z J Psychiatry (in press)

Wassermann E (1998) Risk and safety of repetitive transcranial magnetic stimulation: report and suggested guidelines from the International Workshop on the Safety of Repetitive Transcranial Magnetic Stimulation, June 5–7, 1996. Electroencephalogr Clin Neurophysiol 108:1–16

The Therapeutic Efficacy of Prefrontal Slow rTMS in Major Depression and Schizophrenia

EHUD KLEIN, DANNY KOREN, ANDREI CHYSTIAKOV, and MOSHE FEINSOD

Summary. Recent studies have suggested that repetitive transcranial magnetic stimulation (rTMS) of the dorsolateral prefrontal cortex (DLPFC) might be effective as a treatment for major depression (MD). One line of studies has reported the efficacy of high-frequency rTMS (10–20 Hz) to the left DLPFC, using focal stimulation. Our work has focused on the evaluation of low-frequency (1 Hz) rTMS to the right DLPFC. Using this approach, rTMS has been shown to be significantly more effective than sham stimulation in a double-blind controlled study in 70 subjects with MD. At the end of ten daily rTMS sessions, Hamilton depression ratings (HDRS) were significantly lower in the rTMS group. Also, a significantly larger portion of patients had HDRS ratings <10 and did not need electro convulsive therapy (ECT). In contrast, we failed to show therapeutic efficacy of rTMS in 31 schizophrenic patients using the same treatment protocol. In a third study, 46 normal volunteers were assessed for neuropsychological effects of one session of low-frequency rTMS applied to the right or left DLPFC as compared to sham rTMS. In this double-blind study, rTMS did not appear to have any adverse cognitive effects as assessed by several neuropsychological tests. Taken together, these findings suggest that right prefrontal rTMS may be selectively effective in MD without noticeable neuropsychological adverse effects. These results should be viewed as preliminary, and further studies are necessary to assess the long-term efficacy and the optimal treatment parameters of rTMS in MD and possibly other neuropsychiatric disorders.

Keywords. Magnetic brain stimulation, Major depression, Dorsolateral prefrontal cortex, Schizophrenia, Normal volunteers

Introduction

Transcranial magnetic stimulation (TMS) has been used, since its introduction in 1985 [1], as a means for noninvasive and safe stimulation of the cerebral cortex. Originally, TMS was used mostly for cortical mapping and assessment of motor [2], cognitive,

Departments of Psychiatry and Neurosurgery, Rambam Medical Center, B. Rappaport Faculty of Medicine, Technion—I.I.T, Efron street Bat-Galim Haifa 31096, Israel

and behavioral functions [3]. More recently, repetitive TMS (rTMS) has been tested as a therapeutic tool for psychiatric disorders, primarily major depression. Several studies now suggest that rTMS of the prefrontal cortex can have antidepressant and antimanic effects. In addition, there are preliminary data suggesting that rTMS may be therapeutically beneficial for other conditions such as OCD and PTSD (for a review of these studies, see George et al. 1999 [4]).

The aim of this chapter is to summarize the major findings from a series of three studies, one open [5] and two double-blind sham-controlled [6,7], carried out by our group on the therapeutic efficacy of slow rTMS in major depression and schizophrenia.

Method

Participants

Participants in all three studies were inpatients with a DSM-IV diagnosis of major depression or schizophrenia. Patients were excluded if they had a history of brain trauma, seizures, alcohol or drug abuse, uncontrolled cardiac arrhythmias, or unstable systemic disease or if they had attempted suicide in the 3 months before the study. For ethical considerations, patients in all three studies were allowed to remain on their ongoing medications throughout the treatment protocol.

Treatment

All three studies employed the same treatment protocol using a Cadwell MES-10 magnetic stimulator (Cadwell, Kennewick, WA, USA) with a 90-mm-diameter circular coil. Initially, motor threshold was determined over the right motor cortex by finding the minimal intensity that produced a motor response in the left distal wrist muscles. For the treatment itself, the coil was placed over the right prefrontal area (without crossing the midline) at a point 6 cm anterior to the scalp position at which the motor threshold was determined.

Stimulation parameters were frequency of 1 Hz, 0.1-ms pulse duration, and field intensity 10% above motor threshold (average, 0.95 ± 0.1 tesla). At each treatment session, a train of 60 stimuli was delivered over 1 min followed by a 3-min interval and another train of 60 stimuli. The entire protocol consisted of 10 daily sessions given on consecutive days except weekends. For the sham treatment group, stimulation parameters were identical; however, the stimulation coil was placed perpendicular to the scalp surface, thereby minimizing the flow of energy into the skull.

Clinical Ratings

Clinical ratings in all three studies were carried out at baseline (before treatment), after five treatment sessions (1 week), and after the last treatment (2 weeks). Depressive symptoms were assessed using the Hamilton Depression Rating Scale (HDRS) and the Montgomery-Asberg Depression Rating Scale (MADRS). Schizophrenia symptoms were evaluated with the Positive and Negative Symptoms Scale (PANSS).

General psychiatric symptoms were assessed with the Brief Psychiatric Rating Scale (BPRS), and overall level of psychopathology was rated with the Clinical Global Impression (CGI).

Results

Open Study in Major Depression and Schizophrenia

A total of 24 subjects were enrolled in the study, 14 with MD (9 women, 5 men; mean age, 58.4 ± 14.0 years) and 10 with schizophrenia (5 women, 5 men; mean age, 30.2 ± 9.5 years). Overall, 58% of the patients experienced clinical improvement of marked (reduction of 50% or more on the relevant rating scale) or moderate (20%–50% reduction) degree. However, marked improvement seemed to be more evident in depressed patients compared to patients with schizophrenia.

Double-Blind Sham-Controlled Study in Major Depression

Seventy patients (53 women and 17 men; mean age, 58.7 ± 17.2 years, range, 27–88 years) meeting diagnostic criteria for MD (mostly recurrent) were enrolled in the study. Patients were randomly assigned to receive either rTMs or sham rTMS. The two groups were matched for age and gender and did not differ significantly on most of the clinical variables such as duration of illness and number of previous episodes. Of the 70 patients who initially started the study, 67 completed the entire treatment protocol. Generally the treatment was well tolerated, and no serious adverse effects were reported by any of the patients.

Table 1 presents the scores (means and SD) on the clinical rating scales over time in the two groups. A clear difference between the two groups was noted after the first week and became robust after the second week, with the rTMS group showing a greater reduction in depression scores. The overall MANOVA revealed a significant group × time interaction for HDRS (Wilks' lambda $F_{(2,64)} = 3.29$, $P < 0.03$) and for MADRS (Wilks' lambda $F_{(2,64)} = 3.2$, $P < 0.05$). These results remained significant after controlling for medications effects.

Seventeen rTMS patients (49%) but only 8 (25%) sham rTMS patients had a reduction of 50% or more on at least one of the depression scales ($\chi^2 = 4.0$, $df = 1$, $P < 0.05$). In addition, 16 subjects (46%) in the rTMS group but only 6 (19%) in the placebo group reached a final HDRS score of 10 or less ($\chi^2 = 5.5$, $df = 1$, $P < 0.02$). Furthermore, 15 patients in the rTMS group and 13 in the placebo group were initially considered for electro convulsive therapy (ECT). Eventually, only 7 patients in the rTMS group (47%) but all 13 subjects in the placebo group went on to receive ECT (Fisher exact $P = 0.002$).

Double-Blind Sham-Controlled Study in Schizophrenia

The study sample comprised 35 inpatients meeting DSM-IV criteria for schizophrenia ($n = 30$) or schizoaffective disorder ($n = 5$). All patients were on antipsychotic medications for 2 to 4 weeks before entering the study without evidencing sufficient improvement. On entering the study, patients were randomized to receive rTMS or

TABLE 1. Scores (means and SD) on the clinical rating scales of the two groups over time in the major depression (MD) study

	Baseline		Week 1		End of treatment		ANOVA (group × time)	
	TMS ($n = 35$)	Placebo ($n = 32$)	TMS ($n = 35$)	Placebo ($n = 32$)	TMS ($n = 35$)	Placebo ($n = 32$)	F (2, 64)	P
HDRS	25.8 (5.6)	25.3 (6.4)	16.6 (7.8)	20.8 (9.7)	13.7 (9.2)	19.7 (10.3)	3.3	0.03
MADRS	34.5 (5.4)	34.0 (7.6)	21.8 (10.3)	28.8 (11.4)	19.5 (12.2)	27.3 (11.5)	3.2	0.05
CGI	4.9 (0.8)	4.9 (0.8)	3.9 (1.1)	4.4 (1.4)	3.5 (1.4)	4.2 (1.5)	2.4	0.09

HDRS, Hamilton Depression Rating Scale; MADRS, Montgomery-Asberg Depression Rating Scale; CGI, Clinical Global Impression
The numbers in parentheses are SD
Only subjects who completed the entire study are included

TABLE 2. Scores (means and SD) on the clinical rating scales of the two groups over time in the schizophrenia study

	Baseline		Week 1		End of treatment		ANOVA (group × time)	
	TMS ($n = 16$)	Placebo ($n = 15$)	TMS ($n = 16$)	Placebo ($n = 15$)	TMS ($n = 16$)	Placebo ($n = 15$)	F (2, 28)	P
PANSS								
Positive	13.6 (3.2)	14.9 (7.7)	12.4 (4.4)	13.6 (8.3)	12.4 (5.5)	10.9 (5.4)	2.7	<0.1
Negative	16.5 (5.6)	14.1 (5.0)	17.1 (6.3)	14.2 (3.9)	17.6 (6.8)	15.5 (5.0)	0.59	n.s.
General	34.3 (9.6)	25.6 (8.2)	31.8 (10.3)	24.7 (7.1)	29.8 (10.7)	24.0 (7.0)	1.0	n.s.
BPRS	34.1 (8.9)	30.5 (6.5)	32.5 (10.0)	27.2 (4.5)	29.9 (13.7)	26.8 (4.5)	0.7	n.s.
HDRS	11.4 (6.1)	10.2 (3.8)	9.6 (3.5)	8.2 (3.9)	8.6 (3.5)	6.9 (4.0)	0.1	n.s.
CGI	5.1 (1.0)	4.6 (0.7)	4.8 (1.1)	4.3 (0.6)	4.6 (1.3)	4.0 (0.8)	0.1	n.s.

PANSS, Positive and Negative Syndrome Scale; BPRS, Brief Psychiatric Rating Scale; HDRS, Hamilton Depression Rating Scale; CGI, Clinical Global Impression
The numbers in parentheses are SD
Only subjects who completed the entire treatement are included

sham treatment without changing their medications for the duration of the trial. The groups were similar in their demographic and clinical characteristics.

Thirty-one patients (16 rTMS and 15 sham) completed the 2-week treatment protocol. In general the treatment was well tolerated, and no serious adverse effects were reported. In the rTMS group, however, 2 (11%) patients reported worsening of preexisting akathesia and 2 other patients reported worsening of preexisiting obsessive compulsive symptoms.

Table 2 presents the scores (means and SD) on the clinical rating scales over time in the two groups. Both groups showed similar patterns of slight improvement over time on the various rating scales. In accordance, the set of repeated measures analysis of variance (using the MANOVA approach) failed to reveal significant treatment × time interactions for any of the clinical ratings.

Concluding Comment

The results of this series of studies provide supporting evidence for the therapeutic efficacy of right prefrontal slow rTMS in major depression. The effect of rTMS does not appear to be related to concomitant use of medications and is evident as early as 1 week after initiation of treatment. On the other hand, the same treatment protocol did not produce similar improvement in patients with schizophrenia, suggesting that the effect of rTMS as administered in these studies may be specific for depression.

Unlike previous studies [4] in depressed patients that used high-frequency rTMS, therapeutic efficacy in the current study was seen with slow rTMS. This finding may be important because rapid rTMS has been shown to have a seizure-producing potential, whereas slow rTMS appears to be safer and requires less expensive equipment.

Further evaluation of the therapeutic efficacy of rTMS should assess the importance of various treatment parameters such as frequency, intensity, pulse duration, and stimulation site for its optimal outcome. In addition, longer and preferably medication-free follow-up studies of its outcome are needed. The suggestion that rTMS may become, in some cases, an alternative treatment to ECT seems promising but requires further investigation.

References

1. Barker AT, Jalinous R, Freeston H (1985) Non-invasive stimulation of the human motor cortex. Lancet 1:1106–1107
2. Barker AT, Jalinous R, Freeston H, Jarratt JA (1985) Motor responses to non-invasive brain stimulation in clinical practice. Electroencephalogr Clin Neurophysiol 61:570–574
3. Pascual-Leone A, Grafman J, Cohen LG, et al (1995) Transcranial magnetic stimulation: a new tool for the study of higher cognitive functions in humans. In: Boller F, Grafman J (eds) Handbook of Neuropsychology, vol 9. Elsevier, Amsterdam
4. George MS, Lisanby SH, Sackeim HA (1999) Transcranial magnetic stimulation: applications in psychiatry. Arch Gen Psychiatry 56:300–314
5. Feinsod M, Kreinin B, Chistykov A, Klein E (1998) Preliminary evidence for a beneficial effect of low frequency repetitive transcranial magnetic stimulation in patients with major depression and schizophrenia. Depression 7:65–68
6. Klein E, Kreinin B, Chistyakov A, et al (1999) Therapeutic efficacy of right prefrontal slow repetitive transcranial magnetic stimulation in major depression; a double blind controlled study. Arch Gen Psychiatry 56:315–320
7. Klein E, Kolsky Y, Puyerovsky M, et al (1999) Right prefrontal slow repetitive transcranial magnetic stimulation in schizophrenia; a double blind sham-controlled pilot study. Biol Psychiatry 46:1451–1454

Repetitive Transcranial Magnetic Stimulation (rTMS) for Psychiatric Disorders: The Sydney Studies

PERMINDER SACHDEV, COLLEEN LOO, PHILIP MITCHELL, SIMON GANDEVIA, JANET TAYLOR, RICHARD MCBRIDE, GIN MALHI, WEI WEN, VANESSA CROKER, and HAMADA EL-SAYED

Summary. The authors report a series of studies of repetitive transcranial magnetic stimulation (rTMS) for the treatment of psychiatric disorders and some pilot work using animal models performed by their group. The first is a previously published double-blind sham-controlled study of rTMS for the treatment of resistant major depression, which is noteworthy for being the only published negative study in which, even though all subjects improved during the 2 weeks of treatment, there was no significant difference between real and sham treatments. The authors could not exclude the possibility that the sham used in this study was partially active. The authors then report preliminary results from a sham-controlled study of bilateral prefrontal rTMS for major depression, which again shows no significant differences between the two groups. The authors are currently performing a study comparing the effects of right and left prefrontal rTMS on obsessive-compulsive disorder, with a preliminary analysis showing significant improvement in these subjects but no right–left difference. Last, using the Forced Swim Test model in rats, the authors show that rTMS at high frequency (15 and 25 Hz) has a significant antidepressant effect when compared to lower frequencies.

Keywords. TMS, Depression, Obsessive-compulsive disorder, Animal models

Introduction

Transcranial magnetic stimulation (TMS) is a technique by which a time-varying magnetic field of high intensity is created by a coil placed over the scalp, and this is used to generate a current flow in neural tissue, resulting in cortical stimulation (George et al. 1999). Since the mid-1980s, TMS has been used to stimulate the motor cortex. With the development of technology to deliver TMS at a rapid rate, referred to as repetitive TMS (rTMS), it became possible to produce behavioral and emotional changes in individuals. The investigation of rTMS as possible treatment of neuropsychiatric disorders followed, and many such studies have

---

Schools of Psychiatry and Medicine, University of New South Wales, Neuropsychiatric Institute, Mood Disorders Unit and Prince of Wales Medical Research Institute, The Prince of Wales Hospital, Sydney, Australia

now been published. rTMS has also been increasingly used as a probe of neuropsychological function.

The Prince of Wales Hospital TMS group has used TMS in a number of research studies in the past 3 years, and a summary of published and ongoing studies is presented here.

Studies in Affective Disorders

A Double-Blind Controlled Investigation of Transcranial Magnetic Stimulation for the Treatment of Resistant Major Depression

The objective of this study (Loo et al. 1999) was to examine the efficacy and safety of left prefrontal rTMS for treating major depression. Eighteen subjects (9 male) with a DSM-IV diagnosis of major depressive episode (8 with melancholic features, 1 psychotic) were recruited. Subjects had a mean age of 47 years and had been unwell in the current episode for about 10 months. All subjects had had two or more antidepressants. Five were off antidepressant drugs during treatment; of the remaining, 9 were on venalafaxine and 4 on nefazodone.

Subjects were randomly allocated to 2 weeks (ten sessions) of real or sham rTMS in a double-blind fashion. Following this, they were permitted to have up to 4 weeks of real rTMS in an open extension of the study. Effects on mood, neuropsychological function, EEG, and hearing were assessed. TMS was administered with a 70-mm figure-8 coil (Magstim) to the left dorsolateral prefrontal cortex at 10 Hz, 110% of motor threshold, 30 trains of 5 s each, 30 s apart. For sham stimulation, the coil was held at 45° at the same site.

The results on the Hamilton Depression (Ham-D) and Montgomery-Asberg Depression Rating scales (MADRS) are presented in Fig. 1. There was a significant linear improvement over the 2-week double-blind period on the Ham-D ($F = 24.1$, $df = 1,16$, $P < 0.001$) and MADRS ($F = 27.1$, $df = 1,16$, $P < 0.001$), but there was no significant difference between the groups receiving real and sham treatments. During the 4 weeks, the linear trend for improvement continued.

This is the only published negative study of rTMS for depression, although the parameters used were comparable to those used by Pascual-Leone et al. (1996) and George et al. (1997). The sham response in our study was significant; this may have been because these patients had extensive contact with the research team. Alternatively, it is possible that the sham stimulation, which delivered a very weak stimulus, was modestly effective. rTMS over 4 weeks was demonstrated to be safe in our study.

Bilateral rTMS and Depression: A Double-Blind Controlled Study

Considering the greater efficacy of bilateral electroconvulsive therapy (ECT) over unilateral treatment in major depression, it was argued that bilateral stimulation with rTMS may have greater benefit than unilateral treatment. This sham-controlled study is in progress. The design of the study is similar to the unilateral study just described except that two coils are placed on the head, one overlying each dorsolateral prefrontal

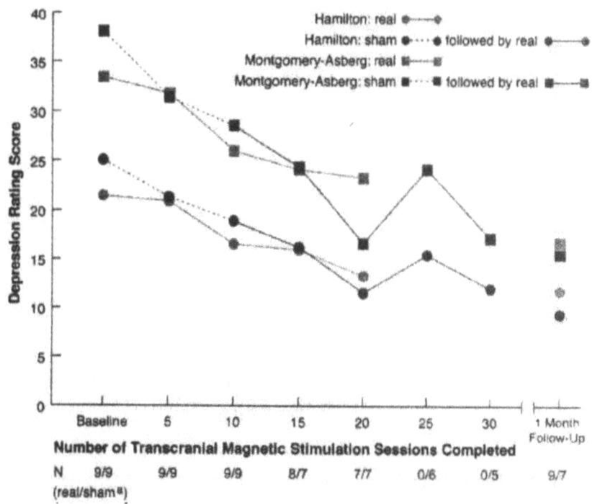

FIG. 1. Mean scores on the Hamilton and Montgomery-Asberg Depression Scales of patient with resistant depression who were treated with real (*solid lines*) or sham (*dotted lines*) transcranial magnetic stimulation (TMS) [Adapted from Loo et al. 1999]

cortex. The parameters of stimulation are identical to the unilateral study and the same for each coil. In the sham situation, no current is passed through the coils, but a third coil is held behind the head and discharged at the the same frequency to produce the acoustic artifact.

Preliminary results on 12 patients (Fig. 2) show no significant difference between real and sham TMS. Even though the study is still in progress, these results suggest that bilateral prefrontal rTMS is ineffective as an antidepressant treatment.

Obsessive-Compulsive Disorder (OCD)

A Comparison of Right and Left Prefrontal rTMS for the Treatment of OCD

This comparison is a pilot study to examine the effect of TMS in OCD and to determine if there is a lateralised effect. A preliminary study by Greenberg et al. (1997) reported significant decreases in compulsive urges for 8 h after right but not left lateral prefrontal stimulation.

We studied nine patients with OCD, allocated randomly to right or left prefrontal rTMS for ten sessions (10 Hz, 30 trains of 5 s each at 110% motor threshold), with the rater blind to the allocation. Subjects were examined using the Yale–Brown Obsessive Compulsive Scale (Y-BOCS) at 1 and 2 weeks and at 1 month. In the total group, there was a significant improvement in compulsions (12.01, $df = 1,9$, $P < 0.01$), obsessions ($F = 8.4$, $df = 1,9$, $P < 0.05$), and total Y-BOCS score ($F = 14.75$, $df = 1,9$, $P < 0.05$), but left- and right-sided stimulation did not show a significant difference (Fig. 3). On close examination of the results, it became apparent that while all right-sided stimulation

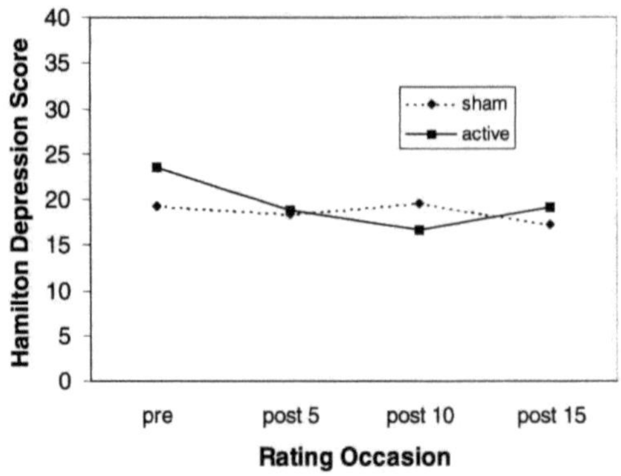

FIG. 2. Mean scores on the Hamilton Depression Scale before TMS and after 5, 10, or 15 treatments with real (*solid*) and sham (*dotted*) bilateral prefrontal TMS in resistant depression [n = 12]

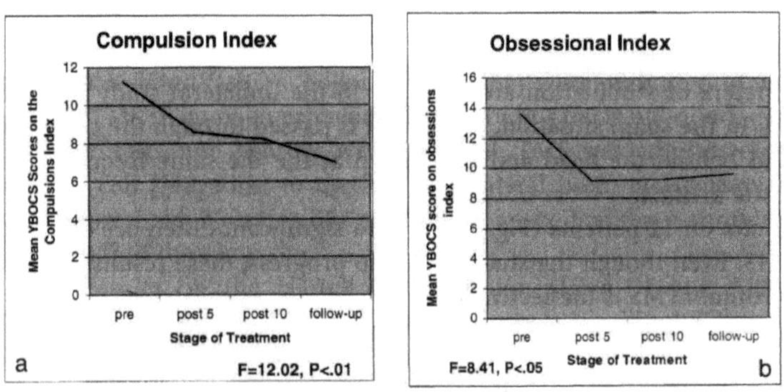

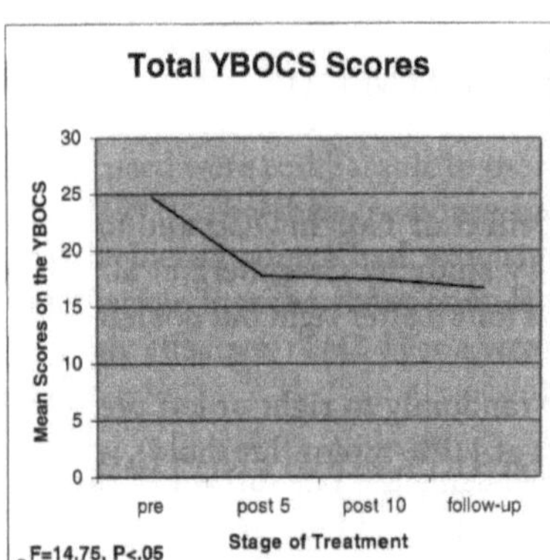

FIG. 3**a–c.** The effect of rTMS on compulsion (**a**), obsession (**b**), and total (**c**) Y-BOCS scores at baseline and after 1 week (5 sessions–post 5) and 2 weeks (10 sessions–post 10) of rTMS, and at 1 month follow-up (*n* = 9). The left- and right-sided stimulation patients are pooled in this figure. Improvement was significant for both compulsions and obsessions

subjects had shown some improvement, the improvement with left-sided stimulation occurred in two of five subjects, with the other three showing no change (two) or worsening (one). The depression scores did not show a significant change and could not account for the improvement in OC scores.

The study showed promise for the application of rTMS in OCD, but does not resolve the issue of right versus left stimulation, even though right-sided stimulation appears to have greater promise.

Animal Models

The Effect of Different Frequencies of rTMS on a Rat Model of Depression

The rat study was designed to examine the differential effects of various frequencies of rTMS, with the hypothesis that only higher frequencies would produce an antidepressant effect. Naïve male Wistar rats weighing 200–300 g were allocated to the following groups (eight each): sham control, restraint control, imipramine treated (IMI), 1-Hz TMS, 5-Hz TMS, 15-Hz TMS, and 25-Hz TMS. A total of 1000 stimuli was administered, using different frequencies, over a period of 20 min daily during 1 week (five sessions). For sham stimulation, the rats are immobilized in the same manner and exposed to the audible artifact of the TMS from a distance of 10 cm. The IMI group were administered imipramine at 10 mg/kg s.c daily for 1 week (five injections). The Porsolt Forced Swim Test was used as a model for the antidepressant effect.

The TMS groups showed significantly lower immobility times than the control groups ($F = 16.63, P < 0.001$). Rapid TMS groups (15 and 25 Hz) had significantly lower immobility times than the slow TMS (1 and 5 Hz) ($F = 7.59, P < 0.05$). There was no significant difference between TMS and imipramine groups. The results suggest an advantage for high-frequency stimulation.

Acknowledgments. The studies were supported by grants from the National Health and Medical Research Council, Australian Research Council, Schizophrenia Fellowship of New South Wales, and the Rebecca Cooper Foundation, and donations by two private benefactors. The authors are grateful to Prof. G. Parker for support and D. Hadzi-Pavlovic for statistical advice.

References

George MS, Lisanby SH, Sackheim HA (1999) Transcranial magnetic stimulation: applications in neuropsychiatry. Arch Gen Psychiatry 56:300–311

Loo C, Mitchell P, Sachdev P, et al (1999) Double-blind controlled investigation of transcranial magnetic stimulation for the treatment of resistant major depression. Am J Psychiatry 156:946–948

Loo C, Taylor JL, Gandevia SC, et al (2000) Transcranial magnetic stimulation in controlled studies: are "sham" forms active? Biol Psychiatry 47:325–331

Mechanisms of Inositol Effects on Behavior

HAIM EINAT and ROBERT H. BELMAKER

Summary. Inositol is a second-messenger precursor that can be given orally and enters the brain. Clinical studies find it therapeutic in depression, panic disorder, and obsessive-compulsive disorder. In rat models of depression and anxiety, inositol is active. Activity of inositol in animal models of depression is blocked by ritanserin, suggesting that inositol works distal to a 5-HT-2 receptor.

Keywords. Inositol, Depression, Panic, Serotonin, Obsessive-compulsive disorder

Introduction

Inositol is an polyol that is a precursor in the phosphatidylinositol (PI) cycle, a source of two second messengers: diacylglycerol (DAG) and inositol-1,4,5,-triphosphate (IP_3). Phosphoinositides involvement in signal transduction was demonstrated for a number of neurotransmitter systems including the noradrenergic, serotonergic, dopaminergic, and cholinergic systems. Recently, inositol supplementation was demonstrated to have clinical therapeutic effects in a number of mental disorders including depression, anxiety disorder, obsessive-compulsive disorder, and bulimia but not schizophrenia, Alzheimer's disease, attention-deficit disorder with hyperactivity, and autism (Levine 1997). The studies presented here used behavioral methodology to investigate the range and mechanism of action of inositol in psychiatric disorders.

Studies

Schizophrenia-Related Studies

Possible effects of inositol were evaluated in two models of schizophrenia: amphetamine-induced hyperactivity and apomorphine-induced stereotypy. No effects of inositol were demonstrated in these models (Kofman et al. 1993), and results are consistent with the lack of inositol effect in schizophrenic patients.

Beer Sheva Mental Health Center, Faculty of Health Sciences, Ben Gurion University of the Negev, Beer-Sheva, Israel

Memory-Related Study

Possible effects of chronic oral inositol on memory were evaluated in rhesus monkeys utilizing spatial discrimination tests that emphasis working and reference memory. Results indicate no inositol effects on any of the behavioral parameters tested in this study (Einat et al. 1998a). These results are consistent with the lack of effects of inositol in Alzheimer's patients.

Anxiety-Related Studies

The elevated plus-maze serves to model anxiety-like behavior in rodents. It is frequently used in psychopharmacology and had been validated in numerous studies (for review, see File 1993). Cohen et al. (1997) examined the effects of a variety of acute inositol doses injected peripherally (i.p.) or intracerebroventricular (i.c.v.) and of one dose injected chronically (i.p.) on elevated plus-maze behavior in rats.

Results indicated that a single peripheral injection of inositol had an anxiogenic effect whereas a single i.c.v. injection of 5 mg inositol resulted in reduced anxiety-like behaviors in the elevated plus-maze (we failed to replicate the anxiogenic effect; Einat et al., unpublished observations). Chronic inositol treatment (daily i.p. injections, 1.25 g/kg for 14 days) was demonstrated to reduce anxiety-like behavior, increasing the time spent in the open arms of the maze. The findings regarding the effects of chronic inositol were supported in an elevated plus-maze study of inositol and one of its isomers (*epi*-inositol). Chronic i.p. inositol treatment produced anxiolytic-like effects, as shown by increased time spent and number of entries to the open arms of the maze. Interestingly, *epi*-inositol appeared to be even more potent than *myo*-inositol in that model (Einat et al. 1998b), but we failed to replicate the *epi*-inositol effect (Einat et al., unpublished observations).

In contrast to the previous i.p. findings, oral inositol treatment (5% in food for 2 weeks) did not result in any anxiolytic-like effects in the plus-maze (Kofman et al. 2000). The observation that IP but not oral inositol has anxiolytic-like activity appears unusual because orally administered inositol was reported to increase brain inositol levels and to have behavioral effects in intact rats (Kofman et al. 1998). However, the fact that serotonin specific reuptake inhibitors (SSRIs) are effective in the treatment of patients with anxiety disorders but do not have any anxiolytic effects in normal controls suggested that inositol may be more active in stressed than in unstressed animals. To test this hypothesis, two studies were designed that included (a) an examination of the effects of oral inositol treatment after chronic mild stress and (b) a study of the effects of chronic oral inositol after acute stress (Kofman et al. 2000).

Results indicated that stress had a significant effect on the performance of rats in the elevated plus-maze. The anxiety-like reduction effect of inositol in the plus-maze was a near-significant trend in rats that experienced mild stress (i.p. saline injections) and became significant in rats that experienced acute (exposure to cat) stress (Kofman et al. 2000). These results support to the hypothesis that inositol's anxiolytic-like effect is stronger when the level of anxiety is higher than normal.

Depression-Related Studies

The effects of inositol treatment were tested in two different conditions related to depression-like behavior: reserpine induced hypoactivity in rats, and the Porsolt forced swimming test in two rat strains and in mice.

Reserpine-Induced Hypoactivity

Reserpine-induced hypoactivity is a model for depression, frequently used for purposes of drug screening (Bourin 1990). Our studies indicate that 14 daily inositol injections (1.2 g/kg) were effective in reducing complete immobility time induced by 0.5 or 0.25 mg/kg reserpine. A similar trend was also demonstrated in the 0.25 mg/kg group for increased ambulatory behavior, but it did not reach statistical significance (Einat et al. 1999a).

Forced Swim Test

The forced swim test is one of the leading models of depression (Kirby and Lucki 1997). The effects of inositol in the model were evaluated in Sprague-Dawley rats after subacute (5 g/kg, 2 i.p. injections spaced 24 h apart), chronic (14 daily 1.2 g/kg i.p. injections), and chronic oral (14 days, 10% in food) treatment. All treatment schedules were found to reduce depression-like behaviors (Einat et al. 1999b; Einat et al., in manuscript, a). Chronic i.p. inositol (5 g/kg, 5 daily treatments) was also found to have similar effects in mice (Einat et al., in manuscript, a). Furthermore, chronic inositol (14 daily 1.2 g/kg i.p. injections) was demonstrated to reduce depression-like behaviors in the forced swim test in the Flinders Sensitive Line rats, a genetic animal model for depression (Einat et al., in manuscript, b).

Experiments Targeting Mechanisms of Action

Because standard antidepressant drugs affect monoamine levels, we examined possible changes in brain monoamines after acute and chronic (14 days intraperitoneal [i.p.] or oral) inositol treatment. Dissected portions of the frontal cortex, striatum, hippocampus, and midbrain were homogenized and analyzed with HPLC for levels of norepinephrine, dopamine, dihydroxyphenilalanine, dihydroxyphenylacetic acid, homovanillic acid, serotonin, and 5-hydroxyindolacetic acid. No significant changes in levels of monoamine or their metabolites were detected compared with control animals (Einat et al. 1999b). Unlike most antidepressant drugs that act (at least at the acute level) in the synapse, the action of inositol may be related to postsynaptic activity and therefore may not directly affect neurotransmitter levels.

Because most antidepressants act through either the serotonergic or the noradrenergic systems or both and the PI cycle is involved in neural transduction in both these systems, we used the consistent effects of inositol in the forced swim test in a paradigm of psychopharmacological profiling to examine whether the source of inositol's antidepressant-like activity is related to these systems. Rats pretreated with subacute inositol or placebo were treated with the serotonin metabolism inhibitor DL-*p*-chlorophenylalanine (PCPA) or vehicle in one experiment and with the noradrenergic neurotoxin *N*-(2-chloroethyl)-*N*-ethyl-2 bromobenzylamine (DSP-4) or vehicle in another experiment and then tested in the forced swim test. Results indicate that PCPA but not DSP-4 abolished the antidepressant-like effects of inositol in the model (Einat et al., in manuscript, a). These results suggest that the therapeutic effects of inositol in depression may be related to the serotonergic and not the noradrenergic system.

To further elucidate the interaction of inositol with the serotonergic system, mice were pretreated with subacute inositol or placebo, treated with receptor-specific agonists and antagonists (the 5-HT_{1A} receptor agonist 8-OH-DPAT; the 5-HT_{1A}/5-HT_{1B} beta-adrenergic receptor antagonist pindolol; the 5-HT_{2A}/5-HT_{2C} receptor agonist DOI, and the 5-HT_{2A}/5-HT_{2C} receptor antagonist ritanserin) or vehicle and tested in the forced swim test (5×2 design). No significant effects for any of the specific agonists–antagonist were demonstrated, but a strong trend was visible for the effects of ritanserin to reduce inositol's action. Accordingly, the experiment was repeated with ritanserin alone (Einat et al., in manuscript, a). Results demonstrated that the significant effects of inositol in the test were abolished by ritanserin treatment. It is therefore possible to conclude that the effects of inositol are related to 5-HT_{2A}/5-HT_{2C} receptors.

Discussion

The involvement of inositol in psychiatric disorders is a novel concept that is supported by recent clinical research. Animal studies provide additional evidence that inositol may be an effective agent for the treatment of depression and anxiety, but not schizophrenia or Alzheimer's disease, and indicate that the source of these effects may be related to 5-HT_{2A} or 5-HT_{2C} receptors of the serotonergic system.

References

Bourin M (1990) Is it possible to predict the activity of a new antidepressant in animals with simple psychopharmacological tests? Fundam Clin Pharmacol 4:49–64

Cohen H, Kotler M, Kaplan Z, et al (1997) Inositol has behavioral effects with adaptation after chronic administration. J Neural Transm 104:299–305

Einat H, Levine J, Grauer E, et al (1998a) Effects of inositol treatment on the behavior of rhesus monkeys: preliminary results. Prog Neuro-Psychopahrmacol Biol Psychiatr 22:999–1005

Einat H, Elkabaz-Shwortz Z, Cohen H, et al (1998b) Chronic epi-inositol has an anxiolytic-like effect in the plus-maze model in rats. Int J Neuropsychopharmacol 1:31–34

Einat H, Karbovski H, Korik J, et al (1999a) Inositol reduces depressive-like behaviors in two different animal models of depression. Psychopharmacology 144:158–162

Einat H, Belmaker RH, Kopilov M, et al (1999b) Monoamine levels after acute and chronic myo-inositol treatment. Eur Neuropsychopharmacol 10:27–30

File S (1993) The interplay of learning and anxiety in the elevated plus-maze. Behav Brain Res 58:199–202

Kirby LG, Lucki I (1997) Interaction between the forced swimming test and fluoxetine treatment on extracellular 5-hydroxytryptamine and 5-hydroxyindolacetic acid in the rat. J Pharmacol Exp Ther 282:967–976

Kofman O, Bersudsky Y, Vinnitsky I, et al (1993) The effect of peripheral inositol injection on rat motor activity models of depression. Isr J Med Sci 29:580–586

Kofman O, Agam G, Shapiro J, Spencer A (1998) Chronic dietary inositol enhances locomotor activity and brain inositol levels in rats. Psychopharmacology 139:239–242
Kofman O, Einat H, Cohen H, et al (2000) The anxiolytic effect of chronic inositol depends on the baseline level of anxiey. J Neural Transm 107(2):241–253
Levine J (1997) Controlled trials of inositol in psychiatry. Eur Neuropsychopharmacol 7:147–155

Effects of Antidepressants and Lithium on Intracellular Calcium Signaling

SHIGETO YAMAWAKI[1,2], ARIYUKI KAGAYA[1,2], YASUMASA OKAMOTO[1,2], MINORU TAKEBAYASHI[2], and TOSHINARI SAEKI[2]

Introduction

It is well known that calcium ions (Ca^{2+}) play a crucial role in the growth and maintenance of basic cellular functions in the central nervous system (CNS). Several technical developments have contributed to the measurement of cytosolic Ca^{2+} in living cells. Since the most effective fluorescent dye, fura-2, and its acetoxymethyl ester derivative were developed, many studies have been performed to determine if there is an abnormal function in cytosolic Ca^{2+} concentration in living cells. In the field of biological psychiatry, many researchers have investigated intracellular Ca^{2+} concentration ($[Ca^{2+}]_i$) using human platelets, a model of the neuron. In this chapter, we review recent advances in the investigation of Ca^{2+} in bipolar disorders from both clinical and basic perspectives.

Ca^{2+} Changes in Mood Disorders

In 1989, Dubovsky et al. first reported an enhanced increase in platelet $[Ca^{2+}]_i$ produced by costimulation with thrombin and platelet-activating factor in both bipolar manic and bipolar depressed patients but not in monopolar depressed patients [1]. The authors also found that patients with mood disorders have an increased level of resting $[Ca^{2+}]_i$ in platelets and lymphocytes [2]. Tan et al., in 1990, reported that both the resting $[Ca^{2+}]_i$ and thrombin-induced $[Ca^{2+}]_i$ rise are enhanced in platelets of bipolar manic patients [3]. Kusumi et al. also found that thrombin-stimulated cytosolic Ca^{2+} rise is facilitated in platelets of bipolar depressed patients [4].

From another perspective, serotonin (5-HT)-2A receptor in platelets has been considered a peripheral model for 5-HT-2A receptor in the CNS because of the similarities in the pharmacological properties. We have observed 5-HT-2A receptor function by measuring $[Ca^{2+}]_i$ in platelets of patients with mood disorders, and found that

[1] Core Research for Evolutional Science and Technology (CREST) of Japan Science and Technology (JST), Japan
[2] Department of Psychiatry and Neurosciences, Hiroshima University School of Medicine, Hiroshima, Japan

intracellular Ca^{2+} mobilization in response to 5-HT was significantly greater in platelets of patients with bipolar disorder than in those of healthy subjects [5,6]. Other laboratories have reported similar findings: 5-HT-induced Ca^{2+} mobilization is facilitated in the platelets of patients with bipolar disorder [7,8].

Some other recent studies also showed that basal cytosolic Ca^{2+} or thapsigargin-induced Ca^{2+} release to cytosol is greater in lymphocytes of bipolar disorder patients [9,10]. Furthermore, intracellular phosphatidylinositol turnover appears to be facilitated in platelets of bipolar disorder patients [11], which is consistent with hyperactivity of cytosolic Ca^{2+} movement in bipolar disorder, as already described. Taken together, these studies strongly suggest that cytosolic Ca^{2+} function is enhanced in patients with bipolar disorder.

Antiepileptic Drugs and Ca^{2+} Channel Antagonists for Bipolar Disorder

In recent decades, there has been increasing recognition that antiepileptic drugs, for instance, carbamazepine and valproate, are effective alone or in combination with lithium in patients with bipolar illness, especially acute mania [12]. Lamotrigine is a new antiepileptic agent that is approved for treatment of partial complex seizure. A series of clinical studies for bipolar illness suggests that lamotrigine may have a therapeutic efficiency in bipolar patients, including rapid cycling and mixed states. Calabrese and coworkers have reported that lamotrigine was examined in 75 bipolar disorder patients, and they suggest that it has moderate to marked efficacy in 68% of depressed patients and in more than 80% of manic patients with bipolar illness [13].

Lamotrigine, which is a clinically useful antiepileptic drug with a property of sodium channel blockade, also inhibits the voltage-operated Ca^{2+} channel (VOCC) [14]. The Ca^{2+} channel blocking action of lamotrigine may contribute to its effectiveness in treating bipolar patients. In fact, several reports suggest the effectiveness of other VOCC blockers for the treatment of patients with mood disorders. Several recent studies also suggest that verapamil is as effective as lithium or other treatment in dozens of manic patients [15–17]. Nimodipine, another Ca^{2+} antagonist, also appears to be effective for treating patients with bipolar disorder [12]. These investigations suggest that the regulation of cytosolic Ca^{2+} has an important role in bipolar disorder treatment.

Basic Statement About Cytosolic Ca^{2+}

Cytosolic Ca^{2+} increases via three major routes—VOCC, agonist-operated Ca^{2+} channel (AOCC), and inositol-1,4,5-tris phosphate (IP3) receptor. VOCCs are divided into four major types, T (transient), L (long-lasting), N (neuronal), and P (on Purkinje cells). The N and P types are mainly distributed to presynaptic nerve endings in the CNS whereas T and L types exist in peripheral tissues as well as in the CNS. AOCCs include NMDA receptor, 5-HT-3 receptor, and nicotinic acetylcholine receptor. The IP3 receptor is stimulated by IP3, which is produced by an activation of Gq/11-coupled receptors, for example, 5-HT-2A receptor, thrombin receptor, α_1-adrenergic receptor, muscarinic acetylcholine receptor, and endothelin receptor. Thus, the modulation of these molecules would change cytosolic Ca^{2+} distribution.

Increased cytosolic Ca^{2+} influences many of the molecular and cellular functions. Cytosolic Ca^{2+} activates and modulates several enzymes, for example, protein kinase C, calmodulin-dependent protein kinases, proteinases such as calpain, and neuronal nitric oxide synthase. It also regulates transmitter release from nerve terminals, growth and differentiation of neuronal cells, and neuronal cell death.

Effect of Antidepressants on Ca^{2+}

Not a few studies have indicated that mood disorders show dysfunction of intracellular Ca^{2+} mechanisms. Therefore, it is important to investigate the effect of mood stabilizers on the intracellular Ca^{2+} signaling system. We have investigated the effect of drugs for mood disorders on intracellular Ca^{2+} movement using the fura-2 method in primary cultured rat neuronal cells, adult rat hippocampal slices, and rat glioma-derived C6 cells. We found that imipramine, at 10–200 μM, acutely reduced depolarization-induced Ca^{2+} increase in primary cultured neuronal cells [18]. Similar inhibitory effect was observed by imipramine, desipramine, and mianserin on acetylcholine-evoked Ca^{2+} increase. NMDA-stimulated Ca^{2+} influx in primary cultured neuronal cells was also attenuated by an acute application with imipramine. A recent study by our laboratory indicated that γ-aminobutyric acid (GABA) produced a transient increase in $[Ca^{2+}]_i$ through the pathway including VOCC [19], and the GABA-induced Ca^{2+} entry was also inhibited by imipramine. This antidepressant also inhibited spontaneous oscillations in these cultured cells.

Effect of Mood Stabilizers and Ca^{2+} Channel Blockers on Ca^{2+}

Questions arise as to why and how Ca^{2+} channel blockers are useful for treatment of mood disorders. Several important studies have shown the effect of verapamil on the CNS or intracellular signaling systems such as neurotransmitter release and Na^+–Ca^{2+} exchanger [20]. To determine the common effect of verapamil and other mood stabilizers, we observed the effect of verapamil, carbamazepine, and valproate in C6 rat glioma cells, which possess a 5-HT-2A receptor, and their intracellular signaling systems. Verapamil (100 nM) attenuated the plateau phase after stimulation with 5-HT as well as the peak amplitude, and a similar inhibitory effect was observed when the cells were acutely exposed to carbamazepine or valproate. However, with carbamazepine and valproate, investigations have been focused on other messengers such as adenylyl cyclase and protein kinase C [21].

Effect of Lithium of Ca^{2+} and Ca^{2+}-Related Cellular Function

Our recent study indicates that lithium has an effect on Ca^{2+} signaling in rat hippocampus slices. Acute treatment with lithium attenuated the plateau phase after norepinephrine-induced $[Ca^{2+}]_i$ rise without an inhibition of the spike amplitude. This effect of lithium on the plateau phase may be at least partly mediated by the Na^+–Ca^{2+} exchanger [22]. This result suggests that lithium also may stabilize intracellular Ca^{2+} signaling systems.

In another recent investigation by our laboratory, we observed that long-term pretreatment with lithium attenuated thrombin-stimulated intracellular Ca^{2+} mobilization in C6 glioma cells [23]. Lithium does not appear to act as a direct antagonist for thrombin receptor-mediated Ca^{2+} response because lithium did not change the response to thrombin by short-time pretreatment or by acute application. It should be noted that lithium blunted the thrombin-evoked response that is often reported to be facilitated in bipolar disorder. Thrombin receptor is activated following proteolytic cleavage of a certain peptide bond of the receptor by the serine proteinase activity of thrombin. Lithium may cleave the same site more slowly to internalize a part of the thrombin receptors, attenuating the subsequent thrombin-evoked Ca^{2+} mobilization. There is a report suggesting that lithium has the activity of enhancement of calpain [24], another type of proteinase that is regulated by Ca^{2+}.

Thus, drugs for mood disorders can act directly on intracellular components. Several mechanisms for action sites of the drugs can be suggested, for example, VOCCs, AOCCs, Na^+–Ca^{2+} exchanger, Gq/11-coupled 7-transmembrane receptors, and phospholipase C, which regulates most of the intracellular signaling components including Ca^{2+}. Furthermore, lithium and other mood stabilizers also change some cellular functions such as protein kinase C activity, transcription factors, gene expression, cell growth, or neuroprotection [21,25], whose functions are regulated by cytosolic Ca^{2+}. For example, Chuang and coworkers have shown that long-term treatment with lithium inhibits NMDA-induced Ca^{2+} influx and attenuates NMDA receptor-mediated apoptosis in cultured cerebellar granule cells [26–28].

Conclusions

In this chapter, we reviewed the nature of cytosolic Ca^{2+} to clarify the mechanism involved in changing the functions of this signaling system in bipolar disorder. Patients with mood disorders have an enhanced intracellular Ca^{2+} response. Further characterization of mood-stabilizing agents that affect cytosolic Ca^{2+} in cultured rat neuronal cells and glioma cells was discussed. Certain kinds of antidepressant drugs inhibit intracellular Ca^{2+} signaling. Lithium and other mood stabilizers change cytosolic Ca^{2+} function and Ca^{2+}-regulated cellular events. These results suggest that intracellular Ca^{2+} signaling is important in the pathophysiology of bipolar disorder and in treatment of the illness.

References

1. Dubovsky SL, Christiano J, Daniel LC, et al (1989) Increased platelet intracellular calcium concentration in patients with bipolar affective disorders. Arch Gen Psychiatry 46:632–638
2. Dubovsky SL, Murphy J, Thomas M, Rademacher J (1992) Abnormal intracellular calcium ion concentration in platelets and lymphocytes of bipolar patients. Am J Psychiatry 149:118–120

3. Tan CH, Javors MA, Seleshi E, et al (1990) Effects of lithium on platelet ionic intracellular calcium concentration in patients with bipolar (manic-depressive) disorder and healthy controls. Life Sci 46:1175–1180
4. Kusumi I, Koyama T, Yamashita I (1992) Thrombin-induced platelet calcium mobilization is enhanced in bipolar disorders. Biol Psychiatry 32:731–734
5. Okamoto Y, Kagaya A, Shinno H, et al (1995) Serotonin-induced platelet calcium mobilization is enhanced in mania. Life Sci 56:R2
6. Yamawaki S, Kagaya A, Okamoto Y, et al (1996) Enhanced calcium response to serotonin in platelets from patients with affective disorders. J Psychiatry Neurosci 21:321–324
7. Kusumi I, Koyama T, Yamashita I (1994) Serotonin-induced platelet intracellular calcium mobilization in depressed patients. Psychopharmacology 113:322–327
8. Berk M, Bodemer W, van Oudenhove T, Butkow N (1995) The platelet intracellular calcium response to serotonin is augmented in bipolar manic and depressed patients. Hum Psychopharmacol 10:189–193
9. Emamghoreishi M, Schlichter L, Li PP, et al (1997) High intracellular calcium concentrations in transformed lymphoblasts from subjects with bipolar I disorder. Am J Psychiatry 154:976–982
10. Hough C, Lu S-J, Davis C, et al (1999) Elevated basal and thapsigargin-stimulated intracellular calcium of platelets and lymphocytes from bipolar affective disorder patients measured by a fluorometric microassay. Biol Psychiatry 46:247–255
11. Soares JC, Mallinger AG (1997) Intracellular phosphatidylinositol pathway abnormalities in bipolar disorder patients. Psychopharmacol Bull 33:685–691
12. Post RM, Frye MA, Denicoff KD, et al (1998) Beyond lithium in the treatment of bipolar illness. Neuropsychopharmacology 19:206–219
13. Calabrese JR, Rapport DJ, Shelton MD, Kimmel SE (1998) Clinical studies on the use of lamotrigine in bipolar disorder. Neuropsychobiology 38:185–191
14. Grunze H, von Wegener J, Greene RW, Walden J (1998) Modulation of calcium and potassium currents by lamotrigine. Neuropsychobiology 38:131–138
15. Dubovsky SL, Franks RD, Lifschitz ML, Cohen P (1982) Effectiveness of verapamil in the treatment of a manic patient. Am J Psychiatry 139:502–504
16. Giannini AJ, Houser WL, Loiselle RH, et al (1984) Antimanic effects of verapamil. Am J Psychiatry 141:1602–1603
17. Hoschl C, Kozeny J (1989) Verapamil in affective disorders: a double-blind, controlled study. Biol Psychiatry 25:128–140
18. Yamawaki S, Kagaya A, Tawara Y, Inagaki M (1998) Intracellular calcium signaling systems in the pathophysiology of affective disorders. Life Sci 62:1665–1670
19. Takebayashi M, Kagaya A, Hayashi T, et al (1996) Gamma-aminobutylic acid increases intracellular Ca^{2+} concentration in cultured cortical neurons: role of Cl^- transport. Eur J Pharmacol 297:137–143
20. Snyder SH, Reynolds IJ (1985) Calcium-antagonist drugs. Receptor interactions that clarify therapeutic effects. N Engl J Med 313:995–1002
21. Manji HK, Bebchuk JM, Moore GJ, et al (1999) Modulation of CNS signal transduction pathways and gene expression by mood-stabilizing agents: therapeutic implications. J Clin Psychiatry 60(suppl 2):27–39
22. Okamoto Y, Kagaya A, Motohashi N, Yamawaki S (1995) Inhibitory effects of lithium on intracellular Ca^{2+} mobilization in the rat hippocampal slices. Neurochem Int 26:233–238
23. Kagaya A, Okada A, Tawara Y, et al (1999) Lithium chloride inhibits thrombin-induced intracellular calcium mobilization in C6 glioma cells. Prog Neuro-Psychopharmacol Biol Psychiatry 24:85–95
24. Greenwood AF, Jope RS (1994) Brain G-protein proteolysis by calpain: enhancement by lithium. Brain Res 636:320–326
25. Jope RS (1999) Anti-bipolar therapy: mechanism of action of lithium. Mol Psychiatry 4:117–128

26. Nonaka S, Hough CJ, Chuang D-M (1998) Chronic lithium treatment robustly protects neurons in the central nervous system against excitotoxicity by inhibiting *N*-methyl-D-aspartate receptor-mediated calcium influx. Proc Natl Acad Sci USA 95:2642–2647
27. Chalecka-Franaszek E, Chuang D-M (1999) Lithium activates the serine/threonine kinase Akt-1 and suppresses glutamate-induced inhibition of Akt-1 activity in neurons. Proc Natl Acad Sci USA 96:8745–8750
28. Chen RW, Chuang D-M (1999) Long term lithium treatment suppresses p53 and Bax expression but increases Bcl-2 expression. A prominent role in neuroprotection against excitotoxicity. J Biol Chem 274:6039–6042

The Neuropsychiatry of Schizophrenia and Related Conditions

Neuroimaging and Neurobiology of Schizophrenia

Nancy C. Andreasen

Summary. Identifying the neural substrates of the symptoms of schizophrenia has been substantially facilitated through the use of in vivo neuroimaging techniques. Magnetic resonance (MR) and positron emission tomography (PET) studies have permitted us to identify distributed nodes on neural networks that implicate an abnormality in neural circuitry in schizophrenia. Evidence is converging to suggest that this neural circuitry may consist of distributed cortical regions that may be functionally abnormal in a task-specific way, with more consistent and persistent abnormalities in the thalamus and cerebellum. We have proposed that abnormalities in this circuit lead to a "cognitive dysmetria," or poor coordination of mental activity, that arises from a dysfunctional cortical-cerebellar-thalamic-cortical-circuit (CCTCC) and is expressed symptomatically in the diverse clinical presentation of schizophrenia.

Keywords. Schizophrenia, Cognition, Neural circuits, Thalamus, Cerebellum

Introduction

Despite nearly a century of research, the relationship between the clinical presentation of schizophrenia and its underlying neural mechanisms remains a riddle. The phenomenology of schizophrenia involves a potpourri of cognitive and emotional symptoms. These symptoms include almost every domain of human experience: perception, thinking, language, motor behavior, volition, emotional expression, and hedonic capacity. No single domain or no single symptom can be used to define the disorder.

Two major European thinkers, Eugen Bleuler and Kurt Schneider, have attempted to identify a phenomenological core. Bleuler emphasized thought disorder and cognition. In accordance with the associated psychology that prevailed at the time, he argued that the fundamental abnormality might involve a loosening of the associative threads that form the fabric of thought (Bleuler 1911). Approaching schizophrenia from another perspective, Kurt Schneider identified the core experience of schizophrenia as a loss of personal autonomy and control over thoughts and emo-

The University of Iowa Hospitals and Clinics, MHCRC, Room 2911, JPP, 200 Hawkins Drive, Iowa City, IA 52242, USA

tions. Schneider's "first rank symptoms" typically involve a blurring of the boundaries between "self" and "not-self," such as "made thoughts," "made volition," or voices commenting on the person's behavior (Mellor 1970). In seeking a core or pathognomic symptom or group of symptoms that could be used to define schizophrenia, Bleuler and Schneider were attempting to identify a unifying theme within the midst of this disorder's symptomatic diversity.

The advent of modern neuroimaging techniques provides investigators with an opportunity to visualize directly the anatomical and physiological substrates of the signs and symptoms of schizophrenia. To date, most investigators have pursued clinical/neuropathological correlates in a piecemeal fashion. That is, most investigators have attempted to link a single symptom (e.g., auditory hallucinations) to a single brain region (e.g., superior temporal gyrus) (Barta et al. 1990). Similar relationships have been sought between negative symptoms and prefrontal regions or "thought disorder" and language regions (Andreasen and Grove 1986; Andreasen et al. 1990a; Shenton et al. 1992). Although our group has been one of the original proponents of this type of piecemeal strategy (Andreasen et al. 1986), we are also currently exploring an alternate approach that attempts to explain diversity of symptoms of schizophrenia based on a single primary brain abnormality and a single core phenomenological deficit (Andreasen et al. 1994a). The primary brain abnormality involves midline reticular/thalamic/cingulate/cortical circuitry whereas the primary clinical or cognitive abnormality involves a defect in filtering or processing information. An ability to filter, to process, and to focus attention could explain the full range of symptoms that characterize schizophrenia. An individual who cannot prioritize information and exclude the relevant from the irrelevant will experience a Schneiderian loss of autonomy or "ego boundaries," as well as a Bleulerian loosening of associations. A defect in information processing could lead to the experience of hallucinations in multiple modalities as well as delusions, disorganized speech, disorganized behavior, and the full range of negative symptoms.

MR Studies

We have now completed four MR studies of schizophrenia, all of which provide some support for an abnormality in midline circuitry, probably caused by a neurodevelopmental abnormality. Our work with MR must be evaluated within the overall context of the enormous body of structural imaging studies that have been completed in patients suffering from schizophrenia. The majority of these studies demonstrated enlargement of the ventricular system (Pearlson and Marsh 1993; Gur and Pearlson 1993). It has not been clear whether ventricle enlargement represents a more regional tissue loss in structures surrounding ventricles (or possibly both). As the ventricular system is itself a midline structure, the consistent findings of ventricular enlargement at least raise the possibility that there may be selective tissue loss in structures surrounding the ventricles. These structures include the reticulo-thalamic-cingulate-cortical circuitry, as well as other subcortical structures such as the basal ganglia.

Our first MR study (MR1), published in 1986, was the first large, controlled study to be conducted (Andreasen et al. 1986). Thirty-eight schizophrenic patients and 49 normal controls were included in this circuitry disruption; different types of symptoms would be more prominent, but a thalamic defect could explain the co-occurrence of all types of schizophrenic symptoms.

PET Studies

The strongest support for abnormalities in the full cortical-cerebellar-thalamic-cortical-circuit (CCTCC) arises from our recent PET studies. The initial clues concerning the importance of this circuit occurred in our studies of normal cognition, including a variety of memory tasks (Andreasen et al. 1995a, b, c) involving both words and faces. Subsequently, as we began to apply these tasks to study patients, it became evident that components of the circuit were frequently disrupted, finally leading to the formation of a hypothesis that cognitive dysmetria could be fundamental to schizophrenia (Andreasen et al. 1996a). We have now observed a pattern of abnormalities in components of the CCTCC in multiple studies involving a variety of cognitive tasks.

Our earliest report of PET data supporting the concept of cognitive dysmetria was derived from our studies of recall memory for complex narrative material (Andreasen et al. 1995a). When we studied patients with this memory task, we equalized task performance in patients and controls by providing the patients with multiple practice sessions before the PET study, thereby permitting them to achieve near-perfect recall (Andreasen et al. 1996b). In this way, we could be sure that any observed abnormalities were caused by primary abnormalities in circuitry, rather than the secondary effects of poor task performance. The regions used by the normal controls during recall included prefrontal, thalamic, and cerebellar areas. On the other hand, the patients showed minimal or no activation in these key nodes of the CCTCC. Although the design (involving perfect performance by the patients) ensures that the failure to activate the CCTCC is not caused by poor task performance, the possibility remained that the difference could be the result of greater variance in the patients. Therefore, we conducted a newly and locally developed statistical test to compare the two groups, a nonparametric randomization analysis (Arndt et al. 1996) that is not affected by between-group differences in variance. The same regions (i.e., frontal, thalamic, and cerebellar) were found to be different between patients and controls.

Subsequently, we have extended this functional imaging work by comparing patients and controls using a variety of different tasks. Initially, we explored other aspects of memory. We examined both practiced and novel recall of word lists (Crespo-Facorro et al. 1999), and we again observed that patients had decreased flow in frontal, cerebellar, and thalamic regions. Because both these studies examined recall, an effortful and demanding form of memory, we then studied recognition memory for a word list as an additional comparison. Again, using randomization analysis to compare patients and controls with a well-practiced and equal performance on the memory task, we observed decreased flow in the patients in frontal and cerebellar regions (Wiser et al. 1998), although thalamic flow was not decreased in this particular study (perhaps reflecting lower attentional demands). We then shifted our memory studies to another input modality to explore whether the abnormalities were specific to verbal material. In this study, we have examined recognition memory for faces (Paulsen et al., in manuscript). Again, decreased flow was observed in frontal and cerebellar regions, as well as regions that are more specific for visual material and specifically for faces (e.g., precuneus, fusiform gyrus, and hippocampus). Finally, we turned to a completely different type of mental system, the subjective experience and attribution of pleasant and unpleasant visual stimuli, because hedonic capacity is also disturbed in schizophrenia; in a study that is as yet unpublished, we compared patients and controls while they observed a series of pleasant, neutral, and unpleasant pictures that were presented on a video monitor. Again, we noted decreased flow in the patients in the cerebellum and thalamus, as well as specific cortical and subcortical regions that were appropriate to this particular task (amygdala, fusiform gyrus, straight gyrus). We have also examined directed visual attention and found evidence for CCTCC abnormalities as well (O'Leary et al., submitted).

Although additional work is needed to continue to dissect the abnormalities in functional circuitry that characterize schizophrenia, the results of this series of PET studies strongly suggest that patients with schizophrenia have abnormalities in neural connectivity and that this appears to affect the circuitry that is used to integrate information from cortical and subcortical regions. The cerebellum has been abnormal in all these studies and the thalamus has been abnormal in the majority. The cortical regions vary depending on the task. In future work, we plan to expand the range of tasks to further define regional specificity, to focus in particular on the tasks that challenge the cerebellum, and to use techniques such as diffusion imaging to measure connectivity.

The Concept of Cognitive Dysmetria

We have developed a model that proposed cognitive dysmetria to be the fundamental deficit in schizophrenia (Andreasen et al. 1996a, b, 1998). Dysmetria is defined in neurology as a disruption in the fluid coordination of motor activity leading to observed abnormalities such as dysdiadokokinesia or inability to perform tandem gait. Cognitive dysmetria is the cognitive or mental equivalent of motor dysmetria: a disruption in the fluid coordination of mental activity that is the hallmark of normal cognition (Schmahmann 1991). The basis of the "poor coordination" may be a defect in timing or sequencing the flow of information as required during normal "thought" and speech. Most previous work studying cognition in schizophrenia has examined the various traditionally defined cognitive systems (e.g., memory, attention) or subsystem (e.g., working memory, encoding, facilitation/inhibition). The concept of dysmetria refers to a more basic process that is behind these systems and subsystems and should therefore be considered a metaprocess. We have chosen to use the term synchrony to refer to the normal process and dysmetria to refer to its disturbance.

Although schizophrenia is not usually considered to be a "motor disease," many indicators of motor dysfunction are present, suggesting that the basic abnormality in the disorder could be a brain system that mediates both motor and cognitive functions. Kraepelin described a variety of motor abnormalities in his classic textbook (Kraepelin et al. 1919). Slowed reaction time is one of the oldest and most robust tests showing differences between schizophrenic patients and normal controls (Shakow and Huston 1936). More recent studies of premorbid indicators and neurological soft signs also implicate the motor system, broadly defined (Flashman et al. 1996; Gupta et al. 1995; Walker and Green 1982). These mild indicators of poor coordination provide a clue that the underlying mechanisms may reflect an abnormality in a basic process that regulates the synchrony of both thought and action. If the synchrony is "off," much like sending signals at the incorrect baud rate between two nodes in a computer network, the signals become garbled. As a consequence, the individual with mistimed information transfer may incorrectly connect perceptions and associations and misinterpret both external and internal processes, leading in turn to delusions or hallucinations. (For example, a neutral perception will be associated with a frightening affective association, internal thoughts, or vocalizations that may be attributed to others.) Defects in coordinating language production will lead to "thought disorder." In addition, the flow of information through the system may become paralyzed, leading to "negative symptoms" such as alogia or affective blunting.

Schizophrenia may be conceptualized as a disease that is characterized by poor coordination, or dysmetria, in all domains of functioning, including both motor and cognitive. The role of the CCTCC is to facilitate the smooth planning and execution of both motor and cognitive activities. When these activities become dysmetric, the vast range of symptoms that characterize schizophrenia may occur.

References

Andreasen NC (1988) Brain imaging: Applications in psychiatry. Science 239:1381–1388

Andreasen NC (1994) The mechanisms of schizophrenia. Curr Opin Neurobiol 4:245–251

Andreasen NC, Grove WM (1986) Thought, language, and communication in schizophrenia: Diagnostic and prognostic significance. Schizophr Bull 12:348–359

Andreasen NC, Nasrallah HA, et al (1986) Structural abnormalities in the frontal system in schizophrenia: a magnetic resonance imaging study. Arch Gen Psychiatry 43:136–144

Andreasen NC, Flaum M, et al (1990a) Positive and negative symptoms in schizophrenia: a critical reappraisal. Arch Gen Psychiatry 47:615–621

Andreasen NC, Ehrhardt JC, et al (1990b) Magnetic resonance imaging of the brain in schizophrenia: the pathophysiological significance of structural abnormalities. Arch Gen Psychiatry 47:35–44

Andreasen N, Flaum M, et al (1993a) Intelligence and brain structure in normal individuals. Am J Psychiatry 150(1):130–134

Andreasen NC, Cizadlo T, et al (1993b) Voxel processing techniques for the antemortem study of neuroanatomy and neuropathology using magnetic resonance imaging. J Neuropsychiatry Clin Neurosci 5:121–130

Andreasen NC, Arndt S, et al (1994a) Thalamic abnormalities in schizophrenia visualized through magnetic resonance image averaging. Science 266:294–298

Andreasen NC, Harris G, et al (1994b) Techniques for measuring sulcal/gyral patterns in the brain as visualized through MR scanning: BRAINPLOT AND BRAINMAP. Proc Natl Acad Sci USA 90(1):93–97

Andreasen NC, Flashman L, et al (1994c) Regional brain abnormalities in schizophrenia measured with magnetic resonance imaging. JAMA 272:1763–1769

Andreasen NC, O'Leary D, et al (1995a) I. PET studies of memory: novel and practiced free recall of complex narratives. NeuroImage 2(4):284–295

Andreasen NC, O'Leary D, et al (1995b) II. PET studies of memory: novel versus practiced free recall of word lists. NeuroImage 2(4):296–305

Andreasen NC, O'Leary DS, et al (1995c) Short-term and long-term verbal memory: a positron emission tomography study. Proc Natl Acad Sci USA 92(11):5111–5115
Andreasen NC, O'Leary DS, et al (1996a) Schizophrenia and cognitive dysmetria: a positron-emission tomography study of dysfunctional prefrontal-thalamic-cerebellar circuitry. Proc Natl Acad Sci USA 93:9985–9990
Andreasen NC, O'Leary DS, et al (1996b) Neural substrates of facial recognition. J Neuropsychiatry Clin Neurosci 8:139–146
Andreasen NC, Paradiso S, et al (1998) Cognitive dysmetria as an integrative theory of schizophrenia: a dysfunction in cortical-cerebellar circuitry? Schizophr Bull 24(2):203–218
Arndt S, Swayze V, et al (1994) Evaluating and validating two methods for estimating brain structure volumes: tessellation and simple pixel counting. NeuroImage 1:191–198
Arndt S, Cizadlo T, et al (1996) Tests for comparing images based on randomization and permutation methods. J Cereb Blood Flow Metab 16:1271–1279
Barta PE, Pearlson GD, et al (1990) Superior temporal gyrus volume in schizophrenia. Schizophr Res 3:22
Bleuler E (1911) Dementia praecox or the group of schizophrenias. (transl. Zin kin, 1950). International Universities Press, New York
Cizadlo T, Andreasen NC, et al (1994) Image registration issues in the analysis of multiple-injection $^{15}OH_2O$ PET studies: BRAINFIT. Proc SPIE Int Soc Opt Eng 2168:423–430
Cohen G, Andreasen NC, et al (1992) Segmentation techniques for the classification of brain tissue using magnetic resonance imaging. Psychiatry Res Neuroimaging 45:33–51
Crespo-Facorro B, Paradiso S, et al (1999) Recalling word lists reveals "cognitive dysmetria" in schizophrenia: a positron emission tomography study. Am J Psychiatry 156(3):386–392
Feinberg I (1982) Schizophrenia: caused by a fault in programmed synaptic elimination during adolescence? J Psychiatric Res 17:319–334
Fish FJ (1962) Schizophrenia. Wright, Bristol
Flashman LA, Flaum M, et al (1996) Soft signs and neuropsychological performance in schizophrenia. Am J Psychiatry 153(4):526–532
Flaum M, Nopoulos P, Cizadlo T, et al (1997) A large MRI follow-up study of ventricular volume in recent onset psychosis. 36th Annual American College of Neuropsychopharmacology
Gupta S, Rajaprabhakaran R, et al (1995) Premorbid adjustment as a predictor of phenomenological and neurobiological indices in schizophrenia. Schizophr Res 16(3):189–197
Gur RE, Pearlson GD (1993) Neuroimaging in schizophrenia research. Schizophr Bull 19:337–353
Kraepelin E, Barclay RM, et al (1919) Dementia praecox and paraphrenia. Livingstone, Edinburgh
Mellor CS (1970) First-rank symptoms of schizophrenia. Br J Psychiatry 117:15–23
Nopoulos PC, Flaum M, et al (1995) Gray matter heterotopias in schizophrenia. Psychiatry Res Neuroimaging 61(1):11–14
Nopoulos P, Swayze V, et al (1997) Cavum septi pellucidi in normals and patients with schizophrenia as detected by MRI. Biol Psychiatry 41:1002–1008
Pearlson GD, Marsh L (eds) (1993) Magnetic resonance imaging in psychiatry. American Psychiatric Association Annual Review of Psychiatry. American Psychiatric Press, Washington, DC
Schmahmann JD (1991) An emerging concept: the cerebellar contribution to higher function. Arch Neurol 48:1178–1187
Shakow D, Huston PE (1936) Studies of motor function in schizophrenia: I. Speed of tapping. J Gen Psychol 15:63–108

Shenton M, Kikinis R, et al (1992) Abnormalities of the left temporal lobe and thought disorder in schizophrenia: a quantitative magnetic resonance imaging study. N Engl J Med 327(9):604–612

Swayze V II, Andreasen N, et al (1990) Developmental abnormalities of the corpus callosum in schizophrenia. Arch Neurol 47:805–808

Walker E, Green M (1982) Soft signs of neurological dysfunction in schizophrenia: an investigation of lateral performance. Biol Psychiatry 17(3):381–386

Willerman L, Schultz R, et al (1991) In vivo brain size and intelligence. Intelligence 15:223–228

Wiser A, Andreasen NC, O'Leary DS, et al (1998) Distributed dysfunction in cortico-cerebellar circuits cause "cognitive dysmetria" in schizophrenia. Neuro Report 9:1895–1899

Positron Emission Tomography in Schizophrenia

JUAN J. LÓPEZ-IBOR JR[1], MARÍA I. LÓPEZ-IBOR[1], and RICARDO MONTZ[2]

Summary. Neuroimaging techniques provide an insight into the workings of the intact living human brain. These techniques have been increasingly used in psychiatric research, especially in the study of neuronal mechanisms involved in the pathophysiology of schizophrenic illness. The application of functional brain imaging methods to the study of schizophrenia has provided an opportunity to establish links between the clinical features and brain function of this illness. It has been possible to find relationships among different behavioral symptoms in schizophrenic illness and the activity in some brain systems. Research in this field has been focused on the study of patterns of brain activity both in a resting condition and during cognitive task performance, and on investigations of neurochemical characteristics (neurotransmitters and neuroreceptors) of schizophrenic patients. Research has also tried to establish correlations between psychopathological aspects of this illness and brain activity measured with neuroimaging techniques. The integration of neuroimaging techniques with other disciplines such as genetics, neuroendocrinology, and psychology will allow a greater understanding of the etiology of schizophrenia and other mental illness.

Keywords. Schizophrenia, Functional neuroimaging, PET, Pathophysiology, Regional cerebral blood flow (rCBF)

Functional Neuroimaging

The use of neuroimaging in psychiatry research has exploded during the past 20 years, and many of the findings have distinct implications for both the etiological basis and the treatment of psychiatric illness.

Neuroimaging involves the collection of data related to the central nervous system and the display of this information in a form that has a direct relationship to the structure and function of the CNS. Although the images and functions are similar, positron

[1] Department of Psychiatry, San Carlos University Hospital, Complutense University, Nueva Zelanda 44, 28035 Madrid, Spain
[2] Instituto PET Dr. Carreras, Clínica López Ibor, Madrid, Spain

emission tomography (PET) differs from single photon emission tomography (SPECT) in several important ways. More labeled tracers are used in PET, but the isotopes (most commonly fluorine-18, carbon-11, nitrogen-13, and oxygen-15) have such short half-lives that they must be synthesized in a cyclotron. The isotopes emit positrons that collide with electrons and thereby produce a pair of gamma photons traveling at 180° to one another. The photons are detected by a ring of detection crystals around the patient's head, which are designed to detect the simultaneous arrival of the two particles. Two particles are emitted at precise angles to one another to allow the computer to provide images with almost twice the resolution of SPECT. The enhanced spatial resolution means that PET can be more easily applied to investigate a suspected functional deficit in a specific area. PET is the research technique of choice for blood flow activation and localization studies.

Neuroimaging Studies in Schizophrenia

When Kraepelin (1919) first described "dementia praecox," he believed that it has an organic basis. Unfortunately, at the beginning of the twentieth century the available measuring tools did not allow pointing out any distinct brain pathology associated with schizophrenia. In pneumoencephalographic investigations in the 1930s and 1950s, it was first noted that in schizophrenic patients there is a lateral ventricular enlargement. Since then, the field of neuroimaging has contributed greatly to the understanding of schizophrenia and has led to a number of neuropathological hypotheses.

The most consistent finding in structural imaging studies in schizophrenia is that of lateral ventricle enlargement. Increased third and fourth ventricle size has also been demonstrated in schizophrenia. Generally, ventricular enlargement is more pronounced in schizophrenic men than in schizophrenic women (Bertollo et al. 1996). Men tend to have larger lateral ventricles than women in both patient and control groups, thus confirming the sexually dimorphic characteristics of this area. The atrophy of the brain tissue is accompanied by a reduction of the bone surrounding it (Messimy et al. 1984). This finding means that what happened to the brain took place early in development, before the final ossification of tha bones of the head.

Reduced volume and loss of asymmetry of the structures surrounding the ventricles have also been demonstrated. These structures include the amygdala, hippocampus, and parahippocampus gyrus. The loss of asymmetry is most marked in the planum temporale, an area that includes the auditory association cortex (Wernicke's area) (Crow 1990). These areas together are concerned with selection, association, and integration of sensory information, memory, and the control of basic drives and emotions, all of which may be disrupted in schizophrenia.

Up to now, no relationships between the duration of illness and structural brain abnormalities have been demonstrated. This lack has led to the hypothesis that brain abnormalities are not degenerative but of long standing and may represent an incomplete brain maturation or dystrophy of surrounding regions. In studies of dyscordant monozygotic twins, the cotwin unaffected by schizophrenia had smaller ventricles than the affected twin but larger ventricles than those of twins from unaffected parents. This finding would tend to suggest that the increase in ventricular size may be secondary to an acquired environmental factor.

Many studies have investigated regional cerebral blood flow (rCBF) and metabolism in schizophrenic patients. Previously, a decrease in frontal blood flow and metabolism (hypofrontality) was believed to indicate schizophrenia; however, only some of the studies have found hypofrontality in all schizophrenic patients, and a variety of other regional abnormalities have been noted. These changes include increased rCBF in the left hemisphere and a similar finding in the globus pallidus. Some studies indicated that the differences in frontal blood flow between patients and controls individuals occur after treatment, and others showed that the changes were persistent.

The application of functional brain imaging methods to the study of schizophrenia has provided an opportunity to establish links between clinical features and brain function of this illness. It has been possible to find relationships among different behavioral symptoms in schizophrenic illness and the activity in some brain systems. These links are based on preclinical research and the observation that there are some symptoms commonly seen in schizophrenia that also occur following brain lesions.

Persistent negative symptoms were initially related to frontal lobe dysfunction, because similar behaviors are evident as sequelae of frontal lobe damage (secondary to brain trauma, cancer, and vascular and other processes). These sequelae include impairment in abstraction, verbal fluency, mental flexibility, and concept formation. Positive, productive symptoms of hallucinations and delusions have been related to the temporolimbic system because this behavior has also been noticed in patients with temporal lobe epilepsy or in persons with evidence of impaired learning and memory. Subcortical regions, with special emphasis on the basal ganglia, have been examined initially in the context of the dopamine hypothesis and other neurotransmitters, and more recent studies have implicated the subcortical nuclei in generation of auditory hallucinations.

Liddle et al. (1992) defined three symptom clusters: psychomotor poverty, disorganization (inappropriate affect, speech content abnormalities), and reality distortion (delusions and hallucinations). They found that reduced rCBF in the left and medial prefrontal cortex correlated with psychomotor poverty, that the severity in disorganization correlated with increased rCBF in the right prefrontal cortex and decreased perfusion in Broca's area, and that the reality disorientation correlated with increased rCBF in the left hippocampal formation.

Metabolism and cerebral blood flow (CBF) in schizophrenia have been measured with a number of methods, both at a resting state and during mental challenges, neurobehavioral tasks, or pharmacological interventions. Several cortical and subcortical regions have been implicated, suggesting abnormalities in the frontal lobes (Weinberger et al. 1986; Andreasen et al. 1992; Buschbaum et al. 1992), temporolimbic structures (DeLisi et al. 1989; Rubin et al. 1991; Tamminga et al. 1992), and basal ganglia (Bushbaum et al. 1987; Resnick et al. 1988; Biver et al. 1995). Liddel et al. (1992) used ^{15}oxygen-labeled water with PET and described abnormal CBF in the parahypocampal gyrus associated with positive symptoms, and Musaleck et al. (1989) found hallucinations to be associated with SPECT changes in the parahippocampus and amygdala.

However, there are conflicting reports of superior temporal gyrus functional changes during active auditory hallucinations. Cleghorn (1990) suggested that patients with hallucinations have significantly lower relative metabolism in Wernicke's region. Anderson et al. (1991) showed asymmetrical temporal lobe perfusion, lower on the left than the right, in schizophrenic patients with auditory hallucinations. DeLisi et al. (1989) and Gur et al. (1989) found that greater metabolism in these area was related to the severity of the symptoms, as we have been able to confirm (Fig. 1).

A recent strategy applied in schizophrenia research that is important in functional neuroimaging is the study of the neuroleptic-naive first-episode patients. In these patients, there are alterations indicating that disruption in normal brain processes already exists at the time of presentation and cannot be attributed to treatment or chronicity. It has been demonstrated in some PET studies that there are differences in CBF in the temporolimbic regions in the initial phases of the illness (Gur 1995; Andreasen et al. 1997; Buschbaum et al. 1996). Earlier studies comparing resting values between patients and controls have noted differences in laterality indices, suggesting relatively higher left-hemispheric compared to right-hemispheric values in patients, and the effect was pronounced in patients with more severe symptoms. An improvement in clinical status correlated with normal CBF (Gur et al. 1989). Different studies reported laterality effects with greater involvement of the left hemisphere, suggesting reduced activity in multiple regions including frontal, temporal, parietal, and basal ganglia.

A variety of neurobehavioral tasks were administered during scanning in studies that examined CBF and metabolism; these have probed attention, language, and memory. One observation that seems to show some consistency is that the temporal lobe of patients is relatively more active, whereas neuroanatomical studies of cortical regions suggested decreased volume in the left temporal lobe. One study by Petty (1999) showed significant positive correlations between brain tissue volume and metabolism in the frontal lobes. This finding suggests that the degree of metabolism

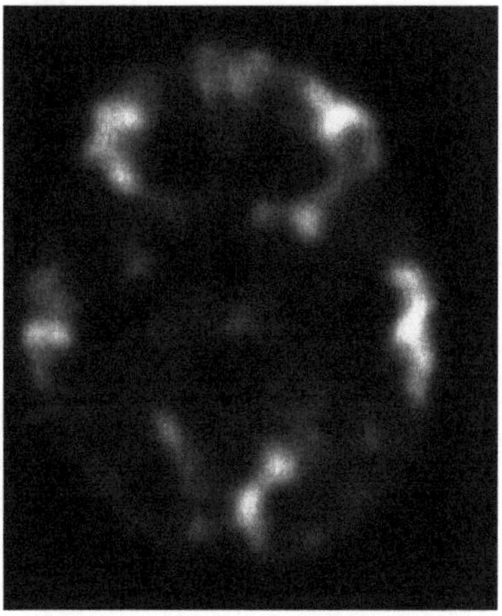

FIG. 1. FDG-PET of a patient with schizophrenia that shows a high metabolism in the Wernicke area (as he is hearing voices) and in the frontobasal cortex (as he is having obsessions about his future)

is higher in patients with atrophy-related changes. This hypothesis could point to pharmacological and neurocognitive rehabilitation strategies.

Pharmacological Strategies

The study of neuroreceptors provides the most direct examination of neuropharmacological alterations and therefore explains the nature of neurochemical abnormalities in schizophrenia. Estimations of receptor density and activity using PET and SPECT techniques have to date focused mainly on the dopaminergic system. The PET ligand [^{11}C]raclopride has been applied in earlier studies (Farde and Nordstrom 1992); sample sized ranged from 4 to 12 patients, and most studies did not include a comparison sample. In studies of patients on medication, radioactively labeled ligands have been used to determine the in vivo receptor occupancy of both typical and atypical antipsychotic drugs, relating these to clinical state. In contrast to the findings in drug-naive patients emission tomography has partially reinforced the accepted theory that the antipsychotic efficacy is related to D_2 blockade. Goyer et al. (1996) evaluated the occupancy of serotonin (5-HT2A) and dopamine (D_2) receptors in five untreated subjects (two healthy controls, two patients with schizophrenia, and one patient with bipolar illness), five patients treated with clozapine, and five patients treated with conventional neuroleptics. The 5-HT2A index separated subjects treated with clozapine from participants in the two other groups, and the D_2 index separated subjects treated with typical neuroleptics from all other participants. In 1997, Wong et al. studied a sample of 22 neuroleptic-naive subjects, and they noted a decline in dopamine receptors associated with B_{max} of D_2-like receptors.

Okuno et al. (1997) studied acute schizophrenic patients without neuroleptic treatment and as a result they found a decreased in D_1-receptor density in the prefrontal cortex. This decrease was positively correlated with the severity in negative symptoms and with poor results in the Wisconsin Card Sorting Test (WCST). In this same study, significant differences in the density of D_2 and D_1 receptors were not found in the striatum. According to these results, Breier et al. (1997) found an abnormal apomorphine sensitivity in dopaminergic receptors in patients with schizophrenia.

Decreased occupancy in GABA/benzodiazepine receptors has been associated with cognitive impairment, specifically in memory and visual attention tests (Ball et al. 1998). Both olanzapine and clozapine have a low incidence of extrapyramidal side effects (EPS), and this is no doubt due to the low striatal D_2 blockade demonstrated in the functional images. EPS have been the focus of several studies, and a threshold of 80% D_2 occupancy has been suggested to be necessary to produce EPS. An intriging finding is that risperidone, with similar D_2 occupancy, produces far less EPS, and it has been suggested that the potent 5-HT2A antagonism of risperidone, also demonstrated by PET, may be protecting aganist EPS (Millner et al. 1997; Pilowsky 1992).

Other groups have investigated the relationship between RCF, receptors, and the predisposition to develop tardive dyskinesia (TD) during neuroleptic treatment. The possibility of alterations in the distribution of D_2 receptors in patients with tardive dyskinesia has not been demonstrated (Anderson et al. 1991). However, it has been described that patients that developed TD had metabolic hyperactivity in the temporolimbic region and cerebellum and reduced metabolic activity in the parietal lobe and cingulum. Receptor occupancy levels are important as a predictor factor to develop extrapyramidal symptoms (Szymansky et al. 1996).

Conclusions

Schizophrenia is probably not the result of a single pathological process. Increasingly, it is viewed as the clinical manifestation of some aspect of brain disease that may be critically influenced by nonbiological events, such as environmental risk factors, the ethnosocial context of the illness, and social outcome. These aspects are being integrated more and more in an attempt to understand this complex and heterogeneous disorder. The brain is the seat of all human emotions and thought and therefore dysfunctions of the brain are the basis of psychiatric disorders. Neuroimaging techniques provide an insight into the workings of the intact living human brain. As the sophistication of technology increases, the quality of these research tools will improve. Identified differences in regional cerebral blood flow, metabolism, or receptor densities between patient groups and control groups would guide the rational development of new pharmacological and nonpharmacological approaches to restore these differences to normal. We can conclude that the integration of neuroimaging techniques with other disciplines such as genetics, neuroendocrinology, and psychology will allow a greater understanding of the etiology of schizophrenia and other mental illness.

References

Anderson J, Fawdry R, Gordon E, Coyle S (1991) SPECT asymmetry of left temporal lobe in hallucinating schizophrenics. Abstr Biol Psychiatry 29:291

Andreasen NC, Rezai K, Alliger R, et al (1992) Hypofrontality in neuroleptic-naive patients and in patients with chronic schizophrenia: assessment with xenon-133 single-photon emission tomography and the Tower of London. Arch Gen Psychiatry 49:943–958

Andreasen NC, O'Leary DS, Flaum M, et al (1997) Hypofrontality in schizophrenia: distributed dysfunction circuits in neuroleptic-naive patients. Lancet 394:1730–1739

Ball S, Bussatto GF, David AS, et al (1998) Cognitive functioning and GABA/benzodiazepine receptor binding in schizophrenia: 123-isomazenil SPECT study. Biol Psychiatry 43:107–117

Bertollo DN, Cowen MA, Levy AV (1996) Hypometabolism in olfatory cortical projection areas of male patients with schizophrenia: an initial positron emission tomography study. Psychiatr Res 60:113–116

Biver F, Glodman S, Luxen A, et al (1995) Altered frontoestriatal relationship in unmedicated schizophrenic patients. Psychiatr Res 60:113–116

Breier A, Su TP, Saunders R, et al (1997) Schizophrenia is associated with elevated amphetamine-induced synaptic dopaminergic concentration: evidence from a novel positron emission tomography method. Proc Natl Acad Sci USA 94:2569–2574

Buschbaum MS, Ingvar DH, Kessler R, et al (1987) Cerebral glucography with positron tomography. Arch Gen Psychiatry 39:251–259

Buschbaum MS, Potking SG, Siegel BV (1992) Striatal metabolic rate and clinical response to neuroleptics in schizophrenia. Arch Gen Psychiatry 49:966–974

Buschbaum MS, Someya T, Teng CY (1996) PET and MRI of the thalamus in never-medicated patients with schizophrenia. Am J Psychiatry 153:191–199

Cleghorn JM (1990) Regional brain metabolism during auditory hallucinations in chronic schizophrenia. Br J Psychiatry 157:562–570
Crow TJ (1990) Temporal lobe asymmetries as the key to the etiology of schizophrenia. Schizophr Bull 16(3):433–443
DeLisi LE, Buschbaum MS, Weinberger DR, et al (1989) Increased temporal lobe glucose use in chronic schizophrenics. Biol Psychiatry 25:853–851
Farde L, Nordstrom AL (1992) PET examination of central D2 dopamine receptor occupancy in relation to extrapyramidal syndromes in patients being treated with neuroleptic drugs. Psychopharmacol Ser 10:94–100
Goyer PF, Berridge MS, Morris ED (1996) PET measurement of neuroreceptor occupancy by typical and atypical neuroleptics. J Nucl Med 37:1122–1127
Gur RE (1995) Functional brain studies in schizophrenia In: Bloom FE, Kupper DJ (eds) Psychopharmacology: the fourth generation progress. Raven Press, New York, pp 1185–1192
Gur Re, Chin S (1999) Laterality in functional imaging studies in schizophrenia. Schizophr Bull 25(1):141–156
Gur RE, Resnick SM, Gur RC (1989) Laterality and frontality of cerebral blood flow and metabolism in schizophrenia: relationship to symptoms specificity. Psychiatr Res 27:325–334
Kraepelin E (1919) Dementia praecox and paraphrenia. Livingstone, Edinburgh
Liddle PF, Friston KJ, Frith CD, et al (1992) Patterns of cerebral blood flow in schizophrenia. Br J Psychiatry 160:179–186
Messimy R, López-Ibor JJ Jr, López-Ibor L, et al (1984) Tomodensitometrie (CT scanner) au cours de la Schizophrénie. Confrontation avec ses résultats avec d'autres investigations. L'Encéphale 10:69–77
Millner DD, Rezai K, Alliger R, Andreassen NC (1997) The effect of antiypsychotic medication on relative cerebral blood perfusion in schizophrenia: assessment with TC-99 m hexametil-propyleneamine oxime single photon emission tomography. Biol Psychiatry 41:550–559
Musaleck M, Podreka I, Walker S, et al (1989) Regional brain function in hallucinations: a study of regional cerebral blood flow in 99 m-Tc-HMPAO-SPECT in patients with auditory hallucinations, and normal controls. Compr Psychiatry 30:99–108
Okuno Y, Suhara T, Suzuki K, et al (1997) Decreased prefrontal dopamine D1 receptors in schizophrenia revealed by PET. Nature (Lond) 385:634–636
Petty R (1999) Structural asymmetries of the human brain and their disturbance in schizophrenia. Schizophr Bull 25(1):121–139
Pilowsky LS, Costa DC, Ell PJ, et al (1992) Clozapine, single photon emission tomography and the D dopamine receptor blockade hypothesis of schizophrenia. Lancet ii:199–202
Resnick SM, Gur RE, Alavi A, et al (1988) Positron emission tomography and subcortical glucose metabolism in schizophrenia. Psychiatr Res 24:1–11
Rubin P, Holm S, Frieberg L, et al (1991) Altered modulation of prefrontal and subcortical brain activity in newly diagnosed schizophrenia and schizophreniform disorder: a regional cerebral blood flow study. Arch Gen Psychiatry 48:987–995
Tamminga CA, Thaker GK, Buchanan R, et al (1992) Limbic system abnormalities identified in schizophrenia using positron emission tomography with fluorodesoxiglucose and neocortical alterations with deficit syndrome. Arch Gen Psychiatry 49:522–530
Weinberger DR, Bernman KF, Zec RF (1986) Physiologic dysfunction of dorsolateral prefrontal cortex in schizophrenia: regional cerebral blood flow evidence. Arch Gen Psychiatry 43:114–125
Wong DF, Pearlson GD, Tune LE, et al (1997) Quantification of neuroreceptors in the human brain: IV. Effect of aging and elevations of D2-like receptors in schizophrenia and bipolar illness. J Cereb Blood Flow Metab 17:331–342

The Genetics of Schizophrenia

DIMITRIS G. DIKEOS

Summary. On the basis of findings from family, twin, and adoption studies, heredity emerges as a major etiological factor in the pathogenesis of schizophrenia. Molecular genetic techniques (mainly genetic association and linkage studies) indicate that area 13q32 on chromosome 13 and, possibly, areas 6p24-22, 6q16-24, 8p, and 22q11-13, as well as the gene of serotonin 2A receptor, may be implicated in the pathogenesis of schizophrenia. As yet, however, no major genes have been identified; this is mainly because of the assumed heterogeneity of the disease, multigenic inheritance, reduced penetrance of genotype(s), and interplay between genetic and environmental vulnerability factors. Identification of genetically homogeneous patient subgroups and carriers of genes with reduced penetrance is based on "soft" neurological signs; deficits in auditory sensory gating and smooth pursuit eye movements; neuroanatomical abnormalities; deviant patterns of cerebral regional blood flow, functional MRI and brain lateralization; and biochemical indices of neurotransmitter abnormalities. The integration of molecular genetics with other fields of neuropsychiatry could provide new advances in our understanding of the interactions among the various genetic and environmental mechanisms leading to schizophrenia and allow the implementation of accurate genetic counseling and more appropriate interventions for the prevention and management of this devastating disease.

Keywords. Schizophrenia, Heredity, Molecular genetics, Biobehavioral markers, Brain imaging.

Introduction

Schizophrenia is a common mental disease with variable clinical expression. Its etiology is considered to be complex, based on the interplay of genetic and environmental (psychosocial and biological) factors. In this chapter, the main results of genetic epidemiology (i.e., family, twin and adoption studies) and the latest findings in molecular genetics of schizophrenia are presented. The mode of genetic transmission in the etiopathogenesis of the disease is also discussed. Moreover, methods of

---

Department of Psychiatry, Athens University Medical School, Athens 11528, Greece

genetic research that are based on advances in neuropsychiatry, particularly neurophysiology and neuroanatomy, are described.

Genetic Epidemiology

Family studies have demonstrated that the rate of schizophrenia and schizophrenia-spectrum disorders is significantly higher among relatives of affected individuals than among the relatives of normal subjects (Gottesman 1991). Whereas the morbidity risk to develop schizophrenia is about 1% for the general population, it is about 10%–15% for siblings or children of affected persons (40%–60% if both parents are affected), and about 3%–4% for second-degree and 2%–3% for third-degree relatives (Gottesman 1991). In twin studies, significantly higher concordance rates have been observed for monozygotic (45%–50%) than dizygotic (about 15%) twin pairs (Kringlen 1995). In adoption studies, a higher prevalence of schizophrenia has been demonstrated in the biological relatives of affected individuals than in their adoptive relatives or in the biological relatives of normal subjects (Schulsinger 1995).

The aforementioned family, twin, and adoption studies show that genetic factors play a major role in the etiology of schizophrenia. Heritability, however, cannot account by itself for the pathogenesis of the disorder; if this were the case, then a diagnostic concordance rate of 100% would be expected regarding schizophrenia in monozygotic twins. In the search for environmental influences that contribute to the etiology of the disorder, consistent results indicate that schizophrenia is more often observed among those (a) who were born during the winter months; (b) whose place of birth was urban; (c) who had suffered from viral infections either in utero or early in life; or (d) whose birth was characterized by perinatal complications (see Tsuang 2000 for review). Among the nonbiological environmental factors, a dysfunctional family environment or early absence of the father have been found to contribute to the development of the disorder (Tsuang 2000). It has been observed, however, that most nongenetic influences exert their action only in the presence of family history of schizophrenia, suggesting that "schizophrenogenic environmental influences" may lead to the development of the disorder only in the presence of genetic risk (Tsuang 2000).

Molecular Genetics

The two main methodological approaches for the identification of genes or chromosomal regions implicated in the pathogenesis of a disorder are linkage and genetic association studies. In the former, the cotransmission of a chromosomal marker and a disorder is examined in families with multiple affected members. In genetic association studies, the distribution of a specific allele of a polymorphic genetic locus is compared between groups of patients and controls, unrelated to each other. The controls are either subjects matched to the patients along sociodemographic and ethnic characteristics or, in the "Transmission Disequilibrium Test," they consist of imaginary individuals bearing the parental alleles that have not been transmitted to the patient (Spielman et al. 1993). Linkage studies are considered more appropriate to identify the major genes responsible for a given disorder and to avoid type I error of false-positive results than association studies, if stringent criteria are used for the interpretation of the statistical findings (Lander and Kruglyak 1995).

On the other hand, linkage methodologies are not considered appropriate or, at least, powerful enough to detect genes with minor effects in the pathogenesis of the disorder, whereas association studies are more advantageous for the identification of such genes (Risch and Merikangas 1996; Karayiorgou and Gogos 1997). Consequently, association studies are valuable for the testing of candidate genes (mainly those coding for development of nervous system, neurotransmitter-synthesizing enzymes, and neurotransmitter receptors) that may have too weak effects to be identified through linkage studies, a case which is considered to be true for many genes that increase vulnerability to schizophrenia (Risch 1990). Additionally, association studies can be used for narrowing regions of interest that are defined by linkage studies. The main drawbacks of association studies are that only previously identified tentative pathogenic genes can be tested and that the probability of a type I error is quite high (Risch and Merikangas 1996).

The most promising chromosomal regions that have been identified, mainly through genome scan linkage studies, as potentially associated with schizophrenia are (a) the area around 6p24-22 on chromosome's 6 short arm and 6q16-24 on the same chromosome's long arm; (b) the whole short arm of chromosome 8; (c) the areas 13q32 and 13q12-14 on chromosome's 13 long arm; and (d) the region 22q11-13 on the long arm of chromosome 22, which is also associated with the velocardiofacial syndrome among the patients of which a higher than expected frequency of schizophrenic morbidity is observed (see Pulver 2000 for review). Of these findings, only that for 13q32 (Blouin et al. 1998) meets the strict criteria for significant linkage (Lander and Kruglyak 1995). The allele 2 of the T102C polymorphism of the gene coding for the serotonin 2A receptor (5-HT2A) has been shown to be more frequent among schizophrenic patients than among controls in a genetic association study on a population large enough to reach a satisfactory statistical significance (Williams et al. 1996). Other weaker findings of association studies have been reported and mainly regard the dopamine receptor genes and their association with schizophrenia or its specific characteristics such as response to treatment and development of side effects (Williams et al. 1998, Okuyama et al. 1999; Jonsson et al. 1999; Scharfetter et al. 1999; Rietschel et al. 2000).

Contribution of Neuropsychiatry to Genetic Research in Schizophrenia

The results of linkage and genetic association studies, by showing that schizophrenia is most probably heterogeneous in its etiology with different genes being potentially pathogenic in different families or, probably, even among different individuals in the same family (Stefanis et al. 1995), point to what was obvious from segregation analyses of multiplex pedigrees, that is, to the understanding that the mode of genetic transmission of schizophrenia is oligogenic. According to this model, a small number of genes, each of which has a low contribution to relative risk and is not involved in all cases, interact among themselves (in additive and/or epistatic patterns) and with environmental factors to lead to the development of the disease phenotype (Risch 1990). It is also possible that, while some of the contributing genes may be "specific" for schizophrenia, others might predispose to some of its characteristics that might be shared by other disorders also, explaining thus the overlap in susceptibility loci of schizophrenia and affective or other mental disorders (Dikeos et al. 1999; Berrettini 2000). As the effect of any gene on the final phenotype of an oligogenic disorder is expected to be relatively weak and, thus, studies of linkage and association with the disorder itself might not have the power to detect it, other approaches have been proposed.

One such approach for the detection of minor genes is to identify their associated phenotypes that are present in patients as well as in their relatives who are "carriers" of these genes. Advances in neuropsychiatry have a significant contribution to this field, because phenotypes that are believed to correspond to genes which might contribute to the development of schizophrenia are mainly the presence of "soft" neurological signs; the neurophysiological deficits in auditory sensory gating and in smooth pursuit eye movements; certain neuroanatomical abnormalities, especially of the periventricular and hippocampal regions; functional deviant patterns as evidenced from studies on cerebral regional blood flow, functional MRI, and studies in brain lateralization; and biochemical indices of increased catecholamine metabolism or other neurotransmitter abnormalities (Stefanis 1990; Spitzer 1997; Toru 1998; Stefanis et al. 1999; Waldo et al. 2000). Positive linkage findings have emerged regarding defective auditory sensory gating and a chromosomal marker corresponding to the α-7 nicotine acetylcholine receptor subunit gene (Coon et al. 1993; Freedman et al. 1997) as well as smooth pursuit eye movement dysfunction and chromosome 6 markers (Arolt et al. 1996). These findings could provide new advances in our understanding of the interactions among genetic mechanisms leading to schizophrenia (Waldo et al. 2000).

Studies of genetic association with the response to antipsychotic treatment are another approach in the effort to identify genes responsible for the disorder in subpopulations of patients. Apart from their contribution in the study of genes with minor effects, pharmacogenetic studies have also the practical utility that they may lead to the identification of genetic characteristics that, according to their presence, predispose a patient to respond favorably or not to a particular therapeutic agent (Tu 1994).

Conclusion

Results from family, twin, and adoption studies have shown that genetic factors play an important role in determining an individual's susceptibility to schizophrenia. Nonetheless, important environmental influences seem also to be involved. It is anticipated that molecular genetics, mainly through linkage and association studies, will help identify the genes that influence susceptibility to schizophrenia and the mechanisms of the biological-environmental interaction that lead to the manifestation of the disorder. Understanding the relationship between genotype and phenotype and identifying the genetic component of schizophrenia will permit the implementation of more accurate genetic counseling and more appropriate and rational approaches not only for the prevention but also for the management of this disabling disease.

Acknowledgments. The author's career in psychogenetics has been partly supported through funding from the STRIDE HELLAS grant 205/92, awarded to the University Mental Health Research Institute, Athens, Greece.

References

Arolt V, Lencer R, Nolte A, et al (1996) Eye tracking dysfunction is a putative phenotypic susceptibility marker of schizophrenia and maps to a locus on chromosome 6p in families with multiple occurrence of the disease. Am J Med Genet 67:564–579

Berrettini WH (2000) Susceptibility loci for bipolar disorder: overlap with inherited vulnerability to schizophrenia. Biol Psychiatry 47:245–251

Blouin JL, Dombroski BA, Nath SK, et al (1998) Schizophrenia susceptibility loci on chromosomes 13q32 and 8p21. Nat Genet 20:70–73

Coon H, Plaetke R, Holik J, et al (1993) Use of a neurophysiological trait in linkage analysis of schizophrenia. Biol Psychiatry 34:277–289

Dikeos DG, Papadimitriou GN, Avramopoulos D, et al (1999) Association between the dopamine D3 receptor gene locus (DRD3) and unipolar affective disorder. Psychiatr Genet 9:189–195

Freedman R, Coon H, Mules-Worsley M, et al (1997) Linkage of a neurophysiological deficit in schizophrenia to a chromosome 15 locus. Proc Natl Acad Sci USA 94:587–592

Gottesman II (1991) Schizophrenia genesis. Freeman, New York

Jonsson EG, Nothen MM, Neidt H, et al (1999) Association between a promoter polymorphism in the dopamine D2 receptor gene and schizophrenia. Schizophr Res 40:31–36

Karayiorgou M, Gogos JA (1997) Dissecting the genetic complexity of schizophrenia. Mol Psychiatry 2:211–223

Kringlen E (1995) Twin studies in mental disorders. In: Mendlewicz J, Papadimitriou GN (eds) Genetics of mental disorders, part I. Theoretical aspects. Bailliere's clinical psychiatry, international practice and research, vol 1. Tindall, London, pp 47–62

Lander E, Kruglyak L (1995) Genetic dissection of complex traits: guidelines for interpreting and reporting linkage results. Nat Genet 11:241–247

Okuyama Y, Ishiguro H, Toru M, Arimani T (1999) A genetic polymorphism in the promoter region of DRD4 associated with expression and schizophrenia. Biochem Biophys Res Commun 258:292–295

Pulver AE (2000) Search for schizophrenia susceptibility genes. Biol Psychiatry 47:221–230

Rietschel M, Krauss H, Muller DJ, et al (2000) Dopamine D3 receptor variant and tardive dyskinesia. Eur Arch Psychiatry Clin Neurosci 250:31–35

Risch N (1990) Linkage strategies for genetically complex traits. I. Multilocus models. Am J Hum Genet 46:222–228

Risch N, Merikangas K (1996) The future of genetic studies of complex human diseases. Science 273:1516–1517

Scharfetter J, Chaudhry HR, Hornik K, et al (1999) Dopamine D3 receptor gene polymorphism and response to clozapine in schizophrenic Pakastani patients. Eur Neuropsychopharmacol 10:17–20

Schulsinger F (1995) US-Denmark adoption studies. In: Mendlewicz J, Papadimitriou GN (eds) Genetics of mental disorders, part I. Theoretical aspects. Bailliere's clinical psychiatry, international practice and research, vol 1. Tindall, London, pp 63–75

Spielman RS, McGinnis RE, Ewens WJ (1993) Transmission test for linkage disequilibrium: The insulin gene region and insulin-dependent diabetes mellitus (IDDM). Am J Hum Genet 52:506–516

Spitzer M (1997) A cognitive neuroscience view of schizophrenic thought disorder. Schizophr Bull 23:29–50

Stefanis CN (1990) On the concept of schizophrenia. In: Kales A, Stefanis CN, Talbott JA (eds) Recent advances in schizophrenia. Springer, New York

Stefanis CN, Dikeos DG, Papadimitriou GN (1995) Clinical strategies in genetic research. In: Mendlewicz J, Papadimitriou GN (eds) Genetics of mental disorders, part I. Theoretical aspects. Bailliere's clinical psychiatry, international practice and research, vol 1. Tindall, London, pp 1–18

Stefanis N, Frangou S, Yakeley J, et al (1999) Hippocampal volume reduction in schizophrenia: effects of genetic risk and pregnancy and birth complications. Biol Psychiatry 46:697–702

Toru M (1998) Biological research on schizophrenia. Psychiatry Clin Neurosci 52(suppl):S170–S172

Tsuang M (2000) Schizophrenia: genes and environment. Biol Psychiatry 47:210–220

Tu JB (1994) Theory and practice of pharmacogenetics. Am J Med Genet (Neuropsychiatr Genet) 54:391–397

Waldo MC, Adler LE, Leonard S, et al (2000) Familial transmission of risk factors in the first-degree relatives of schizophrenic people. Biol Psychiatry 47:231–239

Williams J, Spurlock G, McGuffin P, et al (1996) Association between schizophrenia and T102C polymorphism of the 5-hydroxytryptamine type 2a-receptor gene. European Multicentre Association Study of Schizophrenia (EMASS) Group. Lancet 347:1294–1296

Williams J, Spurlock G, Holmans P, et al (1998) A meta-analysis and transmission disequilibrium study of association between the dopamine D3 receptor gene and schizophrenia. Mol Psychiatry 3:141–149

Deficit and Nondeficit Schizophrenias: Some Neurobiological Correlates and more than 25 Years of Follow-Through Results

Tetsuo Fukuda[1] and Takuji Hayashi[2]

Characteristic deficit features that become manifest in the realm of terminal states of schizophrenia have long been regarded, and still remain, as unique of the schizophrenia (Leonhard 1966; Mitsuda 1975, 1979; Fukuda 1979, 1997, 2000). In contrast, the atypical (nondeficit) schizophrenia, estimated to comprise about one-third of contemporary classification systems, e.g., DSM-IV or ICD-10 (Leonhard 1986; Hayashi et al. 1991, 1998; Suga et al. 1994), has been repeatedly shown to differ beyond doubt: the two phenotypes at issue are distinct one from the other not only at clinicogenetic (Mitsuda 1942, 1968) but also at pathogenetic levels. Thus, the differential imbalance of the central autonomic functions, including the limbic system, was shown in our earlier work (Fukuda and Matsuda 1969). Further, differential brain structure-functions have been shown by brain imaging techniques such as CT, SPECT, and MRI (Hayashi et al. 1992, 1993, 2000). Although the precise cerebral sites or circuits involved await further investigation, recent moves toward prospective longitudinal studies by a few groups as well as the proposal of a paradigm shift to deficit-nondeficit schizophrenia (Carpenter et al. 1999) are promising research approaches in line with those of the present authors and are only welcome and encouraged. The result of more than 25 years in-person follow-through, showing various subtypes of deficit exclusively in the typical group, argues strongly that our typical versus atypical designation could equate with deficit versus nondeficit distinction. It is tempting to conceive of clinical identification of such distinction as early as at the onset of illness, if not even earlier. Impact of the distinction is obvious, as our results indicate.

The present communication has in part been presented elsewhere, as in the list of references.

References

Carpenter WT Jr, Arango C, Buchanan RW, Kirkpatrick B (1999) Deficit psychopathology and a paradigm shift in schizophrenia research. Biol Psychiatry 46:352–360

[1] Yodo-no-mizu Neuropsychiatric Center, Maejima, Takatsuki, Osaka 569-0021, Japan
[2] Department of Neuropsychiatry, Aichi Medical University, Yazako-Karimata, Nagakute, Aichi 480-1195, Japan

Fukuda T (1979) On the diagnostic criteria of schizophrenia: closing remark. In: Fukuda T, Mitsuda H (eds) World issues in the problems of schizophrenic psychoses. Igaku-Shoin, Tokyo, pp 67–76
Fukuda T (1997) Atypical psychoses versus schizophrenia: long-term personal follow-up results. Biol Psychiatry (Suppl) 42:1S, 196S
Fukuda T (2000) Evidence of epileptic involvement in some of the atypical psychoses. In: Franzek E, Ungvari GS, Rüther E, Beckmann H (eds) Progress in differentiated psychopathology. International Wernicke-Kleist-Leonhard Society, Würzburg, Germany, pp 217–222
Fukuda T, Matsuda Y (1969) Comparative characteristics of the slow wave EEG autonomic function and clinical picture during and following EST in typical and atypical schizophrenia. Int Pharmacopsychiatry 3:13–41
Hayashi T, Kitoh H, Kachi T, Suga H, Ohara M (1991) Multivariate analyses of brain imaging data from typical and atypical schizophrenic psychosis. In: Racagni G, et al (eds) Biological psychiatry, vol 1. Elsevier, Amsterdam, pp 452–454
Hayashi T, Watanabe T, Kitoh H, Sekine T (1992) Multivariate analyses of CT findings in typical schizophrenia and atypical psychosis. Jpn J Psychiatr Neurol 46:699–709
Hayashi T, Hotta N, Fukastu N, Suga H (1998) Clinical and socio-demographic studies of atypical psychoses using ICD-10 criteria. Neurol Psychiatr Brain Res 6:147–154
Hayashi T, Hotta N, Andoh T, et al (2000) Magnetic resonance imaging findings in typical schizophrenia and atypical psychoses. In: Franzek E, Ungvari GS, Rüther E, Beckmann H (eds) Progress in differentiated psychopathology. International Wernicke-Kleist-Leonhard Society, Würzburg, Germany, pp 121–127
Leonhard K (1966) Psychopathologische Struktur der chronischen Schizophrenien. In: Panse FR (ed) Problematik, Therapie und Rehabilitation der chronischen endogenen Psychosen. F. Enke-Verlag, Stuttgart, pp 50–62
Leonhard K (1986) Aufteilung der endogenen Psychosen und ihre differenzierte Ätiologie. Akademie-Verlag, Berlin, pp 117–217
Mitsuda H (1968) Clinico-genetic study of schizophrenia (original in Japanese, 1942. Psychiat Neurol Jpn 46:298–362). In: Mitsuda H (ed) Clinical genetics in psychiatry. Problems in nosological classification. Igaku-Shoin, Tokyo, pp 49–90
Mitsuda H (1975) Some notes on the nosological classification of the endogenous psychoses, with special reference to the so-called atypical psychoses. In: Mitsuda H, Fukuda T (eds) Biological mechanisms of schizophrenia and schizophrenia-like psychoses. Thieme, Stuttgart, pp 1–9
Mitsuda H (1979) Clinical-genetic view on the biology of the schizophrenia. In: Fukuda T, Mitsuda H (eds) World issues in the problems of schizophrenic psychoses. Igaku-Shoin, Tokyo, pp 121–124
Suga H, Hayashi T, Ohara M (1994) SPECT findings Using ^{123}I-IMP in schizophrenia and atypical psychosis. Jpn J Psychiatr Neurol 48:833–848

Regional Changes in Brain Gray and White Matter Volumes in Patients with Schizophrenia

MICHIO SUZUKI, SHIGERU NOHARA, HIROFUMI HAGINO,
KENZO KUROKAWA, TAKASHI YOTSUTSUJI, and MASAYOSHI KURACHI

Summary. Thirty-four medicated patients with schizophrenia (19 men and 15 women) (mean age, 27.7 ± 5.2 years) were compared with 31 age- and sex-matched healthy volunteers on magnetic resonance imaging (MRI). Automated volume analysis on three-dimensional MRI was conducted using statistical parametric mapping (SPM) 96. Compared with the controls, relative gray matter volume in the patients was significantly reduced in the left middle and inferior frontal, left superior temporal, left anterior cingulate, medial part of the right superior frontal, and bilateral medial temporal areas. In the white matter, significant volume reduction was found in the bilateral anterior limbs of the internal capsule and the left superior occipitofrontal fasciculus. These findings may imply a morphological substrate for abnormalities in the frontothalamic and frontotemporal connectivity in schizophrenia.

Keywords. Schizophrenia, Magnetic resonance imaging (MRI), Statistical parametric mapping (SPM), Gray matter, White matter

Introduction

Enlargement of the ventricles is one of the most consistent findings in schizophrenia in previous morphological brain imaging studies (Lawrie and Abukmeil 1998). With respect to brain substance, however, results are more inconsistent. Some of the previous magnetic resonance imaging (MRI) studies have suggested that the medial temporal lobe structures may be preferentially affected in patients with schizophrenia. However, other brain regions have also been reported to be abnormal, such as the prefrontal lobe, superior temporal gyrus, and thalamus. In addition, there is relatively little information available on white matter volume in schizophrenia.

In the present study, we assessed the differences in regional gray and white matter volume between patients with schizophrenia and normal controls using a voxel-based method by statistical parametric mapping (SPM).

Department of Neuropsychiatry, Toyama Medical and Pharmaceutical University, 2630 Sugitani, Toyama 930-0194, Japan

Subjects and Methods

Subjects were 34 right-handed patients who fulfilled ICD-10 criteria for schizophrenia; 19 were men and 15 were women, with a mean age of 27.7 ± 5.2 years. All patients were receiving neuroleptic medication. Their mean age at onset of schizophrenia was 21.8 ± 5.1 years, and mean duration of illness was 5.9 ± 4.5 years. Control subjects were 31 healthy volunteers (18 men and 13 women) matched with the patients for age, sex, and handedness. Informed consent was obtained from all subjects.

The subjects underwent brain MRI scans with a Siemens 1.5-T Magnetom Vision system using a three-dimensional gradient-echo sequence (fast low-angle shot, FLASH) yielding high-resolution T_1-weighted images with good contrast between gray and white matter. Image analysis was performed on a Unix workstation using ANALYZE and SPM 96 software running in MATLAB. Image processing was based upon the method reported previously by Shah et al. (1998). Briefly, images were first spatially normalized into the standard space of Talairach and Tournoux, and then segmented into gray matter, white matter, cerebrospinal fluid, and skull/scalp compartments. The spatially normalized segments of gray and white matter were smoothed with a 12-mm full-width at half-maximum isotropic Gaussian kernel to accommodate individual variability in gyral anatomy. Statistical comparison between groups was performed using an ANCOVA model for global normalization that removed global gray or white matter density for each subject. Age was treated as a confounding covariate.

Results

Gray matter volume in the patients was significantly reduced in the left inferior frontal gyrus, left superior temporal gyrus, left anterior cingulate gyrus, medial part of the right superior frontal gyrus, right superior temporal gyrus and insula, left middle frontal gyrus, and bilateral uncus and hippocampus.

In the white matter, significant volume reduction in the patients was found in the bilateral anterior limbs of the internal capsule and the left superior occipitofrontal fasciculus.

Discussion

Our results are consistent with a pathological process in schizophrenia involving distributed volume changes within the brain. In contrast to many of the previous studies employing regions of interest analysis, the present study indicates that regional volume changes are present in various brain regions in the same sample of patients with schizophrenia. In this respect, automated voxel-based methods such as SPM have the advantage and provide a complementary technique to the regions of interest methods for investigating the broader morphological deviation found in schizophrenia (Wright et al. 1999).

It is of interest to note that the white matter volume reductions were found in the anterior limbs of the internal capsule and the superior occipitofrontal fasciculus.

These findings may imply a morphological substrate for abnormalities in the frontothalamic and frontotemporal connectivity suggested in previous studies in schizophrenia (Carlsson 1988; Weinberger 1987).

References

Carlsson A (1988) The current status of the dopamine hypothesis of schizophrenia. Neuropsychopharmacology 1:179–186

Lawrie SM, Abukmeil SS (1998) Brain abnormality in schizophrenia: a systematic and quantitative review of volumetric magnetic resonance imaging studies. Br J Psychiatry 172:110–120

Shah RJ, Ebmeier KP, Glabus MF, Goodwin GM (1998) Cortical grey matter reductions associated with treatment-resistant chronic unipolar depression: controlled magnetic resonance imaging study. Br J Psychiatry 172:527–532

Weinberger DR (1987) Implications of normal brain development for the pathogenesis of schizophrenia. Arch Gen Psychiatry 44:660–669

Wright IC, Ellison ZR, Sharma T, et al (1999) Mapping of grey matter changes in schizophrenia. Schizophr Res 35:1–14

Cognitive Dysfunction and Exploratory Eye Movements in Patients with Schizophrenia

MIÉ MATSUI[1], YASUHIRO TONOYA[2], and MASAYOSHI KURACHI[2]

Summary. The effect of figure size and a direct instruction on exploratory eye movements and the fixation duration in schizophrenic patients were examined using an infrared eye-mark recorder. Fifteen schizophrenic patients and 15 normal controls were shown the S-shaped figure at original size and at half-size for 15 s each. The patients showed lower search scores than controls even for the half-sized figure. The subjects were also shown a figure slightly different from the original and required to compare the figure with the original. Patients showed lower search scores than normal controls, not only for the original-sized figure but also for the half-sized figure. The direct instruction had the effect of improving the visual performance in patients. Furthermore, the study of tracking eye movements on predetermined stationary targets revealed that the patients showed fewer correct scores than controls at the 200-ms, but not at the 100-ms, setting. These results suggest that limited visual search in schizophrenia patients is due to their cognitive strategy unrelated to the size of the object or the additional question, but that direct instruction has an effect. Moreover, some patients view the targets too quickly.

Keywords. Schizophrenia, Cognitive dysfunction, Exploratory eye movements, Fixation time, Cognitive strategy

Introduction

Eye-scanning track is the pattern of eye movements that occur when an individual processes a complex stimulus. The analyses provide an important clue for understanding of cognitive impairment in schizophrenic patients. Several studies have indicated that schizophrenic patients showed restricted eye-scanning in comparison with normal controls. However, what factor is involved in such limited eye movement pattern in schizophrenic patients remains unknown. Two possible factors may play a role in this restricted eye-scanning behavior: one is poor oculomotor activity of the patients. If this is the main factor, then the extent of visual search of the patients would improve with reducing the size of the object. The other possibility is visual cognitive

Departments of [1]Psychology and [2]Neuropsychiatry, Toyama Medical and Pharmaceutical University, 2630 Sugitani, Toyama 930-0194, Japan strategy of the patients unrelated to the size of the object. If so, then patients may still show limited visual scanning even though the size of a figure is reduced. In the present study, to investigate the factor relating to restricted eye-scanning in schizophrenic patients, exploratory eye movements while viewing S-shaped figures (Moriya et al. 1972; Kojima et al. 1986) differing in size were examined. The second purpose of the present study was to examine the effect of the instruction on restricted viewing pattern of schizophrenic patients. A direct function was given to the subjects while viewing a figure slightly different from the original S-shaped figure. Third, we examined not only fixations longer than 200 ms but also those longer than 100 ms for further investigation of eye-scanning characteristics in schizophrenic patients.

Subjects and Methods

Study 1: Exploratory Eye Movement on Figures Differing in Size

Fifteen patients (9 men, 6 women) who fulfilled Diagnostic and Statistical Manual of Mental Disorders, 3rd edition revised (DSM-III-R) criteria for schizophrenia and 15 normal controls (9 men, 6 women) participated in this study. The mean (SD) age for schizophrenic patients and normal controls was 27.5 (5.2) years (range, 21–38 years) and 25.0 (1.7) years (range, 23–28 years). The schizophrenic patients including 14 inpatients and 1 outpatients were recruited from the Toyama Medical and Pharmaceutical University Hospital, and their mean (SD) duration of illness was 5.0 (5.3) years (range, 0.3–19.0 years). The control subjects were healthy volunteers recruited from college students. Informed consent was obtained from all the subjects.

The subject sat on a chair 1.2 m in front of a screen, and an infrared eye-mark recorder (Nac, type-V) was attached to their head. Two geometric figures of the same shape but differing in size were individually projected from the rear on the screen: one was an original S-shaped target figure (Kojima et al. 1986) of which the angle of sight was 33° horizontally and 27.5° vertically, and the other figure is half size at each angle. Each subject was shown a figure of original size for 15 s and asked to draw the figure after viewing it. Next, the subject was shown a figure of half-size for 15 s and asked to draw the figure. To assess the extent of visual scanning, each figure was divided into seven sections according to the study by Kojima et al. (1986). The number of sections on which the eye fixed once or more during the 15-s viewing period for each figure was counted and scored for 1 to 7 points as Search Score.

Study 2: Exploratory Eye Movement After a Question and an Instruction

The test procedure, which was obtained by modifying the procedure described by Kojima et al. (1986), was conducted. Subsequently after study 1, the subject was shown for 15 s a figure slightly different from the original of which one bump was in a different position. The subject was asked to compare it with the original and answer how it differed. After the subject had finished replying and while still being shown the figure, the question, "Are there any other differences?" (Kojima et al. 1986), was then asked. Following this, the subject was asked to draw the figure based on the memory.

Next, in the present study, the subject was again shown the figure, which this time was slightly different from the original, and was given the instruction, "Please look at all the parts and make sure," and then asked to reproduce it again. The search score on seven sections was analyzed for the first 5 s immediately after each question and instruction.

Study 3: Examination of the Elementary Motor Aspects of Saccadic Eye Movements

Twenty-three schizophrenic patients (10 men and 13 women) were recruited from inpatient and outpatient clinics. Their mean age was 27.9 ± 8.6 (SD) years (range, 15–43 years), and their mean duration of illness was 7.3 ± 5.3 years. The control subjects consisted of 23 healthy volunteers (14 men and 9 women) with a mean age of 25.4 ± 3.9 years (range, 23–40 years). Eight black points of 1 angular degree in size were placed on the circumference of a circle having a diameter of 20 angular degrees. The subject was first instructed to look at the center (+) of each figure. Then he or she was asked to scan each of the 8 points once in clockwise order by moving the eyes. Each task was self-paced. When a fixation hits a target, a one-point score (Target Hitting) is given. The maximum possible score is eight points.

Results

Study 1

Figure 1 shows representative examples of the eye-scanning tracks of a normal control and a patient while viewing the original and half-sized figures for 15 s. The 2 (group) × 2 (size) repeated-measure ANOVAs, employing search scores as the dependent variable, yielded a significant main effect of group ($F = 9.52$; $df = 1{,}28$; $P = 0.005$). There

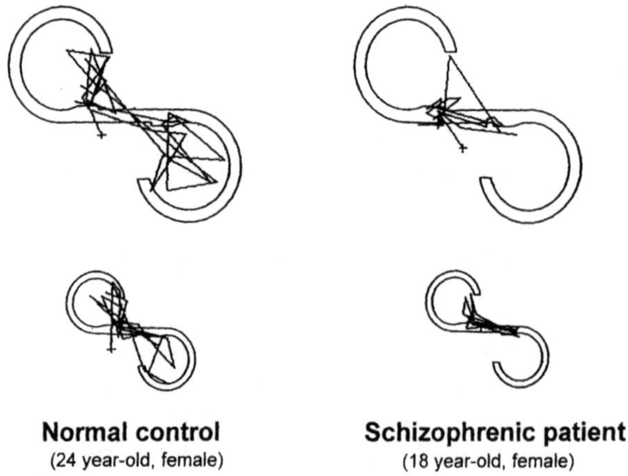

FIG. 1. Eye-scanning tracks on the original-sized figure (*top*) and the half-sized figure (*bottom*) for 15 s

were no significant effects of figure size ($F = 0.83$; $df = 1{,}28$; $P = 0.37$) or of group-by-size interaction ($F = 0.03$; $df = 1{,}28$; $P = 0.86$). Schizophrenic patients showed lower search scores than normal controls for the half-sized figure ($P < 0.01$) as well as for the original ($P < 0.01$).

Study 2

Figure 2 displays representative examples of the eye-scanning tracks and the search scores in study 2. The 2 (group) × 2 (condition) × 2 (setting level) repeated-measure ANOVAs were conducted with search scores as the dependent variable. No significant effect of group was observed ($F = 4.05$; $df = 1{,}28$; $P = 0.054$). The main effect of setting level (100 ms versus 200 ms) was significant ($F = 32.16$; $df = 1{,}28$; $P < 0.0001$), but no significant effect of condition (question versus instruction) was observed ($F = 0.11$; $df = 1{,}28$; $P = 0.74$). At the 200-ms setting, the responsive search score of the patients was siginificantly lower than normal controls ($P < 0.01$). At the 100-ms setting, however, the difference between the responsive search score of the patients and that of normal controls was not significant. In contrast, no significant difference was observed between the instructed search score of the patients and normal controls at both the 100-ms and the 200-ms setting.

Study 3

Table 1 shows the number of subjects who achieved full target hitting score (8 points) and who did not attain full target hitting score. At the 200-ms setting, 21 of the 23

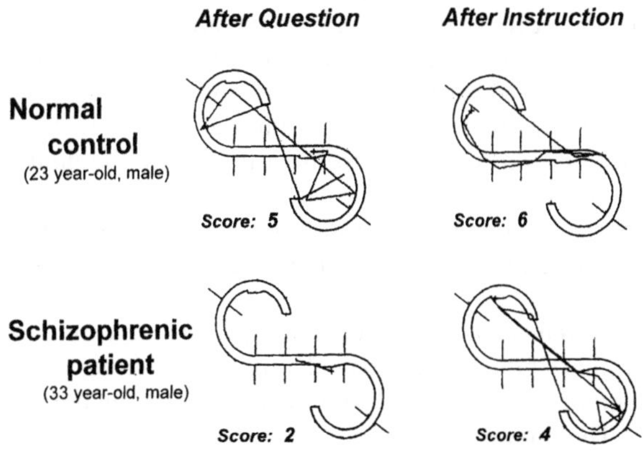

FIG. 2. Eye-scanning tracks and the scoring of search scores for 5 s in a normal control (23-year-old man) and a schizophrenic patient (33-year-old man). *Left*, sequences of eye movements for 5 s after the question; *right*, after the instruction. A normal control showed a wide extent of eye movements after the question, and the search score was 5. After the instruction, the search score was 6 in the normal control. A schizophrenic patient had limited area of visual search after the question, and the search score was 2. After the instruction, a patient showed a wider extent of eye movement, and the search score was 4

TABLE 1. Numbers of subjects with full target hitting score and less than full target hitting score

Score	Full (8 points)	Less than full (<8)
200-ms setting		
Controls	21	2
Patients	10**	13
100-ms setting		
Controls	23	0
Patients	21	2

** $P < 0.01$ (Fisher's exact test on scores for controls and patients)

normal controls attained full target hitting score, while only 10 of the 23 patients attained full target hitting score ($P = 0.0361$). On the other hand, there was no significant difference between patients and controls at the 100-ms setting.

Discussion

In the present study, the main effect of figure size and the interaction between group and size were nonsignificant. Moreover, patients showed lower search scores than normal controls, not only for the original-sized figure but also for the half-sized figure. These results suggest a stable pattern of restricted eye-scanning in schizophrenic patients unrelated to the size of the object. This finding supports the hypothesis that limited visual search of the patients is not the result of poor eye movement per se, but may be related to their cognitive strategy.

As in most previous studies investigating exploratory eye movement, the patients showed lower search scores than normal controls after the confirmative question. Moreover, in the present study the direct instruction was given, and then no significant difference was observed between the patients and normal controls. One possible and likely interpretation of these results is that normal controls understand the implication of the question, which suggests to them to explore the figure all around to confirm their own conclusion, whereas the patients were not fully aware of it and need to be given a direct instruction to initiate an adequate plan of action. The instruction may have facilitated in generating plans of action or taken the place of a willed intention in the patients.

In saccadic eye movement on the stationary target, we found there were two groups of patients: an ordinary group who obtained a full target hitting score at the 200-ms setting and a fast group who obtained the full score at 100 ms but not at 200 ms (Matsui et al. 1995, 1997). The typical duration of an eye movement cycle is estimated to be 230 ms, with 110 ms required for cognitive operations, and the briefest duration of minimum movement automatized without cognitive operation is assumed to be about 70 ms (Russo 1978). Thus, about 200 ms or more should be required for the fixations in which the cognitive system is adequately operated. Therefore, the present result seems to provide evidence of a neurocognitive deficiency in schizophrenic patients because the patients reached the normal performance level only when fixations longer than 100 ms were applied to the analyses of eye-scanning tracks.

In conclusion, the present study suggests that the findings in patients result from cognitive strategy rather than poor oculomotor functions per se, and that neither the size of the figure, nor the additional question, but the direct instruction has an effect to improve the visual performance of schizophrenic patients. In addition, some schizophrenic patients view the object too quickly.

Acknowledgments. This work is partly supported by the 1998 Satow's Research Fund for Behavioral Science.

References

Kojima T, Matsushima E, Iwama H, et al (1986) Visual perception process in amphetamine psychosis and schizophrenia. Psychopharmacol Bull 22:768–773

Matsui M, Kurachi M (1995) Impaired saccadic eye movements on stationary targets in patients with schizophrenia spectrum disorder. Eur Arch Psychiatry Clin Neurosci 245:129–134

Matsui M, Kurachi M, Yuasa S, et al (1997) Saccadic eye movements and regional cerebral blood flow in schizophrenic patients. Eur Arch Psychiatry Clin Neurosci 247:219–227

Moriya H, Ando K, Kojima T, et al (1972) Eye movements during perception of pictures in chronic schizophrenia. Folia Psychiatr Neurol Jpn 26:189–199

Russo JE (1978) Adaptation of cognitive processes to the eye movement system. In: Senders JW, Fisher DF, Monty RA (eds) Eye movements and the higher psychological functions. Wiley, New York, pp 89–112

Discriminant Analysis Between Schizophrenics and Nonschizophrenics Using Exploratory Eye Movements

TAKUYA KOJIMA[1], EISUKE MATSUSHIMA[2], SHIGERU OBAYASHI[2], KATSUYA OHTA[2], KAZUNORI NAKAJIMA[2], HARUNOBU ANDO[2], and KATSUMI ANDO[2]

Summary. To extract a common feature from schizophrenics, we discriminated schizophrenics from nonschizophrenics using exploratory eye movements. Eye movements while viewing a stationary figure were recorded using an eye-mark recorder. Subjects were 60 schizophrenics and 140 nonschizophrenics, consisting of six patient groups with various psychiatric diseases and normal controls. Of five indicators of eye movements available, the responsive search score (RSS), which is eye movements in response to repeated questions in a comparison task and number of eye fixations (NEF) in memory tasks, were selected by stepwise selection. The schizophrenics were discriminated from nonschizophrenics with a sensitivity of 73.3%–76.7% and a specificity of 81.4%–84.3%. The obtained discriminated function in this study was applied to the data of a WHO collaborative project including 167 schizophrenics, 144 depressed patients, and 154 normal subjects in six countries. In total, the sensitivity was 88% and specificity was 83.9%. It was found that we could extract a common feature from many schizophrenics using the RSS and NEF of exploratory eye movements.

Keywords. Exploratory eye movements, Responsive search score, Schizophrenia, Nonschizophrenia, Discriminant analysis

Introduction

In daily practice, we observe the facial expressions and eye movements of patients to understand their mental state. These eye movements are considered to play a role not only in perceiving the environment but also in reflecting behavior to gather new information. To record these eye movements in psychiatric patients, we utilized an eye-mark recorder. In our previous studies we reported that schizophrenics and the parents of schizophrenics had less frequent eye movements and a more limited area of inspection than normal controls [1,2,5]. Using these eye movements, we also examined an interpersonal response for a patient with schizophrenia between the patient

[1] Department of Neuropsychiatry, Nihon University School of Medicine, 30-1 Oyaguchi-kamimachi, Itabashi-ku, Tokyo 173-0032, Japan
[2] Department of Neuropsychiatry, Tokyo Medical and Dental University, Tokyo, Japan

and the investigator that is called the responsive search score [1–7]. From the results of many subsequent studies, eye movements have come to be regarded as being one of the specific findings of schizophrenia.

In this chapter I show if we can extract a common feature from schizophrenics using the exploratory eye movements. To clarify this aim, we performed discriminant analysis between schizophrenics and nonschizophrenics using the exploratory eye movements. We also applied the obtained discriminant function to subjects of several countries.

Method

The subject is seated on a stool in a relatively dark and quiet room, fitted with nac, the fifth type of eye-mark recorder, and shown S-shaped figures projected on a screen 150 cm from his or her eyes. The eye movements of the subject were recorded on a videotape as they looked at the S-shaped figures. The examination procedure was as follows.

Step 1. The target S-shaped figure is shown for 15 s. This step is a memory task.
Step 2. Immediately afterward, the subject is asked to draw the target figure from memory.
Step 3. Each of the two figures different from the target is shown for 15 s. These figures are partially different from the target; one has a bump in a different place and the other has no bumps. After 15 s have passed, and with the figure still showing, the subject is asked if it differs from the target figure and, if different, how it differs. After the subject finishes replying, he or she is asked: "Are there any differences?" This step is a comparison task.

We analyzed three indicators of exploratory eye movements, that is, the number of eye fixations and the mean eye scanning length of the target figure for 15 s in the memory task, and the responsive eye movements that occurred in the 5 s following the question: "Are there any other differences?" in the comparison task. The responsive eye movements of the two figures partially different from the target are counted as a responsive search score (RSS).

We performed discriminant analysis between schizophrenics and nonschizophrenic subjects [4]. There were 60 schizophrenics, consisting of 20 acute, 20 chronic, and 20 remitted schizophrenics. The number of the nonschizophrenics, 140, consists of 20 depressed patients, 20 amphetamine psychotics, 20 alcoholics, 20 neurotics, 20 temporal lobe epileptics, 20 patients with frontal lobe lesion, and 20 normal controls. These subjects were divided into two groups, A and B. We first performed discriminant analysis on group A. The obtained discriminant function in group A was applied to group B to confirm cross-validity.

Results

Discriminant Analysis

First, discriminant analysis in group A was performed.

Of five indicators of eye movements available, the RSS and the number of eye fixations were selected by using stepwise selection. The *F*-value for the RSS was 45.61 and that for eye fixations was 3.55. It was found that the RSS was more effective in discrimination than the number of eye fixations (NEF). The discriminant function was $[D = 10.265 - (0.065 \times NEF + 0.871 \times RSS)]$. The NEF and the RSS of each subject were substituted into this function, and a negative result for D indicated that the subject was not schizophrenic, whereas a positive result for D indicated that the subject was schizophrenic. All subjects were assessed using this discriminant function.

The power of discrimination in group A was as follows: 76.7% of the schizophrenics were assessed as being schizophrenic and 81.4% of nonschizophrenic group subjects were assessed as nonschizophrenic. As for the schizophrenics, 90% of acute schizophrenics, 80% of chronic schizophrenics, and 60% of remitted schizophrenics were assessed to be schizophrenic. For the nonschizophrenic group, 70% of depressed patients, amphetamine psychotics, and neurotics were assessed to be nonschizophrenic, and 80% of alcoholics, 90% of temporal lobe epileptics and normal controls, and 100% of patients with frontal lobe lesions were also assessed as being nonschizophrenic. The sensitivity was 76.7% and the specificity was 81.4%.

The discriminant function was applied to the other subject group, group B, to confirm cross-validity. The power of discrimination in group B was as follows: 73.3% of schizophrenics were assessed to be schizophrenic and 84.3% of nonschizophrenic subjects were classified as nonschizophrenic.

These results confirm the validity of the discriminant function. The results also suggest that the RSS and the NEF play an important role in distinguishing between schizophrenics and nonschizophrenics.

WHO Collaborative Project

A World Health Organization (WHO) collaborative project on exploratory eye movements in schizophrenics was performed [3,6]. The purpose of the WHO collaborative project is to evaluate the replicability of these results of eye movements by ethically and culturally different countries. Seven WHO centers (Beijing, Casablanca, Montreal, Munich, Prague, Sapporo, and Tokyo) in six countries joined in this project. The results of discriminant analysis of this project using the discriminant function obtained in the aforementioned study was reported. The total number of the schizophrenia group was 167, that of the depression group 144, and that of the normal control group 154. Of 167 schizophrenia patients, 147 were discriminated as schizophrenia, and 115 of 144 depressed patients and 135 of 154 normal controls were discriminated as nonschizophrenic. In total, the sensitivity was 88.0% and the specificity was 83.9%.

The value of the discrimination was high as a rating, and this method and formula could be used in practice to diagnose schizophrenia. It was also found that we could extract a common feature in many schizophrenics using the RSS and NEF of exploratory eye movements.

Conclusions

1. Schizophrenics were discriminated from nonschizophrenic subjects with 73%–88% of sensitivity and 81%–83% of specificity using the RSS and number of eye fixation of exploratory eye movements.
2. It was found that we could extract a common feature in many schizophrenics using the RSS and NEF of exploratory eye movements.

References

1. Kojima T, Matsushima E, Moriya H, et al (1986) Visual perception process in amphetamine psychotics and schizophrenics. Psychopharmacol Bull 22:768–777
2. Kojima T, Matsushima E, Nakajima K, et al (1990) Eye movements in acute, chronic and remitted schizophrenics. Biol Psychiatry 27:975–989
3. Kojima T, Matsushima E, Ohbayashi S, et al (1992) WHO project on eye movements in patients with schizophrenia. Clin Neuropharmacol 15(suppl 1A):489–490
4. Matsushima E, Kojima T, Ohta K, et al (1998) Exploratory eye movement dysfunctions in patients with schizophrenia: possibility as a discriminator for schizophrenia. J Psychiatr Res 32:289–295
5. Xia ML, Takahashi S, Tanabe E, et al (1996) Eye movement studies on schizophrenics and their parents. Eur Neuropsychopharmacol 6(suppl 3):64
6. Kojima T, Matsushima E, Ohta K, et al. Stability of exploratory eye movements as a marker of schizophrenia—A WHO multi-center study. Schizophrenia Research (in press)
7. Kojima T, Matsushima E, Ando K (2000) Eyes and the mind—psychophysiological approach to psychiatric disorders through visual, and ocular functions. KARGER, Basel

Exploratory Eye Movements as a Trait Marker of Schizophrenia

EISUKE MATSUSHIMA[1], KATSUYA OHTA[2], SHIGERU OBAYASHI[2], MASAMICHI HAGIWARA[2], SAKAE TAKAHASHI[3], KAZUO YARA[3], and TAKUYA KOJIMA[3]

Summary. To clarify a genetic factor in the development of schizophrenia from a psychophysiological point of view, the exploratory eye movements that we have shown to be specific to schizophrenia in healthy families of schizophrenics were investigated. Eye movements of parents, siblings, and healthy cotwins of monozygotic discordant pairs were examined while they looked at S-shaped figures. The responsive search scores (RSSs) of both parents and siblings were similar to those of schizophrenics. In the RSS, there was a relationship between each pair in discordant twins. These results suggest that RSS shown in schizophrenics may be a trait marker for schizophrenia. Furthermore, eye movements of schizophrenics with schizophrenic family members in their first-degree relatives were measured. As the number of schizophrenic family members of schizophrenics increased, their RSS became lower. This result also indicates that RSS can be related to the genetic factors of schizophrenia.

Keywords. Schizophrenia, Exploratory eye movements, Trait marker, Family study, Twin study

Introduction

Much discussion has taken place concerning the etiology of schizophrenia. Studies carried out on family, twins, and adopted individuals have indicated that factors of genes and environment contribute to the occurrence of schizophrenia. However, from the large amount of data derived from family studies, the conclusion has been reached that the lifetime risk of developing schizophrenia for family members of schizophrenics is greater than 1% of the general population (Gottesman 1991), and that the closer the degree of genetic relatedness with a schizophrenic (meaning the greater the ratio of commonly held genes), the higher that risk becomes. These results strongly indicate that there is some genetic factor contributing to the cause of schizophrenia.

Sections of [1] Liaison Psychiatry and Palliative Medicine and [2] Psychiatry and Behavioral Science, Graduate School of Tokyo Medical and Dental University, Tokyo, Japan
[3] Department of Neuropsychiatry, Nihon University School of Medicine, Tokyo, Japan

On the other hand, using exploratory eye movements in the S-shaped figure test (Kojima et al. 1986, 1989, 1990, 1992), schizophrenics could be discriminated from nonschizophrenics such as patients with depression, amphetamine psychosis, alcohol psychosis, anxiety disorder, frontal lobe lesions, temporal lobe epilepsy, and healthy normal controls, with a sensitivity of 76.7% and a specificity of 81.4% (Matsushima et al. 1998). This finding indicates that exploratory eye movements can be a specific marker for schizophrenia.

In this chapter, we extrapolate the exploratory eye movements that we have shown to be specific to schizophrenia to family members of schizophrenics and discuss a genetic factor in the development of schizophrenia from the psychophysiological point of view.

Methods

Examination Procedure

The subject is fitted with a nac, the seventh type of eye-mark recorder, and shown S-shaped figures on a screen, which consist of the target figure (top of Fig. 1) and two figures partially different from the target; one has a bump in a different place and the other has no bumps. The eye movements of the subject are recorded on a videotape as he or she looks at the S-shaped figures. The examination procedure is as follows:

Step 1. The target figure is shown for 15 s.
Step 2. Immediately afterward, the subject is asked to draw the target figure from memory.
Step 3. Each of the two figures different from the target is shown for 15 s. After 15 s have passed, and with the figure still showing, the subject is asked if it differs from

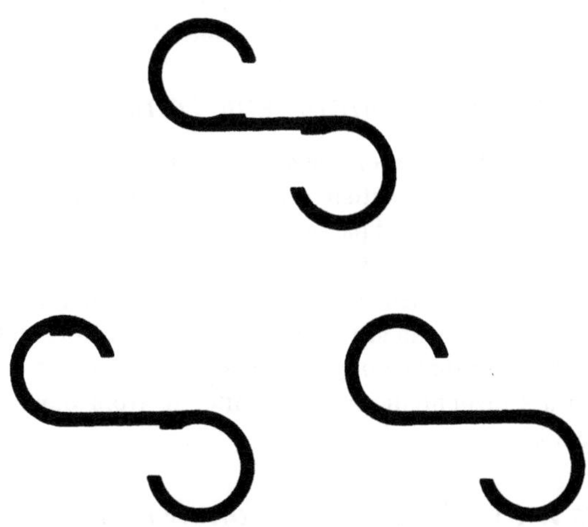

FIG. 1. Three S-shaped figures used in the examination. The two at the *bottom* are slightly different from the target figure at the *top*

the target figure and, if different, how it differs. After the subject finishes replying, he or she is asked: "Are there any other differences?"

Measurement

The responsive eye movements that occurred in the 5 s following the question: "Are there any other differences?" are analyzed. The responsive eye movements are counted related to the two figures partially different from the target as a responsive search score, RSS.

Family and Twin Studies

We considered whether it is possible to derive a marker for genetic vulnerability in schizophrenics from the exploratory eye movements, based on the family studies of schizophrenics, such as healthy siblings and parents of schizophrenics, depressed patients with schizophrenic family members and schizophrenics with schizophrenic family members, and on twin studies such as with monozygotic twin pairs.

Healthy Siblings and Parents of Schizophrenics

Takahashi et al. (1999) compared the responsive search scores (RSSs) among three subject groups, 23 proband-sibling pairs in which were included 23 schizophrenic probands and 23 their healthy siblings, and 43 unrelated normal controls who had no history of psychotic illness in their first-degree family members. The probands had significantly lower RSS than their siblings and the normal controls. In addition, the siblings showed significantly lower RSS than the normal controls. Namely, the results show that not only the schizophrenic probands but also their siblings had a low RSS, falling into values that lie between those of the probands and normal controls.

Also, the responsive search scores of healthy parents of schizophrenics (Kojima et al. 1996) were the same as those of healthy siblings of schizophrenics.

Depressed Patients with Schizophrenic Family Members

Yara et al. (1999) compared the responsive search scores among five subject groups, 26 schizophrenics, three depressed patient groups, and 26 normal controls. Depressed patient groups included 15 depressed patients with schizophrenic family members, 17 depressed patients with depressed family members, and depressed patients without psychiatric family members in their first-degree relatives. The RSSs of schizophrenics and the depressed patients with schizophrenic family members were significantly lower than those of the other three groups. The results indicate that, among depressed patients, those with a schizophrenic trait are different from those without schizophrenic trait in the RSS.

Schizophrenics with Schizophrenic Family Members

Hagiwara et al. (1999) compared the responsive search scores among 50 schizophrenics with schizophrenics in their first-degree relatives, which were divided into three groups by the number of schizophrenic family members; that is, 30 schizophrenics with 1 schizophrenic family member, 13 schizophrenics with 2 schizophrenic family members, and 7 schizophrenics with 3 or more schizophrenics in their first-degree relatives. As the number of schizophrenic members that schizophrenics had increased, their RSS became significantly lower.

The results of four family studies suggest that responsive search score could be related to genetic factors.

Twins

Matsushima et al. (1997, 1999) examined the responsive search scores in 28 monozygotic twin pairs, which consisted of 12 pairs discordant and 8 pairs concordant for schizophrenia, and 8 normal control pairs. The relationship between monozygotic twin pairs was observed in the RSS. There was a significant relationship between each twin pair in the RSS, even including discordant twins. The result suggests that low RSS shown in schizophrenics may be a trait marker for schizophrenia. Furthermore, they compared the RSSs among these three groups. The RSSs of discordant twin group were higher than those of the concordant twin group but were lower than those of the normal twin group. The results suggest that concordant twins are more strongly related to genetic factors of developing schizophrenia than discordant twins.

Conclusion

The family studies suggest that low RSS shown in schizophrenics and their family members can be a trait marker for schizophrenia. Furthermore, the twin study suggests that concordant twins are more strongly related to trait factors of developing schizophrenia than discordant twins.

References

Gottesman II (1991) Schizophrenia genesis: the origins of madness. Freeman, New york

Hagiwara M, Matsushima E, Ohkura T, et al (1999) The relationship between exploratory eye movements in schizophrenia and gene factor. In: Abstracts of the 21st annual meeting of the Japanese Society of Biological Psychiatry, p 103

Kojima T, Matsushima E, Iwama H, et al (1986) Visual perception process in amphetamine psychosis and schizophrenia. Psychopharm Bull 22:768–773

Kojima T, Potkin SG, Kharazmi M, et al (1989) Limited eye movement patterns in chronic schizophrenic patients. Psychiatry Res 28:307–314

Kojima T, Matsushima E, Nakajima K, et al (1990) Eye movement in acute, chronic and remitted schizophrenics. Biol Psychiatry 27:975–989

Kojima T, Matsushima E, Ando K, et al (1992) Exploratory eye movements and neuropsychological tests in schizophrenic patients. Schizophr Bull 18:85–94

Kojima T, Takahashi S, Tanabe E, et al (1996) Eye movements in family of schizophrenia. In: Toru M (ed) Annual report '90 of the National Project Team (Basic and clinical studies on the onset mechanism and pathophysiology of schizophrenia). Tokyo, pp 5–8

Matsushima E, Ohta K, Obayashi S, et al (1997) Exploratory eye movements in patients with schizophrenia: a monozygotic twin study, 2nd report. Psychiatr Clin Neurosci 51:S84

Matsushima E, Kojima T, Ohta K, et al (1998) Exploratory eye movement dysfunctions in patients with schizophrenia: possibility as a discriminator for schizophrenia. J Psychiatr Res 32:289–295

Matsushima E, Kubo H, Kojima T, et al (1999) Exploratory eye movements in patients with schizophrenia—a monozygotic twins study. In: Abstracts II of the XI world congress of psychiatry, Hamburg, p 11

Takahashi S, Tanabe E, Kojima T, et al (1999) Exploratory eye movement dysfunctions in schizophrenic patients and their siblings. In: Abstracts II of the XI world congress of psychiatry, Hamburg, p 15

Yara K, Takahashi S, Tanabe E, et al (1999) Exploratory eye movements in mood disorder with family history of schizophrenia. In: Abstracts of the 21st annual meeting of the Japanese Society of Biological Psychiatry, p 105

No Differences Between Bipolar Patients and Normal Controls in Inositol Levels and Inositol Monophosphatase Activity in Postmortem Brain

Galit Shaltiel, Joseph Shapiro, and Galila Agam

Summary. The discovery of inositol monophosphatase (IMPase) activity inhibition by lithium (Li) ions led to Berridge's inositol depletion hypothesis, and brain inositol levels have been studied in relation to psychiatric disorders. We have previously reported low *myo*-inositol levels in the frontal cortex of bipolar and schizophrenic patients and low IMPase activity in lymphocyte-derived cell lines from this group of patients. In the present study, *myo*- and *scyllo*-inositol levels and IMPase activity were measured in the Stanley Brain Consortium postmortem brain specimens from bipolar patients and normal controls. No differences were found between the diagnostic groups in any parameter in any brain area studied. There was a positive correlation between *myo*- and *scyllo*-inositol in frontal and occipital cortex. We could not replicate our previous report of low *myo*-inositol levels in the frontal cortex of bipolar patients. In subjects treated with neuroleptic drugs, there was no correlation between *myo*-inositol levels and estimated chlorpromazine equivalents administered peri mortem.

Keywords. Postmortem brain, Frontal cortex, Occipital cortex, Inositol monophosphatase, Myo-inositol, Scyllo-inositol

Introduction

Brain inositol levels have been studied in relation to psychiatric disorders. Free inositol is both produced and taken up in mammalian brain [1]. It is an intermediate in the phosphatidylinositol (PI) cycle that serves as a signal transduction system for numerous neurotransmitters, e.g., muscarinic cholinergic. Inositol is produced downstream to the generation of two second messengers, diacylglycerol and inositol triphosphate (IP_3), and their degradation. The last dephosphorylation step of IP_3 is carried out by inositol monophosphatase (IMPase). Inositol, an IMPase product, is utilized for the resynthesis of phosphatidylinositol bisphosphate, the precursor of these two second messengers. In addition, it is a precursor of other inositol phospholipids involved in PI-related signaling cascades, such as PI-3-kinase [2,3].

Among the nine stereoisomers of inositol, the two inositol transport systems — from plasma to the cerebrospinal fluid (CSF) and from the CSF into the brain — transport only *myo*- and *scyllo*-inositol [1]. An epimerase activity has been reported

Stanley Center for Bipolar Research, Ben-Gurion University of the Negev, Beer-Sheva, Israel

capable of exchanging between *myo-* and *scyllo*-inositol [4]. This exchange could lead to an equilibrium between levels of these two naturally occurring inositol stereoisomers. The saturable transport system of *myo*-inositol through the blood–brain barrier [5] and the sodium-dependent uptake of *myo*-inositol into mouse astroglia-rich primary cultures [6] were shown to be inhibited by *scyllo*-inositol.

We have previously reported that *myo*-inositol is reduced in postmortem frontal cortex of bipolar patients [7]. Moore et al. [8] found a decreased *myo*-inositol concentration in the right frontal cortex of bipolar patients.

Methods

Postmortem Brain Samples

Postmortem frontal and occipital cortex tissue specimens of bipolar patients and normal controls were obtained from the Stanley Foundation Brain Collection [9].

Gas Chromatographic Measurement of Inositol Levels

Human brain free inositol levels were analyzed as trimethylsilyl (TMS) derivatives by gas-liquid chromatography (GC), as previously described [10], using a capillary column. The correlation coefficients of the daily standard curves were always above 0.987. Replicate reliability was tested in rat brain. When two different specimens from four rat brains were sampled, the correlation coefficients were 0.80 and 0.99 for *myo-* and *scyllo*-inositol, respectively. When a single brain extract was devided into ten separate samples, each assayed individually, the coefficients of variation were 23.5% for both *myo-* and *scyllo*-inositol. Each sample extract was assayed on two consecutive days, at least in duplicate/day. The results presented are the average of the replicates. The correlation coefficients between the results obtained on the first and second days were 0.99 for frontal cortex *myo-* and *scyllo*-inositol and for occipital cortex *scyllo*-inositol and 0.97 for occipital cortex *myo*-inositol. Assays were performed in a blind and balanced design such that each run included samples from both groups. Frontal and occipital cortex from the same donor were run on separate days.

IMPase Activity

IMPase activity was assayed by measuring inorganic phosphate liberated from inositol-1-phosphate, quantified spectrophotometrically in an ELISA reader (iEMS, Labsystems) using the malachite green color reagent. To distinguish IMPase activity from nonspecific phosphatases, the reaction was carried out in the presence and absence of 30 mM LiCl. LiCl is a specific inhibitor of this enzyme and at these concentrations totally inhibits IMPase activity. The enzyme activity was calculated as the difference between the value in the absence minus the activity in the presence of lithium.

Statistical Analysis

Statistical analyses of the data were performed by the software STATISTICA for Windows.

Results

No differences were found between the diagnostic groups in any parameter in either brain area studied (Table 1). *Myo-* and *scyllo*-inositol and the *myo-/scyllo*-inositol ratio in frontal or occipital cortex did not correlate with age, age of onset of the disease, or postmortem interval. In subjects treated with neuroleptic drugs, none of the parameters measured correlated with estimated chlorpromazine equivalents (CPZE) administered perimortem. There was a positive correlation between *myo-* and *scyllo*-inositol ($r = 0.465$, $n = 54$, $P = 0.004$ and $r = 0.43$, $n = 60$, $P = 0.0006$ in frontal and occipital cortex, respectively).

Discussion

The results of IMPase activity confirm our previous finding in a different postmortem brain collection [7]. The lack of difference in IMPase activity does not corroborate our recent reports of reduced activity in Epstein–Barr virus (EBV) transformed lymphoblastoid cell lines derived from bipolar patients [11] (Shaltiel et al., in manuscript). The discrepancy may stem from the apparent different relative expression of the two inositol monophosphatase human genes (IMPA) in brain and leukocytes. IMPA-1 and IMPA-2 are similarly expressed in brain, but IMPA-2 is dominant in neutrophils. If the latter is also the case in B lymphocytes that dominate EBV-transformed lymphoblastoid cell cultures, and if only IMPA-2 is reduced in bipolar patients, total IMPase activity measurement may detect a reduction in the cell lines but not in brain.

In recent years, the search for the mechanism of action of lithium (Li) has been aided by studies in model organisms such as the slime mold *Dictyostelium* and the

TABLE 1. Brain inositol levels and IMPase activity in bipolar patients versus control subjects

	Frontal cortex			
	Inositol (nmoles/kg wet weight)			IMPase activity
	myo-	*scyllo-*	*myo/scyllo*	(nmoles/min × mg protein)
Bipolar patients ($n = 15$)	4.7 ± 1.4	0.13 ± 0.06	43.5 ± 24.3	1.52 ± 0.41
Control subjects ($n = 15$)	4.2 ± 1.2	0.17 ± 0.09	26.6 ± 11.7	1.62 ± 0.39
	Occipital cortex			
	Inositol (nmoles/kg wet weight)			IMPase activity
	myo-	*scyllo-*	*myo/scyllo*	(nmoles/min × mg protein)
Bipolar patients ($n = 15$)	4.9 ± 1.2	0.17 ± 0.09	35.2 ± 21.0	1.54 ± 0.41
Control subjects ($n = 15$)	4.7 ± 0.9	0.20 ± 0.06	28.4 ± 7.8	1.59 ± 0.55

Results are means ± SD

yeast *Saccharomyces cerevisiae*. An IMPA-1 null mutant of *Saccharomyces cerevisiae* was not found to be an inositol auxotroph, consistent with a claim that IMPase activity of IMPA-2 may compensate for the lack of IMPA-1 expression [12]. A Li-resistant mutant of *Dictyostelium* exhibits disrupted prolyl oligopeptidase (POase) and elevated IP_3 concentrations. Increased IP_3 levels are also evident in wild-type cells treated with a POase inhibitor [13]. Apparently, loss of POase activity counteracts Li-induced reduction in IP_3. Interestingly, abnormal POase activity is reported to be associated with manic and depressive episodes [14]. In conclusion, IMPA-2 rather than IMPA-1 is more likely involved in the etiology of bipolar disorder and in the mechanism of action of Li.

Interest in the role of brain inositol levels began with the discovery that lithium inhibits the enzyme inositol monophosphatase [15], which indeed leads to brain *myo*-inositol depletion [8]. We originally hypothesized that brain *myo*-inositol levels in Li-responding bipolar patients are higher than in control subjects but surprisingly found them to be reduced [7]. Considering the possible interrelationship between *myo*- and *scyllo*-inositol, we were interested to compare their levels. No differences between the groups were found for *scyllo*-inositol in either the frontal or occipital cortex.

We also aimed to test the hypothesis that brain *scyllo*-inositol levels regulate brain *myo*-inositol levels by competing with the active transport of the latter through the blood–brain barrier [16]. In agreement with the finding of Lien et al. (1994) in hepatic encephalopathy [16], and with the ^{1}H-NMR study of Michaelis et al. [17] comparing a healthy volunteer and a Leigh's disease patient, a positive, rather than negative, correlation between *myo*- and *scyllo*-inositol levels was obtained in both frontal and occipital cortex. This finding contradicts the hypothesis that *scyllo*-inositol might be the endogenous inhibitor of *myo*-inositol uptake and supports a metabolic interrelationship between the two isomers, perhaps via the intermediate of their epimerization, *myo*-inosose-2 [4].

The present study does not replicate our previous report of low *myo*-inositol levels in the frontal cortex of bipolar patients [7]. The Stanley's brain collection control group showed mean levels of *myo*-inositol in the frontal and in the occipital cortex that are ~40% lower than the values in the previously studied collection [7]. It is possible that the previous control specimens had high *myo*-inositol levels because of perimortem agonal state effects [18]. For example, hypernatremia results in elevated brain *myo*-inositol levels [19].

The present study does not offer an explanation for the beneficial effect of 12–18 g/day *myo*-inositol in unipolar patients [20] nor does it suggest a role of brain *scyllo*-inositol levels in the psychiatric disorders studied.

Acknowledgments. Postmortem brains were donated by the Stanley Foundation Brain Consortium courtesy of Drs. Llewellyn B. Bigelow, Juraj Cervenak, Mary M. Herman, Thomas M. Hyde, Joel E. Kleinman, Jose D. Paltan, Robert M. Post, E. Fuller Torrey, Maree J. Webster, and Robert H. Yolken.

References

1. Spector R, Lorenzo AV (1975) The origin of myo-inositol in brain, cerebrospinal fluid and choroid plexus. J Neurochem 25:353–354
2. Michell RH (1997) The multiplying roles of inositol lipids and phosphates in cell control processes. Essays Biochem 32:31–47
3. Toker A, Cantley LC (1997) Signalling through the lipid products of phosphoinositide-3-OH kinase. Nature (Lond) 387:673–676
4. Hipps PP, Holland WH, Sherman WR (1977) Interconversion of myo- and scyllo-inositol with simultaneous formation of neo-inositol by an $NADP^+$ dependent epimerase from bovine brain. Biochem Biophys Res Commun 77:340–346
5. Spector R (1988) Myo-inositol transport through the blood-brain barrier. Neurochem Res 13:785–787
6. Wiesinger H (1991) Myo-inositol transport in mouse astroglia-rich primary cultures. J Neurochem 56:1698–1704
7. Shimon H, Agam G, Belmaker RH, et al (1997) Reduced frontal cortex inositol levels in postmortem brain of suicide victims and patients with bipolar disorder. Am J Psychiatry 154:1148–1150
8. Moore GJ, Bebchuk JM, Parrish JK, et al (1999) Temporal dissociation between lithium-induced changes in frontal lobe myo-inositol and clinical response in manic-depressive illness. Am J Psychiatry 156:1902–1908
9. Torrey EF, Webster M, Knable M, et al (2000) The Stanley Foundation brain collection and Neuropathology Consortium. Schizophr Res 44:151–155
10. Shapiro J, Belmaker RH, Beigon A, et al (2000) Scyllo-inositol in post-mortem brain of suicide victims, bipolar, unipolar and schizophrenic patients. J Neural Transm 107:603–607
11. Shamir A, Ebstein RP, Nemanov L, et al (1998) Inositol monophosphatase in immortalized lymphoblastoid cell lines indicates susceptibility to bipolar disorder and response to lithium therapy. Mol Psychiatry 3:481–482
12. Murray M, Greenberg ML (2000) Expression of yeast INM1 encoding inositol monophosphatase is regulated by inositol, carbon source, and growth stage and is decreased by lithium and valproate. Mol Microbiol 36:651–661
13. Williams RS, Eames M, Ryves WJ, et al (1999) Loss of a prolyl oligopeptidase confers resistance to lithium by elevation of inositol (1,4,5) trisphosphate. EMBO J 18:2734–2745
14. Maes M, Goossens F, Scharpe S, et al (1994) Lower serum prolyl endopeptidase enzyme activity in major depression: further evidence that peptidases play a role in the pathophysiology of depression. Biol Psychiatry 35(8):545–552
15. Hallcher LM, Sherman WR (1980) The effects of lithium ion and other agents on the activity of myo-inositol-1-phosphatase from bovine brain. J Biol Chem 255:10896–10901
16. Lien YH, Michaelis T, Moats RA, Ross BD (1994) Scyllo-inositol depletion in hepatic encephalopathy. Life Sci 54:1507–1512
17. Michaelis T, Helms G, Merboldt KD, et al (1993) Identification of scyllo-inositol in proton NMR spectra of human brain in vivo. NMR Biomed 6:105–109
18. Hardy JA, Wester P, Winblad B, et al (1985) The patients dying after long terminal phase have acidotic brains; implications for biochemical measurements on autopsy tissue. J Neural Transm 61:253–264
19. Lien YH, Shapiro JI, Chan L (1990) Effects of hypernatremia on organic brain osmoles. J Clin Invest 85:1427–1435
20. Levine J, Barak Y, Gonzalves M, et al (1995) Double-blind, controlled trial of inositol treatment of depression. Am J Psychiatry 152:792–794

Establishment of the First Systematic Brain Bank Network for Psychiatric Disorders in Japan

Izuru Matsumoto, Masayuki Ito, Takeshi Iwasaki, Isao Shibata, and Shin-ichi Niwa

Summary. It is our intention to establish the first systematic brain bank for schizophrenia in Japan and, in so doing, develop innovative collaborative research programs between neuroscience and psychiatry researchers, based on the shared premise that the biological basis of brain function is the key to understanding the cause of this mental illness. Specimens of schizophrenia brain tissue for research will be collected and appropriately preserved to interact with diagnostic assessment to ensure appropriate identification and documentation of tissue held. We have established a strong network between our department and 42 associated hospitals, precise protocols for brain collection, and the site to store the materials. We predict at least ten schizophrenia and ten control brains will be collected annually. This project represents a unique opportunity to explore the biologically and socially important question of the changes associated with schizophrenia in the human brains. It brings together the resources contained in the brain tissue collection maintained by a team of enthusiastic psychiatrists and pathologists, and the expertise of experienced neurochemists, to promote and increase current Japanese schizophrenia research projects to internationally competitive levels, thus leading to the development of new therapeutic agents.

Keywords. Human Brain Bank, Schizophrenia, CNS

Background

Although various animal models have been developed and studied to understand the pathogenesis of schizophrenia, delineating this human-specific brain disorder has been largely dependent upon the availability of postmortem human brains. However, despite the emphasis placed on establishing brain banks, no systematic brain bank exists in Japan. Considering the lack of availability of human schizophrenic brain samples, during the last 2 years we have been working to establish a brain bank in Fukushima prefecture. Fukushima prefecture is a relatively large state, located 250 km north from Tokyo, with a population of 2 126 000. Compared with other prefectures in

Department of Neuropsychiatry, School of Medicine, Fukushima Medical University, 1 Hikarigaoka, Fukushima 960-1295, Japan

Japan, there are a large number of psychiatric hospitals established in Fukushima prefecture (total, 39), holding more than 8000 psychiatric beds (Table 1). The total number of inpatients in these hospitals is 7944, and of that number 4658 are schizophrenic patients (male, 2802; female, 1856) (Table 2). This large catchment area creates an ideal situation for establishing a brain bank. Our department of neuropsychiatry plays a significant role in improving the collaboration between these psychiatric hospitals and pathology and other departments of Fukushma Medical University (FMU) involved in biologically oriented psychiatric research. We have established a strong network system and precise protocols for collecting brain samples.

Research Proposal

Establishment of a Human Brain Bank for Schizophrenia

To establish and maintain a human brain bank, the following issues need to be addressed.

Recruitment and Information of Donors and Controls

By educating and informing the family support groups that exist in the majority of the hospitals (the total number of families registered is approximately 1500) and by

TABLE 1. Number of psychiatric hospitals and beds in northeast Japan

Prefecture	Population (×1000)	No. of psychiatric hospitals	No. of psychiatric beds	No. of psychiatric beds/10 000	No. of inpatients
Aomori	1 482	26	4 929	33.3	4468
Iwate	1 420	22	4 915	34.6	4678
Miyagi	1 358	20	3 578	26.3	3410
Akita	1 214	26	4 458	36.7	4357
Yamagata	1 257	18	3 226	25.7	3089
Fukushima	2 133	39	8 600	40.3	7942
Tokyo	11 772	117	26 428	22.4	4130

TABLE 2. Disease category of psychiatric inpatients in Fukushima

Schizophrenia	4658 (58.6%)
Organic mental disorders	1228 (15.5%)
Mood disorders	557 (7.0%)
Other psychotic disorders	467 (5.9%)
Mental retardation	418 (5.3%)
Substance-related disorders	376 (4.7%)
Anxiety disorders	113 (1.4%)
Personality disorders	26 (0.3%)
Others	99 (1.3%)
Total	7944

placing a qualified and authorized brain bank coordinator in each hospital, we have established a strong network for brain collection. In addition to caring for these families and patients, brain bank coordinators are responsible for educating both patients and families to understand the necessity and importance of the bank. The consent form to comply with the proceedings of the bank, which will also include storage of personal data, will be given in written form and will be signed by the next of kin and if possible by patients, and witnessed by caregivers and coordinators.

Clinical and Pathological Documentation of Disease Status

We have obtained a Diagnostic Instrument for Brain Studies, Psychosis and Mood Disorder "version," through our established relationship with the Mental Health Research Institute of Victoria, Australia, which is actively engaged in schizophrenia research using more than 60 human brain specimens. The instrument includes autopsy summary, patient's background (sociodemographics), substance use, psychotic symptoms, affective symptoms, and diagnostic summary. Using a modified version of this instrument, it is possible to give a precise diagnosis, following the diagnostic criteria of DSM-III-R, DSM-IV, ICD-10, RDC, and Schneider and Feighner (multidiagnostic evaluation). On completion of the neuropathological report, all the necessary information is entered into the database.

Provisions in Case of Death of a Donor and Tissue Preparation

In case of death of a donor, the responsible brain bank coordinator will be notified immediately and initiate the proper handling of the body. We have established a hot line directly to the hospital, and outside of working hours, switchboard operators will answer calls and page the brain bank staff member on call. The staff member then contacts the caller to arrange for the donation.

The body will be refrigerated at 4°C within the first 4h after death. The brain will be removed within 48h in the autopsy room of the pathology department of the FMU. The brain will be cut midsagittally in half. Coronal, whole-hemisphere slices cut at standardized landmarks are frozen with a cooling device at –80°C. The hemi-brainstem and hemi-cerebellum from half of the brain are detached from the cerebral hemisphere. The brainstem and cerebellar slices are then frozen with the cooling device. Each frozen slice is transferred to a prelabeled plastic bag and stored at –80°C. For neuropathological examination, the other half is immersed in 10% formalin. After 3 weeks, a macroscopical examination will be carried out. The brain is serially sectioned in the coronal plane using the same landmark for fresh brains. Sections are routinely taken from various regions. Blocks are processed through paraffin and sectioned at 10 μm. Routine staining with haematoxyline and eosin is undertaken on all sections. Several silver stains and cresyl violet for cellular evaluation are performed on the temporal lobe, frontal cortex, and caudal hippocampal sections as a routine.

Transport and Storage of Tissue to the Bank

The brain bank coordinator will supervise the process of brain removal, intermediate storage, and transport. The brain tissue is then put into storage in the bank established in our department. The freezers have already been set in a large, well-ventilated room. Freezers have been connected to an automated alarm system, and in case of power failure an emergency generator will be activated so that a security guard can alert the person in charge of the freezers. As important as proper tissue storage is for prospective studies, so too is proper data banking. Data will be both stored in written form on file and digitized in a computer databank.

Ethics and Public Relations Program

Our research proposal described in this paper has been ethically approved by a research ethics committee organized within the FMU and an independent assessment committee made up of individuals representing the patients, their families, and various interest groups. During the past years, our department has greatly expanded its Public Relations program. We have established a close relationship with each hospital's family support group through periodical meetings and lectures, which are coordinated by the bank coordinator. Furthermore, our proposed research programs have been reported in plain form and are well understood by the wider community through newsletters.

Conclusion

To develop postmortem human brain studies of psychiatric illnesses following the recent movement in Western countries, there is an urgent necessity for all users, caregivers, and researchers in Asian countries to recognize the need for intensive collaboration to establish systematic brain banks. Our medical staff must give strong support and education to patients and families so that they can understand the significance of the research and spontaneously join the research projects without being afraid of social discrimination against the mentally ill. We should be sensitive to the opinions and needs of the donor and family at all times during the process. The Mitsubishi Foundation grant awarded to our department this year emphasizes all these matters, and funding will be available to promote further collaboration between Asian countries for the purpose of establishing a Brain Bank Network.

Increased $5HT_{2A}$ Receptors and Impaired Phosphoinositide Signaling in the Postmortem Brain of Suicide Victims

GHANSHYAMA N. PANDEY, YOGESH DWIVEDI, XINGUO REN, ROSALINDA C. ROBERTS, ROBERT CONLEY, and CAROL TAMMINGA

Summary. Abnormalities in the serotonergic system have been implicated in suicidal behavior; however, the neurobiology of teenage suicide is relatively unexplored. We have studied $5HT_{2A}$ receptors, phospholipase C (PLC), and protein kinase C (PKC), which are important components of the phosphoinositide (PI) signaling system and to which $5HT_{2A}$ receptors are linked, in the postmortem brain of teenage suicide victims and nonpsychiatric controls. We found that the number of binding sites (B_{max}) for the $5HT_{2A}$ receptor were increased without any change in the affinity in the membrane fraction and that [^{3}H]PDBu binding to PKC was decreased in the membrane and cytosol fractions of prefrontal cortex of teenage suicide victims as compared to nonpsychiatric control subjects. We also found that the mean PI-PLC activity was significantly decreased in both the membranal and cytosolic fractions of the prefrontal cortex of teenage suicide victims as compared to nonpsychiatric control subjects, and this decrease was accompanied with selective decrease in the immunolabeling of PLC β_1 isozyme without any significant change in PLC-δ_1 or PLC-γ_1. These studies thus indicate that the $5HT_{2A}$ receptors, PKC, and PLC are altered in teenage suicides such that the phosphoinositide signaling system to which $5HT_{2A}$ receptors are linked appear to be impaired in these individuals.

Keywords. $5HT_{2A}$ receptors, Phosphoinositide signaling, Phospholipase C, Protein kinase C, Suicide, Postmortem brain

Introduction

Dysregulation of the serotonergic system has been implicated in depression and suicidal behavior. This concept is based primarily on observations of decreased 5-hydroxy-indoleacetic acid in the cerebrospinal fluid of depressed suicidal patients and on decreased serotonin uptake and decreased serotonin transporter sites in platelets and postmortem brain of depressed or suicidal subjects (Tuomisto and

Psychiatric Institute, Department of Psychiatry, University of Illinois at Chicago, 1601 West Taylor Street, Chicago, IL 60612, USA

Tukiainen 1976; Meltzer et al. 1981; Rausch et al. 1986; Asberg 1997; Arango et al. 1999). Of the serotonin receptor subtypes, $5HT_{1A}$ and $5HT_{2A}$ receptors have been widely studied in depression and suicidal behavior. Some recent studies suggest that $5HT_{2A}$ receptors are increased in platelets of depressed patients and of depressed/suicidal patients (Biegon et al. 1987; Cowen et al. 1987; Arora and Meltzer 1989). In a recent study, we observed that the increase in platelet $5HT_{2A}$ receptors is independent of diagnosis, such that patients with bipolar, schizophrenia, or schizoaffective disorders who exhibit suicidal behavior have increased $5HT_{2A}$ receptors compared with nonsuicidal patients and normal control subjects (Pandey et al. 1995). Postmortem brain studies also suggest increased $5HT_{2A}$ receptors in the brain of suicide victims, although this observation is not replicated in all studies (reviewed by Gross-Isseroff et al. 1998). Nonetheless, these studies suggest an abnormality of $5HT_{2A}$ receptors.

Teenage suicide is a major public health concern. Although several studies have shown neurobiological abnormalities in the postmortem brain of adult suicide victims, virtually no neurobiological studies have been conducted in postmortem brain of teenage suicide victims. It has been suggested that the driving factor for teenage suicidal behavior could be impulsive aggressive behavior (Brent et al. 1993; Apter et al. 1995). Because impulsive aggressive behavior has been shown to be related to an abnormality in the serotonergic system, it is possible that teenage suicide may also be associated with abnormalities in the serotonergic system, specifically the upregulation of $5HT_{2A}$ receptors. To examine if such abnormalities exist in suicide, we studied $5HT_{2A}$ receptors and the receptor-linked phosphoinositide signaling system (PI) in postmortem brain of teenage suicide victims.

In the PI signaling system, activation of receptors by agonists causes the hydrolysis of phosphatidyl inositol 4,5-bisphosphate (PIP_2) by the PI-specific phospholipase C (PLC) enzyme, resulting in the formation of two second messengers, diacylglycerol (DG) and inositol 1,4,5-trisphosphate (IP_3). DG activates a calcium-dependent enzyme known as protein kinase C (PKC), whereas IP_3 mobilizes Ca^{2+} from intracellular stores (Nishizuka 1988; Berridge et al. 1998). To examine if the $5HT_{2A}$ receptor-linked signaling system is altered in teenage suicide, in addition to the $5HT_{2A}$ receptors we also studied the effectors, namely PLC and PKC, in the postmortem brain of teenage suicide victims.

These studies were performed in the prefrontal cortex (Brodmann's areas 8/9) obtained from 18 teenage suicide victims and 18 matched control subjects. The brain samples were obtained from the Brain Collection Program at the Maryland Psychiatric Research Center in Baltimore, MD, USA, in collaboration with the Medical Examiner's Office of the State of Maryland. These samples were free of neuropathological abnormalities and HIV antibodies. Toxicology data were obtained by analyzing urine and blood samples. The subjects were diagnosed on the basis of an interview conducted using the Diagnostic Evaluation After Death (DEAD) and the Structural Clinical Interview for DSM-III-R criteria. Cases were considered to be suicide only if the manner of death was determined to be suicide by the Medical Examiner. The mean age of the suicide subjects was 15.5 ± 1.8 years and that of the control subjects 16.7 ± 1.7 years. The age range was between 12 and 19 years.

$5HT_{2A}$ Receptors in the Prefrontal Cortex of Teenage Suicide Victims

We determined the density and the affinity of $5HT_{2A}$ receptors in Brodmann's areas 8/9 of teenage suicide victims and control subjects by using [^{125}I]LSD as the ligand. Binding was carried out at several concentrations of [^{125}I]LSD (0.25–3.0 nM). Ketanserin (1 μM) was used as the displacer, and B_{max} and K_D were calculated by Scatchard analysis. When we compared the B_{max} values of [^{125}I]LSD binding, we found that B_{max} of [^{125}I] LSD binding was significantly increased in suicide victims compared with control subjects, without any significant differences in K_D values (Fig. 1). To examine if there was a relationship between the presence or absence of mental disorders and B_{max} of $5HT_{2A}$ receptors, we subdivided the teenage suicide subjects into those who had a history of mental disorders and those without a history of mental disorders. We did not find any significant differences between these groups, and B_{max} in both groups was significantly higher than in control subjects. Our studies thus indicate that $5HT_{2A}$ receptors are significantly increased in the prefrontal cortex of teenage suicide victims.

PLC in the Prefrontal Cortex of Teenage Suicide Victims

PLC, one of the major components of the PI signaling cascade, hydrolyzes PIP_2 into the second messengers IP_3 and DG. PLC is predominantly present in the cytosol, but its presence in the membrane has also been demonstrated (Lee et al. 1987). PLC isoforms have been classified into three major families and further subdivided into several subtypes. The major families are PLC-β, PLC-γ, and PLC-δ (Cockcroft and Thomas 1992). We determined PI-PLC activity and the immunolabeling of PLC-β_1, -γ_1, and -δ_1 isozymes in both the cytosol and the membrane fraction of prefrontal cortex from teenage suicide victims and matched normal control subjects. PI-PLC activity and the immunolabeling of PLC isozymes were determined according to the methods published by us earlier (Dwivedi and Pandey 1999a). We found that the mean PI-PLC activity was significantly lower in both the membrane and the cytosol fraction of the prefrontal cortex of teenage suicide victims as compared with normal subjects (Fig. 2). As was determined in the case of $5HT_{2A}$ receptors, we also examined the effects of a history of mental disorders on PI-PLC activity. Among the 18 suicide sub-

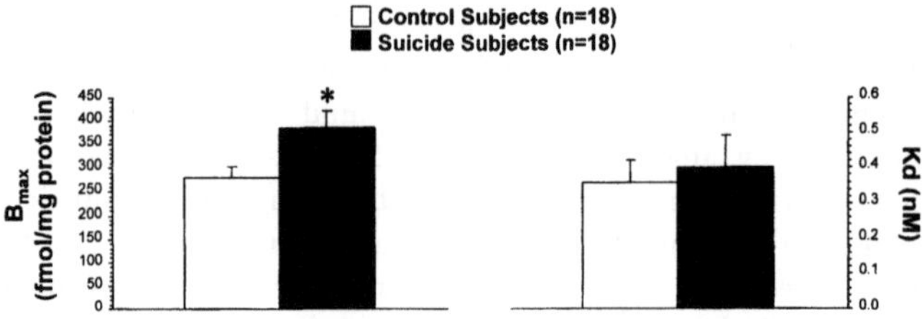

FIG. 1. [^{125}I]LSD binding to $5HT_{2A}$ receptors in prefrontal cortex of suicide (*black bars*) and normal control (*white bars*) subjects. Values are mean ± SD. *$P < 0.001$

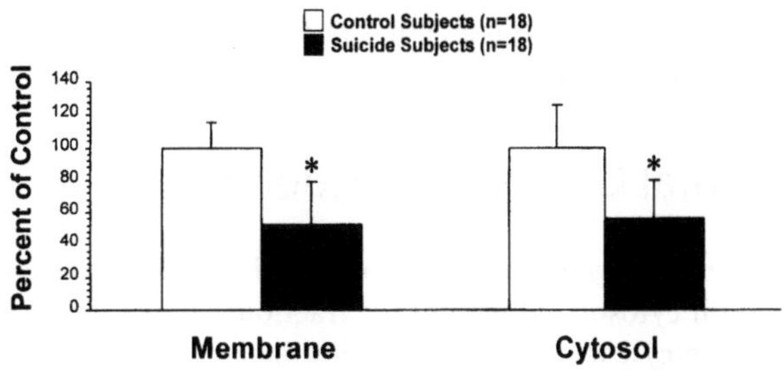

FIG. 2. PI-PLC activity in membrane (*left*) and cytosol (*right*) fractions of prefrontal cortex of suicide (*black bars*) and normal control (*white bars*) subjects. Values are mean ± SD. $^{*}P < 0.001$

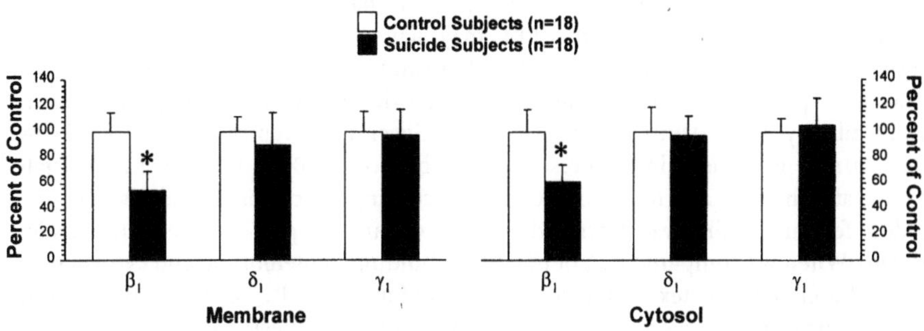

FIG. 3. Immunolabeling of PLC isozymes in membrane (*left*) and cytosol (*right*) fractions of prefrontal cortex of suicide (*black bars*) and control (*white bars*) subjects. Values are mean ± SD. $^{*}P < 0.001$

jects, 6 had no known history of mental disorders, 10 had a history of mental disorders, and 2 had a history of alcohol abuse but not mental disorders. We found that the mean PI-PLC activity in both the membrane and the cytosol fraction in suicide subjects with a history of mental disorder was not significantly different from that of suicide subjects with no history of mental disorders. However, PI-PLC activity in suicide subjects with or without a history of mental disorders was significantly lower than in normal control subjects.

To examine if the decrease in PI-PLC activity in both cytosol and membrane fractions of the prefrontal cortex was related to changes in a specific PI-PLC isozyme(s), we determined the immunolabeling of PLC-β_1, -γ_1, and -δ_1 in both the membrane and the cytosol fraction. We found that the immunolabeling of PLC-β_1 was significantly lower in both the membrane and the cytosol fraction of teenage suicide subjects compared with the normal control subjects, whereas no significant differences were found in the immunolabeling of either PLC-δ_1 or PLC-γ_1 (Fig. 3). We again examined the effect of the presence of mental disorders in the suicide subjects, and as with PI-PLC activity, no significant differences were found in any of the PLC isozymes between suicide subjects with or without a history of mental disorders. These results suggest that the presence or absence of mental disorders has no significant effect on PI-PLC activity or on any of the PLC isozymes, but that PLC-β_1 levels are significantly lower in suicide subjects than in normal controds.

PKC in Prefrontal Cortex of Suicide Victims

PKC is a key regulatory enzyme that is present in various tissues and has been shown to be present in both cytosol and membrane fractions. Activation of PKC results in its translocation from cytosol to membrane (Nishizuka 1988). It has been suggested that the association of PKC with the membrane is required for any subsequent physiological responses. The majority of nonactivated PKC is located in the cytosol fraction and tends to relocate on activation. PKC has been shown to be involved in many neuronal and physiological functions (Nishizuka 1988). The role of PKC in mental disorders, and particularly in suicide, is unclear and has not been extensively studied; however, a few studies suggest that PKC may play a crucial role in mental disorders (Friedman et al. 1993; Masliah et al. 1990; Manji and Lenox 1999). We therefore studied PKC in the postmortem brain of teenage suicide victims by determining [^{3}H]phorbol 12,13-dibutryrate (PDBu) binding to PKC. Several concentrations of [^{3}H]PDBu (0.8–3.0 nM) were used in the presence and absence of 10 μM phorbol 12-myristate 13-acetate, and B_{max} and K_D were calculated according to Scatchard analysis. The procedure for the binding was described by us in an earlier report (Dwivedi and Pandey 1999b). When we compared B_{max} of [^{3}H]PDBu binding in membrane and cytosol fractions of prefrontal cortex of suicide subjects, we found that B_{max} of [^{3}H]PDBu binding was significantly decreased in both fractions of suicide subjects as compared to with normal control subjects; however, no changes were observed in K_D values between control and suicide subjects (Fig. 4). Similarly, as was observed in the case of PLC and $5HT_{2A}$ receptors, there were no significant differences in [^{3}H]PDBu binding, either in the membrane or the cytosol fraction, between suicide subjects with a history of

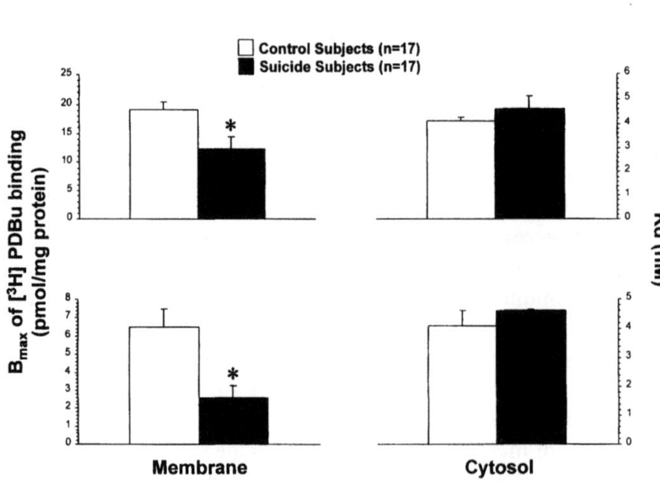

Fig. 4. [^{3}H]PDBu binding to PKC in membrane (*left*) and cytosol (*right*) fractions of prefrontal cortex of suicide (*black bars*) and control (*white bars*) subjects. Values are mean ± SD. *$P < 0.001$

mental disorders and suicide subjects with no such history, although suicide subjects with or without mental disorders had significantly lower [^{3}H]PDBu binding in both the membrane and the cytosol fraction of the prefrontal cortex. These results thus suggest that PKC binding sites are significantly decreased in the postmortem brain of teenage suicide victims.

Discussion

Our present studies of the $5HT_{2A}$ receptor subtype and of the PI signaling system in postmortem brain of teenage suicide victims indicate that teenage suicide may be associated with an increase in $5HT_{2A}$ receptors and that this increase may also involve abnormalities in the PI signaling system, such that the activities of the effector enzyme PI-PLC are decreased, and that this decrease is associated with a decrease in the expression of a specific isozyme, PLC-β_1. Further, there appears to be a decrease in [^{3}H]PDBu binding to PKC, both in the membrane and in the cytosol fraction of the prefrontal cortex of teenage suicide victims.

As mentioned earlier there are some studies of postmortem brain of adult suicide victims that indicate an increase in the number of $5HT_{2A}$ receptors, although these studies are not consistent (Gross-Isseroff et al. 1998). Our studies indicate an increase in B_{max} of $5HT_{2A}$ receptors in the prefrontal cortex of teenage suicide subjects as determined by binding techniques using [^{125}I]LSD as a ligand. The inconsistencies in the literature in regard to $5HT_{2A}$ receptors may be related to several factors, such as the type of radioligand used in studies of $5HT_{2A}$ receptors, differences in methodology, differences in postmortem interval, and other variables. Nonetheless, our studies of teenage suicide victims suggest an upregulation of $5HT_{2A}$ receptors in suicide.

$5HT_{2A}$ receptors are linked to the PI signaling system through G_q protein, which is coupled with PLC-β_1. There are few studies of PI-PLC in postmortem brain of adult suicide victims, and these studies are mostly negative. For example, Jope et al. (1996) did not find any significant abnormalities in calcium-stimulated PI-PLC activity in postmortem brain tissue obtained from adult bipolar patients. Also, Pacheco et al. (1996) did not observe any significant abnormalities in PI-PLC activity or in PLC-β_1 immunolabeling in prefrontal or occipital cortex of postmortem brain obtained from depressed adult suicide subjects. However, in the present investigation we observed that immunolabeling of the specific PLC-β_1 isozyme and the activity of PI-PLC are decreased in both cytosol and membrane fractions of prefrontal cortex of teenage suicide victims. In addition, [^{3}H]PDBu binding to PKC was also decreased in the prefrontal cortex of these subjects, although we do not know whether this decrease is associated with a decrease in PKC activity and/or in expression of any specific PKC isozyme(s). Thus, overall our study suggests an increase in $5HT_{2A}$ receptors in postmortem brain of teenage suicide subjects that is associated with decreased functional responses, as indicated by decreased PI-PLC and PKC.

Another important aspect of this study is that the abnormalities in $5HT_{2A}$ receptors, PLC-β_1, and [^{3}H]PDBu binding to PKC are not restricted to or associated with major mental disorders. We observed that there were no significant differences in $5HT_{2A}$ receptors, PLC-β_1, or PKC binding sites in suicide victims with or without the presence of major mental disorders, although these levels were abnormal in suicide subjects compared with normal control subjects. However, to further evaluate these abnormalities in $5HT_{2A}$ receptors, PI-PLC, or PKC isozymes in relation to specific mental disorders, a larger number of suicide subjects with various mental disorders should be studied.

The mechanisms by which $5HT_{2A}$ receptors are increased and PLC and PKC are decreased in postmortem brain of teenage suicide victims are not clear at the present time; however, several studies suggest that manipulation of the HPA axis may cause upregulation of $5HT_{2A}$ receptors (Chaouloff 1995) and decreased expression of PKC and PLC isozymes (Dwivedi and Pandey 1999a, 1999b). Further, overactive HPA function has been shown to be associated with depression and suicide (Nelson and Davis 1997). It is quite possible that the HPA axis may be regulating $5HT_{2A}$ receptors and PKC and PLC in suicide subjects.

In summary, it appears that serotonergic abnormalities, specifically upregulation of $5HT_{2A}$ receptors and abnormalities in the PI signaling system at the level of PKC and PLC, may be associated with the pathophysiology of teenage suicide. These abnormalities appear to be specific to suicidal behavior rather than to the presence of specific or general mental disorders.

References

Apter A, Gothelf D, Orbach I, et al (1995) Correlation of suicidal and violent behavior in different diagnostic categories in hospitalized adolescent patients. J Am Acad Child Adolesc Psychiatry 34:912–918

Arango V, Underwood MD, Bakalian MJ, et al (1999) Reduction in serotonin transporter sites in prefrontal cortex is localized in suicide and widespread in major depression. Soc Neurosci Abstr 25:1798

Arora RC, Meltzer HY (1989) Increased serotonin-2 ($5HT_2$) receptor binding as measured by [^{3}H]-lysergic acid diethylamide [^{3}H]LSD in the blood platelets of depressed patients. Life Sci 44:725–734

Asberg M (1997) Neurotransmitters and suicidal behavior. The evidence from cerebrospinal fluid studies. Ann NY Acad Sci 836:158–181

Berridge MJ, Bootman MD, Lipp P (1998) Calcium—a life and death signal. Nature (Lond) 395:645–648

Biegon A, Weizman A, Karp L, et al (1987) Serotonin 5-HT2 receptor binding on blood platelets—a peripheral marker for depression? Life Sci 41:2485–2492

Brent D, Kolko D, Wartella M, et al (1993) Adolescent psychiatric inpatients risk of suicide attempt at 6-month follow-up. J Am Acad Child Adolesc Psychiatry 32:95–105

Chaouloff F (1995) Regulation of 5HT receptors by corticosteroids: where do we stand? Fundam Clin Pharmacol 9:219–233

Cockcroft S, Thomas GM (1992) Inositol-lipid-specific phospholipase C isoenzymes and their differential regulation by receptors. Biochem J 288:1–14

Cowen PJ, Charig EM, Fraser S, Elliott JM (1987) Platelet 5HT receptor binding during depressive illness and tricyclic antidepressant treatment. J Affect Disord 13:45–50

Dwivedi Y, Pandey GN (1999a) Repeated administration of dexamethasone increases phosphoinositide-specific phospholipase C β_1 activity and mRNA and protein expression of the phospholipase C β_1 isozyme in rat brain. J Neurochem 73:780–790

Dwivedi Y, Pandey GN (1999b) Administration of dexamethasone upregulates protein kinase C activity and the expression of γ and ε protein kinase C isozymes in the rat brain. J Neurochem 72:380–387

Friedman E, Wang HY, Levinson D, et al (1993) Altered platelet protein kinase C activity in bipolar affective disorder, manic episode. Biol Psychiatry 33:520–525

Gross-Isseroff R, Biegon A, Voet H, Weizman A (1998) The suicide brain: a review of postmortem receptor/transporter binding studies. Neurosci Biobehav 22:653–661

Jope RS, Song L, Li PP, et al (1996) The phosphoinositide signal transduction system is impaired in bipolar affective disorder brain. J Neurochem 66:2402–2409

Lee K-Y, Ryu SH, Suh P-G (1987) Phospholipase C associated with particulate fractions of bovine brain. Biochemistry 84:5540–5544

Manji HK, Lenox RH (1999) Protein kinase C signaling in the brain: molecular transduction of mood stabilization in the treatment of manic depressive illness. Biol Psychiatry 46:1328–1351

Masliah E, Cole G, Shimohama S, et al (1990) Differential involvement of protein kinase C isozymes in Alzheimer's disease. J Neurosci 10:2113–2124

Meltzer HY, Arora RC, Baber R, Tricou BJ (1981) Serotonin uptake in blood platelets of psychiatric patients. Arch Gen Psychiatry 38:1322–1326

Nelson JC, Davis JM (1997) DST studies in psychotic depression: a meta-analysis. Am J Psychiatry 154:1497–1503

Nishizuka Y (1988) The molecular heterogeneity of protein kinase C and its implications for cellular regulation. Nature (Lond) 334:661–665

Pacheco MA, Stockmeier C, Meltzer HY, et al (1996) Alterations in phosphoinositide signaling and G-protein levels in depressed suicide brain. Brain Res 723:37–45

Pandey GN, Pandey SC, Dwivedi Y, et al (1995) Platelet serotonin 2A receptors: a potential biological marker for suicidal behavior. Am J Psychiatry 152:850–855

Rausch JL, Janowsky DS, Risch SC, Huey LY (1986) A kinetic analysis and replication of decreased platelet serotonin uptake in depressed patients. Psychiatry Res 19:105–112

Tuomisto J, Tukiainen E (1976) Decreased uptake of 5-hydroxytryptamine in blood platelets from depressed patients. Nature (Lond) 262:596–598

Neurochemical Changes in Postmortem Brain Tissue from Subjects with Schizophrenia: Implications for the Illness

BRIAN DEAN

Summary. The underlying neurobiology of schizophrenia remains to be elucidated. However, there is now a growing body of information from the study of tissue obtained postmortem that suggests changes in the serotonergic systems of the brain are involved in the pathology of this illness. The evidence implicating differential changes in the serotonergic systems of the frontal cortex and hippocampus of subjects with schizophrenia is reviewed.

Keywords. Schizophrenia, Serotonin, Postmortem, Frontal cortex, Hippocampus

Serotonin and the Pathology of Schizophrenia

Schizophrenia is a serious psychiatric illness affecting approximately 1% of the population worldwide [1]. Given the relatively high incidence of schizophrenia, it is surprising that little is known about the pathological processes that precipitate the illness. This lack of knowledge means that most of the hypotheses concerning schizophrenia are, in the main, based on neuropharmacological findings [2]. Abnormalities in the serotonergic system in schizophrenia are suggested by the observation that lysergic acid diethylamide, a serotonin (5HT) receptor agonist, causes or exacerbates schizophrenic-like symptoms [2]. The improved therapeutic outcomes using antipsychotic drugs that antagonize 5HT receptors also suggest a role for 5HT in the pathology of schizophrenia [3]. Together, the apparently opposing effects of agonists and antagonists on schizophrenic-like symptoms suggest that the symptoms of schizophrenia are due, at least in part, to overactive serotonergic neurons.

The Rebecca L. Cooper Research Laboratories, The Mental Health Research Institute of Victoria and The University of Melbourne Department of Psychiatry, Parkville, Victoria, 3052, Australia

Evidence for Abnormalities in Serotoninergic Systems from the Study of Postmortem Brain Tissue

In addition to neuropharmacological evidence, there is now a growing body of data from the study of tissue obtained post mortem to support a role for serotonergic abnormalities in the pathology of schizophrenia. The most consistent change in serotonergic markers is a decrease in the density of $5HT_{2A}$ receptors in the prefrontal cortex from subjects with schizophrenia [4–10]. The consistency of this finding on the $5HT_{2A}$ receptor does not appear to be as predominant in other brain regions. For example, one study has reported an increase in the density of $5HT_{2A}$ receptors in the hippocampus from subjects with schizophrenia [11], but another reported a decrease in that receptor in the parahippocampal gyrus with no change in the hippocampus [10]. Thus, more studies are needed to determine the extent of changes of $5HT_{2A}$ receptors in schizophrenia.

Since the cloning of the $5HT_{2A}$ receptor, studies have attempted to gain further information on the mechanism by which this receptor is changed in schizophrenia. One such study showed a decreased level of the $5HT_{2A}$ receptor binding and its mRNA in BA 46 from subjects with schizophrenia [10]. Decreased levels of mRNA for $5HT_{2A}$ receptors have also been measured in another study of other areas of the prefrontal cortex from antipsychotic-free schizophrenic subjects [12], but that study did not report the binding data on the same brain tissue. However, it would seem likely that the decrease in density of cortical $5HT_{2A}$ receptors in schizophrenia is caused by decreased expression of that receptor. Studies are now needed to determine which factors may be causing this decreased expression of cortical $5HT_{2A}$ receptors in schizophrenia.

The study that showed a decrease in $5HT_{2A}$ receptor density in BA 46 from subjects with schizophrenia also reported an increase in the density of $5HT_{1A}$ receptors in that brain region [10]. There was no change in the levels of mRNA for the $5HT_{1A}$ receptor in that tissue. This result could suggest that the increased density of the $5HT_{1A}$ receptor in schizophrenia is not caused by an increase in the rate of expression. Other studies have also reported an increase in $5HT_{1A}$ receptors in other areas of the cortex [13–15], indicating that there are widespread changes in this receptor in the brains of subjects with schizophrenia. Results from the study of the hippocampus from subjects with schizophrenia seem to be less consistent with two studies reporting no change in the $5HT_{1A}$ receptor [10,13] and one reporting a decrease in that receptor [11].

It has been reported that the density of 5HT transporter (SERT) was decreased in the prefrontal cortex from subjects with schizophrenia [9,11]. This finding raised the possibility that changes in 5HT receptors in schizophrenia were a result of changes in the prevailing concentrations of 5HT caused by decreased 5HT uptake by the SERT. More recent studies have failed to show a change in SERT in the prefrontal cortex from subjects with schizophrenia [16–18], placing the findings from the earlier studies in doubt. Given the importance of SERT in maintaining serotonergic function, more studies are needed to clarify whether there is a change in cortical SERT in schizophrenia.

In the hippocampus from subjects with schizophrenia, it has been suggested that a change in the affinity of [^{3}H]paroxetine binding has resulted from a conformational change in SERT [16,19]. Moreover, in studies of SERT in the human platelet, a change in the affinity of [^{3}H]paroxetine binding of the same order of magnitude as seen in the hippocampus from subjects with schizophrenia was associated with a decrease in the capacity of SERT to take up 5HT [20]. As neuronal and platelet SERT are the same gene product, it would seem likely that the same relationship between the affinity of [^{3}H]paroxetine binding and 5HT uptake would hold in both environments. This would therefore suggest that the conformational change in SERT in subjects with schizophrenia would result in decreased hippocampal 5HT uptake and hence a relatively hyperserotonergic state in that brain region. Extending this hypothesis into the clinical arena, it could be that it is by blocking overactive serotonergic neurotransmission in the hippocampus that antipsychotic drugs which antagonize serotonin receptor gain their improved therapeutic outcomes when used in the treatment of schizophrenia.

In summary, studies using postmortem tissue clearly support a role for changes in serotonergic function in schizophrenia. From studies on the frontal cortex and hippocampus, the mechanisms underlying such changes seem likely to differ between brain regions. Understanding these different changes and how they can generate some of the symptoms of schizophrenia will be a high priority for those studying both tissue obtained post mortem and those attempting to understand the basic mechanism of serotonergic function.

Acknowledgments. Brian Dean is a recipient of a NARSAD Young Investigator Award. This work was supported by NH&MRC Project Grant 11425. Finally, my thanks to Dr. Elizabeth Scarr for her editorial assistance in preparing this chapter.

References

1. Goldstein G, Hall W, Andrews G (1984) The incidence of schizophrenia in New South Wales, Australia. Acta Psychiatr Scand 70:220–227
2. Meltzer HY (1987) Biological studies in schizophrenia. Schizophr Bull 13:77–107
3. Huttunen M (1995) The evolution of the serotonin-dopamine antagonist concept. J Clin Psychopharmacol 15(suppl 1):4S–10S
4. Dean B, Hayes W (1996) Decreased frontal cortical serotonin 2A receptors in subjects with schizophrenia. Schizophr Res 21:133–139
5. Dean B, Hussain T, Hayes W, et al (1999) Changes in serotonin 2A and GABA(A) receptors in schizophrenia: studies on the human dorsolateral prefrontal cortex. J Neurochem 72:1593–1599
6. Arora RC, Meltzer HY (1991) Serotonin 2 (5-HT2) receptor binding in the frontal cortex of schizophrenic patients. J Neural Transm Gen Sect 85:19–29
7. Bennett JP, Enna SJ, Bylund DB, et al (1979) Neurotransmitter receptors in frontal cortex of schizophrenics. Arch Gen Psychiatry 36:927–934
8. Mita T, Hanada S, Nishino N, et al (1986) Decreased serotonin S2 and increased dopamine D2 receptors in chronic schizophrenics. Biol Psychiatry 21:1407–1414
9. Laruelle M, Abi-Dargham A, Casanova MF, et al (1993) Selective abnormalities of prefrontal serotonergic receptors in schizophrenia: a postmortem study. Arch Gen Psychiatry 50:810–818
10. Burnet PW, Eastwood SL, Harrison PJ (1996) 5-HT1A and 5-HT2A receptor mRNA and binding site densities are differentially altered in schizophrenia. Neuropsychopharmacology 15:442–455

11. Joyce JN, Shane A, Lexow N, et al (1993) Serotonin uptake sites and serotonin receptors are altered in the limbic system of schizophrenics. Neuropsychopharmacology 8:315–336
12. Hernandez I, Sokolov BP (2000) Abnormalities in 5-HT2A receptor mRNA expression in frontal cortex of chronic elderly schizophrenics with varying histories of neuroleptic treatment. J Neurosci Res 59:218–225
13. Hashimoto T, Nishino N, Nakai H, Tanaka C (1991) Increase in serotonin 5-HT1A receptors in prefrontal and temporal cortices of brains from patients with chronic schizophrenia. Life Sci 48:355–363
14. Sumiyoshi T, Stockmeier CA, Overholser JC, et al (1996) Serotonin 1A receptors are increased in postmortem prefrontal cortex in schizophrenia. Brain Res 708:209–214
15. Simpson MDC, Lubman DI, Slater P, Deakin JFW (1996) Autoradiography with [^{3}H]8-OH-DPAT reveals increases in 5-HT1A receptors in ventral prefrontal cortex in schizophrenia. Biol Psychiatry 39:919–928
16. Dean B, Opeskin K, Pavey G, et al (1995) [^{3}H]Paroxetine binding is altered in the hippocampus but not the frontal cortex or caudate nucleus from subjects with schizophrenia. J Neurochem 64:1197–1202
17. Dean B, Tomaskovic-Crook E, Opeskin K, et al (1999) No change in the density of the serotonin 1A receptor, the serotonin 4 receptor or the serotonin transporter in the dorsolateral prefrontal cortex from subjects with schizophrenia. Neurochem Int 34:109–115
18. Gurevich EV, Joyce JN (1997) Alterations in the cortical serotonergic system in schizophrenia: a postmortem study. Biol Psychiatry 42:529–545
19. Naylor L, Dean B, Opeskin K, et al (1996) Possible conformational changes in the serotonin transporter in the hippocampus of subjects with schizophrenia identified using [^{3}H]paroxetine. J Neural Transm Gen Sect 103:749–757
20. Maguire K, Tuckwell V, Pereira A, et al (1993) Significant correlation between ^{14}C-5-HT uptake by and ^{3}H-paroxetine binding to platelets from healthy volunteers. Biol Psychiatry 34:356–360

Brain Banking in Psychiatric Disorders: The Amsterdam Experience

Rivka Ravid[1], Wouter Kamphorst[2], Marina Kahlmann[1], and Anne Holtrop[1]

Summary. The growing number of sophisticated neurobiological techniques that can be applied on postmortem brain obtained from psychiatric patients increases the pressure on brain banks to supply autopsy material to the scientific community. Brain banks that collect postmortem tissue from patients with psychiatric disorders form an important link between clinicians, scientists, and neuropathologists. The rapid autopsy system we set up in Amsterdam for collecting brain specimens for research on depression, bipolar disorders, and schizophrenia includes matching for several factors, both antemortem and postmortem. Antemortem factors include age, sex, agonal state, seasonal alterations, circadian variation, clock time of death, and medication. Postmortem factors include postmortem delay, fixation and storage time, and lateralization. The material and data collected by the Netherlands Brain Bank as presented in this chapter illustrate the wide variety of potentialities and pitfalls in the use of autopsy tissue for research on psychiatric disorders.

Keywords. Brain bank, Autopsy, Postmortem, Affective disorders, Schizophrenia

The possible causes and underlying pathologies of most psychiatric disorders are still unknown, and current scientific research is focusing on the neurobiological entities and the possible changes occuring in the brains of affected patients. The Netherlands Brain Bank (NBB) was established in 1985 to support neurobiological and medical research by supplying clinically and neuropathologically well-characterized postmortem specimens from patients with neurological and psychiatric disorders. The NBB is part of the European Brain Bank Network and works also in close collaboration with other brain banks worldwide. The NBB's unique procedures of rapid autopsy with a short postmortem delay and fresh dissection protocol provide high-quality specimens for research (Fig. 1). We use the pH of the brain as a measure for agonal state and the quality of the tissue for scientific research (Ravid et al. 1992; Kingsburry et al. 1995; Schram et al. 1999).

The availability of postmortem material has remained small over the years, while the interest from the international scientific community is ever growing. To provide a solution to this problem, the NBB, in collaboration with several psychiatric depart-

[1] Netherlands Brain Bank, Meibergdreef 33, 1105 AZ, Amsterdam, Netherlands
[2] Department of Pathology, Free University Hospital, Amsterdam, Netherlands

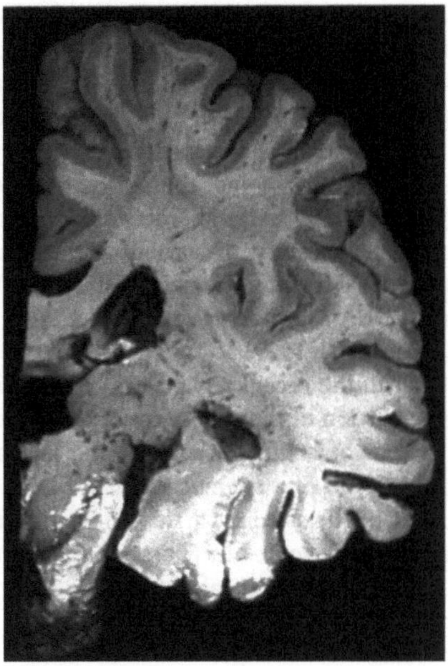

FIG. 1. Coronal section of cerebral left hemisphere of a 48-year-old schizophrenic patient, obtained via the rapid autopsy system of the Netherlands Brain Bank (case 99-037). (Courtesy of G. van der Meulen)

ments and institutions, started to implement a postmortem research program for depression, bipolar disorders, and schizophrenia, including the possibility of genetic research through simultaneously approaching patients and their relatives. The psychiatrist approaches the potential candidates and conducts the antemortem and retrospective diagnostics. The NBB established a national donor program based on informed consent of the patients and their next of kin obtained during life. The NBB makes all possible effort to operate a well-functioning autopsy system that works within a well-defined ethical code of conduct in addition to the essential internationally accepted safety measures against hazardous agents for brain bank personnel and researchers using the tissues.

Postmortem research of schizophrenia has not progressed rapidly, partly because of the development of several techniques that enabled scientists to do in vivo research on patients by applying computerized tomography (CT) and magnetic resonance imaging (MRI), which proved to be successful, noninvasive, and fast techniques to investigate the morphology of the brain. The development of neuroleptica and the lack of clear histopathological markers for the disease as well as a lack of consistent findings from the neuropathological studies were other contributing factors to the loss of interest in postmortem research (Kromkamp et al. 1998). Several structural imaging studies showed subtle changes in the brain structure, for example, enlargement of the ventricles and the cortical sulci, as well as smaller hippocampi. These findings imply a neurobiological substrate for schizophrenia.

Minor tissue abnormalities were also reported in limbic structures. Limbic dysfunction may lead to a dissociation between cognitive activities and basic emotional reactions, which may account for several aspects of the psychopathology of the disease. MRI studies revealed a decrease in the size of the thalamus in schizophrenia, which may in turn account for hallucinations and delusions (Andreasen et al. 1994). Postmortem studies of the thalamus indicated a reduction of neurons in the mediodorsal nucleus (MDN) as well as a volume reduction of MDN (Pakkenberg 1990). Other findings such as cortical asymmetry indicated that schizophrenia is a disorder in the early neurodevelopmental stage of brain growth, an argument against the notion of the disease being a degenerative brain disorder (Bogerts 1993, 1999). Interest in postmortem research increased as a result of the applicability of various modern neurobiological techniques on postmortem material. Immunocytochemistry, in situ hybridization, receptor autoradiography, and DNA microarrays are all leading to a better understanding of disease processes (Kahn et al. 1999).

With the recent advances in molecular biology and with the availability of a large proportion of the sequences of human genes, it is possible to start to study the pathogenesis of schizophrenics at the level of gene expression. Enhanced or decreased expression of a specific gene may indicate molecular changes underlying functional deficits observed in patients suffering from schizophrenia. Thus, the study of gene expression profiles in postmortem brain tissue from schizophrenic patients will be our approach to reveal potential drug targets; radioactive DNA probes prepared from polyA + RNA extracts from subdivisions of the thalamus and cortex that display neuroanatomical changes will be used for screening.

We are currently putting continuous effort in recruiting more patients to our donor program and have a better collaboration with the various psychiatric institutions to convince psychiatrists that basic research is timely and essential for the development of appropriate therapies. Investigating the biological basis of psychiatric diseases requires a professional battery of techniques applied by brain banks that collect the tissues; dissection, handling, storage, and dissimination of samples should be standardized. Supplying clinically and neuropathologically well-documented material can significantly contribute to the understanding of the causes and pathologies of the various disorders and lead to new targets for therapeutic agents.

References

Andreasen NC, Arndt S, Swaze V, et al (1994) Thalamic abnormalities in schizophrenia visualized through magnetic resonance image averaging. Science 266:294–298

Bogerts B (1993) Recent advances in the neuropathology of schizophrenia. Schizophr Bull 19(2):431–445

Bogerts B (1999) The neuropathology of schizophrenic disease: historical aspects and present knowledge. Eur Arch Psychiatry Clin Neurosci 249(suppl 4):2–13

Kahn J, Bittner ML, Chen Y, et al (1999) DNA microarray technology: the anticipated impact on the study of human disease. Biochim Biophys Acta 1423:M17–M28

Kingsburry AE, Foster OJ, Nisbet AP, et al (1995) Tissue pH as indicator of mRNA preservation in human post-mortem brain. Brain Res Mol Brain Res 28:311–318

Kromkamp M, Ravid R, Swaab DF, et al. Protocol for the initiation of a post mortem research programme in schizophrenia in the Netherlands. Netherlands Brainbank, Annual Report 1998–2000, (in press)

Pakkenberg B (1990) Pronounced reduction of total neuron number in mediodorsal thalamic nucleus and nucleus accumbens in schzoiphrenics. Arch Gen Psychiatry 47:1023–1028

Ravid R, van Zwieten EJ, Swaab DF (1992) Brain banking and the human hypothalamus: factors to match for, pitfalls and potentials. In: Swaab DF, Hofman MA, Mirmiran M, et al (eds) The human hypothalamus in health and disease. Progress in brain research, vol 93. Elsevier, Amsterdam, pp 83–95

Schramm M, Falkai P, Tepest R, et al (1999) Stability of RNA transcripts in post-mortem psychiatric brains. J Neural Transm 106(3–4):329–335

Escalating Dose-Binge Exposure to Amphetamine and Methamphetamine: Behavioral and Neurochemical Characterization

David S. Segal and Ronald Kuczenski

Summary. We have used an escalating dose-binge (ED-B) regimen in rats to simulate a pattern of drug intake typically displayed by high-dose stimulant abusers. ED-B treatment results in the progressive emergence of a unique behavioral profile that could not be produced by any acute or single daily injection stimulant dose tested. Corresponding to this emergent behavioral profile, in vivo microdialysis revealed that the caudate-putamen dopamine response is significantly diminished whereas the nucleus accumbens dopamine response is unchanged or slightly increased. To further assess the relevancy of this model in the context of available neurochemical markers associated with various patterns of stimulant abuse, we determined how a methamphetamine ED-B treatment affects striatal dopamine integrity. Our data revealed a pattern of change in striatal dopamine levels, as well as in measures of the dopamine transporter and vesicular monoamine transporter that paralleled the findings in postmortem brain tissue from methamphetamine abusers. During the 30 days after the last binge exposure, the reduced dopamine levels and the altered behavioral response to subsequent methamphetamine challenge significantly recovered, suggesting that the functional consequences of the ED-B treatment may not be permanent.

Keywords. Methamphetamine, Binge, Neurotoxicity, Animal models, Dopamine transporter

Introduction

Our recent research has involved the use of an escalating dose-multiple binge (ED-B) treatment as a model of stimulant psychosis [18]. This model represents a significant departure from the typical sensitization procedures we and others have used to study chronic stimulant effects. In particular, this treatment was developed to more closely simulate the drug exposure patterns most frequently associated with the induction of stimulant psychosis. The rationale for the ED-B paradigm is based on several characteristics of the use patterns in stimulant abusers. For one, stimulant psychosis reflects a qualitative change in the stimulant response after high doses are gradually

Department of Psychiatry, School of Medicine, University of California, 9500 Gilman Drive, San Diego, La Jolla, CA 92093, USA achieved, often during the course of frequent high-dose drug administrations over relatively long periods of time (i.e., binges) [1]. It also appears that the psychosis becomes progressively more pronounced within and between successive binges [1,15]. Moreover, high-dose patterns of stimulant abuse are virtually always preceded by some period of gradually increasing dosage; i.e., as many of the toxic effects subside with repeated drug exposures, individuals can survive the otherwise lethal high doses frequently administered during repeated binges and associated with the induction of psychosis [1,4–6,16,17]. Therefore, it is important to note that in our treatment model animals are initially exposed to an ED-B pretreatment regimen.

Results

Our previous findings revealed that the ED-B treatment results in the progressive emergence of unique behavioral and dopamine response profiles (Fig. 1) [11,18,19,21]. The behavioral characteristics include a decrease in the duration of the stereotypy phase (tolerance) (Fig. 1B), and then a profound qualitative change in the subsequent

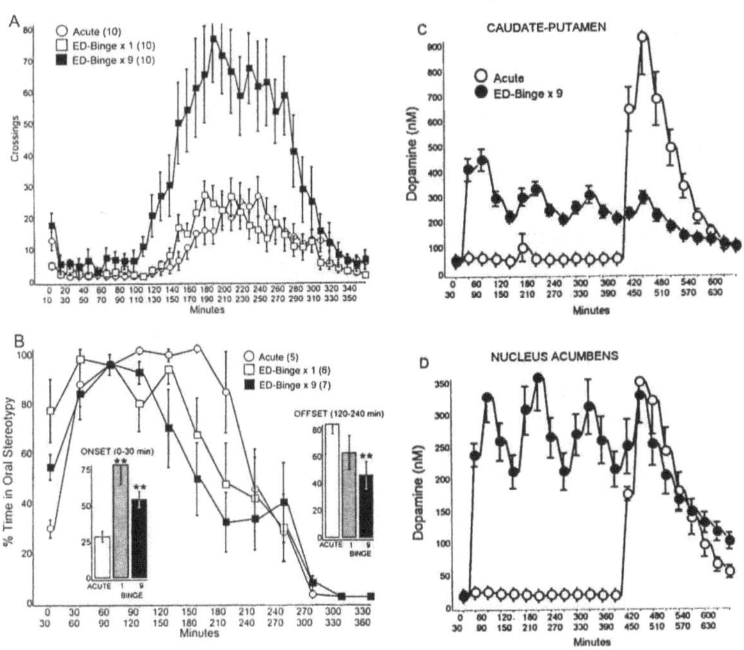

FIG. 1A–D. Effects of an ED-B amphetamine treatment on the behavioral and neurochemical responses to a subsequent amphetamine binge (8 mg/kg). **A** Locomotor responses and **B** stereotypy responses to the fourth 8 mg/kg amphetamine injection of a 1st or 9th binge compared to an acute drug administration. **C** Caudate-putamen and **D** nucleus accumbens dopamine responses to the 9th amphetamine binge compared to an acute drug administration

period of locomotor activation (Fig. 1A). During this latter phase the animals appear to be highly "agitated" and engage in a repetitive burst pattern of locomotion. This behavioral profile gradually develops over multiple binge exposures, and the number of binges required is inversely related to the stimulant dose.

Concurrently, there are differential changes in the dopamine (DA) response profile: the caudate-putamen DA response is significantly diminished (Fig. 1C), whereas the nucleus accumbens DA response is unchanged or slightly increased (Fig. 1D) [11,18,21]. These behavioral and neurochemical effects persist in response to an acute stimulant challenge for at least several days after the last binge. Furthermore, our results from a series of studies indicate that ED-B administration of all stimulants tested, including both DA releasers and uptake blockers like methylphenidate [20], result in the gradual development of the unique emergent behavioral profile and the regionally differential DA response patterns. Importantly, these effects could not be produced by any acute or single daily injection stimulant dose tested.

One major problem in assessing the relevancy of these disparate animal models to the various patterns of stimulant abuse that are apparent from the available literature [8–10,22] is the difficulty in equating drug exposure conditions in humans and experimental animals such as rats. For one, with some of the stimulants, especially amphetamine (AMPH) and methamphetamine (METH), there are pronounced species-related pharmacokinetic differences [2,3,13,14]. Furthermore, it is extremely difficult to establish actual drug parameters in stimulant abusers. Accurate data relating to the amount and frequency of intake are not available, and therefore estimates of dose are largely based on anecdotal information. There is typically little reliable quantitative evidence to corroborate the retrospective self-reports of abusers whose veracity is often questionable. Even when abusers attempt to be truthful, they may not know the drug purity. In addition, pharmacokinetic interactions with other coadministered drugs may also significantly influence effective dose.

Despite these limitations, some potentially useful comparison criteria have emerged recently from both postmortem and neuroimaging studies. Since each stimulant may be associated with different abuse characteristics, in large part because of their respective pharmacokinetic and pharmacodynamic profiles as well as the accessible forms of the drug, it is important to focus on a particular stimulant for comparison of its effects in humans and animals. Currently, perhaps the best comparative data are available for METH.

Wilson and her colleagues [23] recently reported reduced levels of a number of DAergic nerve terminal markers, including striatal levels of DA and the DA transporter (DAT), in postmortem studies of chronic METH abusers. However, they observed no changes in levels of the vesicular monoamine transporter (VMAT2), a marker for neuronal terminal loss. These data led those authors to conclude that the observed changes reflect compensatory adaptational processes and that chronic METH abuse did not cause permanent degeneration of DA terminals in their subjects. In contrast, Ricuarte and coworkers, using positron emission tomography (PET) to examine the density of DAT, found a significant decrement in DAT–ligand binding in 3-year-abstinent METH users [12]. Based on the persistence of the decreased DAT density, as well as on results of their PET and postmortem studies in baboons [22], these researchers concluded, in contrast to Wilson, that METH abuse is capable of producing striatal DAergic nerve terminal degeneration, at least in binge-pattern abusers.

We designed a study to determine how the ED-B treatment affects striatal DA integrity indices including DA content and radioligand-binding measures of DAT and VMAT2 to further assess this model in the context of available neurochemical markers associated with various patterns of stimulant abuse.

The results of our study revealed that after animals received acute high-dose binge administration of METH (10 mg/kg/2 h ×4), there was a marked decrement in both DAT (1.03 ± 0.04 versus 0.56 ± 0.03; $P < 0.001$) and $VMAT_2$ (2.22 ± 0.08 versus 1.22 ± 0.04; $P < 0.001$) levels (as measured by [^{3}H]WIN 35,428 and [^{3}H]dihydrotetrabenazine binding, respectively). These results are consistent with previous reports and demonstrate the neurotoxic effects of this type of treatment, including evidence of structural damage to DA terminals. In contrast, no evidence in the literature suggests that sensitization protocols produce effects on either DAT or VMAT2 or any other evidence of structural damage (Fig. 2) [7]. However, our data revealed that the ED-B METH (4.0 mg/kg) exposure resulted in a distinct pattern of neurochemical changes. As with the short-term binge treatment, both DA levels (Fig. 2) and [^{3}H]WIN 35,428 binding (1.05 ± 0.02 versus 0.78 ± 0.02; $P < 0.001$) were reduced by about 32% and 25%, respectively, 1–3 days after the last drug exposure. In contrast, [^{3}H]dihydrotetrabenazine binding was not significantly altered at 3 days after treatment (2.88 ± 0.25 versus 2.76 ± 0.31; $P = 0.78$).

In a related series of studies, we examined the behavioral response to AMPH (2.5 mg/kg) challenge on various days after the ED-B (METH, 4.0 mg/kg) treatment (Fig. 2A,B). One day after the last binge, the typical emergent behavioral profile appeared; i.e., the stereotypy phase is reduced and the poststereotypy activation is enhanced and qualitatively changed. Both behavioral features were attenuated in response to AMPH challenge after 7 days of withdrawal, and by 30 days the only resid-

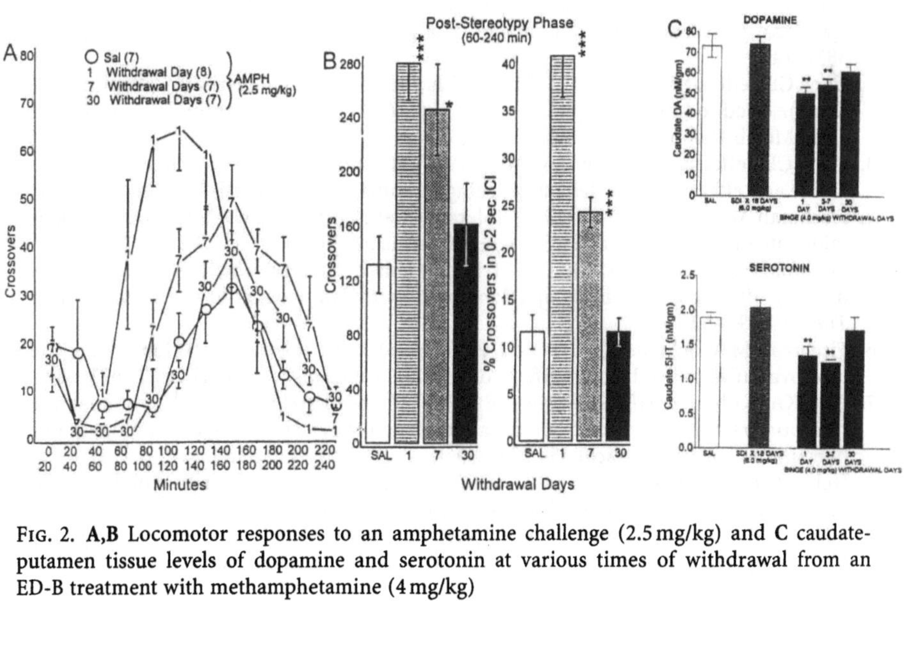

FIG. 2. **A,B** Locomotor responses to an amphetamine challenge (2.5 mg/kg) and **C** caudate-putamen tissue levels of dopamine and serotonin at various times of withdrawal from an ED-B treatment with methamphetamine (4 mg/kg)

ual effect was a more rapid onset of stereotypy (i.e., evidence of sensitization). In a separate group of animals similarly treated, caudate-putamen tissue levels of DA and serotonin were determined at times corresponding to the METH challenge injections. There was a decrease in both neurotransmitters that persisted for at least 3–7 days, but this level significantly recovered by day 30. This time course paralleled the behavioral recovery (Fig. 2C).

Discussion

In summary, it is apparent that the various patterns of stimulant abuse may be associated with different DA responses and behavioral profiles, and that time courses of recovery may correspondingly differ. One approach to assessing the relevancy of various animal models for these different abuse patterns is to establish neurochemical as well as behavioral and pharmacokinetic markers in humans. Although only limited data are currently available, we suggest that the ED-binge paradigm compares more closely with respect to relative changes in DA level, [^{3}H]WIN 35,428 binding to DAT, and [^{3}H]DTBZ binding to VMAT2, than do other animal models for which these markers have been assessed. Thus, ED-B treatment appears to simulate the effects produced in recreational or maintenance METH abusers. More intense drug exposure, especially including more frequent administrations during periods of prolonged binge exposures, may be required to reproduce the effects associated with repeated binge-crash METH abuse.

References

1. Angrist B (1994) Amphetamine psychosis: clinical variations of the syndrome. In: Cho AK, Segal DS (eds) Amphetamine and its analogues. Academic Press, San Diego, pp 387–414
2. Cook CE, Jeffcoat AR, Hill JM, et al (1993) Pharmacokinetics of methamphetamine self-administered to human subjects by smoking S-(+)-methamphetamine hydrochloride. Drug Metab Dispos 21:717–723
3. Cook CE, Jeffcoat AR, Sadler BM, et al (1992) Pharmacokinetics of oral methamphetamine and effects of repeated daily dosing in humans. Drug Metab Dispos 20:856–862
4. Fischman MW, Schuster CR (1974) Tolerance development to chronic methamphetamine intoxication in the rhesus monkey. Pharmacol Biochem Behav 2:503–508
5. Fischman MW, Schuster CR (1977) Long-term behavioral changes in the rhesus monkey after multiple daily injections of *d*-methylamphetamine. J Pharmacol Exp Ther 201:593–605
6. Fischman MW, Schuster CR, Javaid J, et al (1985) Acute tolerance development to the cardiovascular and subjective effects of cocaine. J Pharmacol Exp Ther 235:677–682
7. Frey KA, Kilbourn MR, Robinson TE (1997) Reduced striatal vesicular monoamine transporters after neurotoxic but not after behaviorally-sensitizing doses of methamphetamine. Eur J Pharmacol 334:273–279
8. Huber A, Ling W, Shoptaw S, et al (1997) Integrating treatments for methamphetamine abuse: a psychosocial perspective. J Addict Dis 16:41–50
9. Jaffe JH (1995) Amphetamine (or amphetaminelike)-related disorders. In: Kaplan J (ed) Comprehensive textbook of psychiatry. Williams and Wilkins, Baltimore, pp 791–799

10. Konuma K (1994) Use and abuse of amphetamines in Japan. In: Cho AK, Segal DS (eds) Amphetamine and its analogs. Academic Press, San Diego, pp 415–435
11. Kuczenski R, Segal DS (1997) An escalating dose-high dose binge pattern of amphetamine administrations results in differential changes in the extracellular dopamine response profiles in caudate-putamen and nucleus accumbens. J Neurosci 17:4441–4447
12. McCann UD, Wong DF, Yokoi F, et al (1998) Reduced striatal dopamine transporter density in abstinent methamphetamine and methcathinone users: evidence from positron emission tomography studies with [^{11}C]WIN-35,428. J Neurosci 18:8417–8422
13. Melega WP, Williams AE, Schmitz DA, et al (1995) Pharmacokinetic and pharmacodynamic analysis of the actions of D-amphetamine and D-methamphetamine on the dopamine terminal. J Pharmacol Exp Ther 274:90–96
14. Riviere GJ, Byrnes KA, Gentry WB, Owens SM (1999) Spontaneous locomotor activity and pharmacokinetics of intravenous methamphetamine and its metabolite amphetamine in the rat. J Pharmacol Exp Ther 291:1220–1226
15. Sato M (1992) A lasting vulnerability to psychosis in patients with previous methamphetamine psychosis. Ann NY Acad Sci 654:160–170
16. Schmidt CJ, Gehlert DR, Peat MA, et al (1985) Studies on the mechanism of tolerance to methamphetamine. Brain Res 343:305–313
17. Schuster CR, Fischman MW (1996) Amphetamine toxicity: behavioral and neuropathological indexes. In: Current status of behavioral pharmacology. ASPET, Rockville, MD, pp 1845–1851
18. Segal DS, Kuczenski R (1997b) An escalating dose "binge" model of amphetamine psychosis: behavioral and neurochemical characteristics. J Neurosci 17:2551–2566
19. Segal DS, Kuczenski R (1997a) Repeated binge exposure to amphetamine and methamphetamine: behavioral and neurochemical characterization. J Pharmacol Exp Ther 282:561–573
20. Segal DS, Kuczenski R (1999b) Escalating dose-binge treatment with methylphenidate: role of serotonin in the emergent behavioral profile. J Pharmacol Exp Ther 291:19–30
21. Segal DS, Kuczenski R (1999a) Escalating dose/binge stimulant exposure: relationship between emergent behavioral profile and differential caudate-putamen/nucleus accumbens dopamine responses. Psychopharmacology 142:182–192
22. Villemagne V, Yuan J, Wong DF, et al (1998) Brain dopamine neurotoxicity in baboons treated with doses of methamphetamine comparable to those recreationally abused by humans: evidence from [^{11}C]WIN-35,428 positron emission tomography studies and direct *in vitro* determinations. J Neurosci 18:419–427
23. Wilson JM, Kalasinsky KS, Levey AI, et al (1996) Striatal dopamine nerve terminal markers in human, chronic methamphetamine users. Nat Med 2:699–703

Involvement of G-Protein βγ-Subunit-Mediated Signal Transduction in Methamphetamine-Induced Behavioral Sensitization

Shuichi Kikuchi[1,2], Hiroto Iwasa[3], Mio Sato[1], Chizu Ishida-Hiraiwa[1], Sigeru Ozaki[1], Akiko Kikuchi[1], and Kiyoshi Wada[1]

Summary. Heterotrimeric guaninenucleotide-binding protein (G protein) plays an obligatory role on a biochemical basis in psychostimulant-induced psychosis. However, little is known about the contribution of G-protein beta/gamma-subunit-mediated signal transduction. We investigated the expression and function of beta/gamma subunits, especially the beta-1 subunit, using in situ hybridization, immunohistochemistry, and the antisense knockdown technique, to clarify the molecular basis of methamphetamine (MAP)-induced behavioral sensitization. Expression in beta-1 subunit mRNA and protein transiently increased in the ventral tegmental area (VTA) of animals acutely treated with MAP. However, after a challenge injection, this increased response was not observed in VTA of animals repeatedly administered MAP. Antisense knockdown of the beta-1 subunit in VTA revealed an increase in the intensity of stereotypy, and an acceleration in the development of behavioral sensitization. These results suggest that G-protein beta-1 in VTA plays an inhibitory role in the establishment of MAP-induced behavioral sensitization. Furthermore, a lack of response in the expression of beta-1 may lead to a decreased inhibition of the development of behavioral sensitization.

Keywords. G-protein β1 subunit, Methamphetamine, Antisense oligonucleotide, Ventral tegmental area, Behavioral sensitization

Introduction

Repeated administration of psychostimulants such as methamphetamine (MAP) [1] and cocaine [2] may cause progressive and long-lasting augmentation of hyperactivity and stereotyped behavior. These behavioral changes, called behavioral sensitization, are regarded as valuable experimental models for searching into the

[1] Department of Drug Dependence Research, National Institute of Mental Health, National Center of Neurology and Psychiatry, Ichikawa, Japan
[2] Department of Psychiatry, Sodegaura Satsukidai Hospital, Sodegaura Satsukidai Hospital, 5-21 Nagaura-ekimae, Sodegaura, Chiba 292-0246, Japan
[3] Department of Neuropsychiatry, Chiba University School of Medicine, Chiba, Japan

neurobiological basis of methamphetamine-induced psychosis and schizophrenic disorders [3].

Many neurochemical changes have been reported as being associated with the pathogenesis of MAP-induced behavioral sensitization. Several researchers reported that alterations of heterotrimeric guanine nucleotide-binding regulatory proteins (G proteins) were observed in the chronic administration of several psychostimulants such as cocaine and amphetamine [2,4].

However G protein consists of three subunits, alpha, beta, and gamma subunits. Although most interest in G protein has concentrated on the alpha subunit, the molecular changes in G protein, especially beta/gamma subunits, remain unknown. Furthermore, it is suggested that abnormalities in the function of various G proteins are implicated in the ventral tegmental area (VTA) [4]. These findings suggest that each subunit of G protein plays a crucial regulatory role in G-protein expression and function in VTA.

In the present study, we examined alteration in the expression and function of G-protein beta 1 subunit in the VTA of MAP-induced behaviorally sensitized rats to elucidate the neurobiological basis of behavioral sensitization.

Materials and Methods

Treatment Schedule in Expression Study

Sprague-Dawley male rats were used. After a week for handling, the rats were injected intraperitoneally (i.p.) with methamphetamine (MAP, 5 mg/kg) once daily for 14 days. Assessment of abnormal behavior was done using the scale of Ujike et al. [5]. Rats received a challenge injection of MAP (MM group) or saline (MS group) over intervals to 8 weeks. Rats in the control group were treated with saline under the same conditions as the chronic treated group. Rats in the acutely treated group (SM group) were administered with saline once daily for 14 days, and MAP (5 mg/kg, i.p.) was challenged once over an 8-week interval.

In Situ Hybridization and Immunohistochemistry

From the brains of the rats, 4-μm paraffinized sections were prepared by perfusion with 4% paraformaldehyde under pentobarbital anesthesia at 6h or 24h after treatment with methamphetamine (5 mg/kg, i.p.). mRNA level was detected using a digoxigenin-labeled cRNA probe of 300 bp and visualized by fluorescence-labeled F(ab) fragment. Immunoreactivity detected by the primary antibody was visualized by an ABC elite system (Vecstatin Elite kit). Immunopositive cells were counted after taking three photographs at 200× and calculated per square millimeter. The data were analyzed statistically with unpaired Student's *t*-test.

Antisense Treatment of the Ventral Tegmental Area

Male Sprague Dawley rats (350–400 g) were used. After anesthesia with pentobarbital, a guide cannula connected with osmotic pumps (Alza, 0.5 μl/h, total 200 μl) containing beta1 antisense (0.5 μg/μl, 5′-TTCACTCATCTTCACGTC) or missense (0.5 μg/μl,

5′-ATCGCTCGTCGTCATCTCGTC) [6] was implanted at midline and 7.0mm caudal from the bregma. After 5-day pretreatment of oligonucleotides, methamphetamine (5mg/kg, i.p.) was injected for 9 days. Behavior was rated on day 1, day 9, and on the day of the challenge injection of methamphetamine treatment according to the criteria of Akiyama and Ujike [5]. Challenge injection was performed 1 week after the last injection. Scores were analyzed with one-way ANOVA followed by Fisher's post hoc test. The suppression of beta 1 protein expression was confirmed 3h after methamphetamine injection on day 9 using the ABC elite system.

Results

Development of Behavioral Sensitization

All animals treated with MAP exhibited the progress of augmentation in hyperactivity followed by stereotypical behavior, i.e., continuous compulsive sniffing without locomotion. All MAP-treated rats exhibited a score of 4 within 10min after the last injection of MAP. No behavioral changes were observed in the saline-treated control group.

Results of In Situ Hybridization and Immunohistochemistry

The mRNA of beta 1 was observed to increase in the VTA of the acutely treated SM group; however, the mRNA did not change at challenge in behaviorally sensitized animals (MM group). An immunohistochemical analysis revealed that the immunopositive cells increased after acute treatment, but the response of an increase in beta 1-positive cells disappeared after the challenge injection in the behaviorally sensitized group (Fig. 1). No alteration was observed in behaviorally sensitized animals that did not receive the challenge injection.

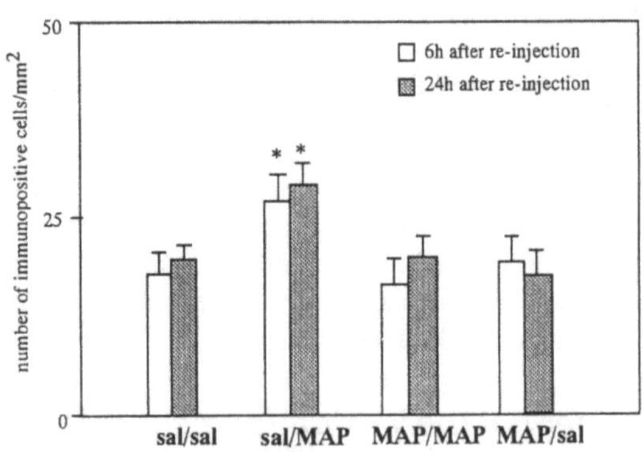

FIG. 1. Changes in number of beta-1 immunopositive cells in ventral tegmental area. *Sal*, saline; *MAP*, methamphetamine. *$P < 0.05$, unpaired *t*-test

Results of Antisense Knockdown of Beta-1 Subunit in VTA

Because the difference in expression of mRNA and protein levels of beta 1 was observed in the ventral tegmental area, the antisense treatment was aimed at VTA. Using immunohistochemical staining, we confirmed that the beta-1 immunopositive cells diminished as much as −90%.

The continuity of stereotypy was prolonged in the antisense-treated animals as compared with the missense-treated group (Fig. 2). On the day of challenge injection, the augmented stereotypy emerged even without the influence of antisense administration.

Discussion

It has been reported that administration of psychostimulants such as amphetamine and cocaine [2,4,7] induce the alteration of levels of G-protein alpha subunits. Furthermore, a previous report showed a pertussis toxin-catalyzed ADP ribosylation decrease in the VTA in repeated cocaine treatment [2,8]. Another report demonstrated that cholera toxin-catalyzed ADP ribosylation accelerates the development of amphetamine-induced behavioral sensitization [4]. These data showed the involvement of heterotrimeric G protein with behavioral sensitization, but the role of the beta/gamma subunit was still unclear.

In this study we examined the changes of G-protein beta-1 subunit mRNA and protein levels in rats with MAP-induced behavioral sensitization. A remarkable increase of beta-1 mRNA and protein was observed in the VTA at 24h after the challenge injection of MAP in acutely treated animals. However, the response of increase in expression disappeared after the establishment of behavioral sensitization; this can be regarded as the relative downregulation or lack of response of transcriptional regulation of beta 1.

Antisense knockdown of beta-1 mRNA revealed that the suppression of beta-1 mRNA promotes the latency and intensity in emergence of stereotypy. Furthermore, because the development of sensitization was accelerated by the antisense, we suppose

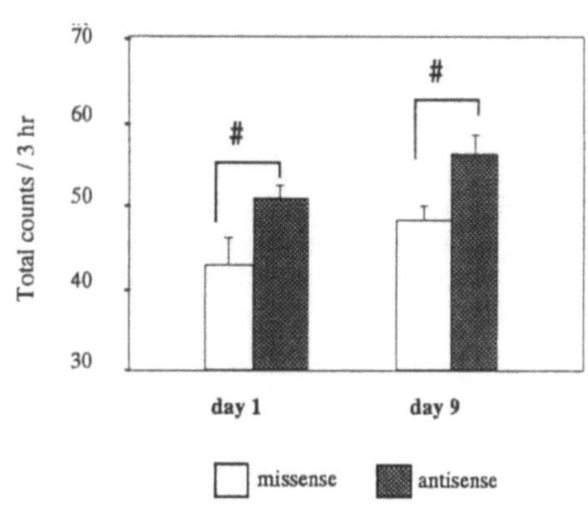

Fig. 2. Cumulative score of stereotypy in the antisense group (*open bars*) and missense group (*stippled bars*). #$P < 0.05$, one-way ANOVA followed by Fisher's post hoc test

that the beta-1 subunit mediates the signal-inhibiting development of the behavioral sensitization.

It is still unknown which receptor and effector are coupled with the beta-1 subunit. Recent research has identified the candidate receptors and effectors, some of which are reported to play an important role in sensitization [9]. Further research is needed to clarify the signaling system.

In conclusion, G-protein beta-1 subunit plays a crucial role in the development of behavioral sensitization, and may be concerned with the neuroadaptational process of behavioral sensitization.

Acknowledgments. We thank Professors Mitsumoto Sato and Youtarou Numachi, Tohoku University, very much for their constant interest and helpful suggestions. This work was supported by the Brain Research Grant from the Ministry of Health and Welfare, and Scientific research grants from the Ministry of Education, Science and Culture, Japan.

References

1. Robinson TE, Becker JB (1986) Enduring changes in brain and behavior produced by chronic amphetamine administration: a review and evaluation of animal model of amphetamine psychosis. Brain Res Brain Res Rev 11:157–198
2. Terwilliger RZ, Beitner-Johnson D, Sevarino KA, et al (1991) A general role for adaptations in G-proteins and the cyclic AMP system in mediating the chronic actions of morphine and cocaine on neuronal function. Brain Res 548:100–110
3. Sato M, Numachi Y, Hamamura T (1992) Relapse of paranoid psychotic state in methamphetamine model of schizophrenia. Schizophr Bull 18:115–122
4. Byrnes JJ, Wallace LJ (1997) Amphetamine-induced sensitization and release of dopamine in slices from the ventral tegmental area of rats is enhanced following administration of cholera toxin into the ventral tegmental area. Neurosci Lett 223:45–48
5. Ujike H, Onoue T, Akiyama K, et al (1989) Effects of selective D-1 and D-2 dopamine antagonists on development of methamphetamine-induced behavioral sensitization. Psychopharmacology 98:89–92
6. Wang X-B, Funada M, Imai Y, et al (1997) rGb1: a psychostimulant-regulated gene essential for establishing cocaine sensitization. J Neurosci 17:5993–6000
7. Iwasa H, Kikuchi S, Suzuki K, et al (1996) Alteration of G proteins subclass mRNA levels in the methamphetamine-induced behavioral sensitization. Ann NY Acad Sci 801:110–115
8. Nestler EJ, Terwilliger RZ, Walker JR, et al (1990) Chronic cocaine treatment decreases levels of the G protein subunits Gi α and Go α in discrete regions of rat brain. J Neurochem 55:1079–1082
9. Kalkbrenner F, Dippel E, Wittig B, Shultz G (1996) Specificity of interaction between receptor and G protein: use of antisense techniques to relate G-protein subunits to function. Biochim Biophys Acta 1314:125–139

A Molecular Approach to Identify Essential Factors for Establishment of Psychostimulant-Induced Behavioral Sensitization

Yasushi Kajii, Shigenobu Toda, Asami Umino, and Toru Nishikawa

Summary. Identification of genes specifically involved in the establishment of psychostimulant-induced behavioral sensitization is quite important to understand the molecular basis for the pathophysiology of stimulant psychoses. The sensitization is a development-dependent phenomenon and is produced in rats only after postnatal week 3. We, therefore, have explored methamphetamine-regulated transcripts in the neocortex of developing rats (postnatal days 8 and 50) by RNA arbitrarily primed-PCR (RAP-PCR) fingerprinting to identify genes that respond to the drug after the critical period. The bands of the candidate transcripts were cloned, and the expression profile of each RAP-PCR clone was reexamined by semiquantitative RT-PCR accompanying competitive amplification of 28*S* ribosomal RNA as an internal standard for the assay. Our unique approach based on the developmental aspect of the drug-induced neuroplastic changes should contribute to understanding of the molecular cascade establishing psychostimulant-induced behavioral sensitization.

Keywords. Methamphetamine, Behavioral sensitization, RAP-PCR, Postnatal development, mRNA

Introduction

Preexposure to psychostimulants, such as methamphetamine (MAP) or cocaine, results in long-lasting behavioral vulnerability to these drugs or stress. This psychostimulant-induced behavioral sensitization has been proposed as a useful model of both drug-induced psychosis and addiction in the human [1,2]. Although psychostimulant-regulated gene expression has been demonstrated to be required in the establishment of this long-lasting neuroplastic adaptation [3], the molecular pathways involved in the sensitization remains unclear [4].

Behavioral response to psychostimulants is observed throughout postnatal development and is believed to be mediated mainly by the mesencephalic dopamine (DA) systems [5]. The hypothetical neuroadaptive changes in the DA systems underlying

Department of Mental Disorder Research, National Institute of Neuroscience, National Center of Neurology and Psychiatry, 4-1-1 Ogawa-Higashi, Kodaira, Tokyo 187-8502, Japan

behavioral sensitization seem to be late developing, because, in the case of rats, young animals before postnatal week 3 are never behaviorally sensitized even if they receive repeated administrations of amphetamine or MAP [6,7]. These observations indicate that there is a critical period of development of behavioral sensitization around postnatal week 3. Some other neuronal systems, whose function should be late developing, appear to modify these dopaminergic systems. We have shown that some corticostriatal system arising from the prefrontal cortex (PFC) is one of the candidates [8–10]. In addition, recent evidence also indicates that the inputs from the PFC contribute to the functional changes in the mesencephalic DA system accompanying behavioral sensitization [11,12].

From these aspects, we have focused on the studies of the relationship between the developmental profile of the behavioral sensitization and MAP-regulated gene expression in the neocortex containing the PFC to identify the specific molecules involved in the cascade establishing psychostimulant-induced behavioral sensitization.

Materials and Methods

Animals

The present animal experiments were performed in strict accordance with the guidance of the National Institute of Neuroscience, National Center of Neurology and Psychiatry, and were approved by the Animal Investigation Committee of the Institute. Male Wistar rats (ST strain, Clea Japan, Tokyo, Japan) at postnatal day (PD) 8 and PD50 were used. The animals were housed at 22.0° ± 0.5°C in a humidity-controlled room under a 12-h light:dark cycle and had free access to food and water.

RNA Arbitrarily Primed (RAP)-PCR

Rats were administered subcutaneously 4.8 mg/kg of MAP or saline and killed by cervical dislocation 1 h later. Equal amounts of the neocortical RNA from four to six individual rats of PD8 or PD50 in MAP- or saline-treated group were pooled. Single-strand cDNAs were synthesized from 0.2 μg of the pooled sample using an RNA Preamplification Kit (Life Technologies, Gaithersburg, MD, USA), and the resulting cDNAs were serially diluted in TE buffer (pH 8.0) followed by being used as a template for PCR with various 12-mer arbitrary primers. PCR amplification was performed in a solution containing 1.5 mM $MgCl_2$, 0.1 mM dNTP (N = A, G, C, or T), 0.2 μM arbitrary primer, 0.1 unit/μl DNA polymerase (Expand Hi-Fi; Roche Diagnostics, Mannheim, Germany) and the supplied reaction buffer (1×) for 40 cycles (94°C for 45 s, 37°C for 45 s, 72°C for 1 min). The resulting PCR product was separated in denaturing polyacrylamide gel containing 50% urea. The gel was stained with SYBR Green I (Molecular Probes, Eugene, OR, USA), and the cDNA bands were visualized and analyzed by a FluorImager SI (Molecular Dynamics, Sunnyvale, CA, USA) or an FM Bio (Takara, Kyoto, Japan).

Semiquantitative Reverse Transcribed (RT)-PCR

Reverse transcription was performed as just described, and the resulting cDNAs were suspended in 10 volumes of TE buffer (pH 8.0). A 10-µl aliquot of the cDNA suspension was used as a template. We used Platinum Taq DNA polymerase (Life Technologies) to perform "hot-start" PCR. PCR amplifications were done with primers for each RAP-PCR clone and those for 28*S* ribosomal RNA (rRNA). The sequences of primers for 28*S* rRNA are 5′-CTCGCTGGCCCTTGAAAATCC-3′ and 5′-CCCAGCCCTTAGAGCCAATCCTTA-3′. Competitor oligomers for 28*S* rRNA phosphorylated at their 3′-ends were also added into the PCR reaction in ratios ranging from 7:3 to 9:1. The PCR product was electrophoresed in agarose gel, and the gel was stained with ethidium bromide followed by visualization and quantification of DNA bands using a Lumi-Imager (Roche Diagnostics).

Results and Discussion

Although it is well known that repeated intermittent treatment with moderate doses of psychostimulants is most effective in inducing behavioral sensitization [13], a single exposure to a stimulant has been found to produce the sensitization phenomenon [14]. This finding suggests that changes in gene expression, which are essential to establishment of the sensitization, should be induced after a single exposure to psychostimulants. The consequence of such pretreatment with the drugs may depend on postnatal development because behavioral sensitization is observed in rats only after postnatal week 3 [6,7] (Fig. 1). Therefore, it seems possible to identify the essential factors of the molecular cascade establishing behavioral sensitization by exploring the transcripts whose expression in the brain is regulated by a single administration of a psychostimulant specifically after the critical period of development. MAP was administered to rats of PD8 and 1 h before being killed by cervical dislocation, and fingerprints of their neocortical RNA were compared. For RNA fingerprinting, we adopted the RAP-PCR technique [15,16]. RAP-PCR is one of the modified methods of differential display PCR [17] and enables us to amplify sequences without a poly(A) tail. It is worth mentioning that poly(A)-negative mRNA exists in the brain and that changes in the mRNA polyadenylation state do occur in response to specific physiological stimuli [18]. In addition, changes in gene expression induced by psychostimulants have some similar properties to those induced by various physiological stimuli [4]. Thus, we selected this technique.

The results of RNA fingerprinting by RAP-PCR revealed that various transcripts were increased or decreased in the rat neocortex 1 h after administration of MAP and that some of them were development dependent (data not shown). The neocortical transcripts that increased specifically in rats of PD50 seemed to be candidates for the molecules closely related to the development-dependent sensitization. We cloned the cDNA bands from the gel of fingerprinting and analyzed their sequences.

Serial dilution of templates for RAP-PCR fingerprinting enabled us to find some bands of candidates whose expression was regulated by MAP in a development-dependent manner. However, the amplification of RAP-PCR was not quantitative, and the results obtained by RAP-PCR remain to be further investigated. In the next step,

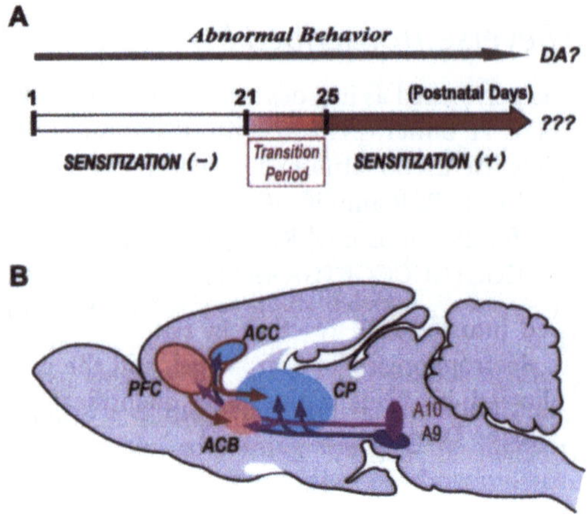

FIG. 1A,B. Schematic representation of the developmental property of psychostimulant-induced behavioral sensitization. **A** In rats, the sensitization is established only after postnatal week 3. **B** A corticostriatal neuronal pathway is a candidate for the hypothetical late-developing modulation system involved in behavioral sensitization. *ACC*, anterior cingulate cortex; *ACB*, nucleus accumbens; *CP*, caudate-putamen; *PFC*, prefrontal cortex; *A*10, ventral tegmental area; *A*9, substantia nigra

we performed a quantitative analysis of each transcript of interest by RT-PCR with a specific primer set under quantitative conditions. To ensure the quantitative condition, 28*S* rRNA was simultaneously amplified with each target transcript as a reference. Because the copy number of 28*S* rRNA was much greater than that of each mRNA, we used the competitive oligomers for the 28*S* rRNA with the phosphorylated 3′-ends to amplify the target transcripts and 28*S* rRNA exponentially under the same conditions. Such competitor oligomers added to the reaction in ratios ranging from 7:3 to 9:1 so effectively modified the PCR kinetics of 28*S* rRNA that both the specific target mRNA and 28S rRNA were exponentially amplified in the same reaction mixture (Fig. 2). As a result, three neocortical transcripts were proven to increase specifically in the rats of PD50 immediately after administration of MAP, as indicated in the RAP-PCR fingerprinting analysis (data not shown).

There are two additional important properties of behavioral sensitization other than the developmental aspect. First, cross-sensitization is observed among various dopamine agonists, and, second, it is a long-lasting phenomenon. We are investigating in detail the expression profile of these candidates according to these views. In addition, to demonstrate the relationship between their expression and the establishment of behavioral sensitization, we plan to adopt an experimental system using antisense oligomers introduced into the lateral ventricle by an osmotic minipump to suppress a specific gene expression in a sequence-specific manner [19]. Although these analyses are still under investigation, the preliminary data suggest that our approach

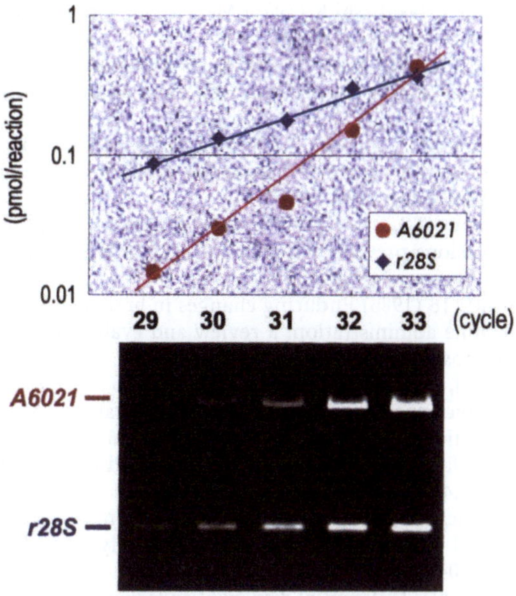

FIG. 2. Simultaneous amplification of a specific transcript and 28S rRNA in the same reaction under quantitative conditions. Transcripts corresponding both to an RAP-PCR clone A6021 (*circles*) and to 28S rRNA (*diamonds*) are exponentially amplified in the same reaction mixture

should shed light on the molecular cascade implicated in psychostimulant-induced behavioral sensitization.

References

1. Sato M (1992) A lasting vulnerability to psychosis in patients with previous methamphetamine psychosis. Ann N Y Acad Sci 654:160–170
2. Robinson TE, Berridge KC (1993) The neural basis of drug craving: an incentive-sensitization theory of addiction. Brain Res Rev 18:247–291
3. Karler R, Finnegan KT, Calder LD (1993) Blockade of behavioral sensitization to cocaine and amphetamine by inhibitors of protein synthesis. Brain Res 603:19–24
4. Kajii Y, Toda S, Hashimoto T, et al (1996) Psychostimulants and gene expression. Jpn J Neuropsychopharmacol 18:557–563
5. Pierce RC, Kalivas PW (1997) A circuitry model of the expression of behavioral sensitization to amphetamine-like psychostimulants. Brain Res Rev 25:192–216
6. Fujiwara Y, Kazahaya M, Nakashima M, Ootsuki S (1987) Behavioral sensitization to methamphetamine in the rat: an ontogenic study. Psychopharmacology 91:316–319
7. Kolta MG, Scalzo FM, Ali SF, Holson RR (1990) Ontogeny of the enhabced behavioral response to amphetamine in amphetamine-pretreated rats. Psychopharmacology 100:377–382
8. Nishikawa T, Umino A, Kashiwa A, et al (1993) Stimulant-induced behavioral sensitization and cerebral neurotransmission. In: Toru M (ed) Neurotransmitters in neuronal plasticity and psychiatric disorders. Excerpta Medica, Tokyo, pp 53–62

9. Umino A, Nishikawa T, Takahashi K (1995) Methamphetamine-induced nuclear c-Fos in rat brain regions. Neurochem Int 26:85–90
10. Hashimoto T, Kajii Y, Nishikawa T (1998) Psychotomimetic-induction of tissue plasminogen activator mRNA in corticostriatal neurons in rat brain. Eur J Neurosci 10:3387–3399
11. Cador M, Bjijou S, Cailhol S, Stinus L (1999) D-Amphetamine-induced behavioral sensitization: implication of a glutamatergic medial prefrontal cortex-ventral tegmental area innervation. Neuroscience 94:705–721
12. Li Y, Hu X-T, Berney TG, et al (1999) Both glutamate receptor antagonists and prefrontal cortex lesions prevent induction of cocaine sensitization and associated neuroadaptations. Synapse 34:169–180
13. Robinson TE, Becker JB (1986) Enduring changes in brain and behavior produced by chronic amphetamine administration: a review and evaluation of animal models of amphetamine psychosis. Brain Res Rev 11:157–198
14. Vanderschuren LJMJ, Schmidt ED, De Vries TJ, et al (1999) A single exposure to amphetamine is sufficient to induce long-term behavioral, neuroendocrine, and neurochemical sensitization in rats. J Neurosci 19:9579–9586
15. Welsh J, Chada K, Dalal SS, et al (1992) Artitrarily primed PCR fingerprinting of RNA. Nucleic Acids Res 20:4965–4970
16. Dalal SS, Welsh J, Tkachenko A, et al (1994) Rapid isolation of tissue-specific and developmentally regulated brain cDNAs using RNA arbitrarily primed PCR (RAP-PCR). J Mol Neurosci 5:93–104
17. Liang P, Pardee AB (1992) Differential display of eukaryotic messenger RNA by means of the polymerase chain reaction. Science 257:967–971
18. Snider BJ, Morrison-Bogorad M (1992) Brain non-adenylated mRNAs. Brain Res Brain Res Rev 17:263–282
19. Kakeyama M, Hashimoto T, Hiraoka S, et al (1998) Inhibition of methamphetamine-induced behavioral sensitization by NMDA receptor subunit antisense oligonucleotide. Annu Rep Pharmacopsychiatr Res Found 29:32–36

Alterations in Corticosterone Receptor mRNA Induced by Methamphetamine in Two Inbred Strains of Rats

Yohtaro Numachi, Sumiko Yoshida, Shigenobu Toda, Hiroo Matsuoka, and Mitsumoto Sato

Summary. A role of the hypothalamo-pituitary-adrenocortical (HPA) axis in facilitating the behavioral and neurochemical effects of psychostimulants has been proposed. Two inbred strains of rats, Fischer 344/N (F-344) and Lewis/N (LEW), have markedly different HPA axes: F-344 rats show a hyperresponsive HPA axis whereas LEW rats display a blunted response. We examined the brain expression of mRNAs for corticosterone receptors (type I, MR; and type II, GR) in methamphetamine (MAP) -treated F-344 and LEW rats using Northern blotting. Chronic MAP significantly increased GR and MR mRNA expression in the striatum of F-344 while decreasing GR mRNA in the striatum of LEW rats. These contrasting differences between F-344 and LEW, in their striatal expression of GR mRNA by chronic MAP, suggest that some striatal genes, whose transcription is regulated by GR and MR, play a crucial role in the development of MAP-induced behavioral sensitization.

Keywords. Methamphetamine, Sensitization, Inbred strain, Corticosterone receptor, Rat

Introduction

Subchronic treatment of psychostimulants including amphetamine (AMP) and methamphetamine (MAP) to rodents often results in a progressive and long-lasting enhancement of stereotyped behavior elicited by a subsequent challenge injection of these drugs. These changes, termed behavioral sensitization, has been widely applied as a model for stimulant-induced psychosis as well as paranoid schizophrenia in humans [1].

Recent studies suggest that corticosterone can facilitate the behavioral and neurochemical effects of psychostimulants and has a critical role in stimulant-induced behavioral sensitization. Two inbred strains of rats, Fischer 344/N (F-344) and Lewis/N (LEW), have markedly different hypothalamo-pituitary-adrenocortical (HPA) axes as well as behavioral responses to psychostimulants. LEW rats have a blunted response

Department of Psychiatry, Tohoku University Graduate School of Medicine, Sendai 980-8574, Japan

in the HPA axis and develop the gradual increase of locomotor activity typically seen following cocaine exposure, whereas F-344 rats show a hyperresponsive HPA axis and display no significant sensitization [2].

Corticosterone exerts its biological effects via intracellular receptors, termed type I (mineralocorticoid receptor, MR) and type II (glucocorticoid receptor, GR), both of which act as ligand-activated transcription factors, binding to specific DNA sequences in the control region of target genes [3]. This study examines the effects of acute and subchronic treatment of MAP on (1) the development of stereotypy sensitization and (2) the brain expression of GR and MR mRNA in F-344 and LEW rats.

Materials and Methods

Animals and Drug Schedule

We conducted all experiments under the guidelines of the animal ethics committee at the Tohoku University School of Medicine. Male Fischer 344/N (F-344) and Lewis/N (LEW) rats, aged 7 weeks [110–130 g (F-344) and 205–220 g (LEW) on arrival], were obtained from Funabashi Farm (Japan) and divided into three groups. One group received a daily intraperitoneal injection of 4 mg/kg MAP (saline solution) for 21 days during the light phase as the chronic group (FC and LC). The other groups received the same amount of saline intraperitoneally for 20 days and 4 mg/kg MAP on the 21st day during the light phase as acute groups (FA and LA). The last groups received the same amount of saline intraperitoneally for 21 days as control groups (FS and LS). For FC and LC rats, changes in stereotyped behavior were rated in the home cage at 0, 1, 2, and 3 h after injection on the 1st, 7th, 14th, and 21st days, according to the scale by Creese and Iversen [4].

Total RNA Extraction and Northern Blot Analysis

Three hours after the last injection, we killed all rats by decapitation and quickly dissected the caudate nuclei, hippocampus, and cerebellum on ice. Extraction of total RNA and Northern blot analysis were done according to our previous report [5].

Statistical Analysis

The behavioral rating scores were analyzed using the Mann–Whitney *U*-test. Rectal temperature was analyzed by unpaired Student's *t*-test. Hybridization signals were analyzed by one-way analyses of valiance (ANOVA) and, if significant, subsequent Scheffe's post hoc tests. In all cases, *P* values less than 0.05 were considered statistically significant.

Results

Behavioral Sensitization in Stereotypy

F-344 and LEW rats developed stereotyped behavior as a result of subchronic MAP treatment (Fig. 1). Behavioral sensitization was manifested as a significant increase in

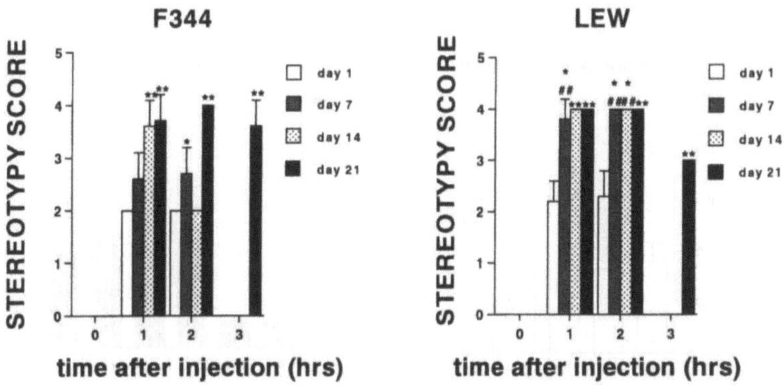

FIG. 1. Development of methamphetamine (MAP) -induced stereotyped behavior in F-344 and LEW rats that received a daily intraperitoneal injection of 4 mg/kg MAP (saline solution) for 21 days during the light phase. Stereotyped behaviors were examined in the home cage at 0, 1, 2, and 3 h after injection on the 1st, 7th, 14th, and 21st days, according to the scale by Creese and Iversen [15]. Each value is the mean ± SD ($n = 6$). *$P < 0.05$, **$P < 0.005$, significantly different from 1st day; ##$P < 0.01$; significantly different from F-344 (Mann–Whitney U-test)

the stereotypy scores from the first MAP treatment after the 7th days for LEW and 14th for F-344, respectively ($P < 0.005$). Stereotypy scores were significantly higher in LEW rats than in F-344 rats on the 7th and 14th day ($P < 0.01$). However, both strains ultimately plateaued at the same stereotypy rating score on the 21st day.

Methamphetamine-Induced GR or MR Expression

An approximately 7-kb GR mRNA, 6-kb MR mRNA, and 2-kb beta-actin mRNA, corresponding to previous reports [6,7], were identified by Northern blot analysis. Figure 2 illustrates striatal, hippocampal, and cerebellar GR and MR mRNA in F-344 and LEW rats by acute or chronic MAP treatment, respectively (standardized by beta-actin mRNA). Acute MAP treatment significantly decreased hippocampal GR and MR mRNA expression in LEW, compared to saline control. Chronic MAP treatment significantly increased striatal and cerebellar GR and MR mRNA in F-344 compared to controls, whereas striatal GR and MR mRNA and hippocampal MR mRNA were significantly decreased in LEW compared to controls.

Discussion

LEW rats developed MAP-induced stereotypy sensitization significantly earlier than F-344 rats, as is consistent with our previous findings [8]. Our result is also consistent with previous reports that LEW rats demonstrated greater locomotor sensitization than F-344 rats as a result of AMP [9] or cocaine [2] administration. However, both F-344 and LEW rats reached the same plateau of stereotypy sensitization, which reflects hyperactivity in the nigrostriatal DAergic pathway. That LEW rats did not acquire tolerance in stereotypy sensitization suggests that the effects of MAP on the nigrostriatal and mesolimbic DAergic system are differentially regulated in F-344 and LEW.

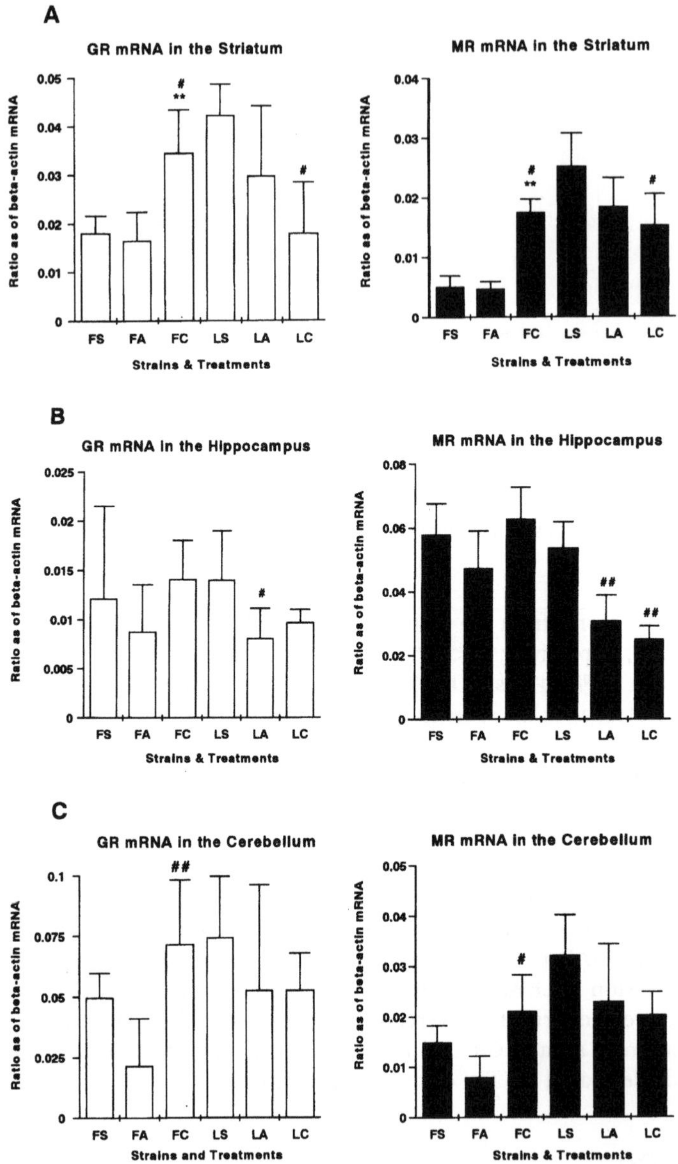

FIG. 2A–C. Striatal (A), hippocampal (B), and cerebellar (C) glucocorticoid receptor (GR) and mineralocorticoid receptor (MR) mRNA in F-344 and LEW rats by acute or chronic MAP treatment. The data represent signal intensity for hybridization signal of GR or MR mRNA, standardized by beta-actin mRNA hybridization signal. Each value is the mean ± SD ($n = 6$). #$P < 0.05$, ##$P < 0.005$, significantly different from saline-treated control; *$P < 0.005$, significantly different from acute MAP-treated group (ANOVA)

Acute administration of AMP or cocaine is known to elevate the level of corticosterone in male Wistar rats for 2h [10]. In LEW, because of blunted negative feedback in the HPA axis, acute and chronic MAP treatment may cause long-lasting elevation in corticosterone level. On the other hand, the duration of MAP-induced elevation in corticosterone may be much shorter in F-344, which have a hyperresponsive negative feedback in the HPA axis. Ortiz et al. [2] reported LEW developed significant locomotor sensitization from treatment with chronic cocaine, but F-344 did not show sensitization without chronic corticosterone pretreatment. Chronic MAP or cocaine possibly reduces the corticosterone level in F-344; thus, F-344 rats might be resistant to sensitizing effects of these drugs.

The hybridization signal of GR or MR mRNA was normalized relative to the signal obtained from beta-actin mRNA, whose expression was not affected by any dose of MAP [11]. Corticosterone receptors can bind to their genes and potently downregulate transcription, while this effect is site specific. Factors other than corticosterone receptor might be involved in this site-specific transcriptional control of corticosterone receptors. Although MAP-induced changes in GR and MR mRNA in F-344 and LEW brain are region specific, we observed increased GR and MR mRNA in F-344 with acute and chronic MAP treatment, and these mRNAs were decreased in LEW by chronic MAP. These results are partly consistent with a previous report [12], in which hippocampal GR mRNA of the Sprague–Dawley rat is upregulated 24h after acute AMP treatment and downregulated by chronic AMP. Differences in the experimental schedule or the HPA axis response of each strain might be the reason for this discrepancy. As discussed, decreased GR and MR mRNA by acute and chronic MAP in LEW might be caused by long-lasting elevation of corticosterone. Conversely, increased GR and MR mRNA by chronic MAP might reflect a reduced corticosterone level in F-344.

Among brain regions examined, we observed marked differences between F-344 and LEW rats in their striatal GR and MR mRNA by chronic MAP: increase in F-344 and decrease in LEW. Striatal genes whose expression is regulated by corticosterone receptors might play an important role in susceptibility to behavioral sensitization.

Acknowledgments. This study was partly supported by grant-in-aid for scientific research (B)(2) #10470200 (Y.N.) and Health Sciences Research Grants for Research on Brain Science from the Ministry of Health and Welfare #100109 (M.S.).

References

1. Sato M, Numachi Y, Hamamura T (1992) Relapse of paranoid psychotic state in methamphetamine model of schizophrenia. Schizophr Bull 18:115–122
2. Ortiz J, Decaprio JL, Kosten TA, et al (1995) Strain-selective effects of corticosterone on locomotor sensitization to cocaine and on levels of tyrosine hydroxylase and glucocorticoid receptor in the ventral tegmental area. Neuroscience 67:383–397
3. Evans RM, Arriza JL (1989) A molecular framework for the actions of glucocorticoid hormones in the nervous system. Neuron 2:1105–1112
4. Creese I, Iversen SD (1973) Blockage of amphetamine induced motor stimulation and stereotypy in the adult rat following neonatal treatment with 6-hydroxydopamine. Brain Res 15:369–382

5. Numachi Y, Yoshida S, Toda S, et al (2000) Two inbred strains of rats, Fischer 344 and Lewis, showed differential behavior and brain expression of corticosterone receptor mRNA induced by methamphetamine. Ann NY Acad Sci 914:33–45
6. Reul JMHM, Pearce PT, Funder JW, et al (1989) Type I and type II corticosteroid receptor gene expression in the rat: effect of adrenalectomy and dexamethasone administration. Mol Endocrinol 3:1674–1680
7. Higashi T, Takeuchi H, Uemura Y, et al (1994) Differential induction of mRNA species encoding several classes of stress proteins following focal cerebral ischemia in rats. Brain Res 650:239–248
8. Yoshida S, Numachi Y, Matsuoka H, et al (1998) Impairment of cliff avoidance reaction induced by subchronic methamphetamine administration and restraint stress: comparison between two inbred strains of rats. Prog Neuropsychopharmacol Biol Psychiatry 22:1023–1032
9. Camp DM, Browman KE, Robinson TE (1994) The effects of methamphetamine and cocaine on motor behavior and extracellular dopamine in the ventral striatum of Lewis versus Fischer 344 rats. Brain Res 668:180–193
10. Budziszewska B, Jaworska-Feil L, Lason W (1996) The effect of repeated amphetamine and cocaine administration on adrenal, gonadal and thyroid hormone levels in the rat plasma. Exp Clin Endocrinol Diabetes 104:334–348
11. Carney JM, Tolliver B, Carney JP, et al (1991) Selective effects of behaviorally active doses of methamphetamine on mRNA expression in the gerbil brain. Neuropharmacology 30:1011–1019
12. Shilling PD, Kelsoe JR, Segal DS (1996) Hippocampal glucocorticoid receptor mRNA is up-regulated by acute and down-regulated by chronic amphetamine treatment. Brain Res Mol Brain Res 38:156–160

Neuroimaging in Chronic MAP Users

Masaomi Iyo, Yoshimoto Sekine, and Norio Mori

Summary. Chronic use of methamphetamine (MAP) produces persistent psychiatric symptoms in some users. Here, we present our four major findings, by using neuroimaging techniques, in the brain of chronic MAP users. ^{99m}Tc-HMPAO/SPECT showed persistent patchy deficits in cerebral blood flow without structural abnormalities on MRI, indicating that persistent functional changes occur in the users. A PET study with ^{11}C-WIN-35,428 indicated significant and persistent reductions in dopamine transporter (DAT) density, which were correlated with both the duration of MAP use and severity of psychotic symptoms, in the striatum, nucleus accumbens, and prefrontal cortex. The DAT reduction may be associated with persistent psychiatric symptoms in the users. An MRS imaging study showed significant elevated choline/creatine but normal level of *N*-acetyl-aspartate/creatine in the striatum, implying altered membrane turnover without neuronal loss. On the other hand, a ^{11}C-*N*-methylspiperone/PET study indicated no change in striatal D_2 receptor density in abstinent MAP users, suggesting reversible changes in D_2 receptors.

Keywords. Methamphetamine, Abuse, PET, SPECT, MRI

Introduction

Methamphetamine (MAP) has been abused worldwide. During chronic use of MAP, some users experience psychotic episodes, called MAP psychosis, and the psychosis easily relapses by reuse of even a low to moderate dose of MAP or by psychological stress. These findings suggest the development of susceptibility to psychosis during chronic use. In Japan, this psychosis is classified from the point of view of the duration into two types, the "early recovery type," in which psychotic episodes disappear within 1 month, and the "prolonged type," in which the psychotic episodes are prolonged longer than 1 month [1]. Although the concept of the prolonged type of MAP psychosis has been established in Japan, this type of psychosis is sometimes considered merely an expression of schizophrenia, i.e., MAP abuse in schizophrenia, in other countries [2]. Therefore, it is necessary to clarify persistent brain dysfunction and its

Department of Psychiatry and Neurology, Hamamatsu University School of Medicine, 3600 Handa-cho, Hamamatsu, Shizuoka 431-3192, Japan

association with prolonged psychosis in MAP users to establish the concept of a prolonged type of MAP psychosis. We have used neuroimaging techniques, single photon emission computed tomography (SPECT), positron emission tomography (PET), and magnetic resonance imaging (MRI) to determine these dysfunctions.

Single Photon Emission Computed Tomography

SPECT using ^{99m}Tc-HMPAO as a tracer and MRI were performed in nine chronic MAP users; six showed prominent cerebral patchy deficits on their SPECT images whereas there was no abnormality, including obvious atrophy and lacunar infarctions, on their MRIs [3]. The period between the last use of MAP and the SPECT study varied from 1.5 months to 10 years in the subjects with abnormal SPECT images. These findings suggest that in chronic MAP users multiple patchy deficits in cerebral blood flow, which are persist for a long period of time after stopping MAP use, are observed with a high rate of incidence. However, we did not find a significant correlation between the severity of deficits and the period of MAP use or severity of psychotic symptoms. Therefore, these deficits may not be responsible for the prolonged psychosis in MAP users.

Positron Emission Tomography

Dopamine D_2 Receptors

MAP induces psychological effects mainly by acting on dopamine nerve terminals. MAP inhibits dopamine transporter (DAT), monoamine transporter, and monoamine oxidase, and then increases the intracellular and extracellular dopamine level. Binding of excessive dopamine to dopamine receptors, in turn, exerts dopaminergic hyperactivity. By using PET and ^{11}C-*N*-methylspiperone, we measured the striatal dopamine D_2 receptor density in six chronic MAP users with a history of psychosis and ten healthy control subjects [4]. As one of the aims of this study was to determine chronic changes in the receptors, the subjects were abstinent from MAP longer than 2 months before the PET study. The results indicated that there was no significant difference in the density between the healthy control and MAP users. It is suggested that the dopamine D_2 receptors may recover when the use of MAP is stopped, although they may transiently reduce with chronic MAP use as a compensation for increased dopamine level in the synaptic cleft by MAP administration. This change might be also related to withdrawal symptoms in chronic MAP use, although it may not be associated with persistent psychosis in chronic MAP users.

Dopamine Transporter Density

The reduction of dopamine transporter (DAT) density was reported in the caudate/putamen or nucleus accumbens of chronic MAP abusers in the postmortem human study [5] and the PET study [6]. However, the relation of the reduction to clinical characteristics is unknown. We studied the DATs in nine MAP users and ten healthy controls by using PET and ^{11}C-WIN35,428. Regions of interest were selected in the caudate/putamen, nucleus accumbens, and prefrontal cortex, which are the terminals of major dopaminergic projections in the brain. The three-compartment model analysis revealed a significant reduction in DAT density in each of the regions observed in chronic MAP users compared to the controls. The three MAP users received second PET scans 6–9 months after the first scan, and no difference in DAT density between the two tests was observed. There was a significant correlation between the duration of MAP use and the severity of positive symptoms evaluated by Brief Psychiatic Rating Scores. The reduction of the DAT density was significantly correlated with the duration of MAP use and the severity of positive symptoms. These findings indicate that DAT density persistently reduces with chronic use of MAP and that this reduction is closely associated with persistent psychotic symptoms. Therefore, it is suggested that reduction in DAT density may actively participate in pathogenesis of prolonged MAP psychosis. Because no change in DAT density in schizophrenia [7] has been reported, the prolonged type of MAP psychosis is a disease independent from schizophrenia.

Proton Magnetic Resonance Spectroscopy

One of the questions is whether the observed reduction in DAT density results from neuronal degeneration. In magnetic resonance spectroscopy, *N*-acetylasparate (NAA) or an *N*-acetyl compound reflects neuronal density and choline reflects membrane turnover [8]. Creatine can be used as a reference. Therefore, we measured the *N*-acetylasparate and choline levels in six MAP users and nine healthy controls. There were no significant differences in the NAA level between the MAP users and controls, whereas MAP users had a significantly higher level in choline than the controls. These findings suggest that the membrane turnover in the striatum is exacerbated in MAP users but that no prominent reduction in neuronal density occurs. These results also suggest that the DAT reduction may not result from merely neuronal degeneration.

Conclusion

^{99m}Tc-HMPAO-SPECT showed persistent patchy deficits in cerebral blood flow without structural abnormalities on MRI, indicating that persistent functional changes occur in the users. A PET study with ^{11}C-WIN-35,428 indicated significant and persistent reductions in DAT density, which were correlated with both the duration of MAP use and the severity of psychotic symptoms, in the striatum, nucleus accumbens, and prefrontal cortex. The eduction may be associated with persistent psychiatric symptoms in the users. An MRS imaging study showed significant elevated choline/creatine but normal level of *N*-acetyl-aspartate/creatine in the striatum, implying altered membrane turnover without neuronal loss. On the other hand, a ^{11}C-*N*-methylspiperone/PET study indicated no change in striatal D_2 receptor density in abstinent MAP users, suggesting reversible changes in D_2 receptors.

References

1. Konuma K, Hirai S, Kasahara M (1994) Use and abuse of amphetamines in Japan. In: Cho AK, Segal DS (eds) Amphetamine and its analogs. San Diego, Academic Press, pp 459–478
2. Angrist B (1994) Amphetamine psychosis: clinical variations of the syndrome. In: Cho AK, Segal DS (eds) Amphetamine and its analogs. San Diego, Academic Press, pp 387–414
3. Iyo M, Namba H, Hirai S, et al (1997) Abnormal cerebral perfusion in chronic methamphetamine abusers: a study using ^{99m}Tc-HMPAO and SPECT. Prog Neuropsychol Biol Psychiatry 21:789–796
4. Iyo M, Nishio M, Itoh T, et al (1993) Dopamine D_2 and serotonin S_2 receptors in susceptibility to methamphetamine psychosis detected by positron emission tomography. Psychiatry Res Neuroimaging 50:217–231
5. Wilson JM, Kalasinsky KS, Levey AI, et al (1996) Striatal dopamine nerve terminal markers in human, chronic methamphetamine users. Nat Med 2:699–703
6. McCann UD, Wong DF, Yokoi F, et al (1998) Reduced striatal dopamine transporter density in abstinent methamphetamine and methcathinone users: evidence from positron emission tomography studies with [^{11}C]WIN-35,428. J Neurosci 18:8417–8422
7. Laakso A, Vilkman H, Alakare B, et al (2000) Striatal dopamine transporter binding in neuroleptic-naive patients with schizophrenia studied with positron emission tomography. Am J Psychiatry 157:269–271
8. Miller BL, Hang L, Booth R, et al (1996) *In vivo* ^{1}H-MRS choline: correlation with *in vitro* chemistry/histology. Life Sci 58:1929–1935

The Genetics of Psychiatric Disorders

Are Monozygotic Twins Discordant for Psychosis Caused by Differential Methylation?

Takahiro Tsujita[1], Tomohiko Kayashima[1,2], Norio Niikawa[2], Yoshibumi Nakane[1], and Yuji Okazaki[3]

Summary. It is known that certain somatic mutations occurring simultaneously with, or after, twinning may cause phenotypic differences between monozygotic twins (MZT). Thus, we hypothesized that cases of MZT discordant for schizophrenia might also be caused by unknown genomic discordance. Genomic differences were detected by using a new technique, restriction landmark genome scanning (RLGS). A detailed comparison of the RLGS patterns detected at least five spots (spots 1–5) showed obviously different autoradiographic intensities between the twins. After trying to clone fragments that produced all the spots, we obtained four clones. Two alternative mechanisms by which the discrepant fragments appear in the twins are possible. First, in either of the twins, a submicroscopic change of DNA, for example, deletion/insertion, substitution, or translocation, may have occurred at *Not*I-flanking sites simultaneously with, or after, twinning. Second, as we used the methylation-sensitive enzyme, *Not*I, the methylation status at *Not*I site(s) may be different between the twins. I think that this possibility might have great significance. If, in this new strategy, differences of transcription level of one or more genes between the twins are shown, this will contribute to a search for the pathogenesis of schizophrenia.

Keywords. Schizophrenia, Monozygotic twins, Restriction landmark genome scanning (RLGS), Methylation, Epigenetics

Introduction

Monozygotic twins (MZT) discordant for psychosis have been analyzed for the prevalence and cause of the disease. Such studies have been based on the premise that MZT are genetically identical but were exposed to different postnatal environments. However, it is known that certain somatic mutations occurring simultaneously with, or after, twinning may cause phenotypic difference between MZT: MZT who are discordant for chromosomal abnormalities and for fragile-X syndrome with different

Departments of [1]Neuropsychiatry and [2]Human Genetics, Nagasaki University School of Medicine, Nagasaki, Japan
[3]Department of Psychiatry, Mie University Faculty of Medicine, School of Medicine, Mie, Japan

triplet repeat expansions in *FMR1*. Moreover, recent studies demonstrated that loss of genomic imprinting or skewed X-inactivation in either of the twins may also cause a discordance. So, I hypothesized that cases of monozygotic twins discordant for schizophrenia might also be caused by unknown genomic discordance. Here, we report differences of genomic DNA between MZT who are discordant for schizophrenia. The difference was detected using a new technique, restriction landmark genome scanning (RLGS).

Subjects

The subjects were 44-year-old male twins. Twin A has been suffering from DSM-III-R schizophrenia, undifferentiated type, since the age of 30. He first entered a catatonic stupor status, then developed hallucination of voices conversing 2 years later, has been confined indoors without a job, and never married. Twin B, an industrial worker, has been healthy and also never married. After complete description of the study to the subjects, written informed consent was obtained. Both the twins have a 46,XY karyotype without any visible chromosomal mosaicism. Monozygosity of the twins was proved using seven blood types and DNA fingerprinting.

Method

RLGS Procedure

Genomic DNA was extracted from peripheral blood leukocytes of each twin, and applied to RLGS analysis as described [1]. In brief, genomic DNA (3.5 μg) was first treated with DNA polymerase I in the presence of dGTPαS, dCTPαS, ddATP, and ddTTP. This step, which is based on the incorporation of the dideoxynucleotide analogue into the nonspecifically damaged sites, such as nicks, gaps, or double-strand breaks, is done to prevent the background. The DNA was then digested with a landmark restriction enzyme, *Not*I, and the cleavage ends were end labeled with a fill-in reaction using Sequenase Ver. 2.0 (USB, Cleveland, Ohio, USA) in the presence of radiolabeled dCTP (6000 Ci/mmol) and dGTP (3000 Ci/mmol). The end-labeled DNA was digested with another enzyme, *Pvu*II, and the DNA was electrophoresed in a 0.8% agarose gel (first dimension). The disk of the gel containing DNA was treated with the third enzyme, *Pst*I, followed by two-dimensional electrophoresis in 6% acrylamide gel. The gels were dried and exposed to Kodak XAR X-ray films at −80°C for several days.

PCR-Mediated Cloning of Target Spot DNA on RLGS Gel

After autoradiography for a few days, the target spots were punched out and their DNA fragments were electroeluted. The DNA fragments were ligated with *Not*I and *Pst*I adaptors, and the eluate was PCR amplified. The PCR products were then inserted into plasmid vectors and subjected to DNA sequencing.

Results

The RLGS analysis revealed approximately 2000 spots on each twin's autoradiogram. A detailed comparison of the RLGS patterns detected at least five spots (spot 1–5) that showed obviously different autoradiographic intensities between the twins [2]. All the spots estimated to be about 300–400 bp were observed only in twin A, while in twin B, spot 1 was lacking and spots 2–5 were very faintly visible. The discrepancies were ascertained consistently by repeated RLGS trials. After trying to clone fragments that produced all the spots, we obtained four clones. Naturally, each of the clones has a *Not*I recognition site at the 5′-end of the fragment.

Discussion

The region, which is abundant in GC bases and is thought to have a transcription regulatory function, is called a CpG island. Usually, a CpG island is present within 2 kb of the 5′-transcriptional end of a functional gene. Furthermore, it is known that 89% of *Not*I recognition sites are located on CpG islands. Thus, the fragments detected in our research have a high probability of reflecting such a mutation, leading to an alteration of the transcription level of a gene.

The RLGS method, developed for a high-speed survey of restriction sites throughout the genome, employs direct end-labeling of genomic DNA digested with a restriction enzyme and high-resolution, two-dimensional electrophoresis. As spot intensity accurately reflects the dose of a *Not*I/*Pst*I restriction fragment, it is evident that twin A's genomic DNA contains five *Not*I/*Pst*I fragments (spots 1–5), while the fragments are in a lower level or are lacking in twin B [2]. Differences derived from variable immunoresponse system genes are generally not detectable because the number of such individual cells to be subjected to RLGS is negligible. Two alternative mechanisms by which the discrepant fragments in the twins appear are possible [2]. First, in either of the twins, a submicroscopic change of DNA, for example, deletion/insertion, substitution, or translocation, may have occurred at *Not*I-flanking sites simultaneously with, or after, twinning. Second, as we used the methylation-sensitive enzyme, *Not*I, the methylation status at *Not*I site(s) may be different between the twins. In general, methylation-sensitive enzymes cannot cleavage methylated recognition sites. I think that this possibility might have great significance.

We would like to emphasize that the understanding of epigenetic regulation of genes as well as sequences of genes may be of epochal value. By definition, epigenetics pertains to mitotically and in some cases meiotically heritable factors that control gene activity and are not directly related to differences in DNA sequence [3]. DNA methylation is one epigenetic mechanism among others. In promoter regions, methylated CpG and its binding proteins usually inhibit transcription of genes by preventing linkage of the transcription factors with the promotor regions. By this mechanism, numerous cellular functions are controlled and mediated, for example, the regulation of gene activity, DNA repair, mutagenesis, and also genomic imprinting [4]. Although previous studies have not supported an association between the etiology of schizophrenia and genomic imprinting, it is reasonable to assume some epigenetic modification, such as DNA methylation, to explain a similar high incidence of schizophrenia among children of schizophrenic monozygotic twins and those of nonaffected co twins [2], because methylation or demethylation usually is reset in the next generation.

The aim of our current research is to clarify the difference of genomic DNA status between the twins at regions near the clones that we obtained. For that purpose, we plan to perform a mutation search and a methylation search using a methylation-specific PCR method or the method of direct sequencing of sodium bisulfite-treated DNA. Interestingly, it appeared that one of the clones that we have has a high homology to the sequence of a gene that expresses widely in the human central nervous system. If, in this new strategy, differences of transcription level of one or more genes between the twins are shown, this will contribute to a search for the pathogenesis of schizophrenia.

References

1. Hayashizaki Y, Watanabe S (1997) Restriction landmark genome scanning (RLGS). Springer, Tokyo
2. Tsujita T, Niikawa N, Yamashita H, et al (1998) Genomic discordance between monozygotic twins discordant for schizophrenia. Am J Psychiatry 155:422–424
3. Riggs AD, Martienssen RA, Russo VEA (1996) In: Russo VEA, Martienssen RA, Riggs AD (eds) Epigenetic mechanisms of gene regulation. Cold Spring Harbor Laboratory Press, Cold Spring Harbor, pp 1–4
4. Russo VEA, Martienssen RA, Riggs AD (eds) (1996) Epigenetic mechanisms of gene regulation. Cold Spring Harbor Laboratory Press, Cold Spring Harbor

Influence of ADH and ALDH2 on Clinical Features of Alcohol Dependence

Susumu Higuchi and Sachio Matsushita

Summary. Alcohol dehydrogenase (ADH) and aldehyde dehydrogenase-2 (ALDH2) play central roles in the metabolism of ethanol and its metabolite, acetaldehyde, in the liver. Genes encoding these enzymes show polymorphisms capable of altering metabolic activities. We have examined the relationship between genetic variations of these enzymes and alcohol-related disorders in Japanese. The results revealed that the less active allele of the ADH2 gene (ADH2*1) is associated with an increased risk for alcohol dependence, alcohol-induced persistent amnestic disorder, and cancers of the upper gastrointestinal (GI) tract, and with the severity of the acute withdrawal syndrome. On the other hand, the inactive allele of the ALDH2 gene (ALDH2*2) is associated with reduced alcohol consumption in the general Japanese population, a decreased risk for alcohol dependence, and an increased risk for the cancers in the same region. Possible mechanisms for these associations are discussed.

Keywords. Alcohol dependence, Genetics, Risk, Alcohol dehydrogense, Aldehyde dehydrogenase-2, Wernicke-Korsakoff syndrome, Upper GI tract cancer

Introduction

Alcohol dependence runs in families. This notion has been consistently supported by family, twin, and adoption studies. To identify genes that alter susceptibility to alcohol dependence, linkage and association studies have been carried out in many laboratories. Despite such enormous efforts, to date there are only two genes whose associations with alcohol dependence are firmly established: class I alcohol dehydrogenase (ADH) and aldehyde dehydrogenase-2 (ALDH2). These enzymes play central roles in the initial stages of alcohol metabolism.

ADH consists of three genes—ADH1, ADH2, and ADH3. Among these genes, polymorphisms with physiological significance exist in the ADH2 and ADH3 loci. Likewise, a functional polymorphism known to cause the flushing response after alcohol ingestion has been identified near the stop codon of the ALDH2 gene. The

Institute of Clinical Research, National Alcoholism Center Kurihama Hospital, 5-3-1 Nobi, Yokosuka, Kanagawa 239-0841, Japan

present study examines genetic variations of ADH2 and ALDH2 with respect to clinical features of alcohol dependence.

ADH2 and ALDH2 and the Risk for Alcohol Dependence

To investigate the effects of the ADH2 and ALDH2 genes on susceptibility to alcohol dependence, we compared the genotype and allele frequencies of these genes between Japanese alcoholics and nonalcoholic controls. The results revealed that the ALDH2*2 allele is strikingly less frequent in alcoholics than in controls. We have examined 3,171 alcoholics and found 322 alcoholics or 10.5% with inactive ALDH2. However, all of them had heterozygous ALDH2*1/2*2, and no alcoholics with homozygous ALDH2*2 have been detected. These results strongly suggest that homozygous ALDH2*2 fully inhibits the development of alcohol dependence because of the severe flushing response it produces, whereas the suppressive effect of heterozygous ALDH2*1/2*2 is incomplete, thus permitting other influences such as sociocultural factors to have an effect (Higuchi et al. 1994). The comparison of the ADH2 gene in Japanese alcoholic samples and normal controls showed that the ADH2*2 allele is significantly less frequent in the former group than in the latter group.

We attempted to quantify the relative risk for alcohol dependence from the results of ADH2 and ALDH2 genotype frequencies. The results showed that inactive ALDH2 is not always associated with a low risk, and active ALDH2 is not always associated with a high risk. In individuals with heterozygous ALDH2*1/2*2 and homozygous ADH2*1, the odds ratio for alcohol dependence was significantly high (Higuchi et al. 1995).

ADH2 and ALDH2 and Clinical Features of Alcohol Dependence

The clinical features examined include the sociofamilial background, comorbid psychiatric disorders, temporal profile of disease development, and comorbid alcohol amnestic disorder and upper gastrointestinal tract cancers. The results should provide information for understanding the mechanisms of the development of dependence and various alcohol-related disorders.

Comorbid Psychiatric Disorders and Disease Course

We examined 409 Japanese alcoholics who were consecutively admitted to the National Institute on Alcoholism, Kurihama National Hospital. A semistructured interview of each subject was conducted to obtain information on family background, social background, drinking history, DSM-III-R criteria for the evaluation of psychiatric conditions, and Feighner's diagnostic criteria for the lifetime diagnosis of alcoholism (Murayama et al. 1998).

Comparison of sociofamilial backgrounds revealed no significant differences between the active (without ALDH2*2 allele) and the inactive (with ALDH2*2 allele) or between the atypical (with ADH2*2 allele) and the usual (without ADH2*2 allele) groups. Likewise, we could not detect any differences in comorbid psychopathologies between the groups. However, the inactive group developed alcohol dependence more slowly than did the other group. The occurrence of every event or symptom related to drinking or drinking problems was delayed from 1 to 5 years in the inactive group compared with the active group (Murayama et al. 1998). Interestingly, the development of alcohol dependence in the atypical group was delayed compared with that in the usual group. These results suggest that the association between the ADH2 gene and alcohol dependence can be explained by the increased acetaldehyde concentration in the blood due to atypical ADH, which is the same mechanism as that of inactive ALDH2.

Alcohol Amnestic Disorder

To test the hypothesis of altered alcohol and aldehyde regulation in the development of Wernicke–Korsakoff syndrome (WKS), we examined the ADH2 and ALDH2 polymorphisms in 47 alcoholics with WKS, 342 alcoholics without WKS, and 175 normal controls (Matsushita et al. 2000). Although the frequencies of the ALDH2 genotypes and alleles did not differ significantly between alcoholics with WKS and those without WKS, the ADH2*1/*1 genotype and the ADH2*1 allele were significantly increased in WKS, suggesting that the ADH2*1 allele is a risk factor for WKS in alcoholic patients.

Upper GI Tract Cancers

We have reported that inactive ALDH2 is a major risk factor for upper GI tract cancers in alcoholics (Yokoyama et al. 1996). We assume that the carcinogenic effect of acetaldehyde is involved in the high incidence of these cancers in alcoholics with inactive ALDH2. Recently, we found that not only ALDH2 but also the ADH2 polymorphism is most likely to confer susceptibility to cancers of the same region in alcoholics.

The study subjects were 169 Japanese male alcoholics aged 40 years or older with upper GI tract cancers. They were systematically screened from 2,456 alcoholics using endoscopy combined with esophageal iodine staining. The control subjects consisted of 526 male alcoholics of the same age who were cancer free. Examination of oropharygolarygeal and esophageal cancers with regard to the ADH2 genotypes revealed that comorbidity is significantly higher in alcoholics with usual ADH2 than in those with atypical ADH2 (Yokoyama et al. 1999).

Summary of the Results

Table 1 presents a summary of the results and the postulated mechanisms for the associations we have obtained. Although we did not show the data, we have found that the acute alcohol withdrawal syndrome was more severe in alcoholics with usual ADH2 than in those with atypical ADH2. Underlying mechanisms of these associations are largely unknown. The exception is the relationship between the ALDH2 polymorphism and drinking behavior, susceptibility to alcohol dependence, and disease

TABLE 1. Summary of the results of association studies with ADH2 and ALDH2 genes and underlying mechanisms for the associations

	ADH2		ALDH2	
Characteristics	Association	Mechanism	Association	Mechanisms
Drinking behavior	No	–	Yes	Adverse reaction due to ACAL
Alcohol dependence	Yes	Adverse reaction due to ACAL (?)	Yes	Adverse reaction due to ACAL
Clinical features				
Disease development	Yes	Adverse reaction due to ACAL (?)	Yes	Adverse reaction due to ACAL
Severity of withdrawal syndrome	Yes	Alcohol consumption (?)	?	
Upper GI cancers	Yes	?	Yes	Carcinogenic effects of ACAL (?)
Wernicke-Korsakoff syndrome	Yes	?	No	

ADH, alcohol dehydrogenase; ALDH2, aldehyde dehydrogenase-2; ACAL, acetaldehyde

development. All these associations can be explained by inactive ALDH2-mediated hyperacetaldehydemia after alcohol intake. We speculate that elucidation of the mechanisms for ADH2-related associations will provide a better understanding of dependence and the withdrawal syndrome. Extensive studies on these issues are warranted.

References

Higuchi S, Matsushita S, Imazeki H, et al (1994) Aldehyde dehydrogenase genotypes in Japanese alcoholics. Lancet 343:741–742

Higuchi S, Matsushita S, Murayama M, et al (1995) Alcohol and aldehyde dehydrogenase polymorphisms and the risk for alcoholism. Am J Psychiatry 152:1219–1221

Matsushita S, Kato M, Muramatsu T, et al (2000) Alcohol and aldehyde dehydrogenase genotypes in Korsakoff syndrome. Alcohol Clin Exp Res 24:337–340

Murayama M, Matsushita S, Muramatsu T, et al (1998) Clinical characteristics and disease course of alcoholics with inactive aldehyde dehydrogenase-2. Alcohol Clin Exp Res 22:524–527

Yokoyama A, Muramatsu T, Ohmori T, et al (1996) Esophageal cancer and aldehyde dehydrogenase-2 genotypes in Japanese males. Cancer Epidemiol Biomark Prev 5:99–102

Yokoyama A, Muramatsu T, Ohmori T, et al (1999) Alcohol and aldehyde dehydrogenase gene polymorphisms influence susceptibility to esophageal cancer in Japanese alcoholics. Alcohol Clin Exp Res 23:1705–1710

Epileptic Psychoses and Anticonvulsants

Schizophrenia-Like Psychosis and Epilepsy: The Status of the Relationship

Perminder Sachdev

Introduction

The association between epilepsy and psychosis has attracted the attention of psychiatrists since the nineteenth century, but most aspects of this relationship remain contentious (Trimble 1991; Sachdev 1998). Some of the controversies relate to a lack of clarity of conceptual issues, while others result from inadequate data. In this chapter, I try to summarize the current state of knowledge about the relationship between epilepsy and schizophrenia-like psychosis (SLP) and to arrive at a synthetic view that may lead to a better understanding in the future. In trying to conceptualize this field, some principles need to be stated at the outset, the relevance of which will become clearer later. These concepts are as follows:

The term psychosis must be strictly and narrowly defined in any analysis. Some of the problems in the literature relate to varying definitions of psychosis. For this analysis, only psychosis with predominantly schizophreniform features and occurring in clear consciousness are included.

It must be appreciated that both epilepsy and schizophrenia are heterogeneous disorders. The question is, therefore, the relationship between which epilepsy and what kind of psychosis?

The similarity between temporal lobe phenomena and psychotic symptoms does not necessarily mean that they have a common origin.

The two themes that have dominated psychiatric thought on the association are (1) they occur together more often than chance ("affinity") and (2) they are "antagonistic" to each other. These seemingly incompatible observations must be reconciled.

The epileptic brain is not normal between clinical seizures. The association is with epilepsy and not seizures alone. Moreover, epilepsy is not a static process, and the brain of the epileptic patient is undergoing structural and neurochemical change, before and after the development of seizures, to which ictal events actually contribute (Engel 1996). The same is probably true for schizophrenia (Olney and Farber 1995).

School of Psychiatry, University of New South Wales, and Neuropsychiatric Institute, The Prince of Wales Hospital, Randwick, Sydney, NSW2031, Australia

Our understanding of the etiopathogenesis of both groups of disorders is incomplete. Consequently, the establishment of a relationship does not automatically lead to new insights.

Classification of SLP with Epilepsy

Such psychoses have traditionally been categorized into *ictal*, *postictal*, or *interictal*, with the latter being either brief or chronic. This distinction is clinically useful but, as is discussed later, the mechanisms underlying these categories probably overlap.

Ictal Psychosis

Prolonged ictal activity can result in symptoms that resemble psychosis. This occurrence is most commonly associated with psychomotor status and less commonly with petit mal status. The disturbance seen in the episode is produced by one of two mechanisms (Gloor 1991): (i) a positive effect of the seizure discharge, i.e., by epileptic activation of a behavioral mechanism represented in the area subjected to the discharge, and (ii) a negative effect whereby either the individual is unable to engage in a certain behavior because the anatomical substrate of that behavior has been temporarily paralyzed, or some behaviors normally suppressed are released by the inactivation of structures that suppress those behaviors. The negative effect may continue postictally, or may initiate then. Experiential phenomena in ictal psychosis are likely to be due to positive effects whereas automatisms may be caused by positive or negative effects.

The question that has generated some degree of controversy is whether more longstanding psychosis in clear consciousness can be produced by continuous subictal electrical activity. The work by Kendrick and Gibbs (1957) and Heath (1962) demonstrated epileptiform discharges on depth recordings that did not spread beyond the amygdala, hippocampus, and septal regions, in both schizophrenic patients and in epileptic patients with psychosis, but this has rarely been examined since.

Postictal Psychosis

Brief psychoses that follow a bout of seizures have received much attention in the past decade (Logsdail and Toone 1988; Umbricht et al. 1995; Kanemoto et al. 1996). The characteristics of postictal psychosis are as follows.

The psychosis usually occurs after an exacerbation in seizure frequency or intensity.
There is usually a nonpsychotic period between the last seizure and the psychosis that ranges from a few hours to a few days.
The psychotic symptoms are pleomorphic, with affective symptoms commonly being present.
There is usually a spontaneous resolution within a few days, and a further seizure may exacerbate the psychosis.
The majority suffer from partial complex seizures that are secondarily generalized. EEG abnormalities persist in the majority during the psychosis.

The pathogenetic mechanisms are not understood. Some findings suggest that ictal activity in the temporal lobe is directly related to this kind of psychosis. Changes in monoamines, in particular that of postsynaptic DA sensitivity, and endogenous opiates have also been suggested as the mediating mechanisms. More recently, the focus has been on GABA and glutamate, as these amino acids are involved in the processes that terminate a seizure. Patients with such psychoses would be ideal candidates for longitudinal studies, using electrophysiological, neuroimaging, and neurochemical techniques to study the chronic course and perhaps the development of chronic psychoses.

Brief Interictal Psychoses

These psychoses are brief, lasting from days to weeks, and occur when seizure activity is relatively quiescent. Separation from postictal psychoses, however, may be difficult. The brief interictal psychoses have received much attention in the context of what has been called paradoxical or forced normalization (Landolt 1953). Paradoxical normalization has been well documented by a number of authors, but not all brief interictal psychoses demonstrate this phenomenon.

Most anticonvulsants have been reported to precipitate psychosis in clear consciousness, in particular, the succinimides and lately vigabatrin. Most authors have considered anticonvulsant-related psychosis to be an example of alternating psychosis. These psychoses may, however, be heterogeneous, as has been shown in relation to vigabatrin (Sander et al. 1991). Many hypotheses have been suggested to explain brief psychosis, none of which is entirely satisfactory. It is possible that the mechanism is not very different from postictal psychosis, with excessive inhibition being a factor.

Chronic Interictal Psychosis

Ever since the seminal work of Slater and colleagues (1963), the chronic psychoses have received a great deal of attention from psychiatrists.

The Evidence for the Association

The primary evidence for an association between epilepsy and schizophrenia-like psychoses must be epidemiological. The prevalence of SLP in epilepsy clinic populations is reported to be high. Mendez et al. (1993) found 9.25% of their patients, by retrospective review, to be suffering from schizophrenia defined by DSM-III R, compared to 1% of migraine patients. Community studies have similarly reported high rates. Gudmundsson (1966), who studied the entire epileptic population of Iceland, reported that 7% had a history of a broadly defined psychosis. The rates of epilepsy in psychotic populations here are also high. Lindsay et al. (1979) reported an overall incidence of 10% of psychosis in temporal lobe epilepsy (TLE) patients followed up over four decades.

TLE and Schizophreniform Psychosis

Suggestions that psychosis in epilepsy might be exclusively or preferentially associated with TLE are supported by the majority of investigations (Sachdev 1998), although this has been disputed by Stevens (1991). For TLE, the psychotic patients are more likely to have a mediobasal spike focus, as recorded on sphenoidal EEG, or an epigastric or "fear" aura.

What About Laterality of Temporal Lobe Focus and Psychosis?

If one examines the EEG studies, the majority opinion is that there is an excess of left temporal foci in the TLE patients with schizophreniform psychosis, as this composite analysis of various studies would suggest. This is not an exclusive relationship, however, and there are a number of studies that are negative for laterality. The neuroimaging data are again inconclusive, with functional but not structural studies pointing to laterality. The functional studies must, however, be considered preliminary as they involved small numbers. The neuropathology data have not supported lateralization (Roberts et al. 1990; Bruton et al. 1994). The laterality issue therefore remains undecided, and the importance of a left-sided focus is not striking. It is possible that the structural abnormality in epileptic psychosis is bilateral but that the functional abnormality may be predominantly left sided. However, right-sided abnormality seems to be sufficient, and generalization of the epileptic disturbance is commonly present in these patients.

Phenomenology of Chronic Epileptic Psychoses

Slater et al. (1963) reported that chronic SLP with epilepsy had a mean age of onset of about 30 years, and the symptomatology was largely paranoid hallucinatory, commonly associated with catatonia, affective blunting, and volitional disturbances. The disorder was indistinguishable from schizophrenia, although the authors reported a better preservation of affect, mood swings, mystical experiences, and visual hallucinations. There is a relative lack of negative symptoms, and a more benign course has been suggested, although supportive data are lacking. In the Slater et al. (1963) study, 45% had a chronic course. In a study by Onuma et al. (1991), 64% had a chronic course.

Risk Factors

The following have been suggested as risk factors: epilepsy starting at an early age and persisting through puberty, severe epilepsy involving multiple seizure types, a history of status epilepticus, and resistance to drug treatment. These patients do not have an increased family history of schizophrenia. Psychosis may sometimes develop following temporal lobectomy for resistant TLE, especially after right-sided surgery.

Possible Mechanisms

Broadly, two mechanisms have been proposed that link epilepsy with schizophrenia-like psychosis: (1) the psychosis is due to the repeated electrical discharges, either directly or through the development of neurophysiological or neurochemical changes, with kindling being proposed as one possible pathomechanism; and (2) both epilepsy and schizophrenia share a common neuropathology that may be localized (emphasis on temporal, but also frontal lobe and the cerebellum) or widespread in the brain. One could also entertain the possibility that both mechanisms are operative, the latter being the primary mechanism, but the former modifying the presentation, determining exacerbations and remissions, or being the proximate cause. The possible role of psychological factors has received much less attention.

The mechanisms by which psychosis may develop as a direct consequence of the epileptiform disturbance are as follows. (a) The psychosis may be related to subictal activity, either continuous or intermittent. There is no direct evidence that chronic psychoses are caused by this mechanism. (b) Recurrent seizures are known to induce homeostatic mechanisms that act to reduce epileptic excitability. This mechanism may explain postictal psychoses and some exacerbations of chronic psychoses but is unsatisfactory for chronic psychoses. (c) Kindling has been proposed as a mechanism. Stevens and Livermore (1978) used electrical and pharmacological kindling of the ventral tegmental area (VTA) to develop a cat model of psychosis, attributing it to mesolimbic dopamine kindling. Amygdaloid kindling by cocaine and apomorphine was used as a model psychosis by Sato. Seizures are known to produce DA subsensitivity downstream and neuroleptics provoke seizures. Kindling may thus explain some aspects of the relationship between epilepsy and psychosis, especially the antagonism. It may not, however, be a satisfactory explanation for chronic psychosis in epilepsy for a number of reasons. First, there is no direct evidence for the abnormality of DA in schizophrenia. Second, it is uncertain whether the effects of kindling can be permanent. Third, the relationship between the duration of epilepsy and psychosis, even though characterized by a delay of many years, is quite variable. Fourth, such patients are usually characterized by seizures that generalize, and neuropathology that is quite widespread, suggesting that more than limbic kindling may be operative. (d) It is known that stimulation of the hippocampus leads to an anomalous axonal sprouting from dentate granule cells before the development of seizures (Sutula et al. 1988). In addition to the presynaptic mossy fiber expansion, there is an increase in perforated postsynaptic densities on granule cell dendrites. These changes are possibly produced by increased expression of mRNA for c-*fos* and NGF (nerve growth factor) by recurrent limbic seizures. The aberrant regeneration and the resultant "miswiring" could contribute to the development of schizophrenia.

The other hypothesis to consider is that both psychosis and epilepsy are symptomatic of the underlying neuropathological or physiological dysfunction: this has taken two forms, the *cortical dysgenesis hypothesis* and the *diffuse brain damage hypothesis*. It is known that a significant proportion of epilepsy patients have dysgenesis, heterotopias, and cellular displacements. A quarter to a third of TLE patients coming to surgery have gliomas, hamartomas, heterotopias, etc., suggesting defective neuroembyogenesis. Heterotopias are also commonly encountered in patients with hippocampal sclerosis. Furthermore, cryptic insults such as childhood viruses, fever, or minor hypoxia may lead to synaptic reorganization in vulnerable brains, thus exacerbating the problem. Thus, dysgenesis is common in epilepsy, in particular TLE, and may be caused by a combination of genetic and environmental factors. There is now considerable evidence that schizophrenia is also a disorder of embryogenesis. More than a decade ago, it was demonstrated that schizophrenic patients had a disorganization of the pyramidal cell layer, especially in the anterior one-third of the pes hippocampus, and at the interface zones between prosubiculum and CA1, and between CA2 and CA3. It was thought that this represented a problem in the migration of primitive neurones into the presumptive hippocampal plate. Heterotopias have been demonstrated in schizophrenic brains. There is also evidence for synaptic reorganisation in schizophrenia. Finally, schizophrenia-like psychoses are more likely to develop in epileptic patients with developmental brain abnormalities, as supported by the analysis by Roberts et al. (1990).

On the other hand, there is evidence that brain abnormalities in the schizophrenic brain are quite widespread. Most neuropathological studies of epilepsy and psychosis have been limited to the examination of resected temporal lobes. In this context, the study by Bruton et al. (1994) is significant. Psychotic epileptic patients had larger cerebral ventricles, excess periventricular gliosis, and more focal cerebral damage compared with the nonpsychotic epileptic patients. Epileptic patients with schizophrenia-like psychoses were distinguished from all other groups by a significant excess of pinpoint perivascular white matter softenings. This excess pathology is unrelated to the pathology commonly associated with epilepsy, but is similar to some of the pathology reported in schizophrenia. This finding argues that schizophrenia may be related to degenerative or regenerative changes in the brain not directly related to the classic epileptic pathology.

A Composite Model

In trying to put the data together, we conceptualize epilepsy and schizophrenia as two heterogeneous syndromes that are distinct but overlapping, both having diverse manifestations, an onset at a young age, and manifesting some electrical storms in the anterior temporal cortex. They are associated with either diffuse brain damage sustained during development or are preceded by neuronal dysgenesis. It is possible that, on the substratum of a vulnerable brain, the occurrence of frank or microseizures leads to further aberrant synaptic reorganization, thus preparing the pathway to schizophrenia. Because the development of medial temporal structures is asymmetrical, it may explain some of the laterality data. Seizures, either by the presence of continuous subictal activity or by their modulation of catecholamine and pre- and postsynaptic GABAergic and glutamatergic activity, modulate the expression of the psychosis. When the vulnerability of the brain is low, the psychotic episodes are brief and largely driven by electrical activity. A more definitive abnormality produces a chronic psychosis that is modified in its expression by the epilepsy. The picture is further complicated by drug therapy and psychosocial factors related to epilepsy.

From this analysis, we can identify a number of areas for future research in relation to epidemiology, clinical features, and neuropathology, thus establishing an exciting agenda for future research. Furthermore, schizophrenia is being studied using a wide range of techniques, and it would be interesting to find out if the same findings hold for schizophrenia associated with epilepsy.

References

Bruton CJ, Stevens JR, Frith CD (1994) Epilepsy, psychosis, and schizophrenia: clinical and neuropathologic correlations. Neurology 44:34–42

Engel J Jr (1996) Introduction to temporal lobe epilepsy. Epilepsy Res 26:141–150

Gudmundsson G (1996) Epilepsy in Iceland: a clinical and epidemiological investigation. Acta Neurol Scand (Suppl) 25:1–124

Heath RG (1962) Common clinical characteristics of epilepsy and schizophrenia. Am J Psychiatry 11:1013–1026

Kanemoto K, Kawasaki J, Kawai I (1996) Postictal psychosis: a comparison with acute interictal and chronic psychoses. Epilepsia 37:551–556

Kendrick JF, Gibbs FA (1957) Origin, spread and neurosurgical treatment of the psychomotor type of seizure discharge. J Neurosurg 14:270–284

Landolt H (1953) Some clinical electroencephalographical correlations in epileptic psychoses (twilight states). Electroencephalogr Clin Neurophysiol 5:121

Lindsay J, Ounstead C, Richards P (1979) Long term outcome in children with temporal lobe seizures III: Psychiatric aspects in childhood and adult life. Dev Med Child Neurol 21:630–636

Logsdail SJ, Toone BK (1988) Postictal psychosis: a clinical and phenomenological description. Br J Psychiatry 152:246–252

Mendez MF, Grau R, Doss RC, Taylor JL (1993) Schizophrenia in epilepsy: seizure and psychosis variables. Neurology 43:1073–1077

Olney JW, Farber NB (1995) Glutamate receptor dysfunction and schizophrenia. Arch Gen Psychiatry 52:998–1007

Onuma T, Adachi N, Hisano T, Uesugi S (1991) 10-year follow-up study of epilepsy with psychosis. Jpn J Psychiatry Neurol 45:360–361

Roberts GW, Done DJ, Bruton C, Crow TJ (1990) A "mock up" of schizophrenia: temporal lobe epilepsy and schizophrenia-like psychosis. Biol Psychiatry 28:127–143

Sachdev P (1998) Schizophrenia-like psychosis and epilepsy: the status of the relationship. Am J Psychiatry 155:325–336

Sander JWAS, Hart YM, Trimble MR, Shorvon SD (1991) Vigabatrin and psychosis. J Neurol Neurosurg Psychiatry 54:435–439

Stevens JR (1991) Psychosis and the temporal lobe. In: Smith D, Treiman D, Trimble M (eds) Neurobehavioural problems in epilepsy. Advances in neurology, vol 55. Raven Press, New York, pp 79–96

Stevens JR, Livermore A Jr (1978) Kindling of the mesolimbic dopamine system: animal models of psychosis. Neurology 28:36–46

Sutula T, He XX, Cavazos J, Scott G (1988) Synaptic reorganization in the hippocampus induced by abnormal functional activity. Science 239:1147–1150

Trimble M (1991) The psychoses of epilepsy. Raven Press, New York

Anticonvulsants in Neuropsychiatry

Moises Gaviria and David Medina

Introduction

The effects that antiepileptic drugs (AEDs) have on the neural membrane and on neurotransmitter receptors give these agents invaluable properties for treatment of a broad variety of neuropsychiatric disorders in addition to seizures and neuropathic pain [17]. Accordingly, AEDs should be more accurately considered as neuromodulatory drugs than strictly as anticonvulsants.

Within the boundaries of neuropsychiatry, the AEDs have been used successfully as mood stabilizers in bipolar disorder, schizoaffective disorder, and cyclothymia. Additionally, they seem to be helpful in the treatment of other major mental problems, such as major depressive disorder and schizophrenia, and in the management of patients with aggressive behavior, disruptive behavior associated with developmental disabilities, affective instability, and impulsiveness. Other possible applications of AEDs are the treatment of patients with personality disorders, and in substance abuse, psychiatric comorbidity of epileptic patients, and other neuropsychiatric conditions [33].

Among the most commonly used AEDs for the management of the neuropsychiatric patients are the "traditional" molecules, including carbamazepine and valproate. Unfortunately, side effects from these drugs are relatively common. Some central nervous system side effects, such as sedation and ataxia, are easily recognized and usually do not represent difficult management problems. More subtle side effects in other areas such as cognition, mood, and personality tend to be more problematic. Among traditional AEDs, there have been reports associating phenobarbital and phenytoin with the occurrence of depression, irritability, and disruptive behavior. Felbamate, ethosuximide, and the new vigabatrin may also generate depression as well as insomnia, agitation, and psychosis. Likewise, older AEDs tend to affect cognitive performance, whereas the new generation of AEDs, such as lamotrigine, gabapentin, and vigabatrin, are proposed to have fewer cognitive effects [28].

This chapter focuses on the newer AEDS, because these agents seem to be generally better tolerated and their utilization has been increasing in both psychiatric and epilepsy patients [17].

Neuropsychiatric Division, Department of Psychiatry, University of Illinois at Chicago, Chicago, IL 60612, USA

Antiepileptic Drugs in Mood Disorders

Only 50% of patients with mood disorders show response to treatment with psychotropic drugs without experiencing troublesome side effects; those patients with rapid cycling bipolar disorder are especially likely to do so [3]. Furthermore, tricyclic antidepressants (TCA) are associated with a high risk of placing patients from the depressive state, in a bipolar depression, to the manic or hypomanic phase or shortening cycle length [7].

For these reasons, AEDs have moved into an important position as an alternative and adjunctive treatment of mood disorders. Traditional mood stabilizers have proven their efficacy in bipolar disorder during either manic or depressive episodes, and their use as prophylactic agents has also been noted [11,12,16,27]. Furthermore, their therapeutic efficacy appears to extend to cyclothymia, schizoaffective disorder, depression, suicide prevention, affective instability related to personality disorders, and other affective features.

Although the rationale for the use of both older and newer AEDs in the treatment of these conditions is based in the fundamental neurobiological basis of mood disturbances and the amygdala kindling concept, none of the new AEDs, including gabapentin, lamotrigine, topiramate, and oxcarbazepine, has received approval from the FDA for any use other than the treatment of seizures. The use of the new AEDs in these conditions has clearly developed because of the need for new therapies for patients with refractory mood disorders, particularly bipolar depression. Although this practice has become quite common, the published literature contains principally anecdotal reports and open-label studies and only a small number of controlled trials [2,8,14,29,32].

Gabapentin

There are several reports of open-label utilization of gabapentin as an adjunctive therapy in the treatment of depressed, hypomanic, manic, or mixed mood states [21,24,31].

In a group of 25 patients with bipolar I disorder or schizoaffective disorder who underwent a 16-week open-label trial of gabapentin (mean dose, 1440 mg/day), 19 patients (76%) showed improvement of manic and hypomanic symptoms with only oversedation as a transient side effect [4]. In another open-label study [36], significant reductions in both depressive and manic symptoms were observed when gabapentin was used as adjunctive therapy for up to 6 months to treat 37 patients with bipolar I or II disorders with or without a rapid cycling course. Also, Erfhurt et al. [13] treated 14 patients with acute mania for up to 3 weeks with gabapentin (1200–4800 mg/day) as adjunctive therapy ($n = 6$) or monotherapy ($n = 8$), and the drug showed efficacy in the 10 patients who completed this open-label trial.

Lamotrigine

Lamotrigine has shown efficacy in the treatment of type I and type II bipolar patients, even if they are rapid cycling (often refractory) or nonrapid cycling patients [3]. In a

48-week, open-label, prospective trial, Calabrese et al. [5], used lamotrigine as adjunctive therapy ($n = 60$) or monotherapy ($n = 15$), in a group of 75 unresponsive/intolerant (to previous medical treatment) bipolar patients whether in the depressed, hypomanic, manic or mixed-states of the illness. In this study, 48% of the depressed patients had a marked response and 20% had a moderate response. Among hypomanic, manic, or mixed-state patients, 81% had significant improvement on the Mania Rating Scale. The most frequent side effects were dizziness, tremor, somnolence, headache, nausea, and rash. The later resulted in a discontinuation of the drug in 9% of the patients, including 1 patient who required hospitalization because of a serious rash.

Finally, the first controlled multicenter study evaluating lamotrigine as monotherapy for outpatients with bipolar I depression ($n = 195$) demonstrated that lamotrigine, at 200 mg/day, had significant antidepressant efficacy compared with placebo without destabilizing mood or precipitating mania and was well tolerated [6].

Topiramate

There are few available data regarding the use of topiramate for mood disorders [15,22]. In a chart review of 58 refractory bipolar patients who received topiramate (mean dose, 200 mg/day), 36 patients (62%) had remarkable or moderate improvement within days or weeks, 16 patients had minimal or no improvement, and symptoms worsened in 6 patients [20].

Oxcarbazepine

The FDA approved oxcarbazepine for antiepileptic monotherapy and as adjunctive therapy for partial seizures in children and adults. Because of its structural similarity to carbamazepine, oxcarbazepine has been used to treat mood disorder in other countries. Several small controlled trials of oxcarbazepine for bipolar disease have shown potential efficacy [1,11,12,35].

Borderline Personality Disorder

Mood symptoms and aggression/impulsiveness associated with borderline personality disorder can respond to the use of anticonvulsivants. In a case report of eight patients who were unresponsive to antidepressants and mood stabilizers and did not have a DSM-IV major mood disorder, three patients showed a sustained response to lamotrigine (75–300 mg/day) for more than a year of treatment, in particular, improvement in impulsive sexual, drug-taking, and suicidal behaviors [25].

Antiepileptic Drugs in Anxiety Disorders

There is a growing amount of information about the use and efficacy of AEDs in the pharmacotherapy of anxiety disorders. The correlations of neurobiological mechanisms of anxiety with the pharmacodynamics of these drugs encourage the rational use of AEDs as anxiolytic agents. Clonazepam has successfully been used in the treatment of several anxiety disorders. In addition, carbamazepine and valproic acid have shown to be beneficial in a wide domain of entities that includes panic disorder, social phobia, generalized anxiety disorder, posttraumatic stress disorder, obsessive-compulsive disorder, and various anxiety symptoms related to other major psychopathologies. Recently, some publications have also reported the efficacy of novel agents such as gabapentin [9,26] and vigabatrin, especially in social phobia [10]. For example, gabapentin, at doses up to 3600 mg, produced a statistically significant reduction of the symptoms of social phobia after a 14-week treatment period compared with placebo [23].

Antiepileptics in Drug Abuse Detoxification

AEDs such as phenytoin, carbamazepine, valproate, gabapentin, and vigabatrin have been reported as effective and safe therapeutic resources for the treatment of acute and chronic intoxication and withdrawal syndrome of cocaine, opiates, alcohol, benzodiazepines, and other drugs. Also, the role of AEDs as a preventive tool and as treatment of comorbid psychiatric conditions of drug abusers has been greatly explored [18].

The available data on the use of AEDs for the treatment of substance abuse disorders integrate the biological basis of drug abuse with the mechanisms of action of these drugs; for example, a case report in which two patients referred diminished alcohol use while they were taking gabapentin, which can be correlated with animal studies showing a protective effect of gabapentin against the anxiogenic component of the alcohol withdrawal [30,34].

Summary

- There are already many data and much clinical experience supporting the use of traditional AEDs for the treatment of major neuropsychiatric disorders.
- Additional controlled studies are needed to prove the efficacy of the new AEDs as monotherapy or adjunctive therapy in the neuropsychiatric patient. These studies should define the appropriate dosing ranges, differential effects on disorder subtypes, and the potential risk of their use.
- Currently published data suggest that lamotrigine and gabapentin are effective for patients with refractory bipolar disorder and anxiety disorders.
- The advantages of lamotrigine over current psychotropic treatment are a low incidence of weight gain and sexual dysfunction. Disadvantages are the need for slow titration, risk of serious rash, and potential for drug interactions [5].
- Gabapentin has advantages over other AEDs because it can be rapidly titrated, tends to be well tolerated, does not require laboratory monitoring, and has little risk of idiosyncratic reactions or drug interactions [19].

References

1. Beijamini V, Skalisz LL, Joca SR, Andreatini R (1998) The effect of oxcarbazepine on behavioural despair and learned helplessness. Eur J Pharmacol 347:23–27
2. Botts SR, Raskind J (1999) Gabapentin and lamotrigine in bipolar disorder. Am J Health Syst Pharm 56:1939–1944
3. Bowden CL, Calabrese JR, Mc Elroy SL, et al (1999) The efficacy of lamotrigine in rapid cycling and non-rapid cycling patients with bipolar disorder. Biol Psychiatry 45:953–958
4. Cabras PL, Hardoy MJ, Hardoy MC, Carta MG (1999) Clinical experience with gabapentin in patients with bipolar or schizoaffective disorder: results of an open-label study. J Clin Psychiatry 60:245–248
5. Calabrese JR, Bowden CL, Mc Elroy SL, et al (1999) Spectrum of activity of lamotrigine in treatment-refractory bipolar disorder. Am J Psychiatry 156:1019–1023
6. Calabrese JR, Bowden CL, Sacks GS, et al (1999) A double-blind placebo-controlled study of lamotrigine monotherapy in outpatients with bipolar I depression: Lamictal 602 study group. J Clin Psychiatry 60:79–88
7. Calabrese JR, Rapport DJ, Kimmel SE, Shelton MD (1999) Controlled trials in bipolar I depression: focus on switch rates and efficacy. Eur Neuropsychopharmacol 9(suppl 4):S109–S112
8. Calabrese JR, Rapport DJ, Shelton MD, et al (1998) Clinical studies on the use of lamotrigine in bipolar disorder. Neuropsychobiology 38:185–191
9. Chouinard G, Beauclair L, Belanger MC (1998) Gabapentin: long-term antianxiety and hypnotic effects in psychiatric patients with comorbid anxiety-related disorders. Can J Psychiatry 43:305
10. Connor KM, Davidson JR, Sutherland S, Weisler R (1999) Social phobia: issues in assessment and management. Epilepsia 40(suppl 6):S60–S65
11. Dilsaver SC, Swann SC, Chen YW, et al (1996) Treatment of bipolar depression with carbamazepine: results of an open study. Biol Psychiatry 40:935–937
12. Emrich HM, Dose M, von Zerssen D (1985) The use of sodium valproate, carbamazepine and oxcarbamazepine in patients with affective disorders. J Affect Disord 8:243–250
13. Erfurth A, Kammerer C, Grunze H, Normann C, Walden J (1998) An open label study of gabapentin in the treatment of acute mania. J Psychiatr Res 32:261–264
14. Ferrier IN (1998) Lamotrigine and gabapentin: alternative in the treatment of bipolar disorders. Neuropsychobiology 38:192–197
15. Gordon A, Price LH (1999) Mood stabilization and weight loss with topiramate [letter]. Am J Psychiatry 156:968–969
16. Grunze H, Erfurth A, Amman B, et al (1999) Intravenous valproate loading in acutely manic and depressed bipolar I patients. J Clin Psychopharmacology 19:303–309
17. Ketter TA, Post RM, Theodore WH (1999) Positive and negative psychiatric effects of antiepileptic drugs in patients with seizure disorders. Neurology 53(5 suppl 2):S53–S67
18. Kosten TR (1998) The pharmacotherapy of relapse prevention using anticonvulsants. Am J Addict 7:205–209
19. Letterman L, Markowitz JS (1999) Gabapentin: a review of published experience in the treatment of bipolar disorder and other psychiatric conditions. Pharmacotherapy 19:565–572
20. Marcotte D (1998) Use of topiramate, a new anti-epileptic as a mood stabilizer. J Affect Disord 50:245–251
21. McElroy SL, Soutullo CA, Keck PE Jr, Kmetz GF (1997) A pilot trial of adjunctive gabapentin in the treatment of bipolar disorder. Ann Clin Psychiatry 9:99–103
22. Normann C, Langosch J, Schaerer LO, et al (1999) Treatment of acute mania with topiramate [letter]. Am J Psychiatry 156:2014

23. Pande AC, Davidson JR, Jefferson JW, et al (1999) Treatment of social phobia with gabapentin: a placebo-controlled study. J Clin Psychopharmacol 19:341–348
24. Perugi G, Toni C, Ruffolo G, et al (1999) Clinical experience using adjunctive gabapentin in treatment-resistant bipolar mixed states. Pharmacopsychiatry 32:136–141
25. Pinto OC, Akiskal HS (1998) Lamotrigine as a promising approach to borderline personality: an open case series without concurrent DSM-IV major mood disorder. J Affect Disord 51:333–334
26. Pollack MH, Matthews J, Scott EL (1998) Gabapentin as a potential treatment for anxiety disorders [letter]. Am J Psychiatry 155:992–993
27. Post RM, Ketter TA, Denicoff K, et al (1996) The place of anticonvulsivant therapy in bipolar illness. Psychopharmacology (Berl) 128:115–129
28. Sackellares JC, Berent S (1996) Psychological disturbances in epilepsy. Butterworth-Heinemann, Boston, 219–245
29. Schaffer CB, Schaffer LC (1999) Open maintenance treatment of bipolar disorder spectrum patients who responded to gabapentin augmentation in the acute phase of treatmen. J Affect Disord 55:237–240
30. Singh L, Field MJ, Ferris P, et al (1996) The antiepileptic agent gabapentin (Neurontin) possesses anxiolytic-like and antinociceptive actions that are reversed by D-serine. Psychopharmacology (Berl) 127:1–9
31. Sokolski KN, Green C, Maris DE, DeMet EM (1999) Gabapentin as an adjunct to standard mood stabilizers in outpatients with mixed bipolar symptomatology. Ann Clin Psychiatry 11:217–222
32. Suppes T, Brown ES, McElroy SL, et al (1999) Lamotrigine for the treatment of bipolar disorder: a clinical case series. J Affect Disord 53:95–98
33. Trimble MR (1998) New antiepileptic drugs and psychopathology. Neuropsychobiology 38:149–151
34. Watson WP, Robinson E, Little HJ (1997) The novel anticonvulsant, gabapentin, protects against both convulsant and anxiogenic aspects of the ethanol withdrawal syndrome. Neuropharmacology 36:1369–1375
35. Windhaber J, Maierhofer D, Dantendorfer K (1997) Oxcarbazepine for panic disorder occurring after two grand mal seizures: a case report [letter]. J Clin Psychiatry 58:404–405
36. Young LT, Robb JC, Hasey GM, et al (1999) Gabapentin as an adjunctive treatment in bipolar disorder. J Affect Disord 55:73–77

Antiepileptic Drugs in the Treatment of Psychiatric Diseases

ANDRES M. KANNER and SUSAN PALAC

Introduction

In the last two decades, antiepileptic drugs (AEDs) have been used for the management of psychiatric disorders. Their greatest use has been in the management of bipolar disorders, although more recent studies have demonstrated the efficacy of AEDs in anxiety disorders, unipolar depression, and the process of detoxifying patients from alcohol and cocaine. In this chapter, we briefly review the evidence in support of the use of AEDs in psychiatric disorders.

Bipolar Disease

Carbamazepine

Carbamazepine (CBZ) was the first AED to be studied for its efficacy in the treatment of affective disorders. After its release in the 1960s, neurologists reported subjective improvements in mood and behavior in patients with epilepsy treated with CBZ. In a literature review of 40 published studies, Dalby [1] reported that about 50% of 2500 patients treated with CBZ for neurological disorders were noted to have positive psychotropic effects from this new AED. Following these reports, Japanese investigators reported improvements in manic symptoms in patients with bipolar disorder treated with CBZ in open clinical trials [2,3]. Eventually, double-blind, placebo-controlled studies of the use of CBZ in the treatment of patients with affective disorders confirmed its efficacy. In one of the earliest such studies, Ballenger and Post [4] reported a statistically significant improvement in mania in five out of nine bipolar manic patients treated with CBZ. A poor response to lithium treatment had previously been seen in seven of these nine patients. Further, the improvement in acute mania was seen within the first week of treatment. Finally in this study, CBZ was reported to be an effective prophylactic treatment of bipolar disorder. In patients followed for up to 22 months of CBZ therapy, two had a complete resolution of symptoms, while three

Department of Neurological Sciences, Rush–Presbyterian–St. Luke's Medical Center, 1653 W. Congress Parkway, Chicago, IL 60612, USA

had a reduction in the severity and/or frequency of manic episodes. More recent placebo-controlled studies have also reported significant reductions (60–65%) in manic episodes in patients with bipolar disease treated with CBZ [5,6].

Numerous studies have compared the efficacy of CBZ to lithium (often considered the gold standard of treatment) as a maintenance treatment for mania in patients with bipolar disease [7–14]. Although some studies [8,13,14] showed a trend that favored lithium over CBZ therapy, especially in alleviating acute manic symptoms and in the less frequent occurrence of adverse side effects, none of these studies found a statistically significant difference in effectiveness between these two therapeutic agents. Approximately two-thirds of patients treated with either drug experienced a decrease in the number of manic episodes compared with the baseline value.

In bipolar patients who had failed previous therapy with antipsychotics and/or antidepressants, Kishimoto et al. [15] reported that 75% of patients had a positive response to the addition of CBZ to their drug regimen. Of 32 patients, 4 were able to discontinue other medications and were successfully treated with CBZ monotherapy. Other studies [16–20] have confirmed the effectiveness of CBZ as adjunctive therapy in patients with refractory bipolar illness. However, in a recent study, Fritze et al. [21] were not able to replicate these results. In their retrospective study of 73 patients who responded poorly to lithium therapy, patients switched from lithium to CBZ had a reduction in manic episodes, but this was not the case with patients switched to combination therapy with lithium and CBZ. The synergistic efficacy of CBZ in the treatment of bipolar disorder refractory to lithium would therefore seem to be an unresolved issue. Prospective studies might help identify which patients with bipolar disorder are good candidates for CBZ therapy.

From all the evidence cited above, it is clear that CBZ is often effective in ameliorating manic episodes, both acutely and prophylactically, in bipolar disorder. The data regarding the responsiveness of depressive symptoms to CBZ therapy in patients with bipolar disorder is less clear. In their study, Ballenger and Post [4] reported that 6 of 13 bipolar depressed patients had a poor antidepressant response to CBZ, while only 4 of the 13 had a good response. In responders, the antidepressant effect was seen 2 weeks after the initiation of CBZ therapy. On the other hand, Okuma [2] found that 33% of patients with acute depression improved with CBZ therapy, and 64% of patients experienced a decrease in the number of depressive episodes. Further studies are needed to clarify the efficacy of CBZ for depressive symptoms in bipolar patients.

In the studies cited above, the doses of CBZ used ranged from 200 to 1200 mg/day, with mean serum levels of about 8.0 μg/ml in studies where levels were attained.

Valproic Acid

In 1995, the Food and Drug Administration officially approved the use of valproic acid (VPA) for the treatment of mania in patients in the United States with bipolar disorder. This approval followed the publication of numerous studies regarding the use of VPA for bipolar illness. Open-label studies reported an improvement in mania in 50%–80% of patients with bipolar disorder treated with VPA [22–26]. In 1991, Pope et al. [27] reported that in a placebo-controlled, double-blind study, 71% of patients with bipolar disorder who were unresponsive to lithium therapy experienced a decrease in mania with VPA therapy. In a large-scale study of 179 patients with acute mania, Bowden et al. [28] reported an improvement in manic symptoms in 48% of patients treated with VPA, which was comparable to the improvement in patients treated with lithium (49%), and better than the 25% response rate seen in patients treated with placebo. Other controlled studies have reported similar improvements in mania in patients treated with VPA [29,30]. Since the introduction of an intravenous preparation of valproic acid (Depacon), scattered case reports have been published [31,32] supporting its efficacy, and reporting faster treatment response times than with oral valproic acid preparations in patients with acute mania.

Fewer studies have investigated the role of VPA as a maintenance therapy for patients with bipolar disorder. Emrich et al. [30] reported that the mean interval between manic episodes increased from 10 ± 4.3 months to 41 ± 18.5 months in patients treated with VPA. In a 1-year trial of 12 bipolar patients, Solomon et al. [33] found that patients treated with VPA and lithium were significantly less likely to have a recurrence of manic episodes than patients treated with lithium and placebo. Bowden et al. [34] recently published the results of a large, multicenter, placebo-controlled study of maintenance therapy with VPA in patients with bipolar disease. Three hundred and sixty-nine patients were randomized to treatment with either VPA, lithium, or placebo, with the primary outcome measure being the time to occurrence of either a manic or a depressive episode. They found no significant difference between treatment groups in time to a mood episode, i.e., neither VPA nor lithium was superior to placebo in preventing manic episodes. The mean serum concentrations of VPA and lithium were 84.8 ± 29.9 μg/ml and 1.0 ± 0.48 mEq/l, respectively. Thus, the utility of VPA in maintenance therapy in patients with bipolar disorder is not as clear as is the utility of CBZ therapy.

No conclusive studies have been published to date regarding the use of VPA for the depressed phase of bipolar disorder.

Other Antiepileptic Drugs

Gabapentin (GBP) has been used as adjunct therapy in the treatment of bipolar disorder for the past 4–5 years. However, reports of its efficacy have been limited to case reports and open-label, uncontrolled trials. These trials [35–38] have reported positive response rates ranging from 39%–92% with GBP, but interpretation of these results is limited by the often diverse diagnoses included in patient selection, and by the lack of objective rating scales in the assessment of patient response to therapy. In a retrospective chart review of 57 patients in which patient diagnoses were defined using DSM-IV criteria, and in which treatment response was assessed using the clinical global impressions of improvement scale (CGI–I), the overall response rate to GBP therapy was 30%. Of note, however, is that the response rate among patients with bipolar disorder I was 2/13, i.e., 15% [39].

The available data regarding the utility of GBP in the treatment of bipolar disorder I depression are conflicting. In the study by Ghaemi et al. [39] cited above, the response rate was 15%–20%. In contrast, Young et al. [40] reported that 8/15 patients with bipolar depression responded to GBP therapy. Clearly, controlled studies of the efficacy of GBP in bipolar disorders are needed.

Open-label trials have also reported positive results in patients with bipolar disease to treatment with lamotrigine (LTG). Most of these studies have focused on the response to LTG therapy of depression, and not mania, in bipolar patients, and report that 50%–72% of patients treated with LTG showed an improvement in depression with this adjunct therapy [41–43]. In a placebo-controlled, double-blind study of 192 patients with bipolar disorder who were actively depressed, about 51% of patients treated with LTG at 200 mg/day experienced an improvement in their depression as measured by three rating scales compared with about 31% of patients treated with placebo. This difference in treatment response was statistically significant, and was seen as early as 3 weeks following the initiation of treatment [44].

There is preliminary data to indicate that topiramate (TPM) may also be effective in the treatment of bipolar disorders. Marcotte [45] has reported that 52% of 44 patients with bipolar affective disorders showed moderate to marked improvement in symptoms following treatment with TPM at a mean dose of 200 mg/day. Further studies are needed to validate these results.

Unipolar Depression

AEDs are sometimes used in the treatment of unipolar depression, but there is little objective data regarding their use for this condition. CBZ is considered by many to have antidepressant effects. Of four patients with unipolar depression included in their study, Ballenger and Post [4] found that only one patient had a significant improvement in depression ratings following treatment with CBZ. In a follow-up study, Post found that 5 of 11 (45%) patients with unipolar depression experienced at least a mild improvement in depressive symptoms with CBZ therapy [46]. The use of CBZ in unipolar depression has not been studied in a large-scale trial.

VPA has also been reported to be effective in the treatment of depression in case reports [47,48] and in an open-label trial [23]. In a study of patients meeting DSM-IV criteria for major depressive disorder, Davis et al. [49] found that 86% showed a significant response in depression after 8 weeks of VPA treatment. The mean VPA dose in this trial was 1460 ± 450 mg/day. Thus, preliminary data regarding the use of VPA in treating depression are encouraging.

No other AEDs have been adequately studied in the treatment of unipolar depression. As previously noted, Ghaemi et al. [39] reported a 20% response rate to gabapentin in patients with unipolar depression. Lamotrigine has been reported to be effective in patients with bipolar disorder depressive state, but no studies regarding its use in major depressive disorders have yet been published.

Anxiety Disorders

Valproate may be effective in the treatment of panic and anxiety disorders. In an open trial, Primeau et al. [50] found that 6 of 10 patients with panic disorder showed moderate to marked improvement after 7 weeks of VPA therapy. Of 12 patients with panic disorder with or without agoraphobia, Woodman and Noyes [51] found that all experienced at least a moderate improvement in symptoms and all were free of panic attacks after 3 weeks of treatment with VPA in doses ranging from 500 to 2000 mg/day. In a small placebo-controlled trial, Lum et al. [52] found that patients with panic and anxiety attacks treated with VPA showed a significant improvement over patients treated with placebo.

Gabapentin also shows some promise as a treatment in anxiety disorders. In a series of 18 patients, Chouinard et al. [53] found significant symptomatic improvements in patients with anxiety-related symptoms treated with GBP at daily doses of 200–1800 mg. Similar findings have been reported by Pollack et al. [54]. In addition, GBP has recently been reported to be superior to placebo in alleviating symptoms in patients with social phobia [55].

There are no published data to date regarding the efficacy of LTG in the treatment of anxiety disorders. CBZ has been shown to have limited value in the treatment of patients with panic disorder with or without agoraphobia in a study of 18 such patients by Uhde et al. [56].

Other Psychiatric Disorders

There are scattered reports throughout the literature describing the use of AEDs in various other psychiatric conditions. For example, AEDs have been used to prevent withdrawal symptoms in patients being treated for substance abuse. In several studies, VPA has been reported to be effective in reducing the severity of withdrawal symptoms in alcohol-dependent patients [57–59]. Rickels et al. [60] found VPA to be superior to placebo when used in the treatment of patients in benzodiazepine withdrawal. CBZ has also been reported to be effective in limiting symptoms during benzodiazepine withdrawal [61]. However, three separate studies failed to find any effect of CBZ on cocaine dependence [62–64].

AEDs have also been used in the treatment of impulse behavior disorders. In children and adolescents age 10–18 years with conduct disorder or oppositional defiant disorder, 80%–86% showed an improvement with VPA treatment in a double-blind, placebo-controlled study by Donovan et al. [65] Kavoussi and Coccaro [66] studied eight patients with personality disorder who also exhibited impulsive aggressive behavior and who were treated with VPA. Six of the eight patients reported significant decreases in irritability and impulsive aggressive behavior after treatment with VPA [66]. Daly and Fatemi [67] recently reported the effective use of lamotrigine therapy in two patients with impulse behavior—one with self-injury and the other with bulimia. It is critical to determine if these results can be verified with larger studies, since these disorders are refractory to other psychotropic medications.

References

1. Dalby MA (1971) Antiepileptic and psychotropic effect of carbamazepine (Tegretol) in the treatment of psychomotor epilepsy. Epilepsia 12:325–334
2. Okuma T (1983) Therapeutic and prophylactic effects of carbamazepine in bipolar disorders. Psychiatr Clin N Am 6:157–174
3. Takezaki H, Hanaoka M (1971) The use of carbamazepine (Tegretol) in the control of manic-depressive psychosis and other manic-depressive states. Clin Psychiatry 13:173–183

4. Ballenger JC, Post RM (1980) Carbamazepine in manic-depressive illness: a new treatment. Am J Psychiatry 137:782–790
5. Okuma T, Kazutoyo I, Otsuki S, et al (1981) A preliminary double-blind study on the efficacy of carbamazepine in prophylaxis of manic-depressive illness. Psychopharmacology 73:95–96
6. Post RM, Uhde TW, Ballenger JC, et al (1983) Prophylactic efficacy of carbamazepine in manic-depressive illness. Am J Psychiatry 140:1602–1604
7. Placidi GF, Lenzi A, Lazzerini F, et al (1986) The comparative efficacy and safety of carbamazepine versus lithium: a randomized, double-blind 3-year trial in 83 patients. J Clin Psychiatry 47:490–494
8. Watkins SE, Callender K, Thomas DR, et al (1987) The effect of carbamazepine and lithium on remission from affective illness. Br J Psychiatry 150:180–182
9. Lusznat RM, Murphy DP, Nunn CM (1988) Carbamazepine vs. lithium in the treatment and prophylaxis of mania. Br J Psychiatry 153:198–204
10. Small JG, Klapper MH, Milstein V, et al (1991) Carbamazepine compared with lithium in the treatment of mania. Arch Gen Psychiatry 48:915–921
11. Coxhead N, Silverstone T, Cookstone J (1992) Carbamazepine versus lithium in the prophylaxis of bipolar affective disorder. Acta Psychiatr Scand 85:114–118
12. Simhandl C, Denk E, Thau K (1993) The comparative efficacy of carbamazepine low and high serum levels and lithium carbonate in the prophylaxis of affective disorders. J Affect Disord 28:221–231
13. Denicoff KD, Smith-Jackson EE, Disney ER, et al (1997) Comparative prophylactic efficacy of lithium, carbamazepine, and the combination in bipolar disease. J Clin Psychiatry 58:470–478
14. Greil W, Ludwig-Mayerhofer W, Erazo N, et al (1997) Lithium versus carbamazepine in the maintenance treatment of bipolar disorders—a randomized study. J Affect Disord 43:151–161
15. Kishimoto A, Ogura C, Hazama H, et al (1983) Long-term prophylactic effects of carbamazepine in affective disorder. Br J Psychiatry 143:327–331
16. Nolen WA (1983) Carbamazepine: a possible adjunct or alternative to lithium in bipolar disorders. Acta Psychiatr Scand 67:218–225
17. Folks DG, King LD, Dowdy SB, et al (1982) Carbamazepine treatment of selected affectively disordered inpatients. Am J Psychiatry 139:115–117
18. Lipinski JF, Pope HA (1982) Possible synergistic action between carbamazepine and lithium carbonate in the treatment of three acutely manic patients. Am J Psychiatry 139:948–949
19. Keisling R (1983) Carbamazepine and lithium carbonate in the treatment of refractory affective disorders. Arch Gen Psychiatry 40:223
20. Warren JA, Crismon ML (1982) Carbamazepine in bipolar disorder-mixed. Clin Pharmacol 1:266–268
21. Fritze J, Beneke M, Lanczik M, et al (1994) Carbamazepine as adjunct or alternative to lithium in the prophylaxis of recurrent affective disorders. Pharmacopsychiatry 27:181–185
22. Calabrese JR, Delucchi GA (1990) Spectrum of efficacy of valproate in 55 patients with rapid-cycling bipolar disorder. Am J Psychiatry 147:431–434
23. Deltito JA, Levitan J, Damore J, et al (1998) Naturalistic experience with the use of divalproex sodium on an inpatient unit for adolescent psychiatric patients. Acta Psychiatr Scand 97:236–240
24. Keck PE, McElroy SL, Tugrul KC, et al (1993) Valproate oral loading in the treatment of acute mania. J Clin Psychiatry 54:305–308
25. McElroy SL, Keck PE, Stanton SP, et al (1996) A randomized comparison of divalproex oral loading versus haloperidol in the initial treatment of acute psychotic mania. J Clin Psychiatry 57:142–146

26. Papatheodorou G, Kutcher SP, Katic M, et al (1995) The efficacy and safety of divalproex sodium in the treatment of acute mania in adolescents and young adults: an open clinical trial. J Clin Psychopharmacol 15:110–116
27. Pope HG, McElroy SL, Keck PE, et al (1991) Valproate in the treatment of acute mania. Arch Gen Psychiatry 48:62–68
28. Bowden CL, Brugger AM, Swann AC, et al (1994) Efficacy of divalproex vs. lithium and placebo in the treatment of mania. JAMA 271:918–924
29. Freeman TW, Clothier JL, Pazzaglia P, et al (1992) A double-blind comparison of valproate and lithium in the treatment of acute mania. Am J Psychiatry 149:108–111
30. Emrich HM, Dose M, Vonzerssen D (1985) The use of sodium valproate, carbamazepine, and oxcarbazepine in patients with affective disorders. J Affect Disord 8:243–250
31. Herbert PB, Nelson JC (2000) Parenteral valproate for control of acute mania (letter). Am J Psychiatry 157:1023–1024
32. Norton JW, Quarles E (2000) Intravenous valproate in neuropsychiatry. Pharmacotherapy 20:88–92
33. Solomon DA, Ryan CE, Keitner GI, et al (1997) A pilot study of lithium carbonate plus divalproex sodium for the continuation and maintenance treatment of patients with bipolar I disorder. J Clin Psychiatry 58:95–99
34. Bowden CL, Calabrese JR, McElroy SL, et al (2000) A randomized, placebo-controlled 12-month trial of divalproex and lithium in treatment of outpatients with bipolar I disorder. Arch Gen Psychiatry 57:481–489
35. Ryback RS, Brodsky L, Munasifi F (1997) Gabapentin in bipolar disorder (letter). J Neuropsychiat Clin Neurosci 9:301
36. Stanton SP, Keck PE Jr, McElroy SL (1997) Treatment of acute mania with gabapentin (letter). Am J Psychiatry 154:287
37. Bennett J, Goldman W, Suppes T (1997) Gabapentin for treatment of bipolar and schizoaffective disorders (letter). J Clin Psychopharmacol 17:141–142
38. Schaffer CB, Schaffer LC (1999) Open maintenance treatment of bipolar disorder spectrum patients who responded to gabapentin augmentation in the acute phase of treatment. J Affect Disord 55:237–240
39. Ghaemi SN, Katzow JJ, Desai SP, et al (1998) Gabapentin treatment of mood disorders: a preliminary study. J Clin Psychiatry 59:426–429
40. Young LT, Robb JC, Hasey GM, et al (1999) Gabapentin as an adjunctive treatment in bipolar disorder. J Affect Disord 55:73–77
41. Sporn J, Sachs G (1997) The anticonvulsant lamotrigine in treatment-resistant manic-depressive illness. J Clin Psychopharmacol 17:185–189
42. Kusumakar V, Yatham LN (1997) An open study of lamotrigine in refractory bipolar depression. Psychiatry Res 72:145–148
43. Fatemi SH, Rapport DJ, Calabrese JR, et al (1997) Lamotrigine in rapid-cycling bipolar disorder. J Clin Psychiatry 58:522–527
44. Calabrese JR, Bowden CL, Sachs GS, et al (1999) A double-blind placebo-controlled study of lamotrigine monotherapy in outpatients with bipolar I depression. J Clin Psychiatry 60:79–88
45. Marcotte D (1998) Use of topiramate: a new anti-epileptic as a mood stabilizer. J Affect Disord 50:245–251
46. Post RM, Uhde TW, Roy-Byrne PP, et al (1986) Antidepressant effects of carbamazepine. Am J Psychiatry 143:29–34
47. Kemp LI (1992) Sodium valproate as an antidepressant. Br J Psychiatry 160:121–123
48. Pies R, Adler DA, Ehrenberg BL (1989) Sleep disorders and depression with atypical features: response to valproate. J Clin Psychopharmacol 9:352–357
49. Davis LL, Kabel D, Patel D, et al (1996) Valproate as an antidepressant in major depressive disorder. Psychopharmacol Bull 32:647–652

50. Primeau F, Fontaine R, Beaclair L (1990) Valproic acid and panic disorder. Can J Psychiatry 35:248–250
51. Woodman CL, Noyes R (1994) Panic disorder: treatment with valproate. J Clin Psychiatry 55:134–136
52. Lum M, Fontaine R, Elie R, et al (1991) Probable interaction of sodium divalproex with benzodiazepines. Prog Neuropsychopharmacol Biol Psychiatry 15:269–273
53. Chouinard G, Beauclair L, Belanger MC (1998) Gabapentin: long-term antianxiety and hypnotic effects in psychiatric patients with comorbid anxiety-related disorders. Can J Psychiatry 43:305
54. Pollack MG, Matthews J, Scott EL (1998) Gabapentin as a potential treatment for anxiety disorders. Am J Psychiatry 155:992–993
55. Pande AC, Davidson JR, Jefferson JW, et al (1999) Treatment of social phobia with gabapentin: a placebo-controlled study. J Clin Psychopharmacol 19:341–348
56. Uhde TW, Stein MB, Post RM (1988) Lack of efficacy of carbamazepine in the treatment of panic disorder. Am J Psychiatry 145:1104–1109
57. Lambie DG, Johnson RH, Vijayasenan ME, et al (1980) Sodium valproate in the treatment of the alcohol withdrawal syndrome. Aust N Z J Psychiatry 14:213–215
58. Rosenthal RN, Perkel C, Singh P, et al (1998) A pilot open randomized trial of valproate and phenobarbital in the treatment of acute alcohol withdrawal. Am J Addict 7:189–197
59. Hammer BA, Brady KT (1996) Valproate treatment of alcohol withdrawal and mania (letter). Am J Psychiatry 153:1232
60. Rickels K, Schweizer E, Garcia Espana F, et al (1999) Trazadone and valproate in patients discontinuing long-term benzodiazepine therapy: effects of withdrawal symptoms and taper outcome. Psychopharmacology 141:1–5
61. Ries RK, Roy-Byrne PP, Ward NG, et al (1989) Carbamazepine treatment for benzodiazepine withdrawal. Am J Psychiatry 146:536–537
62. Montoya ID, Levin FR, Fudala PJ, et al (1995) Double-blind comparison of carbamazepine and placebo for treatment of cocaine dependence. Drug Alcohol Dependence 38:213–219
63. Cornish JW, Maany I, Fudala PJ, et al (1995) Carbamazepine treatment for cocaine dependence. Drug Alcohol Dependence 38:221–227
64. Kranzler HR, Bauer LO, Hersh D (1995) Carbamazepine treatment of cocaine dependence: a placebo-controlled trial. Drug Alcohol Dependence 38:203–211
65. Donovan SJ, Stewart JW, Nunes EV, et al (2000) Divalproex treatment for youth with explosive temper and mood lability: a double-blind, placebo-controlled crossover design. Am J Psychiatry 157:818–820
66. Kavoussi RJ, Coccaro EF (1998) Divalproex sodium for impulsive aggressive behavior in patients with personality disorder. J Clin Psychiatry 59:676–680
67. Daly KA, Fatemi SH (1999) Lamotrigine and impulse behaviour (letter). Can J Psychiatry 44:395–396

Use and Abuse of Anticonvulsants in Neuropsychiatry: Antiepileptic Drugs and Cognition

Santosh K. Chaturvedi

Summary. This chapter summarizes the common cognitive effects of the antiepileptic agents used in neuropsychiatry. The cognitive side effects are likely to compromise the patient's quality of life. The newer antiepileptic drugs appear to be safer in terms of minimal cognitive or other side effects. The risk factors for development of cognitive effects and the management of such cognitive effects due to antiepileptic drugs are discussed. It is also suggested that good seizure control is the best means to maintain cognitive integrity.

Keywords. Anticonvulsants, Neuropsychiatry, Antiepileptic drugs, Cognition, Quality of life

Introduction

This symposium on the use and abuse of anticonvulsants assumes importance because of the large number of patients being maintained on these medications for a number of clinical conditions. This chapter focuses on the cognitive effects of these agents, which can influence not only their work performance and daily living but also their quality of life.

The commonly used antiepileptic drugs (AEDs) in neuropsychiatry are sodium valproate, carbamazepine, phenytoin, phenobarbitone, lamotrigine, topiramate, tiagabine, felbamate, and gabapentin. The indications for use of AEDs in neuropsychiatry are for psychiatric disorders with epilepsy, for affective disorders such as mania, depression, and for prophylaxis of bipolar affective disorders, schizophrenia, alcohol withdrawal states, and some others.

Cognitive Dysfunction due to Antiepileptic Drugs

Some patients develop deficits in attention and concentration, memory, motor speed, and word finding. Cognitive and psychiatric disturbances can interact to aggravate neurobehavioral functioning and affect daily living. Antiepileptic drugs can directly

Department of Psychiatry, National Institute of Mental Health and Neurosciences, Bangalore, India affect cognitive processing and can interact with seizures to disrupt cognition. Cognitive dysfunction can disrupt the patient's life, including work, school, family life, and other aspects of daily living.

Cognitive Effects and Quality of Life

Perceived cognitive deficits are considered a significant problem for people with epilepsy and affect their quality of life (QOL) adversely. In managing patients with epilepsy, it is important to be aware of cognitive and behavioral domains affecting quality of life and of techniques for optimizing neurobehavioral functioning.

AEDs directly affect cognitive processing and can interact with seizures to disrupt cognition. There has been research into the cognitive effects of older AEDs but fewer studies of newer AEDs. However, it is believed that the newer AEDs have less impact on cognitive functions and quality of life than the older antiepileptic drugs.

Cognitive Effects of Phenobarbital

Phenobarbital affects the following functions: psychomotor speed, vigilance, fine motor dexterity, attention, concentration, memory, hyperactivity, irritability, and Intelligence.

Cognitive Effects of Carbamazepine

For carbamazepine, these are sedation and mild memory effects. The neuropsychological functions are similar to that of lithium carbonate. In normal volunteers and epileptics, there were few adverse effects on cognitive process as compared to phenobarbital and phenytoin. On comparing the cognitive effects of phenytoin with those of carbamazepine, it has been found that early studies showed that carbamazepine was better than phenytoin, but later studies conducted after controlling blood levels did not confirm this.

Cognitive Effects of Valproate

Drowsiness was observed in 22% of those on polypharmacy and 0.2% of those on monotherapy. Cognitive functions showed minimal to modest impact. Valproate-induced cognitive effects are less than those seen with phenobarbital, but not less than with phenytoin or carbamazepine.

Cognitive Effects of Lamotrigine

Limited experience with psychiatric patients until now has produced mainly benign effects. Information-processing speed is slightly reduced.

Cognitive Effects of Gabapentin

Limited experience with neuropsychiatric patients until now has suggested gabapentin may not impair performance on neuropsychological tests.

Cognitive Effects due to Topiramate

Cognitive effects due to topiramate are common; for example, cognitive difficulties, impaired attention, and word fluency, which are reversed with reduction of dose. Addition of valproate worsens the cognitive functions.

Regarding cognitive effects of tiagabine, it has been found that it has no significant cognitive effects, although these were noted earlier in 13% with long-term treatment on high doses. There are some more newer and older anticonvulsant medications, but not much information is available about their cognitive effects.

Etiology of Cognitive Deficits

Trauma that initiated seizures
Ongoing cortical disruption caused by seizures
AEDs used for treatment
Etiology of seizure: neoplasm, vascular, head injury, infections, degeneration, etc.
Uncontrolled seizures
CPS of dominant temporal lobe: memory, learning, word retrieval on confrontation naming

Risk Factors for Cognitive Deficits

A number of factors have been found to have a significant effect on cognitive functions when antiepileptic medications are administered: these are structural lesion and diffuse pathology with frontal or temporal focus, especially left temporal. Multiple seizure types, episodes of status, higher blood levels, AED toxicity, polytherapy, and individual variability/tolerance of AEDs are other risk factors. Frequent and generalized seizures, early onset, long duration, high seizure frequency, and greater interictal abnormality are also considered risk factors. AED side effects, AED withdrawal, and refractory patients are also related to cognitive effects of AEDs.

Antiepileptics and Cognition: Research Issues

There have been only a few systematic randomized controlled trials on newer AEDs. The information is based mainly on case reports and narratives. Thus, the knowledge about antiepileptics that we currently have is experience based, not evidence based.

Management of Cognitive Effects due to Antiepileptic Drugs

To minimize negative cognitive effects of antiepileptics, we need to remember that in clinical practice we should try to maintain on monotherapy in therapeutic range.

If a patient still has cognitive deficits, it is suggested to try another antiepileptic medication instead of adding a second one. It should also be noted that good seizure control is the best means to maintain cognitive integrity.

In conclusion, the cognitive effects of the antiepileptic medications should not be ignored, even if they are mild or subtle. Newer antiepileptic medications that are being developed should have nil or minimal impact on cognitive functions and should not impair the person's quality of life.

Acknowledgments. I am grateful to Professor Moises Gaviria, University of Illinois at Chicago, IL, USA, and the Organizers of the 3rd International Congress on Neuropsychiatry for the invitation and assistance.

Treatment of Aggression with Anticonvulsant Drugs

Enrique Probst

Summary. Aggression as an explicit way of violence is common in everyday life and in a large number of psychopathological disorders. Various therapeutic treatments have been put into practice against paroxysmal or permanent expressions of violence. Epilepsy has generated an excellent model in which is possible to carry out studies about the relation between ictal discharges and the rhinencephalic, hippocampus, and cingulate gyrus structures. This chapter discusses the antiaggressive effects of anticonvulsant drugs in psychiatry in relation to the dopaminergic, serotoninergic, and gabaergic receptors. A special emphasis is made in relation to the utilization of certain anticonvulsants according to their pharmokinetic properties. The focus is placed on the modulation of certain psychotherapeutic processes that otherwise would be impossible to be put into practice.

Keywords. Aggression, Violence, Anticonvulsants, Epilepsy, Clonazepam

Violence saturates our everyday life in a unquestionable way. Sometimes it is perceptible and therefore clearly seen by everybody, but frequently it is not discovered because it is hidden and feigned.

The term violence is widely used in everyday language, and it has a profound image and meaning, Nevertheless, there is an aspect that is established in the multiple significance of this behavior. This meaning refers to violence, as in the act of forcing another, in any way, to do precisely what he or she does not want to do. Similarities and differences exist between the terms aggression and violence.

Aggression is an obvious means to show violence that is much less frequent than that which is developed in an unnoticed and hidden way. All violent conduct, manifested or not, is an attempt against human independence. In suppressing the liberty of others, violence plays with their free ideas, sentiments, and conduct. As I have recently said (Probst 2000), violence always expresses intolerance toward the distinct and the different. For the violent person, others cannot be any other way than how he perceives them.

We can all have violent behaviors, but our object here is to analyze certain information on what happens on the biological level of those individuals with paroxysmal or permanent forms of violence. There is exhaustive information about what happens

Department of Psychiatry, School of Medicine, Leyenda Patria 2980, Montevideo 11300, Uruguay to the brain structures involved in aggression, and patients with epilepsy have generated a model in which brain damage and aggression can be correlated.

It is necessary to clarify that the violent behavior of an epileptic patient, when existent, is the result of various factors and it is highly unlikely that a single factor will account for all the incidences of violent and aggressive conduct (Fenwick 1986). Those factors that are found in excess in patients with epilepsy are increased perinatal morbidity, low socioeconomic status, brain damage, and infections.

This is little doubt that multiple seizure types and very specific lesions within the limbic system can lead to poor impulse control and aggressive outbursts. It is also clear that seizure discharges spreading into structures within the brain that are involved with the control of aggression can produce sudden aggressive outbursts in a setting of clouding of consciousness; these episodes are seen in relation to specific factors in the patient's environment and thus seldom in a hospital setting. Sudden aggressive episodes resulting entirely from epilepsy are very rare. What is found is that there is an association between *poor impulse control and brain damage.* There is neurophysiological evidence of the importance of the different circuits of the hypothalamus in aggression. The relationship of the amygdala to aggression is a complex one because there is evidence that it may play an excitatory and an inhibitory role.

The rhinencephalic structures, the hippocampus and cingulate gyrus, are involved with emotions. Coccaro and Sieve (1995) defined impulsivity, which is characteristic of certain personality disorders, as a lowered threshold for psychomotoric action, particularly aggressive behavior, in response to events in the patient's (PE) environment. We have known for a long time that people with a tendency toward impulsivity tend to project their problems and overreact to events in their environment. Coccaro and Sieve also described that sometimes impulsivity is coupled with a great affective instability, as in borderline patients. For this reason, they react with impulsive or aggressive actions to the dysphoria engendered by a frustration such as a loss or separation. In contrast, antisocial personality-disordered patients are much less likely to have affective instability, and for this reason Coccaro and Sieve think that their antisocial and aggressive behaviors are fairly persistent and more likely to result in their being seen in a forensic setting rather than in a psychiatric clinic.

As Shader and Greenblatt (1995) said, neuromodulators that we know play a role in stimulating and inhibiting external behavior are likely candidates for the biological system that underlies impulsivity or aggression, whether directed toward the self or against others. The serotonin reuptake inhibitors might ameliorate aggression in such patients. In contrast to serotonin, the noradrenergic system may play an important and a facilitatory role generating impulsivity and aggression. Heightened noradrenergic activity may then be related to enhanced sensitivity to stimuli in the environment, whereas reductions in noradrenergic activity appear to be more associated with withdrawal from the environment and restitutive functions.

An etiological role for epileptiform activity in the limbic system in patients with personality disorder is suggested by some data related to the presence of certain EEG abnormalities in patients with borderline personality disorder and the response of dyscontrol behaviors to anticonvulsant medications.

We want to focus our approach on the mechanisms of action for the antiaggressive effects of anticonvulsants. It is possible that limbic excitability may underlie the etiology and responsiveness of some patients to anticonvulsants. It is also possible that these anticonvulsive agents work partially through the central 5-HT system.

As Harwey and Champe (1997) said, drugs such as phenytoin and carbamazepine stabilize neuronal membranes to depolarization by decreasing the flux of sodium ions in the neurons in the resting state or during depolarization. These drugs also reduce the influx of calcium ions during depolarization and suppress repetitive firing of neurons. Valproic acid reduces the propagation of abnormal electrical discharge in the brain. It may also enhance GABA action at inhibitory synapses. Clonazepam, as all benzodiazepines, has sedative properties. It is now clear that all benzodiazepines are mediated by benzodiazepine receptors. Moreover, it has also been shown that the benzodiazepine receptor is really a subtype of $GABA_A$ receptor. According to Paul (1995), we know that the $GABA_A$ receptor is a member of a large family of ligand-gated ion channels. Although the exact subunit composition of most $GABA_A$ receptors is unknown, it appears that their composition varies from brain region to region. Type 1 receptors are expressed predominantly in the cerebellum, whereas type 2 are in the hippocampus.

To end this brief exposure, I would like to talk of my experiences over the years in the use of clonazepam in certain psychotherapeutic treatments, which would have otherwise been impossible to manage. Psychotherapy of a psychoanalytical orientation has its indications and contraindications. One of the major difficulties in the psychoanalytical process is the acting—out tendency of certain patients who have a profound intolerance and sensitivity toward their unconscious conflicts. The anxiety generated in these circumstances is perceived by them as a tremendous disorganization of the self. Consequently, treatment is frequently interrupted.

For some time and in these circumstances I have been using a modulating psychopharmaceutical drug for the mobile emotions. Clonazepam is one of these, and utilizing it in daily doses of 1–2 mg permits better psychotherapeutic attention, without diminishing the patient's awareness. The particular pharmacokinetic advantage of this product is that it can be utilized daily, and especially during the night.

References

Coccaro E, Sieve L (1995) The neuropsychopharmacology of personality disorders. In: Bloom F, Kupper D (eds) Psychopharmacology. Raven Press, New York, pp 1567–1581
Fenwick P (1986) Aggression in epilepsy. In: Trimble MR, Bowig T (eds) Aspects of epilepsy and psychiatry. Wiley, London, pp 31–61
Harwey R, Champe P (1997) Drugs used to treat epilepsy in pharmacology. Lippincott-Raven, Philadelphia, pp 143–150
Paul SM (1995) GABA and glycine. In: Bloom F, Kupper D (eds) Psychopharmacology. Raven Press, New York, 87–94
Probst E (ed) (2000) Las fronteras invisibles. Montevideo, Uruguay, pp 75–86
Shader R, Greenblatt D (1995) The pharmacotherapy of acute anxiety. In: Bloom F, Kupper D (eds) Psychopharmacology. Raven Press, New York, pp 1341–1347

Antiepileptic Drugs in Child Neuropsychiatry: A Latin American View

Edgar Belfort

Summary. This chapter provides an overview of anticonvulsant pharmacotherapeutic approaches to understand the treatment of children and the adolescent population in the Latin American context, according to the physician's experience, in the formation process, in classification and diagnosis, and in relation to the ethnic and cultural aspects of Latin American reality.

Keywords. Anticonvulsants, Children, Adolescent, Latin American, Cultural aspects

The endeavor is to give a vision of the most important aspects in the treatment of children and the adolescent population in the Latin American context, especially the anticonvulsant pharmacotherapeutic approaches.

The presence of vulnerable groups, the population of children and adolescents, invites us to look for objective proposals adapted to the Latin-American context. In this sense, the neuropsychiatry the evolutionary development of children and adolescents, based not only in the psychological or behavioral process but also in the complex development, would be of great interest in the proposal of psychotherapeutic approaches.

It is this way that an appropriate understanding and a greater knowledge of this development process, within the sociocultural and geographic interaction context, is translated into the keys to understand not only a great part of the deviations of those evolutionary patterns but also the interpretation and application of pharmacotherapeutic models adjusted to reality and context.

For this reason, some general considerations are presented, according to the experience of the physician, found in the formation process, the diagnosis, the classifications, the relationships, and in the ethnic and cultural aspects of Latin American reality that allow the necessary adjustments for a better understanding of this practice and the use of the available tools for anticonvulsant treatment.

The anticonvulsants provide the doctor with a new vision and the possibility of influencing human development; with early interventions the physician can modify behaviors in children to alleviate psychological disorders, reducing behavior or affec-

Net of Venezuelan Medical Scientific Societies, Edif. Majestic, No. 64, Av. Libertador, Caracas 1010, Venezuela

tive symptoms, to avoid the psychosocial complications of the behavioral dysfunctions, and possibly prevent to illnesses in adult life.

Unfortunately, this growth has been divorced from the physician's educational or formal training in this area. Honoring the truth, in the region formal training programs on psychopharmacology in children are few and far between, found neither in the neurological programs nor in psychiatrics programs, even infantile. As for the possibility of including such training—during the last decade, probably it was not included because there was not a lot to teach. Before the 1960s, the only medication, mostly used on behavioral problems, were psychostimulants to treat hyperactivity; therefore, learning infantile psychopharmacology meant doing so through the stimulants.

Although it is certain that the biological revolution was slow in benefiting children, particularly because of care or cautions due to traditional innovations, it is not less certain that notorious limitations still remain in many parts of the Latin American region; for example, the use of medication incompatible with analytical training and analysis of the transferential aspects. The use of medications was seen as an imposition or as an external intrusion, an assault or violation of the patient's rights.

Learning how to manage all these negative variables helps the physician to incorporate innovations to his practice; he must look for therapy options, and learn the practice and empiric limitations of the new anticonvulsant treatments and how to incorporate the advances of recent research. The training programs must present new models and the integration of these in the patient's treatment. Information about efficient therapeutic pharmacokinetics, doses and regimes, adverse effects and their management, precautions, commercially available formulations and their cost, drug interactions, interference with diagnosis, and toxicity and withdrawal symptoms must be included.

Another aspect to be observed in the region is the consideration regarding the conceptualization of mental status or the term mental disorder, in that people commonly feel that there is some division between the mental and the physical. Also, we can expect that some parents will be surprised and confused by the notion that a mental disorder may be treated with medications, or they will presume that a pharmacological treatment has nothing to do with the cause.

The same situation arises with the terms emotional disorders, behavioral disorder, and developmental problem. All these terms have the disadvantage of not conveying what they mean, and thus these could carry a stigmatizing label and result in refusal of the treatment. The frequent comorbility and coexistence of symptoms in the population diagnosed in the region have implications for the treatment; for example, when the presence of one disorder changes the indications of treatment of another, it can present a special risk or error in the decision making. From this arises the necessity to adjust the diagnoses, such as action preceding the treatment, with the use of models that organize groups of symptoms within concepts of entities or properly categorized phenomena and, with an understanding of the phenomenon more located in its ethnic and cultural context, to establish the treatment priority and to avoid in this way the customary and notable tendency of using two or more medications to treat a single condition.

An additional consideration, in relation to the difficulties or lack of progress in psychiatric epidemiology, is the loss of common analytical, technical, and uniform

TABLE 1. Antiepileptic agent

Class	Agent	Seizure-related indications	Common pediatric doses	Common side effects
Amino acid	Gabapentin	Partial seizure with or without secondary generalization	30–60 mg/kg/d (tib)	Fatigue, somnolence, dizziness, ataxia
Barbiturates	Phenobarbital	Partial seizures, primary or secondary generalized tonic-clonic seizures	<12 yr: 3–7 mg/kg/d (qid-bid); neonates: 3–4 mg/kg/d (qid)	Sedation, dizziness, mood changes, insomnia, hyperkinesis (children, elderly), cognitive dysfunction, osteomalacia Dupuytren's contracture, frozen shoulder, reduced libido
Benzodiazepines	Clonazepan	Partial seizures, generalized tonic-clonic, absence, atonic, myoclonic seizures (Lennox–Gastaut syndrome)	0.01–0.2 mg/kg/d (bid-tid)	Sedation, ataxia, behavior problems, psychosis, hyperactivity, hypersalivation, seizure exacerbation
	Clorazepate	Partial seizures	15–60 mg/d (bid-tid)	Sedation, ataxia, memory disturbances
Hydantoins	Phenytoin	Partial seizures, primary or secondary generalized tonic-clonic seizures	5–10 mg/kg/d (bid)	Nystagmus, ataxia, dizziness, hirsutism, gingival hyperplasia, peripheral neuropathy, osteomalacia, folate deficiency
Other agents	Carbamazepine	Partial seizures, primary or secondary generalized tonic-clonic seizures	10–35 mg/kg/d (bid-qid)	Drowsiness, dizziness, diplopia, ataxia, blurring of vision, osteomalacia, peripheral neuropathy, water retention, hyponatremia
	Valproic acid	Partial seizures; primary and secondary generalized tonic-clonic, typical and atypical absence, atonic, myoclonic seizures	15–60 mg/kg/d (bid-qid)	Nausea, vomiting, drowsiness, dizziness, hair loss/thinning, weight gain, thrombocytopenia

bid, twice daily; tid, three times daily; qid, four times daily
From Graves and Fisher (1999), modified by the author

methods to present the data. For example, the presentation of the prevalence rate for subgroups based on age, sex, socioeconomic and educational status, vulnerability, minority ethnic groups, or rural or urban setting, is of great impact in the Latin region; this weakens even more the possibilities to show the prevalence of the disorders of populations of children and adolescents in the region. This situation prevents us from accurately knowing the possible interventions in specific groups.

We find a similar situation in relation to the safety and efficacy of all the pharmacological agents that frequently have been observed in the clinical practice, where data are extrapolated from little existent information that is not consistent with our reality, with data coming from the effectiveness and safety of adults studies with similar conditions. This is reaffirmed with the more frequent use, every day, of drugs such as the anticonvulsants (Tables 1 and 2), extrapolating data of the FDA based on studies that sometimes include few adolescents and without the approval for their use in children. It seemed that the FDA gives the approval and we, the prescription. We could ask

TABLE 2. Mood stabilizers: anticonvulsants

Agent	Dosage forms	Usual adult dosage form	Therapeutic plasma level	Common adverse effects
Carbamazepine	T, L	10–20 mg/kg/d	6–12 mg/l[a]	Nausea, dizziness, sedation, headache, dry mouth, constipation Children: gastrointestinal distress, neurotoxicity
Valproic acid		15–40 mg/kg/d	50–120 mg/l	Nausea, diarrhea, abdominal cramps, sedation, tremor
		Children initial target dose[b]	Therapeutic plasma level	Common adverse effects
	T, C, L	1.0–2.5 mg (Not recommended for preschoolers	50–100 mg/ml	Nausea, gastrointestinal distress, weight gain, increases hepatic enzymes (hepatotoxicity) Drug interaction: erythromycin, benzodiazepines or salicylates)
Lamorigine Gabapentin	Insufficient information available for use in bipolar disorder in children and adolescents			

[a] Levels are not established for therapeutic efficacy, but rather are used to monitor for toxicity
[b] Treatment of acute mania in children and adolescents
T, tablet; C, capsule; L, liquid
From Puzantian and Stimel (1999), modified by the author

ourselves: must we await studies for their use? will it be ethical? are we in the presence of an iatrogenic act? In any case, the answer would be an act of reflection.

The proposal is to try to identify the obstacles to investigate in children, and to consider specific models related to investigation methods, regulations, ethical aspects, collateral effects, the parent's and community's perspectives, etc., that guide us to a potential solution in which the parents and family interact with all aspects of the investigation design. Without the support and the consent of those parents or the community, such investigations would be hard to implement.

Furthermore, in this region, we know environmental situations, not reported in studies carried out in other realities that differ from ours, which could possibly interfere with the good progress of the medications. Poverty, physical illnesses in comorbility with many psychiatric dysfunctions, malnutrition, dehydration, caloric protein consumption, all could be an obstacle for the metabolization and toxicity of certain antiepileptic drugs and thus be a probable contraindication for the prescription of a medication or others that are seldom considered in the treatment plan.

This information not only can impede or reduce the obstacles in the course of the treatment but also can provide the possibility to elaborate some more appropriate tools for our reality, allowing us to pursue and control the therapeutical proposal.

References

Graves N, Fischer J (1999) Review of psychotropic drugs. CNS (Contemp Neurol Ser) (Spec edn) 1:74–79

Kutcher SP (1997) Child adolescent psychopharmacology. Saunders, London, pp 509

Kutcher SP (1998) Affective disorders in children and adolescents: a clinically relevant review. In: Walsh T (ed) Child Psychopharmacology, American Psychiatric Press, London, pp 91–114

Puzantian T, Stimmel G (1999) Review of psychotropic drugs. CNS (Contemp Neurol Ser) (Spec edn) 1:15–26

Sleep Disorders

Neuropsychiatric Aspects of Disturbed Sleep

Constantin R. Soldatos and Dimitris G. Dikeos

Summary. Various types of sleep disruption or even disorganization are often caused by brain dysfunction secondary to traumatic brain injury, encephalitis, cerebral stroke, etc., depending on the brain regions mainly affected. Thus, lesions of the pontine tegmentum result in reduction of REM sleep, whereas lesions of the lower brainstem cause elimination of slow-wave sleep. Moreover, clinical observation shows that some neurological patients present with somnolence whereas others exhibit sleeplessness and some others a disruption of the normal circadian alternation of sleep and wakefulness. On the other hand, primary sleep disorders such as fatal familial insomnia, narcolepsy, and REM sleep behavior disorder are often associated with neuropathological or neurophysiological alterations and are accompanied by neuropsychological manifestations. Also, organicity, mainly in the form of neurodevelopmental aberrations, is strongly suggested in many cases of sleepwalking and night terrors. Finally, serious cognitive and psychosocial consequences of curtailed or otherwise disturbed sleep are often observed in sleep deprivation, chronic insomnia, obstructive sleep apnea syndromes, and narcolepsy. Therefore, to optimize the management of patients with sleep disorders, it is important to specify the exact nature and the degree of any coexisting neuropsychiatric manifestations.

Keywords. Sleep, Sleep disorders, Neurological diseases, Neuropsychiatry

Introduction

Sleep is a behavioral state that is characterized by reduced responsiveness to environmental stimuli, a high degree of immobility and changes of autonomic functions such as body temperature, heart rate, and blood pressure. The traditional concept of brain inactivity during sleep alternating with brain activation during wakefulness has been disproven since the introduction of the EEG in the study of sleep by Loomis et al. (1937), who was the first to note in the late 1930s the presence of various sleep stages. About 20 years later, a distinct sleep stage characterized by rapid eye movements (REM sleep) was discovered and associated with dreaming and muscle atonia (Aserinsky and Kleitman 1953; Dement and Kleitman 1957; Jouvet and Michel 1959).

Sleep Research Unit, Department of Psychiatry, University of Athens, Athens 11528, Greece

Finally, in 1968 the standardized criteria for the identification of sleep EEG stages, still in use today, were established (Rechtschaffen and Kales 1968).

The main distinction of the sleep stages is between the REM and the non-REM (NREM) sleep. NREM sleep is further subdivided in four stages (stage I to stage IV), mainly on the basis of the progressive synchronization of the EEG that is generally characterized by theta-frequency waves of relatively low amplitude in stages I and II, gradually changing to high-amplitude delta waves in stages III and IV. Because of the preponderance of slow frequencies in the EEG during sleep stages III and IV, these two stages taken together are called slow-wave sleep (SWS). During REM sleep, the EEG is desynchronized to resemble that of wakefulness or stage I. In contrast to wakefulness and stage I, muscle tone in REM is very low and the electro-occulogram (EOG) shows the characteristic rapid eye movements. The sequence of sleep stages during the night follows a periodic pattern that is called a sleep cycle. In the first sleep cycle of nocturnal sleep of a young adult, sleep stages I to IV follow each other progressively and, about 90 min after the onset of sleep, the first REM period occurs. After the first REM period, which lasts about 15 min, stage II reoccurs and subsequent cycles resemble the first, although the duration of SWS is progressively shorter and that of stage II and REM is longer (Kales 1969; Bixler et al. 1986).

Sleep regulation is maintained through two basic mechanisms. One depends on the length of wakefulness and the accumulation of "sleepiness" and the other on the circadian (i.e., within the 24-h period) alternation of light and darkness (Borbely et al. 1983). The main brain region that is associated with the circadian regulation of sleep is the suprachiasmatic nucleus of the anterior hypothalamus, which is directly connected to the retina and is, thus, influenced by the light–dark cycle. Apart from this structure, other regions of the diencephalon are also associated with sleep regulation, whereas REM is mainly influenced by structures in the pontine brain stem (Siegel 1990). The main neurotransmitter systems implicated in sleep–wakefulness regulation are the cholinergic, which is particularly active during REM sleep, and the two aminergic, which are quite active during wakefulness; relative equilibrium between these systems is believed to produce the alternation of REM and non-REM sleep (Hobson 1983). These views, however, can be considered rather simplistic; based on many studies over the years, almost all neurotransmitters and neuromodulators as well as various neuropeptides have been found to be implicated in sleep regulation.

By its proper nature, sleep is a neurobehavioral phenomenon. Thus, as is expected, there is an intimate relationship of disturbed sleep to various neuropsychological manifestations. In this review chapter, the neuropsychiatric aspects of disturbed sleep are briefly presented, with the focus on (a) certain neurological disorders that are frequently associated with disturbances of the sleep–wake cycle; (b) brain dysfunction in specific sleep disorders; and (c) the cognitive and psychological consequences of disturbed sleep.

Neurological Disorders Associated with Disturbances of the Sleep–Wake Cycle

Among the neurological disorders, those frequently associated with sleep disturbances are traumatic brain injury, encephalitis, celebral stroke, dementia, and epilepsy.

Sleep problems are more frequent in patients with brain injury than in general neurological patients (Beetar et al. 1996; Hibbard et al. 1998), particularly if they suffer concomitantly from cognitive disturbances and pain (Beetar et al. 1996). Actually, sleep stage changes in patients with brain injury have been found to be similar to those in remitted depressed patients (Frieboes et al. 1999).

Different types of encephalitis may differently affect sleep, obviously depending on the brain regions that are mostly affected. Encephalitis lethargica and human African trypanosomiasis have been reported to be generally associated with somnolence (Lavie 1993; Buguet 1999). It seems, however, that encephalitis lethargica may result in either somnolence or sleeplessness depending on the exact localization of the lesions (Von Economo 1929). Furthermore, patients with trypanosomiasis do not suffer from hypersomnia proper but rather from a dysregulation of the sleep–wake cycle, which is caused by a presumed dysfunction in the interplay between the serotonergic raphe nuclei and the suprachiasmatic nuclei (Buguet 1999). Patients suffering from other types of encephalitis, such as that associated with *Mycoplasma pneumoniae* infection, have been also reported to present with somnolence accompanied by various sleep EEG alterations (Akaboshi et al. 1998).

Patients with cerebral stroke have been found to demonstrate electrophysiological brain abnormalities, particularly during sleep. Actually, the sleep EEG seems to be more sensitive to detect abnormalities resulting from cerebral vascular lesions than the conventional clinical EEG while the patient is awake (Tamura et al. 1983). In general, during the acute phase, cerebral stroke causes overall sleep disturbance with reduction of sleep efficiency (Tamura et al. 1983; Korner et al. 1986). It also appears that stroke involving the pontine tegmentum leads to marked reduction and even complete elimination of REM sleep as well as to a disorganization of non-REM sleep (Tamura et al. 1983). When the vascular lesions are localized in the lower brainstem, they result in elimination of slow-wave sleep and the occurrence of REM at sleep onset (Tamura et al. 1983). Other findings suggest that strokes of the right hemisphere are associated with a reduction of REM and an increase of non-REM sleep, whereas left-hemisphere strokes are accompanied by a reduction of slow-wave sleep (Korner et al. 1986). Finally, in some cases cerebral stroke can be followed by the development of parasomnias (Schenk and Mahowald 1991).

In patients with Alzheimer's disease, the reduction of phasic events during sleep, i.e., rapid eye movements and K-complexes, has been noted (Hoch and Reynolds 1989). Also, an overall slowing of REM sleep EEG has been found; actually, the amount of slow activity in REM is correlated with the severity of dementia as assessed through the mini mental state examination (Montplaisir et al. 1996). Dementia of vascular origin has been reported to be associated with paradoxical emergence of sleep patterns in the waking EEG (Iyama et al. 1992).

As it is well known, in some patients with epilepsy, epileptic discharges occur mainly or exclusively during sleep. Continuous spike-and-wave activity during SWS may occur either as a separate syndrome or as a pathological EEG pattern of other epileptic conditions (Veggiotti et al. 1999). The Landau–Kleffner syndrome is characterized by interictal epileptiform discharges during sleep; it seems that the mechanism leading to these discharges is strongly associated with neural circuits normally involved in the generation of sleep spindles (Nobili et al. 2000). In some other rare neurological diseases, various sleep parameters may show abnormalities; for example, patients with the Prader–Willi syndrome suffer from excessive daytime somnolence, and their sleep often starts with stage REM (Vela-Bueno et al. 1984).

Brain Dysfunction in Specific Sleep Disorders

The main sleep disorders that are believed to be caused by brain dysfunction are fatal familial insomnia, narcolepsy, sleepwalking, night terrors, and REM sleep disorder.

Fatal familial insomnia (Lugaresi et al. 1998) is a rare disorder characterized by almost complete sleeplessness, agitation, and confusion; its progressive course leads eventually to death. This disorder, which is genetically transmitted, is caused by a prion protein gene mutation. Characteristic neuropsychological abnormalities (e.g., impairment of attention and memory) and specific neuropathological alterations (i.e., gliosis of the thalamic nuclei and, sometimes, of the cortex) are associated with the disease (Gallassi et al. 1996).

Narcolepsy, a disorder characterized by hypersomnolence with daytime sleep attacks, cataplexy (i.e., sudden loss of muscle tone), sleep paralysis, and hypnagogic hallucinations, is associated with dysregulation of the REM-producing mechanisms (Daly and Yoss 1974; Kales et al. 1982a). In narcoleptic patients, sleep usually starts with a REM period, daytime sleep attacks are characterized as brief periods of REM sleep, cataplexy and sleep paralysis reflect the intrusion into wakefulness of the muscle atonia that normally accompanies REM sleep, and hypnagogic hallucinations represent dream phenomena occurring before the onset of actual sleep (Hishikawa et al. 1968; Kales et al. 1982a; Hishikawa and Shimizu 1995). Thus, from a neurophysiological perspective, narcolepsy is an abnormality in which the two main manifestations of REM sleep (dreaming and muscle atonia) are dissociated and may occur unexpectedly at any time of the day or night.

Although a genetic predisposition for the development of narcolepsy has been well established (Mignot 1998), the exact mechanism underlying its pathogenesis is yet unknown. It seems, however, that a major role in the pathophysiology of the REM abnormality in narcolepsy is played by a hyperactivity of the cholinergic muscarinic systems and a hypoactivity of the catecholaminergic ones, mainly the dopaminergic system (Nishino et al. 1994; Guilleminault et al. 1998). Brain structures considered to be involved in narcolepsy are the following: pontine reticular formation, pedunculopontine region, amygdala, locus coeruleus, and nucleus accumbens (Nishino et al. 1994; Hishikawa and Shimizu 1995; Guilleminault et al. 1998). In two published cases of secondary narcolepsy, lesions around the third ventricle and the rostral brainstem were identified; in one case, the lesion was caused by cerebral arteriovenous malformation and in another by a brain tumor (Clavelou et al. 1995; Ma et al. 1996). It is noteworthy that in the former case the involvement of the region around the third ventricle in the production of symptoms of narcolepsy was confirmed when clinical improvement occurred following embolization and radiosurgery of the vascular malformation.

Sleepwalking and night terrors are both characterized by the appearance of certain phenomena of wakefulness during slow-wave sleep. These conditions are considered to share a common genetic substrate. Actually, they are believed to be different expressions of a sole disorder that follows a two-threshold multifactorial mode of inheritance, with sleepwalking being the less severe and more prevalent manifestation and night terrors the more severe and less prevalent one (Kales et al. 1980, 1987). There is also an indication for a developmental component in the etiopathogenesis of sleepwalking and night terrors because some children with sleepwalking show an "immaturity factor" in their EEG characterized by sudden, rhythmic, low-voltage, slow-wave activity (Kales et al. 1966). The organicity of the etiopathogenesis of sleepwalking and night terrors is further supported by their occurence in association with febrile illness (Kales et al. 1979), combined neuroleptic and lithium treatment (Charney et al. 1979), and Gilles de la Tourette syndrome (Barabas et al. 1984). At least in the cases of sleepwalking or night terrors that persist into adulthood, however, environmental factors, personality characteristics, and concomitant psychopathology have been shown to play a major role in the pathogenesis of these two disorders (Kales et al. 1980; Soldatos and Kales 1982).

In the so-called REM sleep behavior disorder (RBD), which affects mostly elderly males, REM sleep is not accompanied by muscle atonia (Shenck et al. 1993; Chiu and Wing 1997; Olson et al. 2000). The absence of muscle atonia results in "dream enactment" and excessive motor activity during sleep that is often seriously injurious for the patients or their bed partners. This disorder has a corresponding experimental animal model that involves dorsolateral pontine tegmental lesions in cats (Schenk et al. 1993). Although transient RBD may occur with the intake of certain drugs or during drug withdrawal, the chronic type is either idiopathic or associated with underlying neurodegenerative diseases involving brainstem structures; the latter is the case for more than 50% of RBD patients (Schenck et al. 1993; Chiu and Wing 1997; Tachibana et al. 1997). The majority of neurological patients with RBD suffer from Parkinson's disease, dementia syndromes without parkinsonism, or multiple system atrophy; it is not uncommon for the symptoms of RBD to develop before other clinical manifestations of these neurological diseases occur (Tachibana et al. 1997; Plazzi et al. 1998; Olson et al. 2000).

Cognitive and Psychosocial Impact of Disturbed Sleep

Practically all sleep disorders may be accompanied by a degree of cognitive impairment and various psychosocial consequences. The cognitive and psychosocial impact of disturbed sleep, however, is of particular clinical importance in patients with insomnia and other sleep deficit states as well as in those with sleep apnea, narcolepsy, and other hypersomnias.

Many studies have demonstrated that sleep deprivation, even of only one night, results in a decline of cognitive performance; the degree of this decline does not differ between the two sexes (Wimmer et al. 1992; Harrison and Horne 1998; Chelette et al. 1998; Caldwell and LeDuc 1998; Linde et al. 1999). Also, night work is often accompanied by severe sleepiness and impaired performance as the result of a degree of sleep deprivation in combination with the need for heightened vigilance during the circadian phase that is least conducive to alertness (Akerstedt 1995). Cumulative sleep debt resulting from restricted sleep over a prolonged period of time (e.g., a week of total sleep time per 24 hours less than two-thirds of the habitual sleep duration) has been also found to increase feelings of sleepiness, fatigue, confusion, and tension and to adversely affect mood and psychomotor vigilance; these effects may last for some time beyond the end of the sleep restriction period (Dinges et al. 1997). The neuropsychological mechanism through which the effects of sleep deprivation are exerted is not well understood; however, the results of studies using event-related potentials and functional MRI suggest that sleep deprivation affects the thalamocortical gating which controls attention, discrimination, and decision making, thus causing a decline in the activity of various cortical regions such as the prefrontal cortex (Corsi-Cabrera et al. 1999; Drummond et al. 1999).

A decline of psychomotor performance may also be observed among patients with primary insomnia. The pattern, however, of neuropsychiatric impairment in primary insomnia differs somewhat from that observed in sleep deprivation, suggesting that insomnia affects psychomotor and cognitive functions through additional mechanisms apart from those resulting from sleep deprivation of the insomniac patient (Hauri 1997). Similarly, insomnia secondary to generalized anxiety disorder has been found to be associated with psychomotor performance deterioration (Saletu-Zyhlarz et al. 1997). Cognitive and psychomotor impairment may also be the result of various pharmacological treatments of insomnia. Hypnotics with long elimination half-lives cause performance decrements due to carryover of their sedative effects during the daytime; on the other hand, short-acting hypnotics with high affinity to the benzodiazepine receptor are associated with serious incidents of next-day memory impairment (Kales and Kales 1984). A degree of REM sleep suppression caused by benzodiazepine hypnotics has been also proposed as a possible mechanism involved in drug-induced memory impairment (Misaki et al. 1998).

Obstructive sleep apnea is a life-threatening disorder characterized by snoring and repetitive breath cessations during sleep, accompanied by excessive daytime sleepiness and sleep attacks (Kales et al. 1985a). This disorder may lead to serious health problems such as hypertension, arrhythmias, and ischemic heart attacks. Moreover, it has important psychosocial consequences, such as interpersonal difficulties, marital and family discord, impaired social functioning, and serious work problems that may even lead to quitting a job or being fired (Kales et al. 1985b). Similar interpersonal, marital, work, and social problems are experienced by patients suffering from narcolepsy and other hypersomnias that are associated with certain psychological reactions including suppression of emotional expressiveness, distress, self-doubt, and formation of negative self-image (Kales et al. 1982b). The psychosocial consequences of narcolepsy are even more pronounced than in other disorders of excessive sleep, because this disorder usually starts at an early age and it is thus also associated with quitting school and the development of personality disorders (Kales et al. 1982b).

Conclusion

Sleep is a neurobehavioral phenomenon characterized by distinct cyclic changes in brain activity that constitute the consecutive transitions from non-REM stages (I, II, III, and IV) to stage REM and back to non-REM stages. Under normal conditions, a solid internal sleep architecture with minimal intervening wakefulness is depicted in the hypnopolygram. In contrast, states of brain dysfunction are frequently associated with sleep disruption, even disorganization, whereas certain neuropsychological manifestations are often part of the clinical picture of various sleep disorders. Thus, it is indeed very relevant to study the neuropsychiatric aspects of disturbed sleep.

A number of neurological disorders (traumatic brain injury, encephalitis, cerebral stroke, dementias, etc.) are accompanied by sleep disturbance. Generally, sleep is differently affected in different patients depending on the brain regions mostly affected. For example, in cerebral stroke, a lesion of the pontine tegmentum results in a drastic reduction of REM sleep, whereas a lesion of the lower brainstem in elimination of slow-wave sleep (i.e., non-REM sleep stages III and IV). From a clinical standpoint, some neurological patients present with somnolence, others with sleeplessness, and some others with a disruption of the normal circadian alternation of sleep and wakefulness.

Sleep disorders associated with neuropathological or neurophysiological alterations and accompanied by neuropsychological manifestations include fatal familial insomnia, narcolepsy, and REM behavior disorder. Also, organicity is strongly suggested in many cases of sleepwalking and night terrors, particularly in childhood. Probably even more interesting from the clinician's point of view are the serious cognitive and psychosocial consequences of curtailed or otherwise disturbed sleep, as is the case in sleep deprivation, chronic insomnia, obstructive sleep apnea syndromes, and narcolepsy.

References

Akaboshi S, Koeda T, Houdou S (1998) Transient extreme spindles in a case of subacute *Mycoplasma pneumoniae* encephalitis. Acta Paediatr Jpn 40:479–482

Akerstedt T (1995) Work hours, sleepiness and the underlying mechanisms. J Sleep Res 4(S2):15–22

Aserinsky E, Kleitman N (1953) Regularly occurring periods of eye motility and concomitant phenomena during sleep. Science 118:273–274

Barabas G, Matthews WS, Ferrari M (1984) Somnambulism in children with Tourette syndrome. Dev Med Child Neurol 26:457–460

Beetar JT, Guilmette TJ, Sparadeo FR (1996) Sleep and pain complaints in symptomatic traumatic brain injury and neurologic populations. Arch Phys Med Rehabil 77(12):1298–1302

Bixler EO, Robertson JA, Soldatos CR (1986) Sleep laboratory assessment of normal sleep and sleep disorders. In: Berlin RM, Soldatos CR (eds) Sleep disorders in psychiatric practice. Ryandic, Longwood, FL

Borbely AA, Tobler I, Groos G (1983) Sleep homeostasis and the circadian sleep-wake rhythm. In: Chase M, Weitzman ED (eds) Sleep disorders: basic and clinical research. SP Medical, New York

Buguet A (1999) Is sleeping sickness a circadian disorder? The serotonergic hypothesis. Chronobiol Int 16:477–489

Caldwell JA Jr, LeDuc PA (1998) Gender influences on performance, mood and recovery sleep in fatigued aviators. Ergonomics 41:1757–1770

Charney DS, Kales A, Soldatos CR, Nelson JC (1979) Somnambulistic-like episodes secondary to combined lithium-neuroleptic treatment. Br J Psychiatry 135:418–424

Chelette TL, Albery WB, Esken RL, Tripp LD (1998) Female exposure to high G: performance of simulated flight after 24 hours of sleep deprivation. Aviat Space Environ Med 69:862–868

Chiu HF, Wing YK (1997) REM sleep behaviour disorder: an overview. Int J Clin Pract 51:451–454

Clavelou P, Tournilhac M, Vidal C, et al (1995) Narcolepsy associated with arteriovenous malformation of the diencephalon. Sleep 18:202–205

Corsi-Cabrera M, Arce C, Del Rio-Portilla IY, et al (1999) Amplitude reduction in visual event-related potentials as a function of sleep deprivation. Sleep 22:181–189

Daly DD, Yoss RE (1974) Narcolepsy. In: Magnus O, DeHaas L (eds) The epilepsies, vol 15. In: Vinken PJ, Bruyn GW (eds) Handbook of clinical neurology. North-Holland, Amsterdam, pp 836–852

Dement WC, Kleitman N (1957) The relation of eye movements during sleep to dream activity: an objective method for the study of dreaming. J Exp Psychol 53:339–346

Dinges DF, Pack F, Williams K, et al (1997) Cumulative sleepiness, mood disturbance, and psychomotor vigilance performance decrements during a week of sleep restricted to 4–5 hours per night. Sleep 20:267–277

Drummond SP, Brown GG, Striker JL, et al (1999) Sleep deprivation-induced reduction in cortical functional response to serial subtraction. Neuroreport 10:3745–3748

Frieboes RM, Muller U, Murck H, et al (1999) Nocturnal hormone secretion and the sleep EEG in patients several months after traumatic brain injury. J Neuropsychiatry Clin Neurosci 11:354–360

Gallassi R, Morreale A, Montagna P, et al (1996) Fatal familial insomnia: behavioral and cognitive features. Neurology 46:935–939

Guilleminault C, Heinzer R, Mignot E, Black J (1998) Investigations into the neurologic basis of narcolepsy. Neurology 50(suppl 1):S8–S15

Harrison Y, Horne JA (1998) Sleep loss impairs short and novel language tasks having a prefrontal focus. J Sleep Res 7:95–100

Hauri PJ (1997) Cognitive deficits in insomnia patients. Acta Neurol Belg 97:113–117

Hibbard MR, Uysal S, Sliwinski M, Gordon WA (1998) Undiagnosed health issues in individuals with traumatic brain injury living in the community. J Head Trauma Rehabil 13:47–57

Hishikawa Y, Shimizu T (1995) Physiology of REM sleep, cataplexy, and sleep paralysis. Adv Neurol 67:245–271

Hishikawa Y, Nan'no N, Tachibana M, et al (1968) The nature of sleep attack and other symptoms of narcolepsy. Electroencephalogr Clin Neurophysiol 24:1–10

Hobson JA (1983) Sleep mechanisms and pathopysiology: some clinical implications of the reciprocal interaction hypothesis of sleep cycle control. Psychosom Med 45:123–140

Hoch CC, Reynolds CF III (1989) Electroencephalographic sleep in late-life neuropsychiatric disorders. Int Psychogeriatr 1:51–62

Iyama A, Inouye T, Ukai S, Shinosaki K (1992) Spindle activity in the waking EEG in older adults. Clin Electroencephalogr 23:137–141

Jouvet M, Michel E (1959) Correlations electromyographiques du sommeil chez le chat decortique et mesencephalique chronique. C R Soc Biol (Paris) 153:422–425

Kales A (ed) (1969) Sleep physiology and pathology. Lippincott, philadelphia

Kales A, Kales J (1984) Evaluation and treatment of insomnia. Oxford University Press, New York

Kales A, Jacobson A, Paulson MJ, et al (1966) Somnambulism: psychophysiological correlates: I. All-night EEG studies. Arch Gen Psychiatry 14:586–594

Kales JD, Kales A, Soldatos CR, et al (1979) Sleepwalking and night terrors related to febrile illness. Am J Psychiatry 136:1214–1215

Kales A, Soldatos CR, Bixler EO, et al (1980) Hereditary factors in sleepwalking and night terrors. Br J Psychiatry 137:111–118

Kales A, Cadieux R, Soldatos CR, et al (1982a) Narcolepsy/cataplexy: I. Clinical and electrophysiologic characteristics. Arch Neurol 39:164–168

Kales A, Soldatos CR, Bixler EO, et al (1982b) Narcolepsy/cataplexy: II. Psychosocial consequences and associated psychopathology. Arch Neurol 39:169–171

Kales A, Cadieux RJ, Bixler EO, et al (1985a) Severe obstructive sleep apnea. I: Onset, clinical course and characteristics. J Chronic Dis 38:419–425
Kales A, Caldwell A, Cadieux R, et al (1985b) Severe obstructive sleep apnea. II: Associated psychopathology and psychosocial consequences. J Chronic Dis 38:427–434
Kales A, Soldatos CR, Kales JD (1987) Sleep disorders:insomnia, night terrors, nightmares and enuresis. Ann Intern Med 106:582–592
Korner E, Flooh E, Reinhart B, et al (1986) Sleep alterations in ischemic stroke. Eur Neurol 25(suppl 2):104–110
Lavie P (1993) The sleep theory of Constantin von Economo. J Sleep Res 2:175–178
Linde L, Edland A, Bergstrom M (1999) Auditory attention and multiattribute decision-making during a 33-h sleep-deprivation period: mean performance and between-subject dispersions. Ergonomics 42:696–713
Loomis AL, Harvey EN, Hobart GA (1937) Cerebral states during sleep as studied by human brain potentials. J Exp Psychol 21:127–144
Lugaresi E, Tobler I, Gambetti P, Montagna P (1998) The pathophysiology of fatal familial insomnia. Brain Pathol 8:521–526
Ma TK, Ang LC, Mamelak M (1996) Narcolepsy secondary to fourth ventricular subependymoma. Can J Neurol Sci 23:59–62
Mignot E (1998) Genetic and familial aspects of narcolepsy. Neurology 50(suppl 1):S16–S22
Misaki K, Nakagawa H, Koshino Y, et al (1998) Effect of flunitrazepam on sleep and memory. Psychiatry Clin Neurosci 52:327–332
Montplaisir J, Petit D, McNamara D, Gauthier S (1996) Comparisons between SPECT and quantitative EEG measures of cortical impairment in mild to moderate Alzheimer's disease. Eur Neurol 36:197–200
Nishino S, Reid MS, Dement WC, Mignot E (1994) Neuropharmacology and neurochemistry of canine narcolepsy. Sleep 17(suppl 8):S84–S92
Nobili L, Baglietto MG, Beelke M, et al (2000) Spindles-inducing mechanism modulates sleep activation of interictal epileptiform discharges in the Landau–Kleffner syndrome. Epilepsia 41:201–206
Olson EJ, Boeve BF, Silber MH (2000) Rapid eye movement sleep behaviour disorder: demographic, clinical and laboratory findings in 93 cases. Brain 123(pt 2):331–339
Plazzi G, Cortelli P, Montagna P, et al (1998) REM sleep behaviour disorder differentiates pure autonomic failure from multiple system atrophy with autonomic failure. J Neurol Neurosurg Psychiatry 64:683–685
Rechtschaffen A, Kales A (eds) (1998) A manual of standardized terminology, techniques, and scoring system for sleep stages of human subjects. NIH no 204. National Institutes of Health, Bethesda, MD
Saletu-Zyhlarz G, Saletu B, Anderer P, et al (1997) Nonorganic insomnia in generalized anxiety disorder. 1. Controlled studies on sleep, awakening and daytime vigilance utilizing polysomnography and EEG mapping. Neuropsychobiology 36(3):117–129
Schenck CH, Mahowald MW (1991) Injurious sleep behavior disorders (parasomnias) affecting patients on intensive care units. Intensive Care Med 17:219–224
Schenck CH, Hurwitz TD, Mahowald MW (1993) Symposium: normal and abnormal. REM sleep regulation. REM sleep behaviour disorder: an update on a series of 96 patients and a review of the world literature. J Sleep Res 2:224–231
Siegel JM (1990) Mechanisms of sleep control. J Clin Neurophysiol 7:49–65
Soldatos CR, Kales A (1982) Sleep disorders: research in psychopathology and its practical implications. Acta Psychiatr Scand 65:381–387
Tachibana N, Kimura K, Kitajima K, et al (1997) REM sleep motor dysfunction in multiple system atrophy: with special emphasis on sleep talk as its early clinical manifestation. J Neurol Neurosurg Psychiatry 63:678–681
Tamura K, Karacan I, Williams RL, Meyer JS (1983) Disturbances of the sleep-waking cycle in patients with vascular brain stem lesions. Clin Electroencephalogr 14:35–46

Veggiotti P, Beccaria F, Guerrini R, et al (1999) Continuous spike-and-wave activity during slow-wave sleep: syndrome or EEG pattern? Epilepsia 40:1593–1601
Vela-Bueno A, Kales A, Soldatos C, et al (1984) Sleep in the Prader-Willi syndrome. Clinical and polygraphic findings. Arch Neurol 41:294–296
Von Economo C (1929) Schlaftheorie. Ergeb Physiol 28:312–339
Wimmer F, Hoffmann RF, Bonato RA, Moffitt AR (1992) The effects of sleep deprivation on divergent thinking and attention processes. J Sleep Res 1:223–230

Biological Aspects of Personality and Behavior

A Behavioral Analysis of Personality

Masaya Sato

Summary. The concept of personality was conceptually analyzed from the standpoint of radical behaviorism. In this attempt, personality was defined as the total behavioral repertoire of a particular individual, and trait was defined as a cluster of respondents or operants that are controlled by common variables. Then, the author attempted to define the main common controlling variable of each of the four temperaments and three characters of TCI and the five traits of NEO. Our empirical data fairly well supported these guesses.

Keywords. Radical behaviorism, Behavior analysis, Personality, NEO, TCI

This chapter intends to analyze the concept of personality from the standpoint of radical behaviorism. Radical behaviorism is a philosophy of psychology founded by B.F. Skinner (Skinner 1974). Radical behaviorism is distinguished from methodological behaviorism, which is accepted by most contemporary experimental psychologists except Skinnerians or behavior analysts.

Although there are several differences between methodological behaviorism and radical behaviorism, the following two are most important. First, methodological behaviorism excludes private events such as consciousness from the direct subject matter of psychology, because methodological behaviorists believe that private events cannot be studied objectively, and objectivity is the essence of science. For methodological behaviorists, any private event that is a cause of behavior must be inferred from observable or public behaviors. On the other hand, radical behaviorism accept private events as legitimate subject matter of psychology, because radical behaviorists believe that private events such as consciousness are not causes of behavior but behaviors themselves and can be studied objectively in the same way as observable or public behaviors. Second, methodological behaviorism accepts inner causes of behavior including intervening variables whereas radical behaviorism rejects all kinds of inner causes of behavior. Radical behaviorists believe that the ultimate causes of behavior are not inside the organism but in the phylogenic and ontogenic environments.

There are many definitions of personality. These can be classified into two types: one is the hypothetical-construct view of personality and the other is the behavioral reper-

---

Department of Psychology, Teikyo University, 359 Otsuka, Hachioji, Tokyo 192-0395, Japan

toire view of personality. Here is Gordon W. Allport's definition of personality: Personality is the dynamic organization within the individual of those psychophysical systems that determine his unique adjustment to his environment (Allport 1937, p. 48).

This definition is an example of the hypothetical construct view of personality. Allport's view of personality assumes personality is something within an individual. Most traditional theorists of personality take this view, and they believe personality can be a cause of behavior. The concept of personality based on this view is a conceptual cause of behavior. So, from the standpoint of radical behaviorism, such a concept of personality is fiction, and behavior analysts cannot accept it.

Here is John B. Watson's definition: Personality is the sum of activities that can be discovered by actual observation of behavior over a long enough time to give reliable information (Watson 1930, p. 274). This is an example of the behavioral repertoire view of personality. Watson's view defines personality not as something within an individual that causes behavior but as behavior itself. Watson was not a radical behaviorist because he excluded private events from the subject matter of psychology, but he denied inner causes of behavior. Behavior analysts can accept this view without hesitation.

The science of behavior based on radical behaviorism is called behavior analysis. A behavior analytical definition of personality might be this: personality is the total behavioral repertoire of a particular individual. Then, the goal of the behavior analysis of personality is to reveal the structure of the behavioral repertoire.

Behavior analysis classifies behaviors into two kinds: one is respondent behavior and the other is operant behavior. Respondent behavior is reflexive behavior, and it is elicited by unconditioned or conditioned stimulus. The unit of respondent behavior is called a respondent. Operant behavior is voluntary behavior, and it is emitted by an organism. The frequency of operant behavior is controlled by its consequences. If the consequences have rewarding or reinforcing value, the operant behavior will increase. If the consequences have punishing value, the frequency of the operant behavior will decrease. The unit of operant behavior is called an operant.

The total behavioral repertoire of a particular individual consists of various respondents and operants. It is probable that there is a cluster of respondents or operants. Such a cluster might be considered as a trait. For behavior analysts, a trait is a cluster of respondents or operants that are controlled by common variables.

In the Keio Twin Project, we are using Temperament and Character Inventory (TCI) and NEO-PI-R. TCI's seven-factor model assumes that there are four temperaments and three characters. The four temperaments are Novelty Seeking (NS), Harm Avoidance (HA), Reward Dependence (RD), and Persistence (P), and the three characters are Self-Directedness (SD), Cooperativeness (C), and Self-Transcendence (ST). Table 1 shows my ideas about the main controlling variables of each temperament and character. NEO's five-factor model assumes that there are five traits: Neuroticism (N), Extraversion (E), Openness (O), Agreeableness (A), and Conscientiousness (C). Table 2 shows my ideas of the main controlling variable of each trait.

If my guesses are correct, high positive correlations are predicted between TCI's Reward Dependence (RD), and Cooperativeness (C), between TCI's Harm Avoidance (HA) and NEO's Neuroticism (N), between TCI's Cooperativeness (C) and NEO's Agreeableness (A), and between TCI's Persistence (P) and NEO's Conscientiousness (C). High negative correlations are predicted between TCI's Harm Avoidance (HA)

TABLE 1. Temperaments and characters of TCI and their main controlling variable

Trait	Main controlling variable
Novelty Seeking (NS)	Rewarding value of trying to obtain stimulus changes
Harm Avoidance (HA)	Punishing value of aversive events
Reward Dependence (RD)	Rewarding value of having intimate relationships with other people
Persistence (P)	Rewarding value of achieving desired goals perfectly
Self-Directedness (SD)	Reflexive insensitivity to aversive events
Cooperativeness (CO)	Rewarding value of other people's positive reactions
Self-Transcendence (ST)	Rewarding value of mysterious experiences

TABLE 2. Traits of NEO and their main controlling variable

Trait	Main controlling variable
Neuroticism (N)	Reflexive sensitivity to aversive events
Extraversion (E)	Rewarding value of the existence of other people
Openness (O)	Rewarding value of novel events
Agreeableness (A)	Rewarding value of other people's positive reactions
Conscientiousness (C)	Rewarding value of performing socially significant acts

TABLE 3. Correlation between TCI's seven factors and NEO's five factors (n = 467)

	NS	HA	RD	P	SD	CO	ST	N	E	O	A
NS											
HA	**−0.41**										
RD	0.10	−0.08									
P	−0.16	−0.20	0.13								
SD	0.07	**−0.52**	0.06	0.22							
CO	0.02	−0.26	**0.49**	0.25	0.32						
ST	0.13	−0.21	0.13	0.22	0.06	0.20					
N	−0.19	**0.65**	0.01	−0.14	**−0.59**	−0.29	−0.03				
E	**0.45**	**−0.61**	**0.41**	0.17	0.31	0.33	0.24	−0.38			
O	0.17	−0.27	0.12	0.22	0.24	0.23	0.39	−0.09	0.32		
A	−0.12	−0.02	**0.44**	0.07	0.13	**0.58**	0.16	−0.12	0.12	0.14	
C	−0.30	−0.23	0.12	**0.57**	**0.40**	0.24	0.11	**−0.40**	0.21	0.18	0.10

and Self-Directedness (SD) and between TCI's Self-Directedness (SD) and NEO's Neuroticism (N). Table 3 shows phenotypic correlation between TCI's seven factors and NEO's five factors in our study. All six of these predictions are fulfilled.

References

Allport GW (1937) Personality: a psychological interpretation. Holt, New York
Skinner BF (1974) About behaviorism. Knopf, New York
Watson JB (1930) Behaviorism (rev edn). University of Chicago Press, Chicago

Genetic Structure of Personality: Comparison Between TCI and NEO (Big Five Model)

Juko Ando

Summary. Although the "Big Five" were recently said to be the "human universals" of personality structure, these five factors are not genetically independent. On the contrary, the Basic Three temperamental dimensions (novelty seeking, harm avoidance, and reward dependence) proposed by C.R. Cloninger are genetically unique and independent. By multivariate genetic analysis with 296 Japanese twins, it was revealed that, among the five big factors, neuroticism, extraversion, agreeableness, and conscientiousness could be genetically explained only by the "Big Three". Openness to experience could be explained by the Big Three as well as by an additional genetic contribution (perhaps intelligence).

Keywords. Genetic structure, Personality, Twins, Big Five Model, Temperament, Character

Introduction

How many dimensions are necessary and sufficient to describe human personality? For many years, psychologists have been arguing about the number of personality dimensions. Recently, it has been claimed that those variations could be summarized by the five-factor model as a comprehensive classification of the major sources of individual differences of personality by recent progress of the factor analytical method. The most common terminology for those five factors is *neuroticism* (N), *extraversion* (E), *openness to experience* (O), *agreeableness* (A), and *conscienciousness* (C). This model of five-factor structure, or the so-called Big Five (B5), has been frequently replicated in different cultures, and McCrae and Costa claimed this to be the "human universal" (McCrae and Costa 1997).

If the Big Five model provides the universal structure of human personality, it is necessary to show any plausible reason why those five factors are necessary and sufficient to describe human personality structure. However, at least up to now, it seems that no reasonable explanations have been proposed. One of the possible reasons could be provided by genetics. Many twin and adoption studies have showed sub-

Faculty of Letters, Department of Education, Keio University, 2-15-45 Mita, Minato-ku, Tokyo 108-8345, Japan

stantial genetic contribution to those five factors (Loehlin 1992). However, when there is a substantial genetic contribution to a certain trait, it does not necessarily mean that this trait is genetically independent or has its own trait-specific genetic origin. Actually, recent multivariate genetic analyses of the Big Five model revealed that these five personality factors are not unique genotypically but rather overlapped with each other, even though they are phenotypically independent, robust, and genetically influenced (Ono et al. 2000). That conclusion means the Big Five model is just a phenotypic structure, not a genetic structure, which might be because these five factors are constructed by mere conceptual categorization of personality descriptions (adjectives and sentences that describe varieties of human personality) and are not based upon any biological or physiological assumptions and mechanisms.

Contrary to the FFM, Cloninger's theory on temperament and character (Cloninger 1986; Cloninger et al. 1993) provides a biologically based structure of personality. On the basis of clinical examples and animal studies, Cloninger originally proposed a tridimensional theory of temperament that contained three genetically independent components: *novelty seeking* (NS), *harm avoidance* (HA), and *reward dependence* (RD) (Cloninger 1986). According to his theory, NS is viewed as the activation or initiation of behavior and is thought to be related to dopamine; HA is viewed as the inhibition of behavior and related to serotonine; and RD is viewed as the maintenance or continuation of ongoing behavior and is related to norepinephrine. Cloninger's latest theory (Cloninger et al. 1993) proposed a fourth temperament dimension, *persistence*, and three other new character dimensions, *self-directedness*, *cooperativeness*, and *self-transcendence*. Those seven factors are measured by the TCI (Temperament and Character Inventory).

An interesting finding is that Cloninger's tridimensional temperament factors might be genetically independent. Heath et al. (1994) indicated that Cloninger's four temperament dimensions are genetically more homogeneous than Eysenck's and Gray's personality factors. Stalling et al. (1996) analyzed the genetic and environmental structure of four temperaments and revealed that those three temperament factors were genetically independent, especially in males. Ando and Ono (1998) verified a mutual genetic independence among them.

It is interesting to compare these two comprehensive personality structure models from a behavioral genetic point of view. If Cloninger's three temperament dimensions provide the fundamental structure of human personality, genetic factors of the Big Five dimensions should be completely explained by those of Cloninger's. If any of the Big Five factors taps unique personality dimensions, there should be some specific genetic contribution other than Cloninger's temperament dimensions. There have been no such comparisons, especially for the Japanese population. In this study, we compared the genetic structures of the Big Five model and Cloninger's temperament model measured by NEO-PI-R and TCI.

Materials and Methods

Materials

The Big Five factors were measured by the Japanese version of NEO-PI-R (Yoshimura et al. 1998; Costa and McCrae 1985). Cloninger's temperament

TABLE 1. Goodness of fit statistics (AIC, Akaike's information criteria) for the three models

	N	E	O	A	C
Only B3	**−120.62**	**−125.00**	−158.98	**−135.31**	***−118.41***
Independent	−75.21	−72.94	−148.04	−103.55	−79.19
Mixed	−113.75	−123.00	**−160.74**	***−134.95***	**−119.41**

N, neuroticism; E, extraversion; O, openness; A, agreeableness; C, conscienciousness
The lowest AIC (bold) indicates the best fit model, and the second lowest AIC (bold/italics) is not significantly different from the best one. The "only the Basic Three (B3) model" assumes that each of the Big Five dimensions overlaps and could be thoroughly explained by NS (novelty seeking), HA (harm avoidance), and RD (reward dependence); the "independent contribution model" assumes that each Big Five dimension is genetically independent from each dimension of the Basic Three and has its own specific genetic contribution; and the "mixed model" assumes that each of the Big Five dimensions contain both the Basic Three and its specific genetic contribution. N and E were explained only by the Big Three; A and C could be explained either by only the three Basic factors or by B3 plus the specific genetic contributions; O could be explained exclusively by the mixed model.

factors were measured by the Japanese version of the TCI (Cloninger et al. 1993; Kijima et al. 1996).

Participants

Participants in this study were 296 pairs of twins including 184 pairs of monozygotic (MZ) twins (124 female and 60 male pairs), 77 pairs of same-sex dizygotic (DZ) twins (49 female and 28 male pairs), and 35 pairs of opposite-sex twins. Zygosity was determined by the twins' physical resemblance (Ooki et al. 1991) and by polymorphism of D4DR and serotonin transporter genes with more than 93% accuracy. The average age of the female sample was 20.2 years (±3.4), ranging from 14 to 29 years, and the average age of the males was 19.4 years (±3.4), ranging from 15 to 28 years.

Results

We made the following comparison by the model fitting analysis of structure equation modeling. The first model is "the only B3 model" in which each B5 dimension could be thoroughly explained by NS, HA, and RD. The second model is the "independent contribution model," which assumes that each B5 dimension is genetically independent of B3 and has its own specific genetic contribution. The third is the "mixed model," which is assumed to contain both B3 and its specific contribution.

Table 1 provides the goodness of fit statistics (AIC) of each of the three models for each B5 factor. For N and E, the only B3 model fit best. For A and C, no significant difference could be found between the only B3 model and the mixed model. We can modestly take the only B3 model for the reason of parsimoniousness. Only for O (openness), however, was the mixed model exclusively the best fit model. Therefore, there must be an additional specific genetic contribution other than B3 factors. Under the best fit models, each of these five factors from B5 could be explained as shown in Fig. 1.

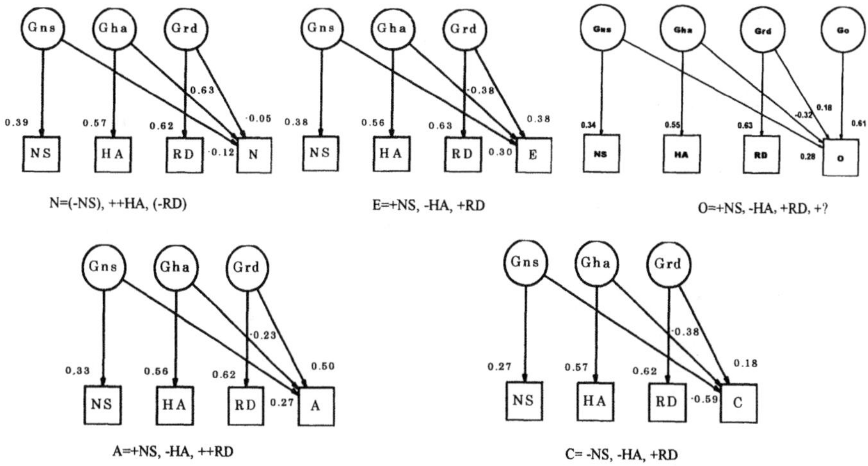

FIG. 1 Genetic relationships between the Basic Three temperamental dimensions (NS, HA, and RD) and four Big Five factors (N, E, O, A, and C). All the Big Five factors, except for O, can be explained by the Basic Three and there are no genetic components specific to the traits. Only O needs an additional specific genetic contribution other than B3. Because the main focus of this chapter is the genetic structure of personality, these pictures do not contain the environmental structures. *Gns*, genetic component of NS; *Gha*, genetic component of HA; *Grd*, genetic component of RD; *Go*, genetic component of O; *NS*, novelty seeking; *HA*, harm avoidance; *RD*, reward dependence; *N*, neuroticism; *E*, extra version; *O*, openness; *A*, agreeableness; *C*, consciensciousness

Discussion

Our conclusion now is that the comprehensive personality structure, the Big Five factors, can be explained mostly by Cloninger's three temperament dimensions. This result indicates that the Basic Three are the fundamental genetic structure of human personality. Only openness (O) needs an additional specific genetic contribution other than B3. We notice that the additive genetic contribution is larger in O than the other four (Loehlin 1992; Ono et al. 2000). Our preliminary analysis showed that phenotypically O and intelligence are significantly correlated, and that the cross-correlation between twin sibling A's O and twin sibling B's intelligence was larger in MZ than DZ, which indicated a genetic overlap between O and intelligence. Therefore, the additional genetic contribution for O could come from intelligence.

If Individual differences of personality can be completely explained by means of only genetic contributions of the Basic Three and intelligence, what is B5? It seems that they are "the socially recognized composites of those four biopsychological resources." Please note that all the B5 factors are labels of social attitude. We recognize an individual's behavioral character as a specific combination of one's behavioral activation (NS), suppression (HA), and maintaining (RD) patterns, plus information processing efficiency, in a social context.

References

Ando J, Ono Y (1998) Keio Twin Project: a preliminary report (abstract of the 9th international congress on twin studies). Twin Res 1:81

Cloninger CR (1986) A unified biosocial theory of personality and its role in the development of anxiety states. Psychiatr Dev 3:167–226

Cloninger CR, Svrakic DM, Przybeck TR (1993) A psychobiological model of temperament and character. Arch Gen Psychiatry 50:975–990

Costa PT Jr, McCrae RR (1985) Comparison of EPI and psychoticism scales with measures of the five-factor model of personality. Pers Individ Differ 6:587–597

Heath AC, Cloninger CR, Martin NG (1994) Testing model for the genetic structure of personality: a comparison of the personality systems of Cloninger and Eysenck. J Pers Soc Psychol 66:762–775

Kijima N, Saito R, Kakeuchi M, et al (1996) Cloninger's seven-factor model of temperament and character and Japanese version of Temperament and Character Inventory (TCI)

Loehlin JC (1992) Genes and environment in personality development: individual differences and developmental series, vol 2. Sage, Newbury Park, CA

McCrae RP, Costa PT Jr (1997) Personality trait structure as a human universal. Am Psychol 52:509–516

Neale MC, Cardon LR (1992) Methodology for genetic studies on twins and families. Kluwer, Boston

Ono Y, Ando J, Onoda N, Yoshimura K (2000) Genetic structure of five factor model among Japanese population. Keio J Med 49:152–158

Ooki S, Yamada K, Asaka A (1991) Zygosity diagnosis of twins by questionnaire for twin's mothers. Shoni Hoken Keikyu 50:71–76

Stalling MC, Hewitt JK, Cloninger CR, et al (1996) Genetic and environmental structure of the Tridimensional Personality Questionnaire: three or four temperament dimensions. J Pers Soc Psychol 70:127–140

Yoshimura K, Nakamura K, Ono Y, et al (1998) Reliability and validity of the Japanese version of the NEO Five-Factor Inventory (NEO-FFI): a population-based survey in Aomori Prefecture. Jpn J Stress Sci 13:45–53

Evolution of Personality-Related Genes in Primates

Miho Inoue-Murayama[1], Youko Niimi[1], Osamu Takenaka[2], and Yuichi Murayama[3]

Summary. Human dopamine receptor D4 (DRD4) and serotonin transporter (5-HTT) genes are polymorphic in terms of the repeat numbers of the GC-rich sequences located in the exon and promoter region, respectively. These genes have attracted special interest as genes related to personality traits. To assess the diversities of these genes in the evolutionary context, we examined the polymorphic regions of these genes in nonhuman primates. Simian primates (apes and monkeys) had four or more repeated sequences in the DRD4 gene polymorphic region, whereas prosimians had one or two repeat units of the 48-bp sequence. These observations imply that the frequency of long-repeated alleles tended to increase during primate evolution. On the other hand, apes and monkeys had relatively longer 5-HTT promoter sequences with an increased number of tandem repeats than human sequences, suggesting that the frequency of short-repeated alleles tended to increase during the process of hominization.

Keywords. Dopamine receptor D4, Primates, Personality, Serotonin transporter, polymorphism

Introduction

Because primates have a highly developed brain and exhibit a variety of psychological and behavioral traits in their elaborate social interactions, an analysis of the genes affecting mental activity may be considered useful for elucidating primate evolution and human origin. Human dopamine receptor D4 (DRD4) is polymorphic in terms of the repeat numbers of the 48-bp sequence located in the third cytoplasmic loop of the receptor [14], and individuals with long repeats (6 or more) in the DRD4 gene have been found to achieve higher scores in a personality test for novelty seeking than do those with shorter repeats [1,4]. Genetic polymorphism has also been reported in the serotonin transporter (5-HTT) gene. A tandem repeated sequence consisting of

[1] Faculty of Agriculture, Gifu University, Gifu 501-1193, Japan
[2] Primate Research Institute, Kyoto University, Kyoto, Japan
[3] National Institute of Animal Health, Tsukuba, Japan

20- to 23-bp units is located in the promoter region of the human 5-HTT gene, and it has been shown that individuals with 14 repeats in the promoter displayed higher scores in a personality test for anxiety/neuroticism than did those with 16 repeats [9].

To assess the changes of the polymorphic region of DRD4 and 5-HTT genes that have occurred during primate evolution, we investigated the allelic variations of these genes in anthropoid apes, Old World monkeys, and prosimians, and determined the DNA sequences of the alleles in each species. Sequence analysis of the DRD4 gene was also performed in tree shrews, a species closely related to primates.

Materials and Methods

Genomic DNA was extracted by the phenol–chloroform method from peripheral blood or tissue samples of tree shrews, prosimians (galagoes, lemurs, and lorises), Old World monkeys (Japanese macaques and patas monkeys), and apes (chimpanzees, gorillas, orangutans, and gibbons). The D4DR and 5-HTT polymorphic regions were amplified by the polymerase chain reaction (PCR) [6,7,8]. The primer sets employed were 5′-TTCTTCCTACCCTGCCCGCTCATG-3′ (D4F) and 5′-GACCACCACCG-GCAGGACCCTCAT-3′ (D4R): 5′-GGCGTTGCCGCTCTGAATGC-3′ (5-HTTF), and 5′-GAGGGACTGAGCTGGACAACCAC-3′ (5-HTTR). Each sample was separated on 2% agarose gel. The PCR products were extracted from the gel and then directly sequenced by the dye termination method using a Perkin Elmer 377 sequencer. Nucleotide sequence was determined in both strands at least twice.

Results and Discussion

As shown in Table 1, 4–8 repeat alleles of the DRD4 gene were found in simian primates as reported previously [11,12]. A sequence homologous to the simian 48-bp sequence does not exist in the rat and mouse D4DR genes [5,13], and the origin of this unit remains unclear. In the present study, we found that the D4DR genes of prosimians consisted of one or two repeat units and that the sequence of the tree shrew contained only one unit that had 71%–75% identities to the prosimian units.

TABLE 1. Allele frequency of polymorphic region in dopamine receptor D4

		Allele (number of repeats)							
	n	8	7	6	5	4	3	2	1
Human[a]	201	0.007	0.138	0.025	0.023	0.684	0.026	0.096	
Chimpanzee	16				1.000				
Gorilla	14			0.680	0.320				
Orangutan	17			0.706	0.176	0.118			
Gibbon	16		0.188	0.375	0.313	0.125			
Japanese macaque	30				1.000				
Patas monkey	14	0.036	0.107	0.107	0.392	0.358			
Prosimians	7							0.786	0.214
Tree shrew	3								1.000

[a] [2]

TABLE 2. Allele frequency of polymorphic region in serotonin transporter gene promoter

		Allele (number of repeats)									
	n	24	23	22	20	18	17.5	17	16	15	14
Human[a]	695				0.006				0.550		0.444
Chimpanzee	16						1.000				
Gorilla	14					0.321		0.143	0.536		
Orangutan	9			0.111	0.778	0.111					
Gibbon	15		0.333	0.067				0.500	0.033	0.067	
Rhesus macaque[b]	154	0.660	0.340								

[a] [3]
[b] [10]

These results indicate that the ancestral primate may have had one 48-bp unit, that duplication of the unit occurred at the stage of prosimians, and that the frequency of long-repeated alleles tended to increase after divergence into simian primates.

Allelic variation of the 5-HTT polymorphic region is given in Table 2. Polymorphism was noted in the gorilla, orangutan, and gibbons, but all chimpanzees examined shared only one genotype with the homozygote of the 17.5-repeat allele. 16- and 20-repeat alleles were most frequent in gorillas and orangutans, respectively. The 5-HTT gene was highly polymorphic in gibbons and the 17- and 23-repeat alleles were frequent among 5 alleles. The polymorphism observed in orangutans and gibbons has strong implications for the origin of 5-HTTLPR in apes. In these Asian apes, extralong-repeat (22 and 23) alleles were recognized, and their sequences were similar to the rhesus macaque 23-repeat sequence. It is inferred that dynamic changes of 5-HTT in its length had occurred at the stage of orangutans and gibbons. The frequency of short repeated alleles in 5-HTT tended to increase during the process of hominization.

In addition to molecular genetic studies, biochemical and behavioral scientific analysis is required if we are to succeed in elucidating the detailed significance of DRD4 and 5-HTT polymorphism in primate societies.

References

1. Benjamin J, Li L, Patterson C, et al (1996) Population and familial association between the D4 dopamine receptor gene and measures of novelty seeking. Nat Genet 12:81–84
2. Chang FM, et al (1996) The world-wide distribution of allele frequencies at the human dopamine D4 receptor locus. Hum Genet 98:91–101
3. Delbrück SJ, et al (1997) A novel allelic variant of the human serotonin transporter gene regulatory polymorphism. Cytogenet Cell Genet 79:214–220
4. Ebstain RP, et al (1996) Dopamine D4 receptor (D4DR) exon III polymorphism associated with the human personality trait of novelty seeking. Nat Genet 12:78–80
5. Fishburn CS, et al (1995) Molecular cloning and characterization of the gene encoding the murine D4 dopamine receptor. FEBS Lett 361:215–219
6. Heils A, et al (1996) Allelic variation of human serotonin transporter gene expression. J Neurochem 66:2621–2624
7. Inoue-Murayama M, et al (1998) Origin and divergence of tandem repeats of primate D4 dopamine receptor genes. Primates 39:217–224

8. Inoue-Murayama M, et al (2000) Allelic variation of the serotonin transporter gene polymorphic region in apes. Primates 41:265–271
9. Lesch KP, et al (1996) Association of anxiety-related traits with a polymorphism in the serotonin transporter gene regulatory region. Science 274:1527–1531
10. Lesch KP, et al (1997) The 5-HT transporter gene-linked polymorphic region (5-HTTLPR) in evolutionary perspective: alternative biallelic variation in rhesus monkeys. J Neural Transm 104:1259–1266
11. Livak KJ, et al (1995) Variability of dopamine D4 receptor (DRD4) gene sequence within and among nonhuman primate species. Proc Natl Acad Sci USA 92:427–431
12. Matsumoto M, et al (1995) Polymorphic tandem repeats in dopamine D4 receptor are spread over primate species. Biochem Biophys Res Commun 207:467–475
13. O'Malley KL, et al (1992) The rat dopamine D4 receptor: sequence, gene structure, and demonstration of expression in the cardiovascular system. New Biol 4:137–146
14. Van Tol HHM, et al (1991) Cloning of the gene for a human dopamine D4 receptor with high affinity for the antipsychotic clozapine. Nature (Lond) 350:610–614

Association Between Novelty Seeking and Dopamine Receptor D_4 (DRD4) Exon III Polymorphism

Shin-ichiro Tomitaka

Summary. In 1996, Ebstein et al. and Benjamin et al. reported significant associations between the long repeat allele of DRD4 exon III and novelty seeking, which is a personality dimension postulated by Cloninger. Because their studies are the first reports that specific genetic polymorphism might influence a normal dimension of personality, a number of replication studies have been conducted to obtain further confirmation of the association. However, it remains unclear whether the initial finding is replicable. The failure to confirm this association is possibly explained by the methodological differences of subsequent studies. Because the estimated size of the DRD4 polymorphism on novelty seeking (NS) explains 3%–4% of the total variance, the noise generated by methodological differences may be sufficient to obscure the small effect of DRD4 on novelty seeking. To clarify these problems, I have reviewed the 14 replication studies from the point of view of demographic and methodological differences. It is suggested that demographic factors might be important to replicate the association between DRD4 exon III polymorphism and novelty seeking.

Keywords. Dopamine receptor D_4, Temperament and character inventory, Novelty seeking, Japanese

Introduction

In 1996, Ebstein et al. and Benjamin et al. reported significant associations between the long repeat allele of dopamine receptor D_4 (DRD4) exon III and "novelty seeking," which is a personality dimension postulated by Cloninger. Because their studies are first reports that specific genetic polymorphism might influence a normal dimension personality, a number of replication studies have been conducted to obtain further confirmation of the association. Table 1 shows the summary of recent replication studies in normal subjects. To my knowledge, over the past 4 years 14 studies have been reported. Of the 14 studies, 7 studies are positive and 6 studies are negative. The

Department of Psychiatry, Tokyo Women's Medical University, Kawada-cho, 8-1, Shinjuku-ku, Tokyo 162-0054, Japan

TABLE 1. Summary of dopamine receptor D_4 (DRD4) studies of personality in normal subjects

Author	Year	Country	Result
Ebstein	1996	Israel	Positive
Benjamin	1996	U.S.A.	Positive
Malhorta	1996	Finland	NS
Jönsson	1997	Sweden	NS
Ebstein	1997	Israel	Positive
Vandenbergh	1997	U.S.A.	NS
Ono	1997	Japan	Positive in NS1
Pogue-Geile	1998	U.S.A.	NS
Jönsson	1998	Sweden	NS
Noble	1998	U.S.A.	Positive
Kühn	1999	Germany	NS
Strobel	1999	Germany	Positive
Ekelund	1999	Finland	2 and 5 repeat, positive
Tomitaka	1999	Japan	Positive

study by Ekelund et al. shows positive association, not in the 7-repeat allele, but in the 2- and 5-repeat allele. In view of these results, it remains unclear whether the initial finding is replicable.

The failure to confirm this association is possibly explained by the methodological differences of subsequent studies. Because the estimated size of the DRD4 polymorphism on NS explains 3%–4% of the total variance, the noise generated by methodological differences may be sufficient to obscure the small effect of DRD4 on novelty seeking. To clarify these problems, we have reviewed the 14 replication studies from the point of view of demographic and methodological differences.

Methods

For demographic differences, we first classified the population of subjects of each study into two groups, homogeneous population or general population. Some studies recruited their subjects from a homogeneous population, such as university students or medical staff. Other studies recruited their subjects from the general population. There are other demographic differences such as age, gender, or ethnicity. Of 14 studies, 7 studies are positive and 6 studies are negative. The study by Ekelund et al. shows positive association not in the 7-repeat allele but in the 2- and 5-repeat alleles. This time we classified Ekelund et al. into the negative group.

Results and Discussion

Figure 1 shows the differences of results between the studies with a homogeneous population and the studies of the general population. Of 14 studies, 7 studies used a homogeneous population, 6 studies used the general population, and 1 study is difficult to classify. Of 7 studies with a specific population, 6 studies had positive results

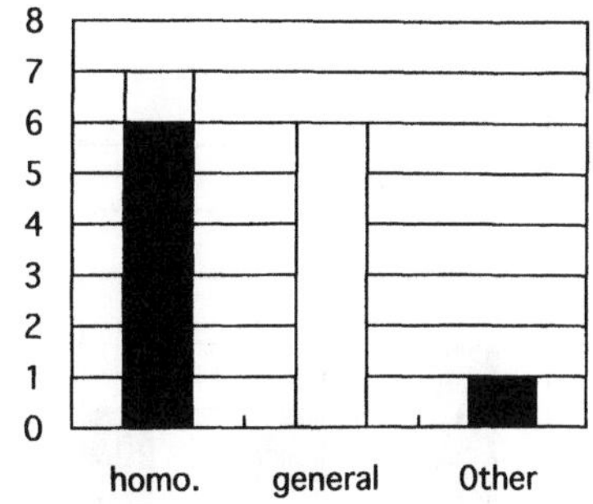

FIG. 1. Differences in results between studies with a homogeneous population and the general population. *Open bar*, negative; *Solid bar*, positive

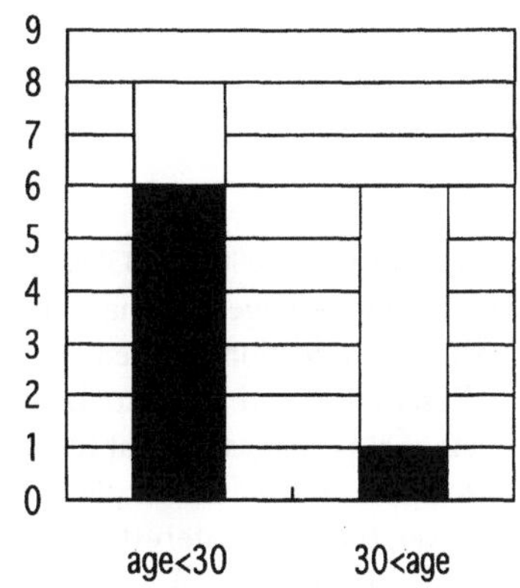

FIG. 2. Differences in results between studies with younger and older subjects. *Open bar*, negative; *Solid bar*, positive

and 1 study negative results. In contrast, of 6 studies with the general population, all 6 studies are negative. These results suggest that, to replicate the association, the choice of subjects is important. It is possible that the choice of homogeneous population may minimize the effects of sociocultural factors.

Figure 2 shows the differences in results between studies with young subjects and studies with older subjects. Of 14 studies, in 8 studies the mean age of the subjects is under 30 and in 6 studies the mean age of the subjects is over 30 years. Of 8 studies that used younger subjects, 6 studies are positive and 2 studies are negative. In contrast, of 6 studies that used older subjects, 1 study is positive and the other 5 studies are negative. These results suggest that, to replicate the association, the age of subjects is also important.

Figure 3 shows the differences in results between studies with differing female percentage. We classified the 14 studies into three groups, those with the percentage of female subjects greater than 67%, those with the percentage of female subjects between 66% and 33%, and those with the percentage of female subjects less than 33%. In 3 studies, the percentage of female subjects is greater than 66%, and these 3 studies are all positive. With regard to the studies whose percentage of female sub-

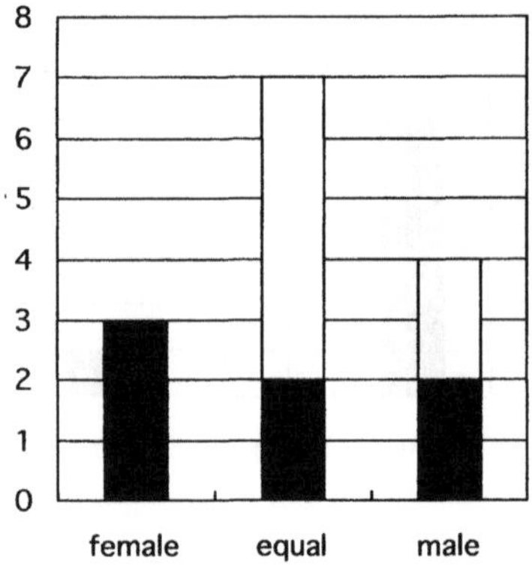

FIG. 3. Differences in results between studies having different female percentages. *Open bar*, negative; *Solid bar*, positive

jects is between 66% and 33%, there are only 2 positive studies of 7 studies. In studies with the percentage of female subjects less than 33%, there are 2 positive studies of 4 studies. In addition, Ebstein et al. reported that, with the combination of their 2 studies, they found the association only in females, not in males. Taking these results together, it is suggested that females may show a greater tendency for this association than males. I have no explanation why females may show this greater tendency. However, there are interesting data that may support this phenomenon. Last year, an analysis of novelty seeking for DRD4 knockout mice was reported by Dulawa et al. They used the emergence test, which is a free exploratory paradigm designed to assess exploratory behavior in rodents. In their experiments, the DRD4 knockout procedure causes female mice to be less responsive to the novel stimuli, but, not males. It is interesting that this interaction of genotype and sex was observed in DRD4 transgenic mice.

With regard to the ethnicity of subjects, although the 7-repeat allele is the second most common in Caucasians, the 7-repeat allele is rare in Japanese and Chinese; instead, the 5-repeat allele is the third most common among Japanese and Chinese. Therefore, in Japanese and Chinese DRD4 association studies, alleles with 5 or more repeats are often grouped with the long allele. The definition of long alleles as 5–7 repeats sometimes differs from that of other analyses with Caucasian populations. Although the 7-repeat allele is rare in Japanese, it is intriguing that two Japanese studies, including ours, replicated the association and two Oriental studies show association between substance abuse and the long repeat allele. However, it is difficult to determine whether the ethnicity of the subjects is an important factor in replicating the association.

In summary, it is suggested that demographic factors might be important to replicate the association between DRD4 exon III polymorphism and novelty seeking.

References

Benjamin J, Li L, Patterson C, et al (1996) Population and familial association between the D4 dopamine receptor gene and measures of novelty seeking. Nat Genet 12:81–84

Dulawa SC, Grandy DK, Low MJ, et al (1999) Dopamine D4 receptor-knock-out mice exhibit reduced exploration of novel stimuli. J Neurosci 19:9550–9556

Ebstein RP, Novick O, Umansky R, et al (1996) Dopamine D4 receptor (D4DR) exon III polymorphism associated with the human personality trait of novelty seeking. Nat Genet 12:78–80

Ebstein RP, Nemanov L, Klotz I, et al (1997) Additional evidence for an association between the dopamine D4 receptor (D4DR) exon III repeat polymorphism and the human personality trait of novelty seeking. Mol Psychiatry 2:472–477.

Ekelund J, Lichtermann D, Jarvelin MR, et al (1999) Association between novelty seeking and the type 4 dopamine receptor gene in a large Finish cohort sample. Am J Psychiatry 156:1453–1455

Jonsson EG, Nothen MM, Gustavsson JP, et al (1997) Lack of evidence for allelic association between personality traits and the dopamine D4 receptor gene polymorphisms. Am J Psychiatry 154:697–699

Jonsson EG, Nothen MM, Gustavsson JP, et al (1998) Lack of association between dopamine D4 receptor gene and personality traits. Psychol Med 28:985–989

Kuhn KU, Meyer K, Nothen MM, et al (1999) Allelic variants of dopamine receptor D4 (DRD4) and serotonin receptor 5HT2c (HTR2c) and temperament factors: replication tests. Am J Med 88:168–172

Malhotra AK, Virkkunen M, Rooney W, et al (1996) The association between the dopamine D4 receptor (D4DR) 16 amino acid repeat polymorphism and novelty seeking. Mol Psychiatry 1:388–391

Noble EP, Ozkaragoz TZ, Ritchie TL, et al (1998) D2 and D4 dopamine receptor polymorphisms and personality. Am J Med Genet 81:257–267

Ono Y, Manki H, Yoshimura K, et al (1997) Association between dopamine D4 receptor (D4DR) exon III polymorphism and novelty seeking in Japanese subjects. Am J Med Genet 74:501–503

Pogue-Geile M, Ferrell R, Deka R, et al (1998) Human novelty-seeking personality traits and dopamine D4 receptor polymorphisms: a twin and genetic association study. Am J Med Genet 81:44–48

Strobel A, Wehr A, Michel A, et al (1999) Association between the dopamine D4 receptor (DRD4) exon III polymorphism and measures of novelty seeking in a German population. Mol Psychiatry 4:378–384

Tomitaka M, Tomitaka S, Otuka Y, et al (1999) Association between novelty seeking and dopamine receptor D4 (DRD4) exon III polymorphism in Japanese subjects. Am J Med Genet 88:469–471

Vandenbergh DJ, Zonderman AB, Wang J, et al (1997) No association between novelty seeking and dopamine D4 receptor (D4DR) exon III seven repeat alleles in Baltimore longitudinal study of aging participants. Mol Psychiatry 2:417–419

Personality as a Vulnerability Factor in Eating Disorders

Hiroko Mizushima, Yutaka Ono, and Masahiro Asai

Summary. We performed a study to distinguish the trigger of and the factors maintaining bulimia nervosa (BN). The subjects were BN patients, normal women without diet experiences, and normal women with diet experiences. We used the Temperament and Character Inventory scales (TCI) as the instrument. As a result, a high Novelty Seeking score (NS) is identified as the main characteristic of BN, and a high Harm Avoidance score (HA) is assumed to contribute to maintaining bulimic symptoms. As the sociocultural background for eating disorders (ED); there may be pressure on women to be thin to be attractive. Also, ED patients have often been pointed out as having problems with interpersonal relationships. We assume that under sociocultural pressure those women having disordered interpersonal relationships with certain contributing personality factors may develop a diet and ED including BN. Our result using TCI may show that women with high NS go on a diet and women whose HA is also high develop BN in our modern culture.

Keywords. Eating disorders, Vulnerability factor, Personality, Temperament and Character Inventory, Interpersonal relationship

Introduction

Personality has been pointed out to be one of the most important vulnerability factors in eating disorders, and many studies have been performed to assess the association between personality and eating disorders. Among others, studies using Cloninger's seven-factor model have provided us with beneficial findings [1–5]. The seven factors consist of four temperamental factors and three character factors. TPQ [6], the Tridimensional Personality Questionnaire, is an instrument to assess the temperamental factors, and TCI [7], the Temperament and Character Inventory, is an extended version of TPQ that involves all the seven factors.

The studies using TPQ or TCI show that anorexia nervosa patients, restricting type (AN-R), are characterized by low novelty seeking (NS), high harm avoidance (HA),

Department of Neuropsychiatry, Keio University School of Medicine, 35 Shinanomachi, Shinjuku-ku, Tokyo 160-8582, Japan

and high persistence (P), and that anorexia nervosa patients, binge-eating/purging type (AN-B), are characterized by high NS and high HA [1–4]. Our data (unpublished data) show that the AN-B patients have lower reward dependence (RD), but this result is not consistent with some of the previous studies [2,3], probably because of comorbid personality disorders. Bulimia nervosa (BN) patients are characterized by high NS and high HA [1–5].

These findings yield a profile of the eating disorder patient's personality traits, but the way in which these traits contribute to the development and maintenance of eating disorders, and how these traits can be related to treatment targets, have yet to be investigated.

Possible Contributions of Personality to the Development of BN

Most BN patients develop their disorders after following a diet, and Fairburn [8] has pointed out that dieting and binging are common among teenage girls, and thus it is important to focus on factors maintaining bulimic symptoms. Thus, we performed a study to distinguish the trigger and the factors maintaining BN [5]. The subjects were BN patients, normal women without diet experiences (N-N), and normal women with diet experiences (N-D). We used the TCI temperamental scales as the instrument.

Only the NS scale, the NS4 subscale, the HA1, and the HA4 subscales showed significant differences, and the results suggest that a high NS score, which has been identified as the main characteristic of BN, may be related to diet experiences rather than chronic bulimic symptoms. Also, the HA is assumed to contribute to maintaining bulimic symptoms, but it must be interpreted with caution because HA scores have been reported to be strongly associated with depression [2].

The possible contributions of personality to the development of BN are shown in Fig. 1, according to the results of our study. BN patients are present only in modern Western culture. The sociocultural background considered to be necessary to the development of BN is the pressure on women to be thin to be attractive. With this pressure, women with high NS go on a diet, and women whose HA is also high develop

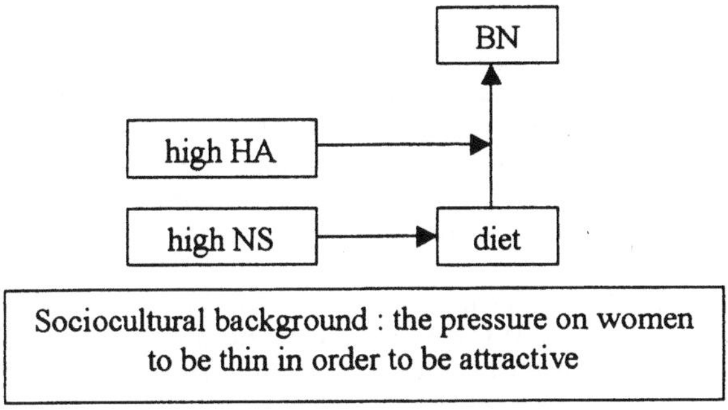

Fig. 1. Possible contributions of personality to the development of bulimia nervosa (BN)

bulimia nervosa following the diet. Thus, women whose NS and HA are both high could be said to be vulnerable to bulimia nervosa in modern Western culture. Character factors, especially low self-directedness (SD), may increase the vulnerability, and specific psychological stress might finally determine the development of the disorder.

Personality as a Vulnerability Factor to Eating Disorders in Terms of Interpersonal Relationships

Eating disorder patients have often been pointed out as having problems with interpersonal relationships. The Eating Disorder Inventory (EDI) [9] contains an item "interpersonal distrust (IPD)," which suggests that disordered interpersonal relationships are one of the core features of eating disorders. Additional evidence that interpersonal relationships are worth investigating in patients with eating disorders is that interpersonal psychotherapy (IPT) has been shown to produce long-term benefits in BN. This finding suggests that interpersonal relationships could be one of the factors maintaining bulimic symptoms.

IPD in the EDI is defined as "reflecting a sense of alienation and a general reluctance to form close relationships," which is considered to be substantially related to development of eating disorders and also to affect the response to treatment. Several studies have shown IPD to be predictive of poor treatment responses in BN [10,11].

Our data show that different personality factors contribute to IPD in each eating disorder subgroup (unpublished data), and these results lead to some discussion on the focus of treatment. In BN patients whose IPD is strongly associated with depression, approaches to modify distorted cognition of others such as those used in IPT are considered to be effective. On the other hand, for AN-B patients whose IPD is related to low RD, therapeutic approaches that mainly focus on attachment bonds may be inappropriate.

We should always take personality into account in determining treatment strategies. From this point of view, investigating personality is not only useful in prevention of eating disorders in vulnerable women, but also is useful in discussing the focus of the treatment.

References

1. Brewerton TD, Hand LD, Bishop ER Jr (1993) The Tridimensional Personality Questionnaire in eating disorder patients. Int J Eating Disord 14:213–218
2. Kleifield EI, Sunday S, Hurt S, Halmi KA (1994) The effects of depression and treatment on the Tridimensional Personality Questionnaire. Biol Psychiatry 36:68–70
3. Kleifield EI, Suncay S, Hurt S, Halmi KA (1994) The Tridimensional Personality Questionnaire: an exploration of personality traits in eating disorders. J Psychiatr Res 28:413–423
4. Anonymous (1995) Temperament in eating disorders. Int J Eating Disord 17:251–261
5. Mizushima H, Ono Y, Asai, M (1998) TCI temperamental scores in bulimia nervosa patients and normal women with and without diet experiences. Acta Psychiatr Scand 98:228–230
6. Cloninger CR (1987) A systematic method for clinical description and classification of personality variants. A proposal. Arch Gen Psychiatry 44:573–588

7. Cloninger CR, Svrakic DM, Przybeck TR (1993) A psychobiological model of temperament and character. Arch Gen Psychiatry 50:975–990
8. Fairburn CG (1993) Interpersonal psychotherapy for bulimia nervosa. In: Klerman GL, Weissman MM (eds) New application of interpersonal psychotherapy. American Psychiatric Press, Washington DC, pp 353–378
9. Garner DM, Olmstead MP, Polivy J (1983) Develpment and validation of a multidimensional eating disorder inventory for anorexia nervosa and bulimia. Int J Eating Disord 2:15–34
10. Olmsted MP, Kaplan AS, Rockert W (1994) Rate and prediction of relapse in bulimia nervosa. Am J Psychiatry 151:738–743
11. Blouin J, Schnarre K, Carter J, et al (1995) Factors affecting dropout rate from cognitive-behavioral group treatment for bulimia nervosa. Int J Eating Disord 17:323–329

The Psychoneuroimmunological Aspect of Eating Disorders

Toshihiko Nagata and Nobuo Kiriike

Summary. Anorexic patients are surprisingly free from infectious complications despite their seriously undernourished state. In a cross-sectional study, compared with controls, a significantly elevated percentage of CD4 and CD4/CD8 ratio in patients with the anorexia nervosa binge eating/purging type (ANBP) was found. Soluble interleukin-2 receptor in patients with anorexia nervosa restricting type (ANR) was significantly lower than that in control group, but not in ANBP. In a longitudinal study, the cytokine productions of interleukin 1, interleukin 6, and tumor necrosis factor-α per monocyte in the patients with ANR recovered only with the start of refeeding, whereas interferon-γ production per lymphocyte were similar to those in controls, and did not change during weight restoration. Only the granulocyte-colony stimulating factor production, even at 75% standard body weight (SBW), did not improve during weight restoration. Between admission and 65%SBW, the increase in percentage of SBW and improvement of total protein level were significantly correlated with the improvement of lymphocyte proliferative response with phytohemoagglutinin. The results suggest that the capacity of cytokine production was dependent on some factor other than the absolute value of body weight, such as the start of refeeding, the neuroendocrine system, or the autonomic nervous system.

Keywords. Anorexia nervosa, Psychoneuroimmunology, Cytokine, Interleukin, Eating disorders

Introduction

Anorexia nervosa is characterized by an individual's refusal to eat sufficiently to maintain minimal healthy weight, intense fear of becoming fat, and having a distorted body image. It is also associated with an increased mortality rate. It is well documented that protein-calorie malnutrition can cause serious immunological deficits, leading to increased susceptibility to infection. However, patients with anorexia nervosa have been anecdotally reported to be relatively free from infections. These observations

---

Department of Neuropsychiatry, Osaka City University Medical School, Asahimachi, Abeno-ku, Osaka 545-8585, Japan

suggest that some kind of compensatory mechanism is working to protect anorexic patients from infection, and that conditions in these patients may differ from those under the usual conditions of nutritional deprivation.

There is extensive evidence that there are "bilateral" communications between the immune and neuroendocrine systems, and between the immune and autonomic nervous systems (Besedovsky et al. 1986). For example, glucocorticoids, which are controlled by pituitary hormones, are well known to be highly immunosuppressive for T cells (Munck and Guyre 1991). An additional route of cytokine-to-brain communication, i.e., an autonomic nervous system route rather than a humoral route, was recently proposed (Watkins et al. 1995). The activation of subdiaphragmatic vagal afferents mediates a wide range of illness responses produced by intraperitoneal lipopolysaccharide (LPS), interleukin 1 (IL-1), and tumor necrosis factor-alpha (TNF-α) administrations in animal models. Lymphocytes (both T- and B cells) and macrophages possess β-adrenergic receptors, and both epinephrine and norepinephrine have been indicated to be able to modulate immune function. Thus, a compensatory mechanism in anorexics might be evoked via either the neuroendocrine system or the autonomic nervous system.

Results of previous studies of cell-mediated immunity such as lymphoproliferative responses and the lymphocyte subset in anorexia nervosa patients are conflicting. For example, lymphocyte proliferative responses in patients with anorexia nervosa were reported to be reduced in most studies (Cason et al. 1986; Polack et al. 1993; Schattner et al. 1990a, 1990b; Vaisman 1990), whereas other investigators reported equal (Brambilla et al. 1993, 1996; Dowd et al. 1984; Emeric-Sauval et al. 1989, 1991) or elevated responses (Golla et al. 1981). These conflicting results are probably due to the heterogeneity of the subjects. Most of these studies did not specify whether the patients underwent refeeding, or whether they were bulimic or restricting-type anorexics.

The present study consists of cross-sectional and longitudinal arms. In the cross-sectional study, the subtype of anorexia nervosa is considered while investigating the relationship of binge and purging behaviors and immunological function in anorexic patients. In the longitudinal study, subjects consisted of patients with restricting-type anorexia nervosa only to maintain a homogenous sample and to better understand the effects of refeeding on immunological functions, and to clarify chronological changes in immunological function during refeeding.

Cross-Sectional Study

Subjects and Method

Subjects consisted of seven patients with anorexia nervosa restricting type (AN-R) and six patients with anorexia nervosa binge-eating/purging type (AN-BP) of DSM-IV (American Psychiatric Association 1994), and eight healthy age-matched female volunteers. Patients had not yet started refeeding at the time of blood sampling, which was confirmed by their daily food logs.

Lymphocyte subpopulations were measured by flow cytometry. The lymphoproliferative response to PHA was measured by the standard producer. The concentrations

TABLE 1. Lymphocyte subsets, lymphoproliferative response to phytohemagglutinin (PHA), and soluble interleukin-2 receptor (sIL-2r) in patients with anorexia nervosa restricting type (AN-R), patients with anorexia nervosa binge eating/purging type (AN-BP), and controls

	AN-R	AN-BP	Controls	Chi-square[a]
N	7	6	8	
%CD4	42.9 ± 5.7	51.8 ± 5.0*	38.9 ± 3.5	10.7***
%CD8	33.1 ± 5.6	29.4 ± 5.0	34.0 ± 4.5	3.3
CD4/CD8	1.3 ± 0.3	1.8 ± 0.6*	1.2 ± 0.2	9.0**
Proliferative response with PHA	36 890 ± 9 153	42 632 ± 22 244	43 936 ± 10 440	2.3
Spontaneous proliferative response	307 ± 194	152 ± 42*	279 ± 98	7.6**
Stimulation index	162 ± 83	295 ± 151	169 ± 59	4.8
sIL-2r (U/ml)	175 ± 46*	282 ± 78	291 ± 95	7.3**

Values are means ± standard deviations
[a] Kruskal–Wallis test
* $P < 0.016$ compared to controls by Mann–Whitney U-test
** $P < 0.05$; *** $P < 0.01$

of soluble interleukin-2 receptor (sIL-2R) were determined using a commercial enzyme-linked immunosorbent assay kit (T-Cell Science, Boston, MA, USA). Intraassay and interassay CVs were both <9% (Table 1).

Results and Discussion

AN-BP patients tended to be older and more chronic than AN-R patients. Although there were no significant differences in lymphoproliferative response among the three groups, sIL-2R in AN-R was significantly lower than that in the C group, but not in AN-BP. Compared with controls, a significantly elevated percentage of CD4 and CD4/CD8 ratio was found in AN-BP. However, the absolute numbers of lymphocytes of anorexic patients were indeed significantly lower than those of controls. These results suggested the presence of some kinds of compensatory mechanisms for cell-mediated immunity, especially in chronically underweight anorexic patients, although their immunological function is indeed impaired.

Longitudinal Study

Subjects and Method

Subjects consisted of 17 inpatients with AN-R and 17 healthy controls. The immune function of patients with anorexia nervosa was assessed three times during weight restoration. The first measurement was within 4 days after their admission (at admission), the second time was when the patients reached 65% of standard body weight (65%SBW), and the third time was when the patient reached 75%SBW. The lymphoproliferative response to phytohemagglutin (PHA) was measured by a standard producer. To measure the capacity of cytokine production, the whole blood was incubated with 10 µg/ml LPS for 24 h at 37°C. The levels of IL-1, IL-6, TNF-α, G-CSF, and IFN-γ in the supernatant of the culture were determined using enzyme-linked immunosor-

TABLE 2. Cytokine production of whole blood and those per monocyte or lymphocyte number of anorexia nervosa patients ($n = 17$) and controls (n = 17)

	At admission	During admission		F(p)	Controls
		65%SBW	75%SBW		
IL-1 α (pg/ml)/monocyte(/μl)	0.6 ± 0.6	1.0 ± 0.7**	1.3 ± 1.2*	5.6 (0.015)	0.9 ± 0.8
IL-1 β (pg/ml)/monocyte(/μl)	2.7 ± 2.1	4.9 ± 2.5**	7.9 ± 6.2**	14 (<0.001)	4.0 ± 2.5
IL-6 (pg/ml)/monocyte(/μl)	0.22 ± 0.12	0.52 ± 0.32**	0.49 ± 0.36**	14 (<0.001)	0.32 ± 0.16
IFN-γ (pg/ml)/lymphocyte(/μl)	0.9 ± 1.7	1.4 ± 1.4	1.4 ± 1.3	1.0 (0.38)	1.1 ± 0.7
G-CSF (pg/ml)/monocyte(/μl)	0.69 ± 0.75	0.70 ± 0.46	0.65 ± 0.52	0.0 (0.97)	0.99 ± 0.75

Values are means ± standard deviations

* $P < 0.05$, ** $P < 0.01$ compared with that at admission by repeated-measures ANOVA with simple contrasts ($df = 2, 15$)

bent assay (ELISA) kits. Intraassay and interassay CVs were within 4.9% and 7.5%, respectively.

Results and Discussion

Numbers of white blood cells and monocytes in anorexic patients did not change throughout refeeding (by repeated-measures ANOVA with simple contrasts). Patient lymphocyte proliferative response with PHA and the stimulation index also did not improve significantly during this study. Cytokine productions of IL-1, IL-6, and TNF-α per monocyte recovered only with the start of refeeding in AN-R patients, whereas IFN-γ production per lymphocyte was similar to that in controls and did not change during weight restoration (Table 2). Only G-CSF production did not improve during weight restoration, even at 75%SBW. These results suggest that the start of refeeding is crucial for recovery of cytokine production by monocytes. However, anorexic patients demonstrated significant anemia and leukopenia even at 75%SBW.

Discussion

Results of cross-sectional study clearly suggest that some kinds of compensatory mechanism are working, especially in chronic and underweight patients, although significant leukopenia indicates reduced immunological function in anorexic patients. Conversely, the results of the longitudinal study suggest that a small increase in body weight rather than the absolute body weight is important in immunological function. Only the capacity to produce G-CSF remained low. CSF is important for the maintenance of basal hematopoiesis. The number of white blood cells in anorexia nervosa patients did not change during this study. Thus, a low capacity to produce G-CSF might be responsible for the continuous leukopenia in anorexic patients. A more detailed study including data on the neuroendocrine system, the autonomic nervous system, and psychological state is needed to clarify these compensatory mechanisms in anorexic patients.

References

Besedovsky H, Del Rey A, Sorkin E, Dinarello C (1986) Immunoregulatory feedback between interleukin-1 and glucocorticocoid hormones. Science 233:652–654

Brambilla F, Ferrari E, Panerai A, et al (1993) Psychoimmunoendocrine investigation in anorexia nervosa. Neuropsychobiology 27:9–16

Brambilla F, Ferrari E, Brunetta M, et al (1996) Immunoendocrine aspects of anorexia nervosa. Psychiatry Res 62:97–104

Cason J, Ainley CC, Wolstencroft RA, et al (1986) Cell-mediated immunity in anorexia nervosa. Clin Exp Immunol 64:370–375

Dowd P, Kelleher J, Walker B, Guillou P (1984) Nutritional and immunological assessment of patients with anorexia nervosa. Proc Nutr Soc 43:90A

Emeric-Sauval E, Bello M, Guitelman A, et al (1989) Anorexia nervosa and bulimia: a model for the study of immune-neuroendocrine interactions in response to human CRH. Neuroendocrinol Lett 11:270

Emeric-Sauval E, Polack E, Finkelman S, et al (1991) Interferon-gamma production-lymphocyte proliferative response in anorexia nervosa patients. Neuroendocrinol Lett 13:204

Golla JA, Larson LA, Anderson CF, et al (1981) An immunological assessment of patients with anorexia nervosa. Am J Clin Nutr, 34:2756–2762

Munck A, Guyre P (1991) Glucocorticoids and immune function. In: Ader R, Felton D, Dohen N (eds) Psychoneuroimmunology, 2nd edn. Academic Press, San Diego, pp 447–474

Polack E, Nahmod VE, Emeric Sauval E, et al (1993) Low lymphocyte interferon-gamma production and variable proliferative response in anorexia nervosa patients. J Clin Immunol 13:445–451

Schattner A, Steinbock M, Tepper R, et al (1990a) Tumour necrosis factor production and cell-mediated immunity in anorexia nervosa. Clin Exp Immunol 79:62–66

Schattner A, Tepper R, Steinbock M, et al (1990b) TNF, interferon-gamma and cell-mediated cytotoxicity in anorexia nervosa; effect of refeeding. J Clin Lab Immunol 32:183–184

Vaisman N, Hahn T, Dayan Y, Schattner A (1990) The effect of different nutritional states on cell-mediated cytotoxicity. Immunol Lett 24:37–41

Watkins LR, Maier SF, Goehler LE (1995) Cytokine-to-brain communication: a review and analysis of alternative mechanisms. Life Sci 57:1011–1026

Long-Term Course and Relapse Prevention in the Treatment of Anorexia Nervosa

Kathleen M. Pike

Summary. Although the problem of relapse in the treatment of anorexia nervosa has been well documented, there has been a paucity of clinical research aimed at developing and evaluating treatment interventions specifically aimed at relapse prevention. In the present study, cognitive behavioral therapy (CBT) was compared to a baseline standard of care that consisted of medical management and nutritional counseling. Findings from this study indicated that CBT was more effective in preventing relapse for individuals who had been hospitalized before participating in this outpatient trial. Overall, individuals in CBT achieved a more satisfactory level of functioning during the year of outpatient treatment. These data provide empirical support for CBT in the relapse prevention of anorexia nervosa. Future efforts aimed at the development and evaluation of additional relapse prevention treatments offer the potential to further improve the long-term outcome of individuals with anorexia nervosa.

Keywords. Anorexia nervosa, Treatment, Relapse prevention, Eating disorders, Outcome

Long-Term Course of Anorexia Nervosa

More than 150 studies examining the long-term course and outcome of anorexia nervosa (AN) have been conducted during the past century (for review, see Pike 1998; Steinhausen et al. 1991). These efforts have failed to identify a single, normative course for this disorder. Instead, the data consistently document quite a variable course, with very limited ability to identify predictors of outcome. Working with the extant data, the best estimates of long-term course and outcome indicate that 20%–25% of individuals with AN remain chronically ill at follow-up, another 20%–25% are symptomatic without meeting full criteria for AN, and the remaining 50%–70% achieve full or partial recovery. The mortality estimate for AN is among the highest rates for any psychiatric disorder: 5% per decade of follow-up (Sullivan 1995).

Department of Psychiatry, Eating Disorders Clinical Research Unit, New York State Psychiatric Institute, Box 98, Columbia University, 1051 Riverside Drive, New York, NY 10032, USA

Relapse Prevention Data

Very few studies specifically assess the course and outcome of AN controlling for initial treatment; however, two recent exceptions are worthy of note (Eckert et al. 1995; Strober et al. 1997a). These studies provide important data regarding rates of relapse and course of illness for individuals 10–15 years following participation in well-documented inpatient programs. The data from both these studies indicate that residual symptoms are the norm following hospitalization. Also, to the extent that individuals remain symptomatic, they are at high risk for relapse within the first year of discharge from the hospital.

In the study conducted by Strober et al. (1997b), nearly 76% of the sample met criteria for full recovery by the end of the follow-up period. However, within the first 2 years of follow-up, individuals remained highly symptomatic: no one met criteria for full recovery and only 10% met criteria for partial recovery. Also, almost 30% of the individuals relapsed at some point during the 10- to 15-year follow-up, with the median time to relapse being 11 months.

Although these data document the need for continuing treatment following hospitalization, in fact very few studies have been conducted to evaluate the efficacy of treatments aimed specifically at relapse prevention. One of the first studies of relapse prevention was published less than 15 years ago (Russell et al. 1987). The findings from this study indicated that family therapy was more helpful than individual supportive therapy for individuals who were 18 years or younger or had a duration of anorexia nervosa of 3 years or less. The data for older patients with a more chronic disorder revealed that neither family therapy nor individual supportive therapy was especially effective.

In terms of medication trials, we have recent but contradictory findings regarding the use of fluoxetine. In a controlled trial comparing fluoxetine to placebo, Kaye and colleagues (1996) found a significant benefit for the use of fluoxetine. However, in a retrospective case-controlled study, Strober and colleagues (1997a) found no benefit for adjunctive fluoxetine. Because these studies employed differing designs and neither controlled for the psychotherapy interventions received, the potential of fluoxetine warrants continuing study.

Columbia Study of Relapse Prevention for Anorexia Nervosa

The Columbia Study of Relapse Prevention for Anorexia Nervosa was a controlled clinical trial conducted on an outpatient basis following the successful completion of initial inpatient treatment for young adult women with AN. For the purpose of the outpatient trial, successful completion of inpatient treatment was defined as achieving a minimum of 90% of recommended weight for a minimum of 2 weeks before discharge.

Participants

The study included 33 women with DSM-IV anorexia nervosa; 15 were randomized to nutritional counseling (NC), and 18 were randomized to cognitive behavioral therapy (CBT).

Randomization

Individuals were randomly assigned to either CBT or NC at the start of the outpatient trial. Everyone in the study received routine medical monitoring. Patients were randomized to one of the two outpatient treatments within 1 week of discharge from the inpatient treatment. Random assignment was stratified for duration of illness, subtype of AN, and medication status.

Treatment Conditions

The structure of the two treatments was identical. CBT and NC were delivered as individual therapy sessions over the course of 1 year. Treatment was delivered twice per week for the first ten sessions and weekly thereafter. The focus of the CBT intervention was on the cognitive and behavioral processes involved in the overvaluation of weight and shape, dysregulation of eating behavior, and deficits in self-esteem that are thought to be central to the maintenance of anorexia nervosa. The NC intervention was based on the core principles of nutritional education and nutritional exchanges. This intervention was psychoeducational and supportive in nature and focused heavily on specific dietary analyses and balanced meal planning.

The rationale for employing NC as the comparison treatment was threefold. First, we wanted to address the first-order research question of whether CBT could be documented to provide additional benefit over standard medical care and nutritional counseling in the relapse prevention of AN. Second, we wanted to provide a comparison treatment that could be manual based. And third, we wanted to provide a comparison treatment that was consistent with a core component of general clinical practice and was consistent with previous studies.

Baseline and Randomization Data

Individuals were not randomized to CBT or NC until they successfully completed the inpatient treatment and were ready for discharge into the outpatient trial. However, to ensure that the two groups were comparable at the time of presentation for treatment (prehospitalization) and at the time of randomization, Mann–Whitney comparisons of means were conducted across all measures of demographic characteristics, eating pathology, associated psychopathology, and social functioning. As indicated in Table 1, at time of presentation for treatment, the two groups did not differ in terms of age, age of onset, duration of AN, weight (BMI), lowest BMI or highest BMI, or number of previous hospitalizations. At time of presentation for treatment and at randomization to the study, the groups also did not differ in eating pathology, comorbid psychopathology, or psychosocial functioning.

Results

The primary comparison of the two interventions was a survival analysis examining rates of premature termination in each condition. Individuals in the treatment trial met criteria for premature termination if weight fell to a BMI of 17.5 or less or they had a sufficiently severe exacerbation of psychopathology requiring alternative care

TABLE 1. Prehospitalization baseline characteristics

Factor	CBT	Nutritional Counseling
Age (years)	26.0 (6.5)	24.3 (6.9)
Age of onset (years)	17.4 (5.3)	16.5 (3.1)
Duration (years)	7.6 (5.9)	7.3 (5.8)
BMI (kg/m^2)	15.9 (2.1)	15.2 (1.5)
Lowest BMI	13.9 (2.4)	14.4 (1.4)
Highest BMI	22.1 (3.8)	21.1 (2.6)

CBT, cognitive behavior therapy; BMI, body mass index

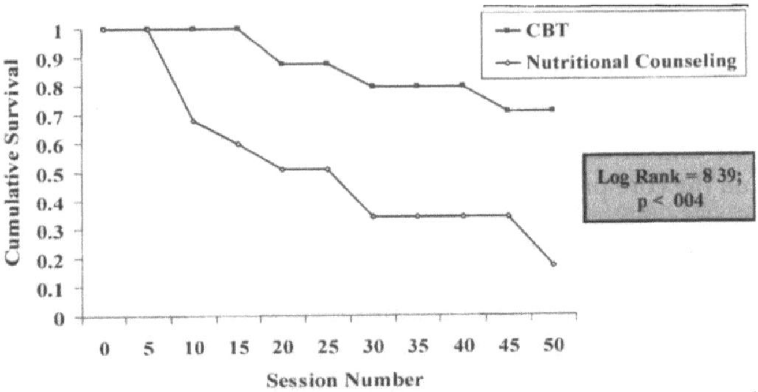

FIG. 1. Survival analysis: time until premature termination (relapse)

(e.g., overdose of laxatives, compromised physical state due to extreme vomiting requiring emergency admission, or suicide). As indicated in Fig. 1, the rate of survival in CBT was significantly better than in the NC Group. The mean survival time for the CBT group was 44 sessions compared to 27 sessions for the NC Group. Four subjects (27%) in CBT compared to eight subjects (53%) in NC met criteria for premature termination.

Figure 2 represents the data utilizing modified Morgan–Russell outcome criteria. "Good Outcome" represents all individuals who both resumed menstrual functioning and maintained their weight above 85% of average (BMI = 18.5) for at least their last 8 weeks before completing treatment; "Fair Outcome" includes individuals whose weight fell below 85% or reported menstrual irregularity for at least their last 8 weeks before completing treatment; and "Poor" Outcome represents individuals whose weight fell below 80% of average (BMI = 17.5) or reported an absence of menstrual functioning. The "Other" category includes both individuals who dropped from the study early without meeting criteria for any of the other outcomes and individuals who met study criteria for premature termination because of an exacerbation of psychopathology. The distribution of individuals in the CBT and NC is quite distinct. A chi-square comparison indicates that a significantly greater percentage of individuals in the CBT condition (44.4%) met criteria specifically for "Good Outcome" compared to the NC group (6.7%; chi-square = 5.89; $P < 0.02$).

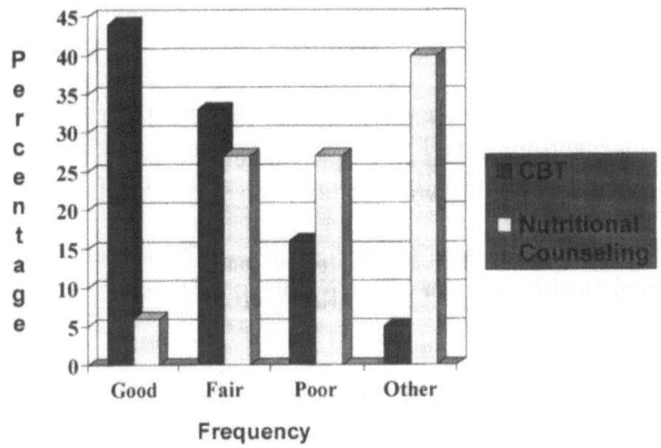

FIG. 2. Categorical outcome: modified Morgan–Russell criteria

In terms of predictors of good outcome, we conducted a hierarchical logistic regression. Because we knew that there were significant treatment effects, we entered treatment in the model first and, in the second step, entered five variables that have been considered significant predictors of long-term outcome in other studies: weight at time of presentation for treatment, duration of illness, highest adult weight, and lowest adult weight. The results of this model indicated that, in addition to treatment, weight at the time of presentation for treatment was the only additionally significant variable in predicting "good outcome," with higher BMI being associated with greater likelihood of achieving "good outcome" ($P < 0.04$).

Summary and Recommendations

The findings from this study suggest that CBT has the potential to be an effective treatment in the relapse prevention for AN. Both in terms of keeping individuals in treatment longer and in terms of clinical functioning, CBT surpassed NC. Nonetheless, there is still substantial room for improvement. Within the CBT condition, a number of individuals achieved full recovery within the first year of discharge from the hospital; however, a larger percentage remained symptomatic in significant ways that may bode poorly for eventual recovery unless they get continuing care. Thus, there is no doubt that we need to consider additional therapies provided either sequentially or in addition to CBT.

Given the complexities of AN, it is important to develop stage-specific interventions. Clinically, we know that both the point in treatment and the state of recovery of the individual influence what treatments we deliver, but there is a paucity of data to guide our decision making regarding treatment delivery. More treatments need to be developed and studied for relapse prevention. Also, given the potentially protracted course of AN and therefore given the multiple treatments that virtually all individuals with severe AN receive, I would argue that immediate outcome data are much more meaningful than long-term, follow-up data in terms of assessing efficacy of specific treatments. Long-term follow-up data are critically important in a number of ways, but they cannot provide information regarding the specific long-term efficacy of a single treatment.

It is incumbent on researchers in the field to continue to work to develop and evaluate treatment interventions aimed at relapse prevention, and it is incumbent on clinicians to heed the data and apply what we have learned thus far with compassion and wisdom.

Acknowledgment. This study was supported in part by a grant from the National Institute of Mental Health awarded to Dr. Kathleen M. Pike.

References

Eckert ED, Halmi KA, Marchi P, et al (1995) Ten-year follow-up of anorexia nervosa: clinical course and outcome. Psychol Med 25:143–156

Kaye WH, McConaha C, Nagata T, et al (1996) Fluoxetine prevents relapse in a majority of patients with anorexia nervosa: a double-blind-placebo-controlled study. Presented at Eating Disorders Research Society Meeting, November 18, 1996, Minneapolis, Minnesota

Pike KM (1998) Long-term course of anorexia nervosa. Clin Psychol Rev 18:447–475

Russell GFM, Szmukler GI, Dare C, Eisler I (1987) An evaluation of family therapy in anorexia nervosa and bulimia nervosa. Arch Gen Psychiatry 44:1047–1056

Steinhausen HC, Rauss-Mason C, Seidel R (1991) Follow-up studies of anorexia nervosa: a review of four decades of outcome research. Psychol Med 21:447–454

Strober M, Freeman R, Morrell W (1997a) The long term course of severe anorexia nervosa in adolescents: survival analysis of recovery, relapse, and outcome predictors over 10–15 years in a prospective study. Int J Eating Disord 22:339–360

Strober M, Freeman RN, DeAntonio MD, et al (1997b) Does adjunctive fluoxetine influence the post-hospital course of anorexia nervosa? a 24-month prospective, longitudinal follow-up and comparison with historical controls. Psychopharmacol Bull 33:425–431

Sullivan PF (1995) Mortality in anorexia nervosa. Am J Psychiatry 152:1073–1074

Psychooncology and Psychoimmunology

Effect of a Structured Intervention on the Immune Function of Cancer Patients and Caregivers of Dementia Victims

Takashi Hosaka

Summary. In the first study, the author developed a structured intervention program for cancer patients, which consisted of five weekly sessions including psychoeducation, problem solving, psychological support, relaxation training, and imagery. Comparing the POMS (Profile of Mood States) scores demonstrated a significant improvement in psychological distress. Because this effect did not persist for patients with adjustment disorders or lymph node metastasis, they received three additional intervention sessions, which demonstrated persisting effects. In the second study, caregivers of dementia victims received a similar structured intervention. Comparing the results of the POMS and the GHQ-30 (General Health Questionnaire-30) revealed a significant improvement in physical and psychological distress. Also, there was a highly significant improvement of natural killer cell activity. The two studies demonstrated that a structured group intervention was effective for physical and psychological distress, and also for immune function. Further study is needed for development of psychoneuroimmunology.

Keywords. Cancer, Caregiver, Immune function, Group intervention, Psychoneuroimmunology

Introduction

Cancer is the most frequent reason for death in Japan, and in 1998 30% of all deaths were caused by cancer. According to various studies in Japan, the psychiatric prevalence among cancer patients ranged from 30% to 40%. Therefore, a psychiatric intervention for cancer patients is needed.

On the other hand, according to many studies, immune function is lowered among caregivers of elderly people, especially of dementia victims. Also, it is demonstrated that these caregivers have a significantly higher prevalence of physical diseases and psychiatric disorders such as depression. Therefore, supportive care for family caregivers is needed.

In this chapter, the author demonstrates the clinical significance of a structured psychiatric intervention for cancer patients and caregivers of dementia victims.

Tokai University School of Medicine, Bohseidai, Isehara, Kanagawa 259-1193, Japan

Methods

Study 1: A Structured Psychiatric Intervention for Cancer Patients

The author developed a structured intervention program for cancer patients. The session was directed by one psychiatrist and one registered nurse. Four to ten patients participated in a series of five sessions once a week. Each session takes 90 min and includes psychoeducation, problem solving, psychological support, relaxation training, and imagery.

In the first study, patients with early stages of breast cancer were assigned to groups of four to ten members to receive a structured psychiatric intervention about 2 weeks after their operation. They were administered the POMS (Profile of Mood States) before and after the interventions, and the same inventory was mailed 6 months after the completion of the intervention. The two sets of scores were compared.

Study 2: A Structured Psychiatric Intervention for Caregivers

Caregivers at home were assigned to groups to receive a structured intervention. The scores of POMS and General Health Questionnaire-30 (GHQ-30), and natural killer (NK) cell activity, were compared for 5 weeks before the intervention program, just before the intervention, just after the intervention, and 2 months later.

The program is a series of five 90-min sessions. Each session includes psychoeducation, problem solving, and relaxation training, which is almost the same as the program for cancer patients.

At 2 months after the end of the program, the participants were asked to fill in two psychological tests by mail.

Results

Study 1: A Structured Psychiatric Intervention for Cancer Patients

Of 57 patients, 47 were analyzed. The mean age was 51 years. Regarding the type of operation, 29 received only mastectomy, 8 had breast reconstruction as well, and 10 had lumpectomy. Fourteen had metastasis to axillary lymph nodes.

A psychiatric interview at the beginning revealed that 12 patients (25.5%) had adjustment disorders with depressed or mixed mood according to the DSM-IV. These disorders clinically improved just after the group intervention.

The scores of the POMS were compared among 40 patients who did not receive chemotherapy, because this treatment might easily produce physical and mental distress. Figure 1 demonstrates a significant improvement in the scores of Depression, Lack-of-Vigor, Fatigue, Tension-Anxiety, Confusion, and Total Mood Disturbances.

To clarify whether a five-session intervention is enough, the POMS data before and after the intervention and 6 months later were compared. The effect persisted 6 months after the intervention among patients who did not have a diagnosis of adjust-

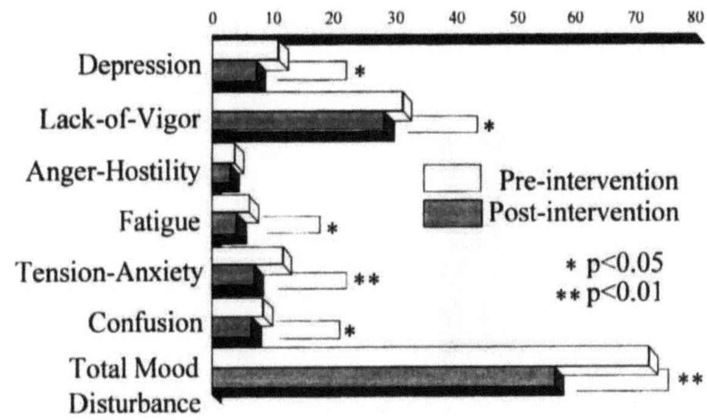

FIG. 1. Effectiveness of intervention ($n = 40$)

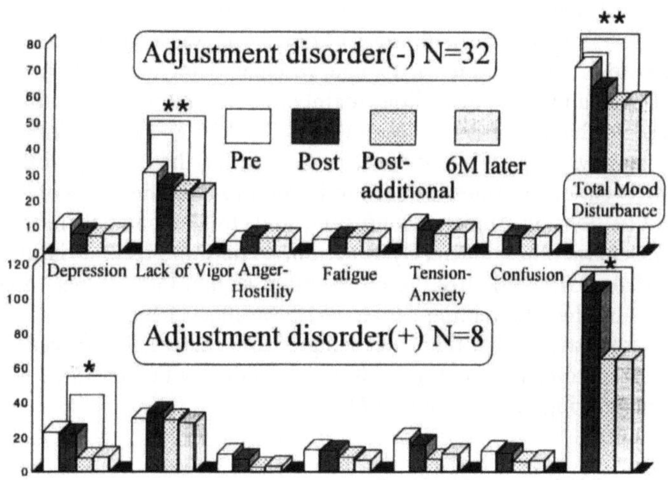

FIG. 2. Effectiveness of additional intervention

ment disorder at entry and among patients without lymph node metastasis. However, for the patients with adjustment disorders at entry or lymph node metastasis, the scores, which lessened just after the intervention, became as high as the preintervention scores after 6 months. Therefore, patients with adjustment disorders or metastasis should be supported by additional interventions after the five-session program.

In the second study, after the regular five-session program, three additional intervention were administered every 2 months to another 40 breast cancer patients. The POMS was mailed 6 months after completion of the additional interventions.

Figure 2 shows the results of the additional interventions among the patients without and with adjustment disorders at entry, which demonstrates that the effectiveness continued 6 months later even for patients with adjustment disorders or lymph node metastasis.

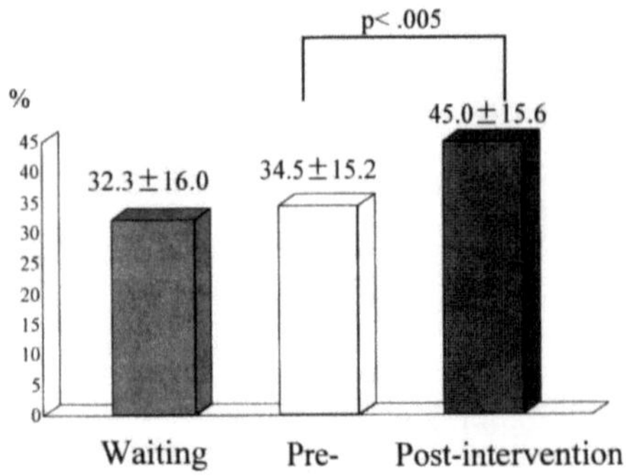

FIG. 3. Effect on natural killer cell activity

Study 2: A Structured Psychiatric Intervention for Caregivers

Of 56 caregivers, 51 were available for analysis. All caregivers were female. The mean age was 57.6 years, and the mean duration of home care was 5.7 years. Concerning the original disease of care recipients, 15 had vascular dementia, 12 had Alzheimer's disease, and 24 had physical disabilities mainly due to cerebrovascular disease.

There were no changes in the scores of POMS,GHQ-30, and natural killer (NK) cell activity during a waiting period of 5 weeks. Comparing the POMS and the GHQ-30 scores preintervention, postintervention, and 2 months later, the scores of Depression, Anger-Hostility, Tension-Anxiety, Confusion, and Total Mood Disturbance (from POMS), and General Illness, Social Dysfunction, Anxiety and Dysphoria, and Suicidal Depression (from GHQ-30) after the intervention significantly decreased compared with those before the intervention. Moreover, these effects persisted 2 months later.

Figure 3 demonstrates that there was a significant increase of NK cell activity in post-intervention compared with pre-intervention data, although there was no significant change during the waiting period.

Discussion and Conclusion

The author demonstrated clinical significance of a group intervention for people in a stressful situation and showed that such an intervention improved immune function among caregivers. Also, the follow-up survey of study 1 revealed that two-thirds of the participants kept contact with the other members, suggesting that group intervention might also be significant for providing a social network.

Further studies including randomized trial are needed.

Acknowledgment. A part of this study was supported by a grant from the Tokai University School of Medicine, Project Research.

Hippocampal Volume, Memory Function, and Reexperience Symptoms of PTSD Among Cancer Survivors

Yosuke Uchitomi and Tomohito Nakano

Summary. Considerable numbers of patients develop symptoms of posttraumatic stress disorder (PTSD) after their cancer experience. There have been several reports of reduced hippocampal volume and decreased memory function in PTSD patients, but no study has been conducted to investigate the association among hippocampal volume, memory functions, and PTSD symptoms in cancer survivors. Patients who had been operated on 3 or more years before and were under the age of 55 years were investigated consecutively. Subjects were evaluated with hippocampal volume measurement by three-dimensional magnetic resonance imaging and memory function measurement by the Wechsler Memory Scale—Revised (WMS-R). Of 142 eligible patients, 67 (47%) subjects participated in the study. The 29 subjects who had histories of reexperience symptoms related to cancer showed 5% smaller left-hippocampal volume and 6% lower visual memory score, both significantly, than 38 subjects without reexperience symptoms. Significance was consistent after adjustment of related factors such as age, height, and years of education. Reduced left-hippocampal volume and decline of visual memory score were associated with a history of reexperience symptoms in cancer survivors. The reduction of hippocampal function may play a role in development of PTSD symptoms in cancer patients, although a prospective study is needed to clarify causality.

Keywords. Reexperience symptoms, Hippocampus, Memory, PTSD, Cancer survivors

Introduction

Several replicated studies have shown that subjects with posttraumatic stress disorder (PTSD) have smaller hippocampi and lower memory function than those without PTSD (Bremner et al. 1995, 1997; Gurvits et al. 1996; Schuff et al. 1997; Stein et al. 1997). Since 1994, when the *Diagnostic and Statistical Manual of Mental Disorders, 4th Edition* (DSM-IV) was established (American Psychiatric Association 1994), it has become possible to evaluate severe traumatic events such as disclosure of cancer diagnosis according to the criteria of PTSD. Some studies indicate that a certain propor-

---

Psycho-Oncology Division, National Cancer Center Research Institute East, 6-5-1 Kashiwanoha, Kashiwa, Chiba 277-8577, Japan

tion of cancer survivors develop PTSD (Heiney et al. 1994; Cordova et al. 1995; Green et al. 1998), although the prevalence of PTSD is not as high as the 8% reported for a population-based study (Kessler et al. 1995). There is also a marked proportion of patients who suffer subclinically from reexperience symptoms in the aftermath of the cancer experience (Alter et al. 1996).

The presence of reexperience symptoms is an essential symptomatic criterion of PTSD. Reexperience symptoms consist of pathological trauma recall and are assumed to be directly related to hippocampal function. Although there is a considerable prevalence of reexperience symptoms among cancer survivors, no study to date has evaluated the relationship between hippocampal volume, memory function, and reexperience symptoms in this population. Therefore, we conducted a cross-sectional investigation of a population of postoperative breast cancer survivors to elucidate whether there is any relationship between reexperience symptoms and hippocampal volume or memory functions.

Subjects

We selected candidates from a list of operation records for patients who had undergone breast cancer surgery more than 3 years before the investigation period. Candidates were eligible if they were women aged 18 to 55 years, were free of residual cancer or recurrence of cancer, and were visiting the follow-up clinic at the National Cancer Center Hospital East, Japan. Of 144 candidates who met the eligibility criteria, 132 were contactable consecutively; 48 subjects refused to participate in the study, and therefore 84 subjects received the Structured Clinical Interview for DSM-IV (SCID)—clinician version (First et al. 1997) for PTSD and major depression.

Before recruitment, all subjects were given a full printed explanation so that written informed consent could be obtained. After the interview, we excluded 2 subjects who had used psychotropic medication within the previous month and 3 left-handed subjects for volumetric analysis of brain structures. Furthermore, we also excluded 12 subjects in whom we detected a history of PTSD or major depression before their cancer experience, because we intended to eliminate any factors that could potentially confound our precise evaluation of the effect due to the cancer experience itself. Finally, 67 subjects underwent magnetic resonance imaging examinations and memory function assessments.

Procedure

By SCID for PTSD, the current and past history of reexperience symptoms and PTSD were obtained. Each participant had her memory function tested using the verbal and visual memory parts of the Wechsler Memory Scale-Revised (WMS-R) (Wechsler 1987). We used all components of verbal and visual memory tests. Finally, 124 magnetic resonance images of coronal brain slices were obtained. Before starting measurements, we established a detailed manual describing the step-by-step procedures for identifying the precise borders of the hippocampus and therefore measuring its volume. The hippocampal borders were traced manually using a pen-tablet-pointing device. The intraclass correlation coefficient (ICC) for intrarater reliability of all measurements was 0.97 and the ICC for interrater reliability for 60 measurements was 0.96.

Results

Of the 67 subjects who completed the investigation, only 1 had an episode that met the full criteria for PTSD. The prevalence of cancer-related reexperience symptoms was 29 (43%). There were no differences between subjects with and without a history of cancer-related reexperience symptoms in any of the demographic and medical factors (Table 1).

Subjects with a history of cancer-related reexperience symptoms had significantly smaller left hippocampal volumes than those without (Table 2). Right hippocampi of subjects with and without reexperience symptoms were not significantly different. After adjustment by multiple linear regression analysis, reexperience symptoms still showed a significant correlation with left hippocampal volume.

The subjects with cancer-related reexperience symptoms presented significantly lower visual memory scores from the WMS-R compared to subjects without (Table 2). Although the difference in verbal memory was not significant, the mean score for subjects with reexperience symptoms was nevertheless 7% lower than that of subjects without. After adjustment by multiple linear regression analysis, there was still a significant effect of the presence of reexperience symptoms on visual memory scores in these subjects.

Discussion

The presence of reexperience symptoms was significantly associated with a smaller left hippocampal volume and a lower visual memory score on the WMS-R among breast cancer survivors even after adjustment of all related factors.

The laterality found in this study is consistent with that observed among sexually abused adults with PTSD (Bremner et al. 1997; Stein et al. 1997), whereas patients with combat-related PTSD showed smaller right (Bremner et al. 1995; Schuff et al. 1997) or bilateral (Gurvits et al. 1996) hippocampal volume. It was assumed that trauma at different stages of development may have differential effects on the hippocampus and therefore on laterality (Bremner et al. 1997). However, this cannot have been the case in this study. There are several possible explanations. Reexperience symptoms might have an effect on hippocampal volume different from that of PTSD, even though reexperience symptoms is a hallmark symptom of PTSD. Also, the traumas of combat and cancer diagnosis are essentially different, so it is not unreasonable that different effects might result. Finally, there may be a differential gender effect on the relationship between PTSD and hippocampal volume because the point in common between the present study and others with similar laterality findings is that the subjects were all women (Stein et al. 1997).

Because of its cross-sectional design, the present study cannot confirm any causality between hippocampal volume, memory function, and reexperience symptoms. To

Table 1. Demographic, medical, and psychological characteristics of subjects

Factors	All participants ($n = 67$)	Cancer-related reexperience symptoms: Present ($n = 29$)	Cancer-related reexperience symptoms: Absent ($n = 38$)	t* or Chi-squared** test	P
Age, mean (±SD) (years)	48.3 (5.3)	48.4 (5.6)	48.2 (5.1)	−0.14*	0.89
Education, mean (±SD) (years)	12.5 (1.8)	12.4 (1.9)	12.5 (1.7)	0.31*	0.76
Days since operation, mean (±SD)	1569 (311)	1622 (357)	1528 (269)	−1.19*	0.24
Height, mean (±SD) (cm)	156.3 (5.6)	156.2 (5.0)	156.3 (6.0)	0.05*	0.96
HADS, mean (±SD)					
Anxiety	5.1 (2.9)	6.0 (2.7)	4.4 (2.9)	−2.18*	0.03
Depression	3.4 (2.2)	3.8 (2.4)	3.1 (1.9)	−1.35*	0.18
Total	8.5 (4.4)	9.8 (4.2)	7.5 (4.5)	−2.09*	0.04
MMS, mean (±SD)	29.2 (1.0)	29.0 (1.0)	29.3 (1.0)	1.13*	0.26
Marital status					
Married	59 (88)	27 (93)	32 (84)	1.24*	0.27
Other	8 (12)	2 (7)	6 (16)		
Occupation					
Full- or part-time	45 (67)	20 (69)	25 (66)	0.75**	0.78
Other	22 (33)	9 (31)	13 (34)		
Alcohol consumption					
More than once a week	29 (43)	13 (45)	16 (42)	0.50**	0.82
Smoking					
Smoker or exsmoker	12 (18)	4 (14)	8 (21)	0.59**	0.44
Surgical procedure					
Total mastectomy	48 (72)	22 (76)	26 (69)	0.45**	0.50
Other	19 (28)	7 (24)	12 (31)		
Menstruation					
Postmenopausal	33 (49)	12 (41)	21 (55)**	1.27	0.26
Premenopausal	34 (51)	17 (59)	17 (45)**		
Pathological stage					
I	16 (24)	5 (17)	11 (29)**	2.85	0.42
II	45 (67)	20 (69)	25 (66)**		
III	5 (8)	3 (10)	2 (5)**		
Other	1 (1)	1 (3)	0 (0)**		
Histological grade					
1	9 (13)	3 (10)	6 (16)**	2.30	0.51
2	21 (31)	8 (28)	13 (34)**		
3	33 (49)	15 (52)	18 (47)**		
Other	4 (6)	3 (10)	1 (3)**		
Lymph node metastasis					
Negative	42 (63)	17 (59)	25 (66)**	0.36	0.55
Positive	25 (37)	12 (41)	13 (34)**		
Hormone therapy received	27 (40)	12 (41)	15 (40)	0.03**	0.88
Chemotherapy					
Oral administration	12 (18)	8 (28)	4 (11)	3.26**	0.07
Intravenous	29 (43)	10 (35)	19 (50)	1.61**	0.20
History of PTSD					
Cancer-related	1 (1)	1 (3)	0 (0)	1.33**	0.25
Other	0 (0)	0 (0)	0 (0)		
History of cancer-related reexperience symptoms	29 (43)	29 (100)	0 (0)	—**	—
History of major depression after cancer	14 (20)	8 (28)	6 (16)	1.39**	0.24

Values are given as number (%) unless otherwise indicated

MMS, mini-mental state; HADS, hospital anxiety and depression scale; PTSD, posttraumatic stress disorder

Statistical analyses were performed by Student's t-test* or Pearson's chi-squared test**

TABLE 2. Hippocampal volumes and memory scores among subjects with and without a history of cancer-related reexperience symptoms

	With ($n = 29$)	Without ($n = 38$)	t	P
Hippocampal volumes (mm^3)				
Right hippocampus	2672 (274)	2711 (262)	0.59	0.56
Left hippocampus	2539 (246)	2668 (245)	2.13	0.04
Scores of WMS-R				
Verbal memory	59.8 (16.7)	64.4 (17.2)	1.08	0.28
Visual memory	56.4 (5.8)	59.7 (4.7)	2.56	0.01

WMS-R, Wechsler memory scale—revised
Values are given as mean (±SD)
Statistical analyses were performed by Student's t-test

elucidate the cause of the difference and clarify the causality between reexperience symptoms and hippocampal alteration, a prospective longitudinal study of cancer survivors is needed.

References

Alter CL, Pelcovitz D, Axelrod A, et al (1996) Identification of PTSD in cancer survivors. Psychosomatics 37:137–143

American Psychiatric Association (1980) Diagnostic and statistical manual of mental disorders, 3rd edn. American Psychiatric Association, Washington, DC

Bremner JD, Randall P, Scott TM, et al (1995) MRI-based measurement of hippocampal volume in posttraumatic stress disorder. Am J Psychiatry 152:973–981

Bremner JD, Randall P, Vermetten E, et al (1997) Magnetic resonance imaging-based measurement of hippocampal volume in posttraumatic stress disorder related to childhood physical and sexual abuse: a preliminary report. Biol Psychiatry 41:23–32

Cordova MJ, Andrykowski MA, Kenady DE, et al (1995) Frequency and correlations of posttraumatic-stress-disorder-like symptoms after treatment for breast cancer. J Consult Clin Psychol 63:981–986

First MB, Spitzer RL, Gibbon M, et al (1997) Structured clinical interview for DSM-IV axis I disorders: clinician version (SCID-CV). American Psychiatric Press, Washington, DC

Green BL, Rowland JH, Krupnick JL, et al (1998) Prevalence of posttraumatic stress disorder in women with breast cancer. Psychosomatics 39:102–111

Gurvits TV, Shenton ME, Hokama H, et al (1996) Magnetic resonance imaging study of hippocampal volume in chronic, combat-related posttraumatic stress disorder. Biol Psychiatry 40:1091–1099

Heiney SP, Neuberg RW, Myers D, et al (1994) The aftermath of bone marrow transplant for parents of pediatric patients: a post-traumatic stress disorder. Oncol Nurs Forum 21:843–847

Kessler RC, Sonnega A, Bromet E, et al (1995) Posttraumatic stress disorder in the national comorbidity survey. Arch Gen Psychiatry 52:1048–1060

Schuff N, Marmar CR, Weiss DS, et al (1997) Reduced hippocampal volume and n-acetyl aspartate in posttraumatic stress disorder. Ann N Y Acad Sci 821:516–520

Stein MB, Koverola C, Hanna C, et al (1997) Hippocampal volume in women victimized by childhood sexual abuse. Psychol Med 27:951–959

Wechsler D (1987) Wechsler memory scale—Revised. Psychological Corporation, New York

Effects of Family Functioning on Psychological Well-Being of Cancer Patients

Toshinari Saeki, Tomoyuki Mantani, Shinichi Inoue, and Shigeto Yamawaki

Summary. In this chapter, first, selected Western literature that attempted to address psychological distress among families of cancer patients is briefly reviewed. Second, some of the findings derived from our research on the relationship between family functioning and psychological distress among breast cancer patients are presented. Because cancer inevitably affects the entire family, the patient and their family members should not be separated in cancer care.

Keywords. Cancer, Psychooncology, Family functioning

Introduction

In recent years, there has been growing recognition in the West that care of a cancer patient should involve treatment of his or her whole family. In Japan, however, medical staff seem to take it for granted that the family would be available as an extended agent of patient care. From the point of view of psychooncology, the experience of a life-threatening illness, such as cancer, is generally believed to cause considerable stress not only to the patient but also to caregivers who share in the associated psychological distress.

Psychological Distress Among Families

Table 1 summarizes the relevant empirical research on family factors in relation to the patient with cancer. Seven studies [3,5,6,7,11–3] have reported a rate of distress in the next-of-kin between 18% and 35%. Moreover, in the longitudinal studies of Ell et al. [5] and Northouse [12], this distress continued for as long as 18 months. Although distress in patients has been found to be maximal at the time of first recurrence [4], Plumb and Holland [13] and Northouse [12] reported that the phases of palliative and terminal care appear to be the most emotionally demanding for the family. They also noted a close relationship between the psychological status of the patient and their

Department of Psychiatry and Neurosciences, Hiroshima University School of Medicine, 1-2-3, Kasumi, Minami-ku, Hiroshima 734-8551, Japan

TABLE 1. Empirical studies of psychological morbidity in families of cancer patients

Study	*n*	Nature of relative	Prevalence of distress in relatives (%)
Buckley (1977) [3]	40	Children	33
Plumb and Holland (1977) [13]	66	Spouses or parents	18
Maguire (1981) [11]	52	Spouses	33
Gotay (1984) [6]	39	Spouses	32
Ell et al. (1988) [5]	143	Spouses and offspring	34
Northouse (1989) [12]	41	Spouses	24
Kissane et al. (1994) [7]	246	Spouses and offspring	35, 28

relatives. Ell et al. [5] have found the perceived degree of social support or personal vulnerability in the spouse predictive of psychological morbidity in the family.

Family Assessment

In today's trend of evidence-based medicine, the serious problem is that there is no consensus on theory or measurement in the field of family assessment. There are many self-report measures of family functioning. Family APGAR, Family Environment Scale (FES), McMaster Family Assessment Device (FAD), Family Assessment Measure (FAM-III), and Family Adaptability and Cohesion Evaluation Scale (FACES-III) are well known in the field of Western family psychiatry, and so far three of these have been validated in Japan. We can say that the situation is chaotic.

Recently, Kissane et al. [10] employed a 12-item self-report questionnaire [Family Relationships Index (FRI)] as a screening instrument to identify at-risk families. The FRI is a shortened version of the 90-item Family Environment Scale and very easy to administrate. It assesses the relationship dimension of the family, and consists of three subscales: Cohesion, Expressiveness, and Conflict. It takes about 5 min to complete.

Melbourne Family Grief Study

In the Melbourne Family Grief Study [8,9], Kissane and his colleagues applied cluster analysis for the longitudinal data from 115 families, a total of 670 individual responses, to develop a typology of perceptions of family functioning during bereavement. Five types of families emerged from dimensions of cohesion, expressiveness, and conflict on the Family Relationships Index: supportive, conflict-resolving, intermediate, sullen, and hostile (Table 2). Half the families were well functioning, either *supportive*, through enjoying high cohesiveness, minimal conflict, and open expressiveness, or *conflict-resolving*, that is, evidently able to handle conflict effectively by dint of their expressiveness and cohesion. Grief waned over 13 months in these families; moreover, their overall psychosocial outcomes were good. By contrast, a third of the families were either *hostile*, distinguished by high conflict, low cohesiveness, and poor expressiveness, or *sullen*, with moderate levels in these three domains. Their outcome was

TABLE 2. Melbourne family grief study

Type of family	Cohesion	Expressiveness	Conflict
Supportive	↑↑	↑↑	↓↓
Conflict-resolving	↑↑	↑↑	↑
Intermediate	↑	↓	↓
Sullen	↓	↓	↑
Hostile	↓↓	↓↓	↑↑

Source: Kissane et al. 1994 [8], 1996a,b [9,10]

poor: sullen families reported high rates of depression whereas hostile families were particularly fractured and chaotic in their adaptation. Intermediate families, a fifth of the sample, exhibited moderate cohesiveness but were still prone to psychosocial morbidity. A randomized controlled trial of brief, focused, family grief therapy for at-risk families is proceeding to confirm the effectiveness of psychotherapeutic intervention on improving the family's outcome longitudinally following the death of a parent.

A Family Study of Breast Cancer Patients in Japan

We introduce here our research data investigating the relationship between psychological distress and family functioning of patients with breast cancer. Subjects consisted of 49 female outpatients with breast cancer after mastectomy and 71 family members including 35 spouses. Perceived family functioning was measured using the Family Relationships Index (FRI) that was mentioned earlier. Perceived depression was measured by the Zung Self-rating Depression Scale (SDS) and perceived anxiety by the Zung Self-rating Anxiety Scale (SAS). Members of dysfunctional families (n = 88) reported a significantly higher SDS score than those of functional families (n = 32) ($P = 0.002$). There were no significant differences in SAS score. Notably, patients of dysfunctional families ($n = 31$) reported significantly higher SDS score than those of functional families ($n = 18$) ($P = 0.017$). There were no significant differences in SAS score. Also, other members of dysfunctional families, excluding patients ($n = 57$), tended to report higher SDS score than those of functional families ($n = 14$) ($P = 0.053$).

Our data suggested that poorer family functioning might relate especially to a higher level of perceived depression, although the level was in the subthreshold range. Therefore, it seems to be useful to consider family functioning as a screening variable when assessing subclinical depression in families of breast cancer patients.

Psychological Well-Being and Family Functioning

Figure 1 shows a theoretical model of various factors influencing the psychological well-being of patients with breast cancer. In this model, the effects of the diagnosis of breast cancer and its treatment are related to physical well-being. Physical well-being affects social well-being, both of which affect psychological well-being. Analyses from a large longitudinal sample conducted by Bloom and her colleagues showed that both

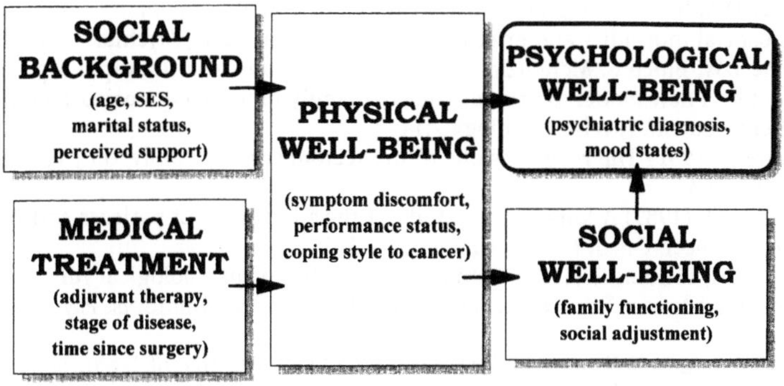

FIG. 1. Theoretical model of factors influencing psychological well-being. SES: socio-economic status. (From Bloom and Kessler 1994 [1], with permission)

family functioning and social adjustment had direct effects on psychological well-being [1,2].

Future Direction of Family Research

Future research will require the accumulation of observational studies of psychological distress in the families of patients with each type of cancer. Furthermore, research on the spouses of breast cancer patients to which psychosocial factors are strongly related, due to the length of time of the disease process, and research on the parents of children with cancer, for whom grief is particularly deep, are also required [14].

References

1. Bloom JR, Kessler L (1994) Emotional support following cancer: a test of the stigma and social activity hypotheses. J Health Soc Behav 35:118–133
2. Bloom JR (1996) Social support of the cancer patient and the role of the family. In: Baider L, Cooper CL, Kaplan-DeNoir A (eds) Cancer and the family. Wiley, Chichester, pp 53–70
3. Buckley IE (1977) Listen to the children: impact on the mental health of children of a patient's catastrophic illness. Cancer Care Inc. and National Cancer Foundation, New York
4. Cassileth BR, Lusk EJ, Strouse TB, et al (1985) A psychological analysis of cancer patients and their next-of-kin. Cancer (phila) 55:72–76
5. Ell K, Nishimoto R, Mantell J, Hamovitch M (1988) Longitudinal analysis of psychological adaptation among family members of patients with cancer. J Psychosom Res 32:429–438
6. Gotay CC (1984) The experience of cancer during early and advanced stages: the views of the patients and their mates. Soc Sci Med 18:605–613
7. Kissane DW, Bloch S, Burns WI, et al (1994) Psychological morbidity in the families of patients with cancer. Psycho-Oncology 3:47–56
8. Kissane DW, Bloch S, Dowe DL, et al (1996a) The Melbourne Family Grief Study. I: Perceptions of family functioning and bereavement. Am J Psychiatry 153:650–658

9. Kissane DW, Bloch S, Onghena P, et al (1996b) The Melbourne Family Grief Study. II: Psychosocial morbidity and grief in bereaved families. Am J Psychiatry 153:659–666
10. Kissane DW, Bloch S, McKenzie M, et al (1998) Family grief therapy: a preliminary account of a new model to promote healthy family functioning during palliative care and bereavement. Psycho-Oncology 7:14–25
11. Maguire P (1981) The repercussions of mastectomy on the family. Int J Fam Psychiatry 6:485–503
12. Northouse L (1989) A longitudinal study of the adjustment of patients and husbands to breast cancer. Oncol Nurs Forum 16:511–516
13. Plumb MM, Holland J (1977) Comparative studies of psychological function in patients with advanced cancer. 1. Self-reported depressive symptoms. Psychosom Med 39:264–276
14. Saeki T, Mantani T, Yamawaki S, Uchitomi Y (2000) The role of Japanese families in cancer care. In: Baider L, Cooper CL, Kaplan-DeNoir A (eds) Cancer and the family, 2nd edn. Wiley, Chichester, pp 111–117

Subject Index

t

MIX
Papier aus verantwortungsvollen Quellen
Paper from responsible sources
FSC® C105338

If you have any concerns about our products,
you can contact us on
ProductSafety@springernature.com

In case Publisher is established outside the EU,
the EU authorized representative is:
Springer Nature Customer Service Center GmbH
Europaplatz 3, 69115 Heidelberg, Germany

Printed by Libri Plureos GmbH
in Hamburg, Germany